Physician Characteristics and Distribution in the US

Derek R. Smart
Jayme Sellers
Division of Survey and Data Resources

2008 Edition

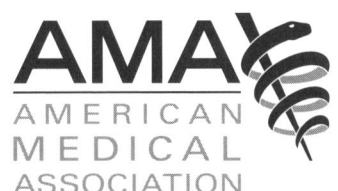

AMA
AMERICAN
MEDICAL
ASSOCIATION

Physician Characteristics and Distribution in the US, 2008 Edition

Additional copies of this book may be ordered by calling 800 621-8335.
Mention product number OP390208.
Secure online orders can be taken at www.amapress.com.

ISBN 978-1-57947-897-1

BP64:07-P-022:12/07

Foreword

Physician Characteristics and Distribution in the US has been published since 1963. As in previous editions of this volume, the 2008 Edition presents extensive statistical information on all physicians located in the United States and Possessions. The growth in physician supply and the focus on primary care physicians coupled with the emphasis on health systems reform have contributed to the rapidly changing health care environment. The current and future supply of physicians has become a significant component in planning for the nation's health care needs. Changes in size and composition of the physician population affect the organization of the US health care system.

To provide necessary statistical data about physician supply, this edition presents a series of summary and detailed tabulations on the professional characteristics of physicians, which can be used as a basis of comparison essential for health manpower planning, policy development, and research studies. In addition, the tabulations in this volume serve as guides for comparing census regions and divisions, states, counties, and metropolitan areas with respect to the distribution of physicians by their specialty and major professional activity.

As in past years, the 2008 Edition includes physician/population ratios for the nation, state of location, and specialty of practice. Also presented are comparative data on the activity, specialty, and location of physicians from 1975 through 2006, along

with information on the school and year of graduation, specialty board certification, and age and sex. The book contains summary and detailed tabulations in six separate chapters of physician data — Physician Characteristics, Physician Distribution, Analysis of Professional Activity by Self-Designated Specialty and Geographic Region, Primary Care Specialties, Osteopathic Physicians, and Physician Trends. The Introduction that follows describes these chapters in more detail and also describes the overall format of the book.

New to this edition is a chapter on Doctors of Osteopathic Medicine. As this segment of the physician populace grows, it becomes more and more important to understand their impact on the overall question of physician supply, as well as how their characteristics compare to their Allopathic colleagues, an issue this chapter strives to address.

As a basic and comprehensive source of data related to the specialty, activity, location, and other characteristics of physicians, this publication serves a wide audience. Hospitals, medical societies, medical schools, specialty boards, government agencies, associations, as well as other health-related organizations have found earlier editions of this book to be significant data sources when conducting research on health care issues, trends in physician supply, and the availability of physician services.

All data in this volume are derived from the American Medical Association's (AMA) Physician

Masterfile and represent the collection, management, and validation efforts of several departments within the Division of Survey and Data Resources.

The Physician Masterfile was established by the AMA in 1906 as a record-keeping system for physician membership and mailing purposes. Today, the AMA Physician Masterfile is the most comprehensive source of information for Doctors of Medicine (MDs) in the United States. The presentation of detailed and summary statistics in this new edition of *Physician Characteristics and Distribution in the US* represents the commitment and historical role of the AMA as a source of physician statistics that will continue to illuminate and shape the changing environment of health care in the United States.

Derek Smart, Manager
Information Management and Data Release

Table of

Contents

Foreword iii

List of Tables viii

List of Figures xii

Introduction xiii

AMA Physician Masterfile xv

Definitions xvii

Major Professional Activity xvii

Self-Designated Practice Specialty xviii

Primary Care Specialties xviii

Board Certification xix

Residency Training Data xix

Other Physician Characteristics xix

Metropolitan Statistical Area Definition xx

Demographic County Classification xx

County Data xx

Acknowledgments xxii

Chapter 1   **Physician Characteristics** 1

Activity by Age and Sex...1

Self-Designated Specialty by Age and Sex...1

Distribution of Detail Specialties by Activity...2

Mean Age by Detail Specialty and Activity 4

International Medical Graduates 4

       Activity by Self-Designated Specialty 4

       Activity by Age and Sex..4

Female Physicians by Self-Designated Specialty and Activity...4

Self-Designated Specialty by Board Certification 5

School of Graduation by Year of Graduation...6

Self-Designated Specialty by Race/Ethnicity 6

Chapter 2 **Physician Distribution** 45

State of Location, Age, and Activity by Sex 45

State of Location and Activity 46

International Medical Graduates (IMGs)...46

Chapter 3 **Analysis of Professional Activity by Self-Designated Specialty and Geographic Region** 59

Total US Physicians..59

International Medical Graduates (IMGs)...59

US Physicians by Geographic Region...60

Metropolitan Data 62

Chapter 4 **Primary Care Specialties** 274

Trends in Primary Care 274

Activity and Sex 274

Age and Sex 275

Board Certification and Sex 276

School and Year of Graduation..276

State of Location and Sex 277

Country of Graduation 277

Metropolitan Areas 278

Chapter 5 **Osteopathic Physicians** 301

Activity by Age and Sex..301

Self-Designated Specialty by Age and Sex.....................................301

Distribution of Detail Specialties by Activity.................................302

Mean Age by Detail Specialty and Activity 302

DOs by Self-Designated Specialty and Activity..............................302

State of Location, Age, and Activity by Sex 303

State of Location and Activity 303

Metropolitan Data 304

Activity and Sex for Primary Care DOs 304

Age and Sex for Primary Care DOs..304

Chapter 6 **Physician Trends** 393

Collection and Classification Systems 393

Total US Physicians..394

    Major Categories 394

    Activity 394

    Specialty 395

    Age and Sex 396

International Medical Graduates (IMGs)...397

    Activity 397

    Specialty 398

Female Physicians 398

    Activity 398

    Specialty 399

Physician-Population Ratios 401

    National Ratios 401

    State Ratios..401

    Specialty Ratios 401

Appendices

Appendix A   Self-Designated Practice Specialties 427

Appendix B   American Specialty Boards 430

Appendix C   List of Metropolitan Statistical Areas (MSAs)..433

Appendix D   List of Regions, Divisions, and States..438

Appendix E   Demographic County Classifications 439

Index 441

List of Tables

Chapter 1   Physician Characteristics

Table 1.1   Total Physicians by Age, Activity, and Sex, 2006 8

Table 1.2   Total Physicians by Age and Self-Designated Specialty, 2006 9

Table 1.3   Male Physicians by Age and Self-Designated Specialty, 2006 10

Table 1.4   Female Physicians by Age and Self-Designated Specialty, 2006 11

Table 1.5   International Medical Graduates by Age and Self-Designated Specialty, 2006 12

Table 1.6   Male International Medical Graduates by Age and Self-Designated Specialty, 2006 13

Table 1.7   Female International Medical Graduates by Age and Self-Designated Specialty, 2006 14

Table 1.8   Physicians' Mean Age by Self-Designated Specialty and Activity (199 Specialties), 2006 15

Table 1.9   Physicians by Self-Designated Specialty and Activity (199 Specialties), 2006 20

Table 1.10   International Medical Graduates by Self-Designated Specialty and Activity, 2006 25

Table 1.11   International Medical Graduates by Age, Activity, and Sex, 2006 26

Table 1.12   Male Physicians by Self-Designated Specialty and Activity, 2006 27

Table 1.13   Female Physicians by Self-Designated Specialty and Activity, 2006 28

Table 1.14   Total Physicians by Self-Designated Specialty and
Corresponding Board Certification, 2006 29

Table 1.15   Male Physicians by Self-Designated Specialty and
Corresponding Board Certification, 2006 30

Table 1.16   Female Physicians by Self-Designated Specialty and
Corresponding Board Certification, 2006 31

Table 1.17   Country and School of Graduation of Total Physicians
by Year of Graduation, 2006 32

Table 1.18   Country and School of Graduation of Male Physicians
by Year of Graduation, 2006 35

Table 1.19   Country and School of Graduation of Female Physicians
by Year of Graduation, 2006 38

Table 1.20   Physicians by Race/Ethnicity, 2006 41

Table 1.21   Male Physicians by Race/Ethnicity, 2006 42

Table 1.22   Female Physicians by Race/Ethnicity, 2006 43

Chapter 2   Physician Distribution

Table 2.1   Total Physicians by Age and State of Location, 2006 47

Table 2.2   Male Physicians by Age and State of Location, 2006 48

Table 2.3   Female Physicians by Age and State of Location, 2006 49

Table 2.4   IMGs by Age and State of Location, 2006...50

Table 2.5   Male IMGs by Age and State of Location, 2006..51

Table 2.6   Female IMGs by Age and State of Location, 2006...52

Table 2.7   Total Physicians by State of Location and Major Professional Activity, 2006 53

Table 2.8   Male Physicians by State of Location and Major Professional Activity, 2006 54

Table 2.9   Female Physicians by State of Location and Major Professional Activity, 2006 55

Table 2.10   IMGs by State of Location and Major Professional Activity, 2006..56

Table 2.11   Male IMGs by State of Location and Major Professional Activity, 2006..................................57

Table 2.12   Female IMGs by State of Location and Major Professional Activity, 2006...............................58

**Chapter 3   Analysis of Professional Activity by Self-Designated Specialty
and Geographic Region**

Table 3.1   Total Physicians in the United States and Possessions by
Self-Designated Specialty and Activity, 2006 63

Table 3.2   International Medical Graduates in the United States and Possessions by
Self-Designated Specialty and Activity, 2006 64

Table 3.3   International Medical Graduates by Census Region,
Self-Designated Specialty, and Activity, 2006...65

Table 3.4   International Medical Graduates by Census Division,
Self-Designated Specialty, and Activity, 2006...70

Table 3.5   Physicians by Census Region, Self-Designated Specialty, and Activity, 2006 80

Table 3.6   Physicians by Census Division, Self-Designated Specialty, and Activity, 2006 85

Table 3.7   Physicians by State, Self-Designated Specialty, and Activity, 2006.....................................95

Table 3.8   Female Physicians by State, Self-Designated Specialty, and Activity, 2006 149

Table 3.9   Physicians by Census Division and County Group, 2006 203

Table 3.10   Physicians by Census Division, State, and County Group, 2006..205

Table 3.11   Physicians by State and County, 2006...213

Table 3.12   Physicians in Metropolitan Areas by Self-Designated Specialty and Activity, 2006 267

Table 3.13   Physicians in Rural Areas by Self-Designated Specialty and Activity, 2006 268

Table 3.14   Physicians by Metropolitan Area, 2006 269

Chapter 4   Primary Care Specialties

Table 4.1   Primary Care Physicians by Self-Designated Specialty
for Selected Years, 1975–2006 279

Table 4.2   Physicians by Self-Designated Primary Care Specialty, Activity, and Sex, 2006 280

Table 4.3   Physicians by Self-Designated Primary Care Specialty, Age, and Sex, 2006.....................281

Table 4.4   Physicians by Self-Designated Primary Care Specialty and Corresponding
Board Certification, 2006 282

Table 4.5   Physicians by Self-Designated Primary Care Specialty
and School of Graduation, 2006 283

Table 4.6   Physicians by Self-Designated Primary Care Specialty,
Year of Graduation, and Sex, 2006..286

Table 4.7   Total Physicians by Self-Designated Primary Care Specialty and State of Location, 2006 287

Table 4.8   Male Physicians by Self-Designated Primary Care Specialty and State of Location, 2006 288

Table 4.9   Female Physicians by Self-Designated Primary Care Specialty
and State of Location, 2006...289

Table 4.10   International Medical Graduates by Self-Designated Primary Care Specialty, Age, and Sex, 2006 290

Table 4.11   International Medical Graduates by Self-Designated Primary Care Specialty and State of Location, 2006 291

Table 4.12   Graduates of US Medical Schools by Self-Designated Primary Care Specialty and State of Location, 2006 292

Table 4.13   Graduates of Canadian Medical Schools by Self-Designated Primary Care Specialty and State of Location, 2006 293

Table 4.14   Metropolitan Physicians by Self-Designated Primary Care Specialty, Activity, and Sex, 2006 294

Table 4.15   Metropolitan Physicians by Self-Designated Primary Care Specialty, 2006 295

Chapter 5   Osteopathic Physicians

Table 5.1   DOs by Age, Activity, and Sex, 2006 305

Table 5.2   DOs by Age and Self-Designated Specialty, 2006 306

Table 5.3   Male DOs by Age and Self-Designated Specialty, 2006 307

Table 5.4   Female DOs by Age and Self-Designated Specialty, 2006 308

Table 5.5   DOs' Mean Age by Self-Designated Specialty and Activity (166 Specialties), 2006 309

Table 5.6   DOs by Self-Designated Specialty and Activity (166 Specialties), 2006 313

Table 5.7   DOs by Self-Designated Specialty and Activity, 2006 317

Table 5.8   Male DOs by Self-Designated Specialty and Activity, 2006 318

Table 5.9   Female DOs by Self-Designated Specialty and Activity, 2006 319

Table 5.10   DOs by Race/Ethnicity, 2006 320

Table 5.11   Male DOs by Race/Ethnicity, 2006 321

Table 5.12   Female DOs by Race/Ethnicity, 2006 322

Table 5.13   DOs by Age and State of Location, 2006 323

Table 5.14   Male DOs by Age and State of Location, 2006 324

Table 5.15   Female DOs by Age and State of Location, 2006 325

Table 5.16   DOs by State of Location and Major Professional Activity, 2006 326

Table 5.17   Male DOs by State of Location and Major Professional Activity, 2006 327

Table 5.18   Female DOs by State of Location and Major Professional Activity, 2006 328

Table 5.19   DOs by State, Self-Designated Specialty, and Activity, 2006 329

Table 5.20   DOs in Metropolitan Areas by Self-Designated Specialty and Activity, 2006 383

Table 5.21   DOs in Rural Areas by Self-Designated Specialty and Activity, 2006 384

Table 5.22   DOs by Metropolitan Area, 2006 385

Table 5.23   DOs by Self-Designated Primary Care Specialty, Activity, and Sex, 2006 390

Table 5.24   DOs by Self-Designated Primary Care Specialty, Age, and Sex, 2006 391

Table 5.25   DOs by Self-Designated Primary Care Specialty and State of Location, 2006 392

Chapter 6   Physician Trends

Table 6.1   Physicians by Activity, 1975–2006 403

Table 6.2   Physicians by Self-Designated Specialty, 1975–2006 404

Table 6.3   Percent Distribution of Physicians by Self-Designated Specialty, 1975–2006 405

Table 6.4   Percent Change of Physicians by Self-Designated Specialty, 1975–2006 406

Table 6.5   Physicians by Age and Sex, 1975–2006 407

Table 6.6   International Medical Graduates by Self-Designated Specialty, 1975–2006 408

Table 6.7   Percent Distribution of International Medical Graduates
by Self-Designated Specialty, 1975–2006 409

Table 6.8   Percent Change of International Medical Graduates
by Self-Designated Specialty, 1975–2006 410

Table 6.9   International Medical Graduates by Activity, 1975–2006 411

Table 6.10   Female Physicians by Self-Designated Specialty, 1975–2006 412

Table 6.11   Percent Distribution of Female Physicians by Self-Designated Specialty, 1975–2006...................413

Table 6.12   Percent Change of Female Physicians by Self-Designated Specialty, 1975–2006..........................414

Table 6.13   Female Physicians by Activity, 1975–2006 415

Table 6.14   Trends in the Distribution of Physicians by Metropolitan/Nonmetropolitan
Status, 1980–2006 416

Table 6.15   Percent Distribution and Change for Physicians
by Metropolitan/Nonmetropolitan Status, 1980–2006 417

Table 6.16   Physicians, Population, and Physician/Population Ratios, 1965–2006...418

Table 6.17   Physicians, Population, and Physician/Population Ratios, 1980–2006...419

Table 6.18   Population Ratios per One Physician by State, 1980–2006 422

Table 6.19   Physician-Population Ratios and Rank by State, 2006..423

Table 6.20   Total and Office-Based Physicians by Self-Designated Specialty, 1980–2006...............................424

Table 6.21   Physician/Population Ratios for Total and Office-Based
Physicians by Self-Designated Specialty, 1980–2006..425

Mini-Tables

Table 1   Percent Distribution of International Medical Graduates
by Age and Self-Designated Specialty Ranked by Size, 2006..3

Table 2   Female Physicians by Self-Designated Specialty and Residency Training, 2006.............................5

Table 3   Percent Distribution of Physicians by Age and Sex, 2006...45

Table 4   Percent Distribution of International Medical Graduates by Age and Sex, 2006 46

Table 5   Percent Distribution of Five Highest Ranking Self-Designated Specialties
by Selected Major Professional Activity, 2006 60

Table 6   Physicians, Population, and Physician/Population Ratios by Census Division, 2006 61

Table 7   Top 10 Schools in Number of Graduates and Self-Designated
Primary Care Specialists, 2006 276

Table 8   Top 10 States With Largest Number of Total Physicians and Percentage
of Self-Designated Primary Care Physicians Compared to Total Physicians in State, 2006 277

Table 9   Country of Graduation of Active Physicians, 2006..277

Table 10   Percent Distribution of DOs by Age and Sex, 2006...303

Table 11   Total US Physicians by Major Categories, 1970-2006..394

Table 12   Physicians by Year and Country of Graduation, 2006 395

Table 13   Total Physicians and International Medical Graduates
by Activity for 1980 and 2006 398

Table 14   Percentage of IMGs in Highest IMG Self-Designated Specialties
Ranked by Size, 2006 400

Table 15   Total Physicians and Female Physicians by Activity for 1980 and 2006 400

List of Figures

Figure 1   Percent Distribution of Total US Physicians by Age and Sex, 2006..2

Figure 2   International Medical Graduates by Age and Major Professional Activity, 2006 5

Figure 3   Percent Distribution of International Medical Graduates Compared With Total Physicians
              by Sex and Year of Graduation, 2006 7

Figure 4   Physicians per 100,000 Civilian Population by Census Division 61

Figure 5   Trends in Self-Designated Primary Care With and Without Subspecialties, 1975–2006 275

Figure 6   Distribution of Self-Designated Primary Care Specialties and Subspecialties, 2006.......................275

Figure 7   Percent Distribution of Total US Physicians by Age and Degree, 2006...302

Figure 8   Physicians by Major Professional Activity, 1975–2006...396

Figure 9   Trends in the Distribution of Physicians
              by Self-Designated Specialty, 1975–2006 397

Figure 10   Percent Change in Total Physicians and International Medical Graduates
              by Major Professional Activity, 1980–2006 399

Introduction

Physician Characteristics and Distribution in the US, 2008 Edition, is the latest in a series begun in 1963 as the *Distribution of Physicians*. It contains historical and current data on the US physician population that provide a basis for comparison essential for health services research, program planning, and policy development. All summary and detailed data on physicians in this edition have been compiled as of December 31, 2006, from the American Medical Association's (AMA) Physician Masterfile, maintained by the Division of Survey and Data Resources. A historical and developmental overview of the Physician Masterfile is provided in the next part of this book. Included in this overview is a description of the structure of the Masterfile, as well as data collection and management procedures.

Data in this publication are presented in six separate chapters: Physician Characteristics, Physician Distribution, Analysis of Professional Activity by Self-Designated Specialty and Geographic Region, Primary Care Specialties, Osteopathic Physicians, and Physician Trends.

Chapter 1 — Physician Characteristics — presents key professional and individual characteristics of the physician population. Cross-tabulations include physicians by age, sex, major professional activity, specialty, and race/ethnicity. The section provides separate tabulations for women physicians and International Medical Graduates (IMGs), for physicians by country, school, and year of graduation, and data on specialty and board certification status.

Chapter 2 — Physician Distribution — focuses on the geographical location of physicians. Tabulations are presented for the states, including statistics for IMG physicians and physicians by age and sex.

Chapter 3 — Analysis of Professional Activity by Self-Designated Specialty and Geographic Region — accents specialty and activity data for the nation, as well as for states, census regions and divisions, MSAs, and counties, including separate tabulations by gender and IMG physicians.

Chapter 4 — Primary Care Specialties — presents data in two groups: (1) the general primary care specialties of Family Medicine, General Practice, Internal Medicine, Obstetrics and Gynecology, and Pediatrics, excluding the subspecialties within these general specialties and (2) the primary care subspecialties including only the subspecialties of those listed in group one. This section presents detailed tabulations about primary care physicians, including the data variables of activity, age, sex, board certification, school and year of graduation, IMGs, state of location, and metropolitan area.

Chapter 5 — Osteopathic Physicians — presents key data on Osteopathic Physicians with table formats taken from each of the first four chapters, allowing for an understanding of what the Osteopathic population looks like both on its own, and when compared to the Allopathic population.

Chapter 6 — Physician Trends — presents data from 1975 through 2006 on the physician characteristics of specialty, major professional activity, age, and sex. National trend data are also displayed for Metropolitan Statistical Areas (MSAs), female physicians, and IMGs. Physician population ratios for selected years 1965–2006 are included, as are ratios by state and specialty.

Five appendices provide easy access to information on geographical locations and categories and include lists of divisions, regions, demographic county classifications, and the county composition for MSAs. Also provided is information on the American Specialty Boards.

Although this publication was designed to address and meet many of the anticipated data requirements concerning the physician population, various users may have specific requests for information from the AMA Physician Masterfile. Such inquiries regarding data contained in this publication, in earlier publications, or from the AMA Physician Masterfile should be directed to the AMA Division of Survey and Data Resources.

This publication is copyrighted, and any use of data contained within this publication is to be referenced as follows: *Physician Characteristics and Distribution, 2008 Edition*, Division of Survey and Data Resources, American Medical Association, 2008.

AMA Physician Masterfile

The American Medical Association (AMA) has continued to develop a unique and comprehensive database of physician and medical student information since the establishment of the Masterfile in 1906. Although initially the Masterfile was primarily used by the Association as a record-keeping device for membership and mailing purposes, today the Masterfile is widely considered to be the most complete and extensive source of physician-related information in the United States.

Current and Historical Information

The Masterfile contains current and historical data on all physicians, including members and nonmembers of the AMA, and graduates of foreign medical schools who are in the United States and meet educational standards for recognition as physicians. International Medical Graduates (IMGs), comprising graduates of foreign medical schools residing in the United States, are included in the Masterfile, generally upon entry into graduate medical training programs accredited by the Accreditation Council on Graduate Medical Education (ACGME). Included also in the Masterfile are IMGs who have been granted a state license to practice medicine but may not have entered ACGME training programs. The Masterfile also includes physicians licensed to practice in the United States but temporarily located abroad.

A record is started on each individual upon entry into medical school or, in the case of international or Canadian medical graduates, upon entry into the United States. A physician's record includes medical school and year of graduation, sex and birthdate. As the physician's training and career develop, additional information is added, such as residency training, state licensure data, and board certification. This information, which comprises the historical portion of the Masterfile, facilitates studies of trends in geographic mobility and medical education.

In addition, the current professional activities portion of each physician's record identifies geographical location and current address, type of practice (Patient Care or Nonpatient Care), specialties (primary and secondary), and present employment (solo, partnership, group practice, medical schools, hospitals, government, and other organizations). These data are particularly useful in manpower planning and research. By definition, the current portion of the record is subject to constant change and must be updated continually through extensive monitoring and data collection activities. Over time, the objectives, collection techniques, and need assessments undergo regular review and change. Quality control, Masterfile expansion, and upgrading of the information collected and analyzed continue to be the major focus of the AMA's Division of Survey and Data Resources.

Data Collection and Updating

A major source of data collection is the Census of Physicians (PPA Questionnaire), which the AMA designed in 1968 in order to collect data under a new classification of physician activities based on "hours worked" criteria. The PPA Questionnaire was sent every four years between 1969 and 1985 to all physicians residing in the United States, as well as to US physicians residing temporarily overseas. Since 1985, the PPA Questionnaire has evolved into a rotating census in which approximately one fourth of all physicians are surveyed each year. New methodologies are periodically tested and implemented to enhance data collection; examples include telephone follow-ups and multi-packet mailings.

Each physician is asked to choose among the categories in each of the following items:

- Professional Activity – Direct Patient Care or Nonpatient Care activities (ie, Administrative Activities, Medical Education, Medical Research, Other Medical Activities)

- Specialization – primary and secondary specialties

- Present Employment – type of employer (ie, Self-Employed, Solo Practice, Two-Physician Practice, Group Practice, HMO, Medical School, Non-Government Hospital, City/County/State Government, US Government, Locum Tenens, Other Patient Care, and Other Nonpatient Care)

All completed questionnaires are passed through a series of computer editing procedures that assign major professional activity, specialty, and employment classifications to each physician's record.

Over the past decade, the PPA Questionnaire has undergone continuous expansion. In addition to the professional activity, specialty, and employment categories, the PPA Questionnaire now includes information about office addresses, principal hospital affiliations, group affiliations, telephone numbers, and other data.

While the data collected from the PPA Questionnaire represent a major source of information to the Masterfile, data also are obtained from several organizations and institutions. These primary sources and the data they provide include:

- Medical schools – name, address, birthdate, birthplace, school, and year of graduation

- Hospitals – physicians in graduate medical training, including IMGs entering US training

- Medical societies – address and membership information

- State licensing agencies – licensure status of physicians

- Educational Commission for Foreign Medical Graduates (ECFMG) – IMGs who are certified or have applied for certification by the ECFMG

- Surgeons general of the US government – physicians in government services

- American Board of Medical Specialties – physicians certified by American Specialty Boards

Data are also extracted from the Masterfile for use by these agencies. In addition, the Masterfile is used by various state and county societies, publishers, and several addressing companies.

Definitions

The following material provides definitions and explanations of the specific physician attributes included in the tabulations of this publication. These materials are presented as a common reference base to facilitate analysis and interpretation of the data.

Major Professional Activity

Major professional activity (MPA) classifications are reported by physicians in the Physicians' Practice Arrangements (PPA) questionnaire. The physician's professional activity is shown in the two categories of Patient Care and Nonpatient care, the latter category being referred to as Other Professional Activity. Patient Care activities include Office-Based practice and Hospital-Based practice. Physicians in Residency training (including Clinical Fellows) and full-time members of Hospital Staffs comprise Hospital-Based practice. Other Professional Activity includes Administration, Medical Teaching, Research, and Other Activities. The subcategory Clinical Fellows is no longer tabulated; physicians formerly counted as Clinical Fellows are now in the category Residents/ Fellows and are tabulated as Residents.

Physicians who are retired, semi-retired, working part-time, temporarily not in practice, or not active for other reasons are classified as Inactive. Physicians are categorized as Not Classified if the American Medical Association (AMA) has not received any recent information as to their type of practice and present employment.

Following are definitions of each of the MPA categories.

Office-Based Practice includes physicians engaged in seeing patients. Physicians may be in solo practice, group practice, two-physician practice, or other patient care employment. This category also includes physicians in patient services such as those provided by pathologists and radiologists.

Hospital-Based Practice includes physicians employed under contract with hospitals to provide direct patient care.

Residents—All Years includes any physician in supervised practice of medicine among patients in a hospital or in its outpatient department, with continued instruction in the science and art of medicine by the staff of the facility. This category also includes clinical fellows in advanced training in the clinical divisions of medicine, surgery, and other specialty fields preparing for practice in a given specialty. These physicians are engaged primarily in patient care.

Medical Teaching includes physicians with teaching appointments in medical schools, hospitals, nursing schools, or other institutions of higher learning.

Medical Research includes physicians in activities (funded or non-funded) performed to develop new medical knowledge, potentially leading to publication. This category also includes physicians in research fellowship programs distinct from an accredited residency program and those primarily engaged in nonpatient care.

Administration includes physicians in administrative activities in a hospital, health facility, health agency, clinic, group, or any similar organization.

Other Activity includes physicians employed by insurance carriers, pharmaceutical companies, corporations, voluntary organizations, medical societies, associations, grants, foreign countries, and the like.

Inactives include physicians who are retired, semi-retired, working part-time, temporarily not in practice, or not active for other reasons and who indicated they worked 20 hours or less per week.

Not Classified includes physicians who did not provide information on their type of practice or their present employment.

Self-Designated Practice Specialty[1]

A physician's self-designated practice specialty (SDPS) is determined, like major professional activity, by the physician from a list of codes included with the PPA Questionnaire. Tables 1.8 and 1.9 provide all specialties listed on the PPA Questionnaire and maintained on the Masterfile. Specialty classifications based on the 40 specialties used by the AMA for statistical purposes are listed in Appendix A.

In the specialty tabulations presented in the Physician Trends, Physician Characteristics (except Tables 1.8 and 1.9), Physician Distribution, and Analysis of Activity by Specialty chapters of the book, the specialties of Family Medicine (FM), General Practice (GP), Internal Medicine (IM), Obstetrics/Gynecology (OBG), and Pediatrics (PD) include both the general primary care specialties and their respective subspecialties as listed in the specialty abbreviations appearing in Appendix A. However, in the primary care chapter, the data are presented separately for the general primary care specialties and the primary care subspecialties.

Primary Care Specialties

As just mentioned in reference to the primary care chapter, detailed statistical data are presented in two separate specialty groupings: (1) the general primary care specialties of Family Medicine, General Practice, Internal Medicine, Obstetrics and Gynecology, and Pediatrics excluding the subspecialties associated with these general specialties and (2) the primary care subspecialties including only the subspecialties of the general specialties listed in group one. The primary care subspecialties are listed in the footnote to Tables 4.5, 4.7-4.9, 4.11-4.13, and 4.15 and include the following:

• FM Subspecialties

Geriatric Medicine (Family Medicine) (FMG) and Sports Medicine (Family Medicine) (FSM)

• IM Subspecialties

Adolescent Medicine (AMI), Critical Care Medicine (CCM), Diabetes (DIA), Endocrinology, Diabetes, & Metabolism (END), Hematology (HEM), Hepatology (HEP), Hematology/Oncology (HO), Cardiac Electrophysiology (ICE), Infectious Diseases (ID), Clinical & Laboratory Immunology (Internal Medicine) (ILI), Geriatric Medicine (Internal Medicine) (IMG), Sports Medicine (Internal Medicine) (ISM), Nephrology (NEP), Nutrition (NTR), Medical Oncology (ON), Pulmonary Critical Care Medicine (PCC), and Rheumatology (RHU)

• OBG Subspecialties

Gynecological Oncology (GO), Gynecology (GYN), Maternal & Fetal Medicine (MFM), Obstetrics (OBS), Critical Care Medicine (Obstetrics & Gynecology) (OCC), and Reproductive Endocrinology (REN)

• PD Subspecialties

Adolescent Medicine (ADL), Pediatric Critical Care Medicine (CCP), Pediatrics/Internal Medicine (MPD), Neonatal-Perinatal Medicine (NPM), Pediatric Allergy (PDA), Pediatric Cardiology (PDC), Pediatric Endocrinology (PDE), Pediatric Infectious Disease (PDI), Pediatric Pulmonology (PDP), Medical Toxicology (Pediatrics), (PDT), Pediatric Emergency Medicine (PEM), Pediatric Gastroenterology (PG), Pediatric Hematology/Oncology (PHO), Clinical & Laboratory Immunology (Pediatrics) (PLI), Pediatric Nephrology (PN), Pediatric Rheumatology (PPR), and Sports Medicine (Pediatrics) (PSM)

The tables in Chapter 4 also include separate statistics for All Other specialties and the Not Classified physicians. In the chapter on primary care, the specialty of Pediatric Cardiology is included in the Pediatrics subspecialty grouping while in the Physician Trends, Physician Characteristics, Physician Distribution, and Analysis of Activity by Specialty, it is listed separately.

Board Certification

Board certification by one or more of the 24 American Specialty Boards listed in Appendix B represents a voluntary effort on the part of the physician. The process of certification entails a complex and rigid series of requirements, including examination and successful completion of an approved residency training program. A licensed physician may practice in any specialty, however, regardless of board certification status. Tables in this publication indicate board certification in the corresponding specialty in which the physician is classified. Although the attainment of certification demonstrates proficiency within a chosen discipline, "Medical specialty board certification is an additional process to receiving a medical degree, completing residency training, and receiving a license to practice medicine."[2]

The terms corresponding board and non-corresponding board in this publication (Tables 1.14 through 1.16) are used to describe the appropriate board certification status of physicians in relation to their SDPS as follows:

• Certified by Corresponding Board Only

Includes physicians in an SDPS who are certified by the respective board having authority to grant certification for that specialty (for example, a physician in the specialty of Family Medicine certified only by the American Board of Family Medicine)

• Certified by Corresponding Board and NonCorresponding Board(s)

Includes physicians in a specialty SDPS who hold two or more certifications: one from the respective board having authority to grant certification in the physicians' SDPS and another from a different board that does not grant certification in the physicians' SDP (for example, a physician in the specialty of Internal Medicine certified by the American Board of Internal Medicine and also the American Board of Surgery)

• Certified by NonCorresponding Board Only

Includes physicians in an SDPS who are certified by a board that does not grant certification in the physicians' SDPS (for example, a physician in the specialty of Emergency Medicine certified by the American Board of Internal Medicine)

• Not Certified

Includes physicians who are not certified by any board

A listing of the American Specialty Boards and information regarding general certification and subspecialty certification are provided in Appendix B.

Residency Training Data

Neither SDPS nor certification by a member board of ABMS should be confused with the fact that a physician has successfully completed a program (or programs) of accredited graduate medical education. Accreditation is the process whereby the Accreditation Council for Graduate Medical Education (ACGME) grants public recognition to a specialized program that meets certain established educational standards as determined through initial and subsequent periodic evaluation by one of the 27 Residency Review committees. AMA collects physicians' residency training data through an annual census of all ACGME accredited residency training programs.

Other Physician Characteristics

The medical education of physicians is grouped into four graduation classifications: (1) US active schools, (2) US inactive schools, (3) Canadian schools, and (4) international schools. Schools of basic medical sciences as well as undeveloped medical schools which, although operational, have not graduated any physicians and therefore are not yet eligible for approval, are excluded from the tabulations. In February 1990, the AMA began using the term International Medical Graduates (IMGs) in place of Foreign Medical Graduates when referring to physicians who graduated from a medical school located outside of the United States, Possessions (Puerto Rico, Virgin Islands, and Pacific Islands), or Canada. Data in prior editions of Physician Characteristics and Distribution refer to this population as Foreign Medical Graduates.

Physician distribution by age is presented in 10-year intervals on a continuum from younger than 35 to 65 and older. Also included are distributions by sex.

Metropolitan Statistical Area Definition

Based on the 1980 decennial census, the Federal Committee on Metropolitan Statistical Areas established a new set of criteria to designate metropolitan areas. The former Standard Metropolitan Statistical Area (SMSA) is now called the Metropolitan Statistical Area (MSA). The MSAs in this edition adhere to the federal government's new revisions and definitions.[3]

An area qualifies as an MSA in one of two ways: (1) if there is a city of at least 50,000 population, or (2) if there is an urbanized area of at least 50,000 population with a total metropolitan population of at least 100,000. In addition to the county containing the central city, an MSA may include additional counties having close economic/social ties to the central county. MSAs comprise entire counties, except for the six New England states, where towns/cities are the units of definition because of the lack of county governments. Except for this base unit, the same criteria are applied to define MSAs in New England as in the rest of the country.

The 280 MSAs tabulated in this edition are listed in Tables 3.14 and 4.15 and in Appendix C. In Tables 3.14 and 4.15, the name of each MSA is the name of the largest city or the first-mentioned of a compound name. In Appendix C, the full name of the MSA is listed. Those MSAs that are located in

more than one state are designated by the state containing the largest city in that particular MSA.

Metropolitan data for 1970 and 1980 reflect variations of the current definition. Descriptions of the earlier SMSA classifications are provided in the *Distribution of Physicians in the United States, 1970,*[4] and *Physician Characteristics and Distribution in the US, 1981.*[5]

Demographic County Classification

The Demographic County Classification that appears in tabulations in this edition is summarized in Appendix E and is referred to as county groups in the publication. The Demographic County Classification is based on physicians' reported preferred professional mailing addresses (PPMAs) rather than office addresses, although PPMAs may refer to offices. The MSAs indicated in county groups 6 through 9 adhere to the federal government's revision of metropolitan areas just described. County groups 1 through 4 comprise nonmetropolitan counties, according to the population in these areas.

The group 5 county classification, which appeared in prior editions, does not appear in the 1990 or later editions. Most of the counties in this group were redistributed to categories 4 or 6 based on population. Because of the elimination of county group 5, the number of counties in the various Demographic County Classifications will not be fully comparable between editions prior to 1990 and 1990 or later editions.

The Demographic County Classification took its present form in 1967 when a prior classification of five county groups was revised. Any conversion of the prior five county groups to the present county groups is not possible because of the different criteria used for each classification.

County Data

Beginning with the 1993 Edition, the independent cities of Virginia are listed separately from the individual counties in Virginia and are designated with the suffix (ic), as shown in Table 3.11. In addition, the independent cities of Baltimore, Maryland, and St. Louis, Missouri, are listed separately from the counties of Baltimore and St. Louis.

The Alaskan Boroughs/Census Areas are listed in Table 3.11 instead of the four Judicial Divisions appearing in editions prior to 1993. Table 3.11 lists only the 21 Boroughs/Census Areas having at least one physician rather than the entire 26 defined by the US Census Bureau. The Boroughs/Census Areas not listed are Bristol Bay, Denali, Lake and Peninsula, Wade Hampton, and Yukon-Koyukuk.

Endnotes

1. The Self-Designated Practice Specialties (SDPS) appearing on the AMA Physician Masterfile and in this publication do not imply recognition or endorsement of any field of medical practice by the AMA.

2. *Graduate Medical Education Directory, 1995-1996.* Accreditation Council for Graduate Medical Education, American Medical Association; p 934.

3. Population Division, US Census Bureau; Internet Release Date: July 1999; Last Revised: January 28, 2006.

4. *Distribution of Physicians in the United States, 1970.* Department of Survey Research, Center for Health Services Research and Development, American Medical Association; 1971.

5. *Physician Characteristics and Distribution in the US, 1981.* Department of Data Release Services, Division of Survey and Data Resources, American Medical Association; 1982.

Acknowledgments

The *Physician Characteristics and Distribution in the US* publication is the result of the combined efforts and participation of a number of staff members within the American Medical Association (AMA).

Gratefully acknowledged is the support provided by Marsha Mildred, Boon Ai Tan, Elizabeth Dudek, and Ronnie Summers from AMA Press in manuscript development and production, and Erica Duke in coordinating the marketing activities for the book.

The publication was greatly improved by Dave Doty, who made sure that the tables were in proper order and incorporated all the figures in the text.

The annual publication of *Physician Characteristics and Distribution in the US* represents the support, commitment, and dedicated efforts of the departments within the Division of Survey and Data Resources that manage ongoing data collection activities of physician-related information, and the planning, survey, and dissemination activities for the AMA Physician Masterfile and other supplementary data files, with particular thanks going to the Department of Database Licensing.

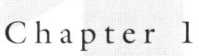

Chapter 1
Physician Characteristics

This chapter provides statistics on several key characteristics of the physician population in the US as of December 31, 2006. These include information regarding (1) major professional activity, (2) primary specialty, (3) specialty board certification status, (4) age and sex, and (5) country, school, and year of graduation. Also presented are separate tabulations for female physicians and International Medical Graduates (IMGs) by their specialty and activity.

Activity by Age and Sex

Table 1.1 indicates that in 2006, nearly two fifths of US physicians were younger than 45 years (38.5%). The 45- to 54-year age interval accounted for the highest percentage of total physicians (24.3%). Of all Office-Based physicians (560,411), the highest percentage was indicated for the 45- to 54-year age group—31.7%. Within the Administration total of 14,575, the largest proportion of physicians comprised the 55- to 64-year age group — more than one third, or 35.8%. Physicians 65 years or older numbered 177,232, or 19.2% of the physicians in the US. Within this group, Patient Care accounted for two-fifths (40.3%), with half (51.9%) listed as Inactive.

Of total female physicians (256,257), the highest percentage (31.1%) was 35 to 44 years of age. Only 7.1% were 65 years or older. Approximately one ninth (11.5%) of Office-Based female physicians were younger than 35 years, compared with 4.7% of Office-Based male physicians. More than one third (34.7%) of all male physicians in Other Professional Activity were in Administration. Administration accounted for 28.4% of all female

physicians in Other Professional Activity. The age interval 35 to 44 years comprised nearly one fifth (18.2%) of female physicians in Medical Teaching but less than one tenth (8.2%) of male physicians. The 45- to 54-year age interval contained the highest percentages of both male (32.8%) and female (34.9%) physicians working in hospitals as full-time staff. Figure 1 displays a percentage distribution of the total US physician population by age and sex.

Self-Designated Specialty by Age and Sex

An analysis of Table 1.2 indicates that at the end of 2006, three fifths (60.0%) of all physicians (553,153) were in the following ten specialty fields:

Internal Medicine (155,705)

Family Medicine (82,866)

Pediatrics (73,208)

Obstetrics/Gynecology (42,333)

Psychiatry (41,385)

Anesthesiology (41,193)

General Surgery (37,556)

Emergency Medicine (29,987)

Diagnostic Radiology (24,624)

Orthopedic Surgery (24,296)

These same specialties (but replacing Diagnostic Radiology with Cardiovascular Diseases) were also highest for all male physicians (Table 1.3), representing 56.4% of the male population. The five disciplines with the most male physicians younger than 35 years were Internal Medicine (21.7% of males younger than 35 years), Family Medicine

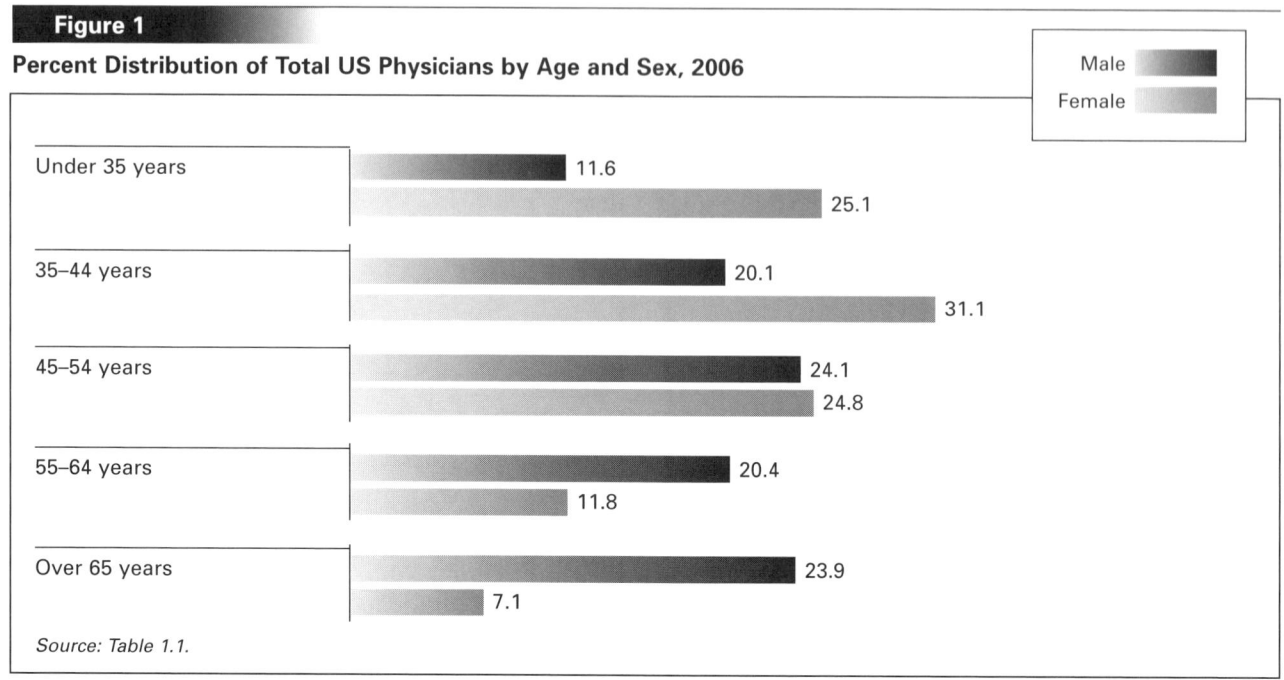

Figure 1

Percent Distribution of Total US Physicians by Age and Sex, 2006

Male
Female

Under 35 years — 11.6 / 25.1

35–44 years — 20.1 / 31.1

45–54 years — 24.1 / 24.8

55–64 years — 20.4 / 11.8

Over 65 years — 23.9 / 7.1

Source: Table 1.1.

(7.7%), General Surgery (7.2%), Pediatrics (6.2%), and Emergency Medicine (5.6%).

For female physicians, the specialties demonstrating the highest numbers differed from the male and overall physician populations. The top 10 disciplines for female physicians (Table 1.4) consisted of the following:

Internal Medicine (49,541)

Pediatrics (39,468)

Family Medicine (28,416)

Obstetrics/Gynecology (18,520)

Psychiatry (14,066)

Anesthesiology (9,369)

Emergency Medicine (6,830)

Pathology (6,620)

General Surgery (5,703)

Diagnostic Radiology (5,524)

For these specialties, the highest percentages of female physicians younger than 35 years were found in Internal Medicine (21.0% of females younger than 35 years), Pediatrics (16.8%), Family Medicine (10.8%), Obstetrics/Gynecology (7.5%), and General Surgery (3.7%).

Table 1 illustrates, for the highest 10 specialties ranked by size, the percentage distribution of total

male and female IMG physicians by age. As Table 1 indicates, Internal Medicine and Family Medicine had the highest proportions of male physicians younger than 35 years. For female physicians, the disciplines with the highest proportions younger than 35 years included Internal Medicine, Family Medicine, and Obstetrics/Gynecology.

Distribution of Detail Specialties by Activity

Detailed specialty data are reported by physicians on the Census of Physicians (PPA Questionnaire) and included on the AMA Physician Masterfile. To meet user needs and requests for more detailed specialty information, Table 1.9 lists the specialties reported by at least one physician. However, care must be exercised in comparing the specialty data displayed in Table 1.9 with the other tables in this publication because it is the only table in this publication that presents the entire list of detail specialties with one or more physicians. For all other tables in this volume, the detail specialties are aggregated into the more generalized specialty categories. For example, the aggregation of detail specialties into general categories can be illustrated by the specialty of Internal Medicine. Table 1.2 shows a total physician count of 155,705 in Internal

Mini-Table 1

Percent Distribution of International Medical Graduates by Age and Self-Designated Specialty Ranked by Size, 2006

Specialty	Rank	Total	Under 35	35-44	45-54	55-64	65 & Over
Total Male IMG's		**165,377**	**10.7%**	**20.8%**	**22.7%**	**21.6%**	**24.2%**
Anesthesiology	4	8,696	5.6%	22.6%	28.5%	26.7%	16.5%
Cardiovascular Diseases	7	6,273	6.5%	23.4%	31.2%	25.4%	13.5%
Family Medicine	2	10,793	14.4%	22.8%	27.9%	21.7%	13.2%
General Practice	9	3,746	0.4%	1.9%	14.8%	34.1%	48.8%
General Surgery	6	6,941	13.4%	12.8%	14.9%	30.7%	28.2%
Internal Medicine	1	39,016	18.3%	28.3%	27.1%	17.3%	9.0%
Obstetrics/Gynecology	8	5,098	6.3%	8.9%	18.6%	38.2%	28.0%
Orthopedic Surgery	10	3,661	5.0%	19.0%	26.6%	21.1%	28.2%
Pediatrics	3	9,721	9.0%	22.0%	30.7%	23.8%	14.4%
Psychiatry	5	8,270	5.5%	16.7%	25.9%	26.1%	25.7%
Total Female IMG's		**71,292**	**19.3%**	**30.0%**	**21.1%**	**16.8%**	**12.7%**
Anesthesiology	5	3,016	6.9%	26.6%	23.4%	28.7%	14.2%
Diagnostic Radiology	10	1,057	7.0%	33.5%	26.3%	20.7%	12.5%
Emergency Medicine	8	1,236	1.4%	3.2%	19.8%	43.0%	32.5%
Family Medicine	3	6,475	26.2%	34.2%	23.0%	11.5%	5.1%
General Surgery	9	1,197	14.5%	39.9%	25.8%	15.0%	4.7%
Internal Medicine	1	18,013	28.6%	37.0%	21.2%	9.5%	3.7%
Obstetrics/Gynecology	7	2,348	19.1%	18.4%	15.3%	29.0%	18.3%
Pathology	6	2,700	8.4%	25.9%	26.1%	24.9%	14.7%
Pediatrics	2	10,597	15.4%	27.3%	26.5%	22.1%	8.7%
Psychiatry	4	4,729	9.5%	23.3%	27.0%	24.5%	15.7%

Note: Percentages may not always add to 100 due to rounding.
Source: Tables 1.6 and 1.7.

Medicine. In Table 1.9, this Internal Medicine count is distributed among the subcategories of Internal Medicine (113,340), Nephrology (7,410), Infectious Diseases (6,342), Medical Oncology (5,386), Endocrinology, Diabetes & Metabolism (5,074), Rheumatology (4,438), Hematology/Oncology (4,317), Geriatric Medicine (Internal Medicine) (2,973), Hematology (Internal Medicine) (2,224), Critical Care Medicine (Internal Medicine) (1,303), Interventional Cardiology (1,068), Clinical Cardiac Electrophysiology (910), Diabetes (317), Nutrition (160), Hepatology (109), Internal Medicine (Emergency Medicine) (94), Internal Medicine/Psychiatry (91), Hospitalist (46), Sports Medicine (Internal Medicine) (43), Internal Medicine (Preventive Medicine) (19), Adolescent Medicine (Internal Medicine) (18), Internal Medicine & Neurology (10), Clinical & Laboratory Immunology (Internal Medicine) (6), Internal Medicine/Dermatology (4), and Nuclear Cardiology (3). The List of Detailed Self-Designated Practice Specialty Codes in Appendix A presents the grouping of the detail specialties into the general specialty categories used throughout this publication.

The 10 specialties showing highest counts of physicians in 2006, in the detail specialties in Table 1.9, included: Internal Medicine (113,340), Family Medicine (81,878), Pediatrics (57,200), Psychiatry (39,423), Anesthesiology (38,858), Obstetrics/Gynecology (37,996), General Surgery (30,932), Emergency Medicine (29,579), Diagnostic Radiology (24,622), and Cardiovascular Disease (22,426). Considering only the category Residents/Fellows, the percentages of Residents/Fellows to total physicians in each of these specialties are Internal Medicine (18.3%), Family Medicine (9.9%), Pediatrics (12.8%), Psychiatry (10.6%), Anesthesiology (11.4%), Obstetrics/Gynecology (11.1%), General Surgery (23.9%), Emergency Medicine (13.4%), Diagnostic Radiology (16.1%), and Cardiovascular Disease (9.3%).

Mean Age by Detail Specialty and Activity

Table 1.8 shows the mean age of physicians in the detail specialties. The 10 specialties with the highest mean ages include the following:

Psychoanalysis (70.6)

General Practice (64.3)

Clinical Molecular Genetics (64.0)

Clinical and Laboratory Immunology (Internal Medicine) (63.3)

Allergy (63.1)

Abdominal Surgery (62.8)

Underseas Medicine (Emergency Medicine) (62.0)

Radiology (61.7)

Gynecology (61.4)

Legal Medicine (61.2)

The table also shows that within the category of Patient Care, Hospital Based physicians are an average of more than two years older than their Office Based counterparts, while physicians in Administration are an average of ten years older than the physician population as a whole.

International Medical Graduates (IMGs)

Activity by Self-Designated Specialty

In 2006, IMGs accounted for 25.7% of the total physician population and 25.6% of the total physicians in Patient Care (Tables 1.10 and 1.1). Within the IMG population itself, 78.2% of physicians were in Patient Care. Of this group of 185,045 physicians, nearly three quarters (74.1%) were in Office-Based practice, representing 24.5% of all Office-Based physicians in the US and Possessions. IMGs accounted for 28.4% of all physicians in residency/fellowship training and nearly one third (31.0%) of all Hospital-Based full-time physician staff. Almost one fifth of all physicians in Research (19.5%) and one out of six physicians in Medical Teaching (16.7%) were IMGs. Only 13.4% of all

physicians in Administration were graduates of international medical schools.

Nearly three fifths (59.6%) of all IMGs were in the specialties of Internal Medicine (57,029), Pediatrics (20,318), Family Medicine (17,268), Psychiatry (12,999), Anesthesiology (11,712), Obstetrics/Gynecology (7,446), General Surgery (7,419), and Cardiovascular Disease (6,822). More than half (57.5%) of all IMGs in residency/fellowship training were concentrated in the Medical Specialties, whereas 18.5% were in Other Specialties. General/Family Medicine represented one eighth of all IMG residents (13.7%), whereas the Surgical Specialties represented 10.3%.

Activity by Age and Sex

Nearly twice as many IMGs (Table 1.11) were in the 35- to 44-year age group in 2006 (23.6%) than in the younger than 35-year age group (13.3%). Female IMGs comprised 30.1% of the IMG complement. Age distribution for female IMGs indicated the highest percentage in the 35- to 44-year age group (30.0%), followed by 21.1% between ages 45 and 54 years. One fourth of male IMGs (22.7%) were in the 45- to 54-year age group, and more than one fifth (21.6%) were in the 55- to 64-year age group. Figure 2 illustrates the distribution of total IMGs by age and activity.

Female Physicians by Self-Designated Specialty and Activity

Representation of female physicians in medicine continues to show steady increases. In 1980, female physicians comprised 11.6% of the physician workforce, but by 2006, they accounted for 27.8% of the total physician population. Female physicians represented two fifths (43.3%) of all residents/fellows in 2006 compared with 21.5% of the resident total in 1980 (Tables 1.13 and 1.1). Of the total female physician population of 256,257, more than four fifths (83.4%) were in Patient Care. Within Patient Care, nearly three quarters (71.4%) were in Office-Based practice. The specialties of Internal Medicine, Pediatrics, Family Medicine, Obstetrics/Gynecology, Psychiatry, and

Figure 2

International Medical Graduates by Age and Major Professional Activity, 2006

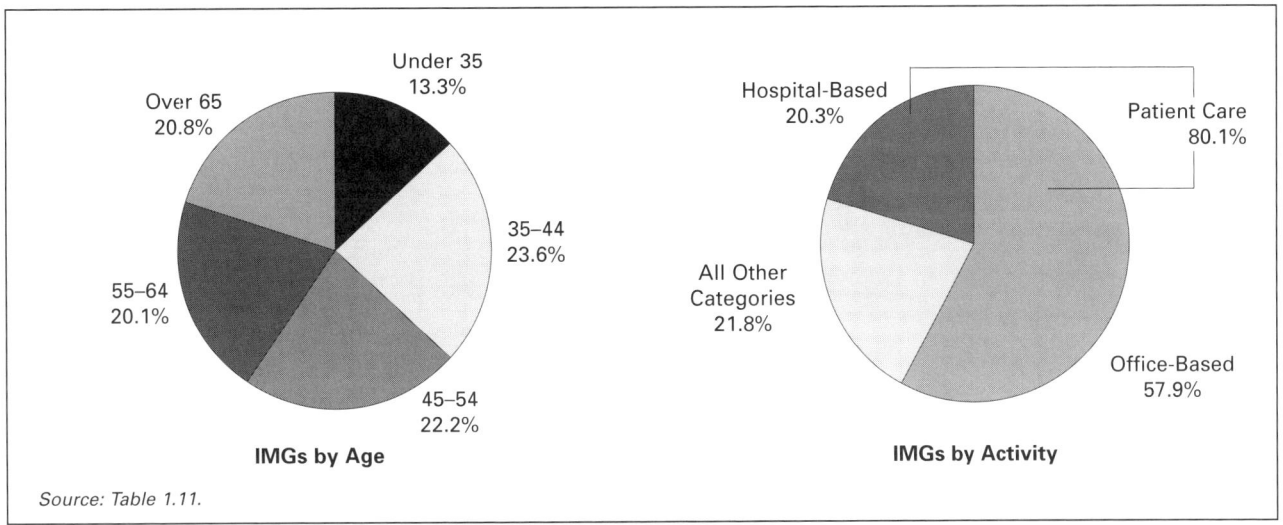

IMGs by Age

IMGs by Activity

Source: Table 1.11.

Anesthesiology accounted for more than three fifths (62.2%) of all female physicians in 2006. Percentages of women in residency training in these specialties are displayed in Table 2.

Other Professional Activity, which includes Administration, Medical Teaching, Research, and Other, accounted for 3.8% of the total female physician population. Female physicians represented 25.8% of all physicians in Medical Teaching, 18.9% of all physicians in Administration, and 21.3% of total physicians in Research (Tables 1.13 and 1.1).

Self-Designated Specialty by Board Certification

Table 1.14 presents data on the specialty board certification status of physicians in the following four categories:

Mini-Table 2

Female Physicians by Self-Designated Specialty and Residency Training, 2006

Specialty	Physicians	Residents	Total (%)
Internal Medicine	49,541	10,779	21.8%
Pediatrics	39,468	7,228	18.3%
Family Medicine	28,416	4,339	15.3%
Obstetrics/Gynecology	18,520	3,119	17.3%
Psychiatry	14,066	2,384	16.9%
Anesthesiology	9,369	1,562	16.7%

Source: Table 1.13.

• Certified by Corresponding Specialty Board Only

• Certified by Corresponding Specialty Board and Other Boards

• Certified by Non-Corresponding Board

• Not Board Certified

These categories can best be illustrated by an example. If a physician reports a specialty of Allergy and Immunology and is certified only by the specialty board for Allergy and Immunology, then the physician falls into the category "Certified by Corresponding Specialty Board Only." If a physician reports the same specialty but is certified by the specialty board of for Internal Medicine as well as the board for Allergy and Immunology, then the physician falls into the category "Certified by Corresponding Specialty Board and Other Boards." If a physician reports the same specialty but is certified by the specialty board for Internal Medicine only, then the physician falls into the category of "Certified by Non-Corresponding Board." See Appendix B for a listing of specialty boards and the subspecialties certified.

In 2006, more than half (53.9%) of all physicians were certified by their corresponding specialty board only, whereas another 2.6% of physicians were certified by their corresponding specialty board and others. Physicians certified only by a board other than that corresponding to their specialty totaled 118,924, or 12.9% of all physicians. More than one quarter (30.7%) of all physicians were not board certified. The greatest proportion of physicians who were board certified (including certification by corresponding board only, certification by corresponding board and others, and certification by noncorresponding board) were physicians in the following 10 specialties:

Radiology (92.5%)

Pediatric Cardiology (92.1%)

Pulmonary Disease (91.6%)

Gastroenterology (90.8%)

Colon/Rectal Surgery (90.7%)

Medical Genetics (89.5%)

Cardiovascular Disease (89.2%)

Thoracic Surgery (89.0%)

Allergy/Immunology (88.1%)

Dermatology (84.3%)

Nearly three fifths of male physicians (56.8%) were certified by a board corresponding to their specialties or certified by a corresponding board and other boards (Table 1.15). The ratio of female physicians similarly accredited was 55.5% (Table 1.16).

Female physicians who were not board certified represented one third (35.3%) of all female physicians. More than one quarter (28.9%) of male physicians were without board certification. The five specialties having the highest percentages of female physicians who were board certified included Vascular Medicine (100.0%), Pediatric Cardiology (90.6%), Radiology (89.2%), Medical Genetics (88.9), and Pulmonary Disease (88.9%). The five specialties with the highest percentages of male physicians who were board certified consisted of Radiology (93.1%), Pediatric Cardiology (92.7%), Pulmonary Diseases (92.1%), Colon & Rectal Surgery (91.9%), and Gastroenterology (91.1%).

School of Graduation by Year of Graduation

Table 1.17 indicates that US active medical schools accounted for 72.8% of all physicians in the US and Possessions. Of the total of 921,904 physicians, three quarters (78.5) received their MD degrees since 1970.

The 10 highest schools, ranked by total number of graduates, included University of Illinois (13,768), Jefferson Medical College (12,688), Indiana University (12,241), University of Minnesota (10,748), University of Michigan (10,468), Medical College of Pennsylvania (10,373), SUNY at Brooklyn (10,300), Wayne State University (10,009), Ohio State University (9,866), and New York Medical College (9,191). These schools graduated 109,652 physicians, who represented one in six (16.3%) of all graduates of US active medical schools.

Tables 1.18 and 1.19 reveal that within the composite physician population, nearly nine tenths (91.5%) of all female physicians graduated from medical schools between 1970 and 2006, whereas 73.5% of male physicians did so. Of the 236,669 IMGs in the US and Possessions in 2006, the highest proportion (25.6%) graduated from 1980 to 1989 (Table 1.17). Figure 3 illustrates these patterns in the data.

Self-Designated Specialty by Race/Ethnicity

Race/Ethnicity was known for more than three fourths (78.2%) of all physicians, 77.2% for male physicians and 80.7% for female physicians (Tables 1.20 through 1.22). Of all physicians for whom race/ethnicity was known, the ten specialties in greatest proportions were Colon/Rectal Surgery (88.1%), Vascular Medicine (87.5%), Forensic Pathology (86.8%), Medical Genetics (86.3%), Dermatology (86.2%), Plastic Surgery (85.6%), Radiation Oncology (84.6%), Otolaryngology (84.5%), Pediatric Cardiology (84.5%), and Physical Medicine and Rehabilitation (84.4%).

Figure 3

Percent Distribution of International Medical Graduates Compared With Total Physicians by Sex and Year of Graduation, 2006

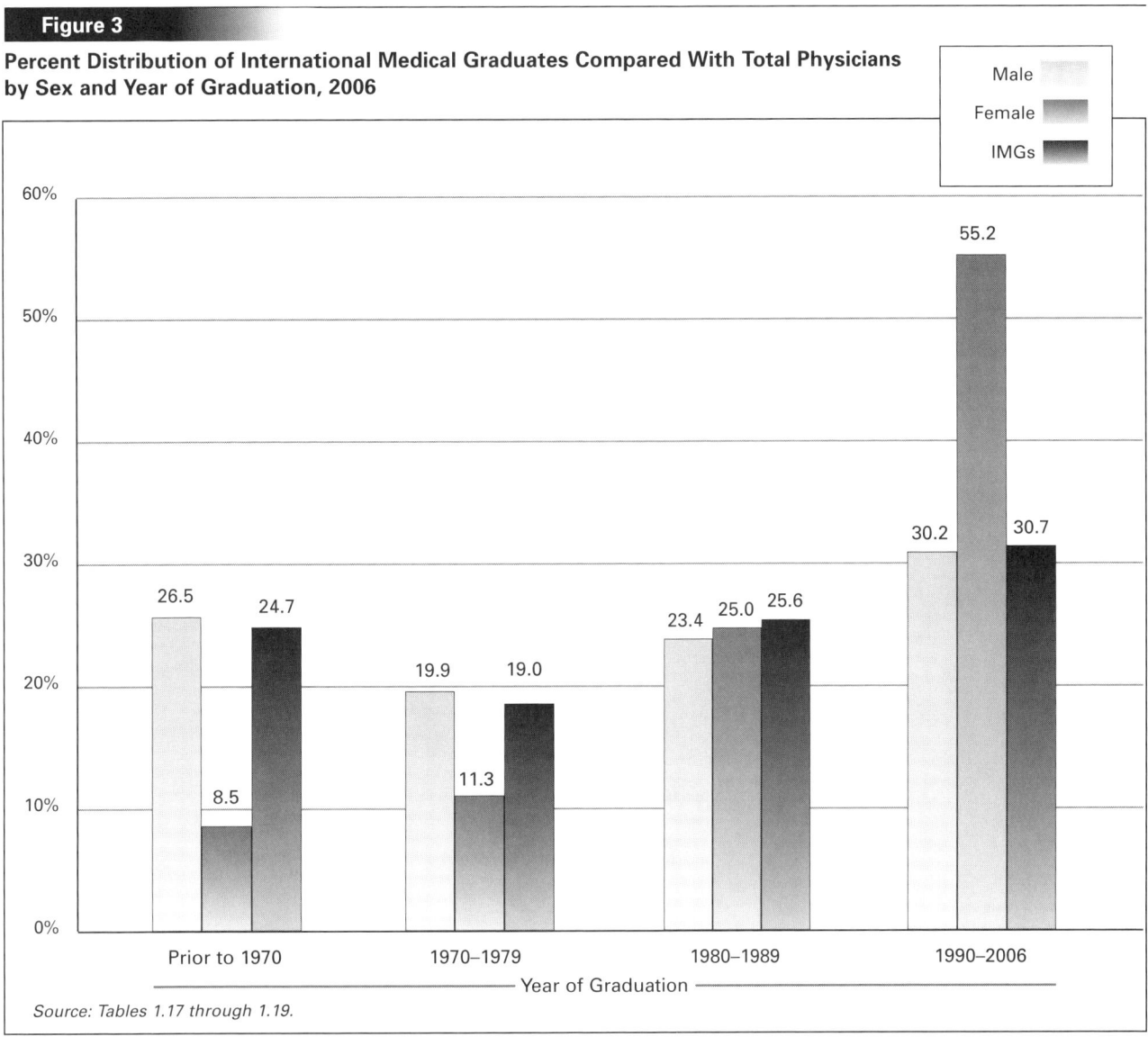

Source: Tables 1.17 through 1.19.

Whites accounted for the largest proportion of all physicians with known ethnicity (71.4%), followed by Asians (15.8%), Hispanics (6.4%), and Blacks (4.5%). The five specialties having the highest proportions of white physicians among those for whom ethnicity was known were Aerospace Medicine (88.7%), Orthopedic Surgery (85.8%), Vascular Medicine (85.7%), Public Health (83.9%), and Occupational Medicine (83.8%). For Asians, the specialties were General Practice (24.7%), Nuclear Medicine (24.3%), Internal Medicine (24.0%), Physical Medicine and Rehabilitation (23.7%), and Radiation Oncology (20.7%). For Hispanics, the specialties were General Practice (12.3%), Pediatrics (8.5%), Child Psychiatry (7.9%), Physical Medicine and Rehabilitation (7.7%), and

Nuclear Medicine (7.3%). For Blacks, the specialties were General Preventative Medicine (11.4%), Obstetrics/Gynecology (8.7%), Public Health & General Preventive Medicine (6.3%), Child Psychiatry (6.2%), and Pediatrics (6.0%).

Table 1.1

Total Physicians by Age, Activity, and Sex, 2006

Activity	Total Physicians	< 35	35-44	45-54	55-64	≥ 65
Both Sexes						
Total Physicians	921,904	141,492	213,311	223,864	166,005	177,232
Patient Care	723,118	120,122	191,190	201,230	139,112	71,464
Office-Based Practice	560,411	36,832	161,189	177,589	122,476	62,325
Hospital-Based Practice	162,707	83,290	30,001	23,641	16,636	9,139
Residents	97,102	80,689	14,554	1,724	127	8
Full-Time Staff	65,605	2,601	15,447	21,917	16,509	9,131
Other Professional Activity	43,718	481	3,674	12,773	14,621	12,169
Administration	14,575	33	626	3,782	5,217	4,917
Medical Teaching	10,273	224	1,108	3,293	3,143	2,505
Research	14,475	170	1,509	4,551	4,970	3,275
Other	4,395	54	431	1,147	1,291	1,472
Inactive	108,344	79	1,342	4,711	10,157	92,055
Not Classified	46,252	20,807	17,104	5,149	2,014	1,178
Address Unknown	472	3	1	1	101	366
Male						
Total Physicians	665,647	77,168	133,515	160,253	135,790	158,921
Patient Care	509,474	65,735	120,185	145,216	114,667	63,671
Office-Based Practice	407,907	19,351	101,312	128,972	102,056	56,216
Hospital-Based Practice	101,567	46,384	18,873	16,244	12,611	7,455
Residents	55,078	45,021	8,995	995	61	6
Full-Time Staff	46,489	1,363	9,878	15,249	12,550	7,449
Other Professional Activity	34,017	244	2,148	8,917	11,869	10,839
Administration	11,817	18	383	2,690	4,339	4,387
Medical Teaching	7,618	123	624	2,179	2,454	2,238
Research	11,394	76	931	3,348	4,099	2,940
Other	3,188	27	210	700	977	1,274
Inactive	94,469	38	677	2,706	7,771	83,277
Not Classified	27,358	11,148	10,505	3,413	1,403	889
Address Unknown	329	3		1	80	245
Female						
Total Physicians	256,257	64,324	79,796	63,611	30,215	18,311
Patient Care	213,644	54,387	71,005	56,014	24,445	7,793
Office-Based Practice	152,504	17,481	59,877	48,617	20,420	6,109
Hospital-Based Practice	61,140	36,906	11,128	7,397	4,025	1,684
Residents	42,024	35,668	5,559	729	66	2
Full-Time Staff	19,116	1,238	5,569	6,668	3,959	1,682
Other Professional Activity	9,701	237	1,526	3,856	2,752	1,330
Administration	2,758	15	243	1,092	878	530
Medical Teaching	2,655	101	484	1,114	689	267
Research	3,081	94	578	1,203	871	335
Other	1,207	27	221	447	314	198
Inactive	13,875	41	665	2,005	2,386	8,778
Not Classified	18,894	9,659	6,599	1,736	611	289
Address Unknown	143		1		21	121

Table 1.2

Total Physicians by Age and Self-Designated Specialty, 2006

Activity	Total Physicians	< 35	35-44	45-54	55-64	≥ 65
			Both Sexes			
Total Physicians	921,904	141,492	213,311	223,864	166,005	177,232
Aerospace Medicine	473	23	52	160	118	120
Allergy/Immunology	4,196	387	790	1,192	1,147	680
Anesthesiology	41,193	5,572	10,807	14,241	7,349	3,224
Cardiovascular Disease	22,426	1,985	4,991	7,365	5,398	2,687
Child Psychiatry	7,260	568	1,950	2,195	1,598	949
Colon/Rectal Surgery	1,340	80	446	391	300	123
Dermatology	10,744	1,696	2,611	2,739	2,457	1,241
Diagnostic Radiology	24,624	4,363	6,310	7,276	4,993	1,682
Emergency Medicine	29,987	6,560	8,522	7,911	5,733	1,261
Family Medicine	82,866	12,898	24,578	25,369	14,620	5,401
Forensic Pathology	657	24	177	227	134	95
Gastroenterology	12,268	1,263	3,081	3,993	2,885	1,046
General Practice	10,493	72	333	1,798	3,391	4,899
General Preventive Medicine	2,161	185	650	714	377	235
General Surgery	37,556	7,936	8,831	8,580	7,143	5,066
Internal Medicine	155,705	30,290	42,356	42,906	27,952	12,201
Medical Genetics	533	60	134	159	123	57
Neurological Surgery	5,425	787	1,398	1,430	1,021	789
Neurology	14,554	1,722	3,603	4,448	3,304	1,477
Nuclear Medicine	1,477	114	271	390	411	291
Obstetrics/Gynecology	42,333	6,166	10,901	11,346	8,967	4,953
Occupational Medicine	2,641	36	187	954	879	585
Ophthalmology	18,058	1,921	4,393	5,336	4,121	2,287
Orthopedic Surgery	24,296	3,863	5,719	6,515	5,132	3,067
Otolaryngology	9,974	1,433	2,565	2,527	2,036	1,413
Pathology-Anatomic/Clinical	19,171	1,987	4,025	5,536	4,364	3,259
Pediatric Cardiology	1,877	268	567	523	304	215
Pediatrics	73,208	15,610	20,861	18,499	12,567	5,671
Physical Medicine & Rehabilitation	7,736	1,070	2,491	2,407	1,211	557
Plastic Surgery	7,063	687	1,712	2,115	1,676	873
Psychiatry	41,385	4,135	7,311	11,123	10,392	8,424
Public Health & General Preventive Medicine	1,434	5	57	378	451	543
Pulmonary Diseases	10,232	1,109	2,898	3,138	2,351	736
Radiation Oncology	4,424	604	1,162	1,370	884	404
Radiology	8,886	540	2,379	1,901	1,897	2,169
Thoracic Surgery	4,807	137	1,068	1,528	1,183	891
Transplant Surgery	151	2	43	72	21	13
Urological Surgery	10,518	1,107	2,428	2,631	2,597	1,755
Vascular Medicine	24	1	7	5	8	3
Other Specialty	5,168	114	543	1,276	1,464	1,771
Unspecified	7,512	3,223	1,656	1,339	774	520
Inactive	108,344	79	1,342	4,711	10,157	92,055
Not Classified	46,252	20,807	17,104	5,149	2,014	1,178
Address Unknown	472	3	1	1	101	366

Table 1.3

Male Physicians by Age and Self-Designated Specialty, 2006

Activity	Total Physicians	< 35	35-44	45-54	55-64	≥ 65
			Male			
Total Physicians	665,647	77,168	133,515	160,253	135,790	158,921
Aerospace Medicine	435	18	45	144	109	119
Allergy/Immunology	3,042	189	448	855	937	613
Anesthesiology	31,824	3,827	8,115	11,319	5,891	2,672
Cardiovascular Disease	20,234	1,613	4,229	6,654	5,131	2,607
Child Psychiatry	3,934	212	909	1,114	1,012	687
Colon/Rectal Surgery	1,155	57	333	350	293	122
Dermatology	6,482	626	1,215	1,545	1,973	1,123
Diagnostic Radiology	19,100	3,148	4,521	5,578	4,291	1,562
Emergency Medicine	23,157	4,314	6,281	6,352	5,072	1,138
Family Medicine	54,450	5,921	13,736	17,787	12,151	4,855
Forensic Pathology	437	15	100	144	97	81
Gastroenterology	10,833	910	2,581	3,567	2,747	1,028
General Practice	8,438	41	220	1,246	2,601	4,330
General Preventive Medicine	1,344	86	369	424	276	189
General Surgery	31,853	5,582	7,080	7,459	6,744	4,988
Internal Medicine	106,164	16,780	25,578	29,972	22,840	10,994
Medical Genetics	280	27	63	81	70	39
Neurological Surgery	5,094	700	1,284	1,326	997	787
Neurology	10,856	995	2,357	3,352	2,802	1,350
Nuclear Medicine	1,179	88	196	292	344	259
Obstetrics/Gynecology	23,813	1,334	4,378	6,589	7,133	4,379
Occupational Medicine	2,099	25	111	688	740	535
Ophthalmology	14,678	1,221	3,211	4,298	3,753	2,195
Orthopedic Surgery	23,133	3,463	5,349	6,231	5,042	3,048
Otolaryngology	8,758	1,076	2,132	2,214	1,942	1,394
Pathology-Anatomic/Clinical	12,551	965	2,281	3,449	3,171	2,685
Pediatric Cardiology	1,336	156	361	391	248	180
Pediatrics	33,740	4,816	7,996	9,000	7,785	4,143
Physical Medicine & Rehabilitation	5,061	629	1,571	1,661	796	404
Plastic Surgery	6,191	524	1,411	1,844	1,565	847
Psychiatry	27,319	1,918	4,089	6,752	7,541	7,019
Public Health & General Preventive Medicine	1,004	1	32	221	338	412
Pulmonary Diseases	8,671	812	2,225	2,713	2,221	700
Radiation Oncology	3,356	409	830	1,055	695	367
Radiology	7,500	424	1,947	1,506	1,590	2,033
Thoracic Surgery	4,620	122	991	1,464	1,154	889
Transplant Surgery	136	2	39	62	20	13
Urological Surgery	9,935	895	2,208	2,513	2,572	1,747
Vascular Medicine	19	1	5	2	8	3
Other Specialty	4,220	75	382	954	1,253	1,556
Unspecified	5,060	1,962	1,124	965	591	418
Inactive	94,469	38	677	2,706	7,771	83,277
Not Classified	27,358	11,148	10,505	3,413	1,403	889
Address Unknown	329	3		1	80	245

Table 1.4

Female Physicians by Age and Self-Designated Specialty, 2006

Activity	Total Physicians	< 35	35-44	45-54	55-64	≥ 65
			Female			
Total Physicians	256,257	64,324	79,796	63,611	30,215	18,311
Aerospace Medicine	38	5	7	16	9	1
Allergy/Immunology	1,154	198	342	337	210	67
Anesthesiology	9,369	1,745	2,692	2,922	1,458	552
Cardiovascular Disease	2,192	372	762	711	267	80
Child Psychiatry	3,326	356	1,041	1,081	586	262
Colon/Rectal Surgery	185	23	113	41	7	1
Dermatology	4,262	1,070	1,396	1,194	484	118
Diagnostic Radiology	5,524	1,215	1,789	1,698	702	120
Emergency Medicine	6,830	2,246	2,241	1,559	661	123
Family Medicine	28,416	6,977	10,842	7,582	2,469	546
Forensic Pathology	220	9	77	83	37	14
Gastroenterology	1,435	353	500	426	138	18
General Practice	2,055	31	113	552	790	569
General Preventive Medicine	817	99	281	290	101	46
General Surgery	5,703	2,354	1,751	1,121	399	78
Internal Medicine	49,541	13,510	16,778	12,934	5,112	1,207
Medical Genetics	253	33	71	78	53	18
Neurological Surgery	331	87	114	104	24	2
Neurology	3,698	727	1,246	1,096	502	127
Nuclear Medicine	298	26	75	98	67	32
Obstetrics/Gynecology	18,520	4,832	6,523	4,757	1,834	574
Occupational Medicine	542	11	76	266	139	50
Ophthalmology	3,380	700	1,182	1,038	368	92
Orthopedic Surgery	1,163	400	370	284	90	19
Otolaryngology	1,216	357	433	313	94	19
Pathology-Anatomic/Clinical	6,620	1,022	1,744	2,087	1,193	574
Pediatric Cardiology	541	112	206	132	56	35
Pediatrics	39,468	10,794	12,865	9,499	4,782	1,528
Physical Medicine & Rehabilitation	2,675	441	920	746	415	153
Plastic Surgery	872	163	301	271	111	26
Psychiatry	14,066	2,217	3,222	4,371	2,851	1,405
Public Health & General Preventive Medicine	430	4	25	157	113	131
Pulmonary Diseases	1,561	297	673	425	130	36
Radiation Oncology	1,068	195	332	315	189	37
Radiology	1,386	116	432	395	307	136
Thoracic Surgery	187	15	77	64	29	2
Transplant Surgery	15		4	10	1	
Urological Surgery	583	212	220	118	25	8
Vascular Medicine	5		2	3		
Other Specialty	948	39	161	322	211	215
Unspecified	2,452	1,261	532	374	183	102
Inactive	13,875	41	665	2,005	2,386	8,778
Not Classified	18,894	9,659	6,599	1,736	611	289
Address Unknown	143		1		21	121

Table 1.5

International Medical Graduates by Age and Self-Designated Specialty, 2006

Activity	Total Physicians	< 35	35-44	45-54	55-64	≥ 65
			Both Sexes			
Total Physicians	236,669	31,451	55,767	52,657	47,656	49,138
Aerospace Medicine	37		2	10	14	11
Allergy/Immunology	1,033	28	207	346	290	162
Anesthesiology	11,712	695	2,776	3,186	3,191	1,864
Cardiovascular Disease	6,822	502	1,671	2,101	1,658	890
Child Psychiatry	2,139	135	639	605	452	308
Colon/Rectal Surgery	263	8	49	60	102	44
Dermatology	645	25	100	145	193	182
Diagnostic Radiology	2,858	229	513	586	1,003	527
Emergency Medicine	2,664	275	351	643	911	484
Family Medicine	17,268	3,255	4,682	4,498	3,080	1,753
Forensic Pathology	152	3	22	51	38	38
Gastroenterology	3,298	244	991	1,039	708	316
General Practice	4,982	32	111	801	1,811	2,227
General Preventive Medicine	309	16	89	95	54	55
General Surgery	7,419	1,114	1,024	1,103	2,197	1,981
Internal Medicine	57,029	12,289	17,718	14,386	8,473	4,163
Medical Genetics	131	21	45	38	14	13
Neurological Surgery	752	61	116	145	238	192
Neurology	4,644	475	1,387	1,431	911	440
Nuclear Medicine	536	38	91	146	156	105
Obstetrics/Gynecology	7,446	769	885	1,308	2,630	1,854
Occupational Medicine	384	3	27	104	140	110
Ophthalmology	1,423	72	243	310	457	341
Orthopedic Surgery	1,610	68	131	216	650	545
Otolaryngology	932	28	57	135	402	310
Pathology-Anatomic/Clinical	6,361	411	1,394	1,680	1,446	1,430
Pediatric Cardiology	466	52	148	127	67	72
Pediatrics	20,318	2,504	5,037	5,799	4,655	2,323
Physical Medicine & Rehabilitation	2,374	167	590	595	678	344
Plastic Surgery	851	27	110	160	345	209
Psychiatry	12,999	903	2,486	3,424	3,319	2,867
Public Health & General Preventive Medicine	168		4	28	42	94
Pulmonary Diseases	3,376	454	1,243	896	558	225
Radiation Oncology	791	12	105	187	317	170
Radiology	1,670	86	281	195	547	561
Thoracic Surgery	1,052	22	173	203	310	344
Transplant Surgery	38	1	8	18	6	5
Urological Surgery	1,588	20	95	258	702	513
Vascular Medicine	5	1	1	2		1
Other Specialty	977	22	79	188	247	441
Unspecified	2,969	343	752	913	552	409
Inactive	22,838	19	211	850	2,517	19,241
Not Classified	21,255	6,020	9,123	3,646	1,565	901
Address Unknown	85	2			10	73

Table 1.6

Male International Medical Graduates by Age and Self-Designated Specialty, 2006

Activity	Total Physicians	< 35	35-44	45-54	55-64	≥ 65
			Male			
Total Physicians	165,377	17,695	34,391	37,589	35,650	40,052
Aerospace Medicine	34		2	9	12	11
Allergy/Immunology	697	11	103	239	212	132
Anesthesiology	8,696	487	1,968	2,479	2,326	1,436
Cardiovascular Disease	6,273	408	1,471	1,955	1,593	846
Child Psychiatry	1,082	61	285	327	233	176
Colon/Rectal Surgery	248	7	41	55	101	44
Dermatology	417	9	47	89	132	140
Diagnostic Radiology	2,206	135	335	444	825	467
Emergency Medicine	2,285	210	275	564	802	434
Family Medicine	10,793	1,558	2,465	3,009	2,337	1,424
Forensic Pathology	106	2	12	38	26	28
Gastroenterology	2,938	180	826	949	674	309
General Practice	3,746	15	71	556	1,279	1,825
General Preventive Medicine	203	10	59	56	39	39
General Surgery	6,941	930	890	1,035	2,128	1,958
Internal Medicine	39,016	7,140	11,054	10,566	6,758	3,498
Medical Genetics	73	13	22	26	7	5
Neurological Surgery	732	55	110	140	235	192
Neurology	3,447	301	909	1,122	731	384
Nuclear Medicine	384	23	61	98	114	88
Obstetrics/Gynecology	5,098	321	454	949	1,949	1,425
Occupational Medicine	293	3	14	76	107	93
Ophthalmology	1,130	48	149	235	393	305
Orthopedic Surgery	1,583	66	126	211	644	536
Otolaryngology	874	21	49	124	378	302
Pathology-Anatomic/Clinical	3,661	184	696	975	773	1,033
Pediatric Cardiology	336	31	87	104	52	62
Pediatrics	9,721	874	2,140	2,989	2,314	1,404
Physical Medicine & Rehabilitation	1,501	103	342	416	411	229
Plastic Surgery	792	24	92	151	324	201
Psychiatry	8,270	456	1,385	2,145	2,161	2,123
Public Health & General Preventive Medicine	107		4	15	25	63
Pulmonary Diseases	2,915	374	1,024	790	521	206
Radiation Oncology	575	4	74	133	221	143
Radiology	1,352	58	209	165	426	494
Thoracic Surgery	1,036	18	169	200	305	344
Transplant Surgery	38	1	8	18	6	5
Urological Surgery	1,573	20	91	257	697	508
Vascular Medicine	4	1	1	1		1
Other Specialty	773	16	54	147	201	355
Unspecified	2,096	195	491	665	415	330
Inactive	18,086	11	112	561	1,672	15,730
Not Classified	13,183	3,309	5,614	2,506	1,084	670
Address Unknown	63	2			7	54

Table 1.7

Female International Medical Graduates by Age and Self-Designated Specialty, 2006

Activity	Total Physicians	< 35	35-44	45-54	55-64	≥ 65
			Female			
Total Physicians	71,292	13,756	21,376	15,068	12,006	9,086
Aerospace Medicine	3			1	2	
Allergy/Immunology	336	17	104	107	78	30
Anesthesiology	3,016	208	808	707	865	428
Cardiovascular Disease	549	94	200	146	65	44
Child Psychiatry	1,057	74	354	278	219	132
Colon/Rectal Surgery	15	1	8	5	1	
Dermatology	228	16	53	56	61	42
Diagnostic Radiology	652	94	178	142	178	60
Emergency Medicine	379	65	76	79	109	50
Family Medicine	6,475	1,697	2,217	1,489	743	329
Forensic Pathology	46	1	10	13	12	10
Gastroenterology	360	64	165	90	34	7
General Practice	1,236	17	40	245	532	402
General Preventive Medicine	106	6	30	39	15	16
General Surgery	478	184	134	68	69	23
Internal Medicine	18,013	5,149	6,664	3,820	1,715	665
Medical Genetics	58	8	23	12	7	8
Neurological Surgery	20	6	6	5	3	
Neurology	1,197	174	478	309	180	56
Nuclear Medicine	152	15	30	48	42	17
Obstetrics/Gynecology	2,348	448	431	359	681	429
Occupational Medicine	91		13	28	33	17
Ophthalmology	293	24	94	75	64	36
Orthopedic Surgery	27	2	5	5	6	9
Otolaryngology	58	7	8	11	24	8
Pathology-Anatomic/Clinical	2,700	227	698	705	673	397
Pediatric Cardiology	130	21	61	23	15	10
Pediatrics	10,597	1,630	2,897	2,810	2,341	919
Physical Medicine & Rehabilitation	873	64	248	179	267	115
Plastic Surgery	59	3	18	9	21	8
Psychiatry	4,729	447	1,101	1,279	1,158	744
Public Health & General Preventive Medicine	61			13	17	31
Pulmonary Diseases	461	80	219	106	37	19
Radiation Oncology	216	8	31	54	96	27
Radiology	318	28	72	30	121	67
Thoracic Surgery	16	4	4	3	5	
Urological Surgery	15		4	1	5	5
Vascular Medicine	1			1		
Other Specialty	204	6	25	41	46	86
Unspecified	873	148	261	248	137	79
Inactive	4,752	8	99	289	845	3,511
Not Classified	8,072	2,711	3,509	1,140	481	231
Address Unknown	22				3	19

Table 1.8

Physicians' Mean Age by Self-Designated Specialty and Activity (199 Specialties), 2006

| Specialty | Total Physicians | Patient Care | | | | Other Professional Activity | | | |
| | | Total Patient Care | Office Based | Hospital Based | | Admin. | Med. Teach. | Research | Other |
				Resid./ Fellows	Phys. Staff				
Total Physicians	50.9	47.7	50.0	31.1	52.1	60.7	56.9	57.2	59.4
A	63.1	63.1	63.1		64.1	61.4	61.0	66.9	67.3
ADL	50.3	48.4	50.3	33.0	54.1	59.9	55.9	52.1	53.7
ADM	59.1	59.2	59.1		59.6	61.1	57.4	54.9	66.0
ADP	46.1	45.1	46.1	38.5	49.6	55.4	53.2	48.8	
AI	50.0	48.4	50.0	32.5	47.5	60.0	56.2	56.0	55.6
ALI	47.7	47.3	47.7		44.8	43.0	63.0	51.5	
AM	57.6	54.2	57.6	37.6	50.0	59.0	55.9	58.1	58.5
AMI	53.8	54.1	53.8		58.0	45.3	69.0	47.0	
AN	49.8	47.8	49.8	31.2	51.8	58.5	56.7	56.0	57.8
APM	44.8	43.7	44.8	33.7	45.7	56.3	51.5	53.5	57.5
AR	38.6	36.6	38.6	33.2	38.3	67.0	69.0		
AS	62.8	62.3	62.8		58.8	70.0	61.8	54.0	53.0
ATP	55.4	55.9	55.4	31.0	57.7	60.4	63.3	56.2	59.2
BBK	48.7	48.4	48.7	38.5	53.8	59.7	60.6	56.8	57.9
CBG	50.0	47.0	50.0		35.0			54.4	
CCA	43.8	42.8	43.8	34.8	43.3	45.0	48.9	40.5	52.5
CCG	50.5	51.6	50.5		52.3				55.0
CCM	45.7	45.5	45.7	35.0	49.6	57.5	55.2	52.2	52.7
CCP	43.2	40.8	43.2	32.8	45.1	53.8	48.2	45.6	48.0
CCS	42.1	41.4	42.1	36.9	44.1	59.8	51.0	54.3	49.0
CD	51.8	50.0	51.8	32.8	53.7	63.4	61.3	58.1	62.9
CFS	40.8	41.9	40.8	37.0	52.0				
CG	56.1	55.6	56.1		54.7	59.8	60.1	55.1	58.0
CHN	50.9	48.3	50.9	33.1	52.3	61.4	62.1	55.3	55.0
CHP	50.9	49.9	50.9	34.8	54.0	60.0	60.1	56.5	61.9
CLP	59.0	59.9	59.0		62.0	62.2	61.7	59.2	61.6
CMG	64.0	64.0	64.0				57.0	46.9	38.0
CN	40.0	38.7	40.0	34.0	40.9		50.7	42.4	66.3
CPP	30.5	30.5		30.5					
CRS	49.7	49.0	49.7	34.4	50.4	63.9	57.4	54.8	54.5
CS	52.4	52.3	52.4		45.0				
CTR	46.0	39.0	46.0	32.0					
D	50.8	48.6	50.8	30.7	48.4	61.1	56.6	56.7	56.6
DBP	50.0	37.6	50.0	34.1	50.0		68.0		
DDL	58.0	58.0	58.0						53.0
DIA	60.5	60.4	60.5		59.7	65.2	65.4	64.2	58.0
DMP	46.1	45.1	46.1	34.4	50.3	59.3	57.3	56.0	50.2
DR	49.4	46.6	49.4	31.0	52.4	58.9	56.8	56.4	56.1
DS	48.0	47.7	48.0		42.6				
EM	46.2	44.7	46.2	30.3	50.6	56.0	51.8	50.3	54.6

A	Allergy	CD	Cardiovascular Disease
ADL	Adolescent Medicine (Pediatrics)	CFS	Craniofacial Surgery
ADM	Addiction Medicine	CG	Clinical Genetics
ADP	Addiction Psychiatry	CHN	Child Neurology
AI	Allergy & Immunology	CHP	Child and Adolescent Psychiatry
ALI	Clinical Laboratory Immunology (Allergy & Immunology)	CLP	Clinical Pathology
AM	Aerospace Medicine	CMG	Clinical Molecular Genetics
AMI	Adolescent Medicine (Internal Medicine)	CN	Clinical Neurophysiology
AN	Anesthesiology	CPP	Pediatric Psychiatry/Child Psychiatry
APM	Pain Management	CRS	Colon & Rectal Surgery
AR	Abdominal Radiology	CS	Cosmetic Surgery
AS	Abdominal Surgery	CTR	Cardiothoracic Radiology
ATP	Anatomic Pathology	D	Dermatology
BBK	Blood Banking/Transfusion Medicine	DBP	Developmental-Behavioral Pediatrics
CBG	Clinical Biochemical Genetics	DDL	Clinical and Laboratory Dermatological Immunology
CCA	Critical Care Medicine (Anesthesiology)	DIA	Diabetes
CCG	Clinical Cytogenetics	DMP	Dermatopathology
CCM	Critical Care Medicine (Internal Medicine)	DR	Diagnostic Radiology
CCP	Pediatric Critical Care Medicine	DS	Dermatologic Surgery
CCS	Surgical Critical Care (Surgery)	EM	Emergency Medicine

Table 1.8

Physicians' Mean Age by Self-Designated Specialty and Activity (199 Specialties), 2006, continued

| Specialty | Total Physicians | Patient Care | | | | Other Professional Activity | | | |
| | | Total Patient Care | Office Based | Hospital Based | | Admin. | Med. Teach. | Research | Other |
				Resid./ Fellows	Phys. Staff				
EMP	30.3	30.3		30.3					
END	49.1	47.5	49.1	32.7	51.3	62.7	60.7	57.2	57.1
EP	38.0	38.0	38.0			53.0		55.5	48.1
ESM	54.2	48.2	54.2	37.3	32.0		51.0		
ESN	42.8	41.3	42.8	33.0	44.0		40.0		
ETX	39.8	37.9	39.8	34.5	42.0	55.0	50.5		54.0
FM	48.0	46.4	48.0	32.4	48.6	56.5	51.9	52.5	54.9
FOP	49.2	48.7	49.2	37.3	51.8	62.3	63.7	61.3	57.4
FPG	47.1	46.5	47.1	35.0	51.6	58.6	52.6	38.7	78.0
FPP	31.9	31.9		31.9					
FPS	50.0	49.8	50.0		44.5		56.0		52.0
FSM	38.7	37.6	38.7	32.0	42.2	48.0	47.5		
GE	50.3	48.7	50.3	32.5	50.9	61.5	58.3	56.6	60.3
GO	53.0	52.7	53.0		51.3	61.3	60.6	59.2	71.0
GP	64.3	64.1	64.3		63.1	66.0	61.6	61.2	64.0
GPM	48.3	46.9	48.3	36.9	48.9	59.1	57.8	55.8	53.3
GS	52.3	47.0	52.3	30.4	54.0	64.5	60.7	57.9	65.5
GYN	61.4	61.3	61.4		61.2	65.4	65.4	57.5	71.9
HEM	53.2	53.0	53.2	34.4	55.1	65.7	62.2	59.1	53.1
HEP	50.6	50.9	50.6		52.1	65.5	60.3	61.8	
HMP	43.8	42.7	43.8	35.0	48.5	57.0	54.6	51.7	46.3
HNS	56.1	56.1	56.1		56.2	60.8	58.5	55.6	43.0
HO	43.1	40.7	43.1	33.0	45.1	56.9	55.5	46.5	48.9
HOS	41.0	40.6	41.0		40.1		55.0		
HS	48.6	48.6	48.6		49.0	64.3	57.8	52.0	68.0
HSO	33.3	33.3		33.3					
HSP	33.7	33.7		33.7					
HSS	34.1	34.1		34.1					
IC	41.2	40.0	41.2	35.3	43.1	57.0	46.4	46.0	
ICE	43.5	42.2	43.5	34.9	44.9	50.3	46.8	55.0	38.0
ID	46.5	45.2	46.5	33.2	49.4	58.4	58.2	55.7	56.9
IFP	31.5	31.5		31.5					
IG	56.4	56.1	56.4		55.1	70.0	63.8	62.5	61.2
ILI	63.3	66.8	63.3		77.0		63.0	54.0	
IM	48.6	45.2	48.6	30.2	50.2	58.8	54.0	55.4	56.9
IMD	27.8	27.8		27.8					
IMG	45.2	45.1	45.2	35.3	50.2	57.6	53.5	53.6	59.1
IPM	32.2	32.2		32.2					
ISM	41.7	41.8	41.7	32.0	47.0		46.0	47.0	
LM	61.2	59.2	61.2		50.1	61.4	66.0	59.5	62.2
MDM	55.8	55.8	55.8			58.6	64.0	59.3	56.0
MEM	29.8	29.8		29.8					

EMP	Pediatrics/Emergency Medicine	HNS	Head & Neck Surgery
END	Endocrinology, Diabetes and Metabolism	HO	Hematology/Oncology
EP	Epidemiology	HOS	Hospitalist
ESM	Sports Medicine (Emergency Medicine)	HS	Hand Surgery
ESN	Endovascular Surgical Neuroradiology	HSO	Hand Surgery (Orthopedics)
ETX	Medical Toxicology (Emergency Medicine)	HSP	Hand Surgery (Plastic Surgery)
FM	Family Medicine	HSS	Hand Surgery (Surgery)
FOP	Forensic Pathology	IC	Interventional Cardiology
FPG	Geriatric Medicine (Family Practice)	ICE	Clinical Cardiac Electrophysiology
FPP	Family Practice/Psychiatry	ID	Infectious Disease
FPS	Facial Plastic Surgery	IFP	Internal Medicine/Family Practice
FSM	Sports Medicine (Family Practice)	IG	Immunology
GE	Gastroenterology	ILI	Clinical and Laboratory Immunology (Internal Medicine)
GO	Gynecological Oncology	IM	Internal Medicine
GP	General Practice	IMD	Internal Medicine/Dermatology
GPM	General Preventive Medicine	IMG	Geriatric Medicine (Internal Medicine)
GS	General Surgery	IPM	Internal Medicine (Preventive Medicine)
GYN	Gynecology	ISM	Sports Medicine (Internal Medicine)
HEM	Hematology (Internal Medicine)	LM	Legal Medicine
HEP	Hepatology	MDM	Medical Management
HMP	Hematology (Pathology)	MEM	Internal Medicine/Emergency Medicine

Table 1.8

Physicians' Mean Age by Self-Designated Specialty and Activity (199 Specialties), 2006, continued

| Specialty | Total Physicians | Patient Care | | | | Other Professional Activity | | | |
| | | Total Patient Care | Office Based | Hospital Based | | Admin. | Med. Teach. | Research | Other |
				Resid./ Fellows	Phys. Staff				
MFM	52.4	52.3	52.4		52.3	58.1	54.0	54.1	62.0
MG	48.3	44.9	48.3	34.6	50.0	58.7	57.8	53.5	69.0
MGP	42.5	36.3	42.5	35.2					
MM	48.6	48.1	48.6	35.4	60.7	58.6	76.0	58.9	52.0
MN	31.0	31.0		31.0					
MP	32.0	32.0		32.0					
MPD	38.0	35.1	38.0	29.6	38.6	43.0	38.5	39.7	46.4
MSR	38.0	36.8	38.0	33.8	37.0	71.0			
N	51.0	49.0	51.0	31.7	52.1	61.8	59.8	56.2	61.7
NC	43.0	40.0	43.0		37.0				59.0
NDN	54.0	39.2	54.0	34.3	44.0				
NDP	50.0	50.0	50.0						
NEP	48.2	46.8	48.2	32.9	52.1	62.4	60.3	57.1	57.7
NM	53.4	52.5	53.4	34.7	57.6	62.2	61.5	61.3	62.8
NMN	34.6	34.6		34.6					
NO	53.0	51.0	53.0	33.8	50.1	55.0	60.5		
NP	50.6	49.7	50.6	36.8	58.5	56.5	67.1	60.1	61.8
NPM	48.9	47.5	48.9	33.4	52.5	59.9	57.3	54.7	58.1
NR	48.6	48.7	48.6	42.2	52.7		53.0	61.5	
NRN	51.0	45.2	51.0	33.3	44.0	59.0		71.0	67.0
NS	51.9	48.8	51.9	31.7	51.8	66.4	59.8	61.8	65.0
NSP	52.6	51.9	52.6		49.3			38.0	
NTR	59.1	58.5	59.1		52.9	63.3	58.1	64.6	59.6
NUP	48.8	50.4	48.8		60.0				72.0
OAR	44.2	43.1	44.2	34.0	46.4		49.5	49.0	
OBG	49.5	47.4	49.5	30.5	50.5	62.1	57.4	55.8	58.4
OBS	56.2	56.4	56.2		57.6	60.3	57.8	65.8	
OCC	51.5	51.5	51.5			69.0		68.5	
OFA	46.8	44.6	46.8	32.8	47.7				
OM	56.8	56.3	56.8	37.1	55.7	60.5	57.7	58.5	61.0
OMF	39.9	39.7	39.9	34.0	38.8	61.0	51.8		
OMM	55.8	55.8	55.8						
OMO	42.8	41.9	42.8	32.2	45.0		50.0		
ON	53.5	53.1	53.5	33.9	55.4	62.2	59.9	56.2	60.4
OP	46.9	46.7	46.9	32.5	50.1	65.3	54.7	69.0	
OPH	51.3	49.9	51.3	30.2	49.4	59.0	54.0	58.6	59.9
ORS	52.4	49.1	52.4	30.0	52.2	63.1	59.8	60.9	67.6
OS	55.4	56.0	55.4	33.0	58.9	66.9	68.9	67.7	62.5
OSM	41.9	41.2	41.9	32.9	44.7	50.0	54.0	51.0	
OSS	46.8	46.2	46.8	34.2	44.8	46.0	46.4	64.0	56.5
OTO	51.4	49.0	51.4	30.2	50.2	61.3	56.9	61.1	61.2
OTR	46.0	45.5	46.0	36.5	45.4		51.8		

MFM	Maternal & Fetal Medicine	NSP	Pediatric Surgery (Neurology)
MG	Medical Genetics	NTR	Nutrition
MGP	Molecular Genetic Pathology (Pathology)	NUP	Neuropsychiatry
MM	Medical Microbiology	OAR	Adult Reconstructive Orthopedics
MN	Internal Medicine/Neurology	OBG	Obstetrics & Gynecology
MP	Internal Medicine/Psychiatry	OBS	Obstetrics
MPD	Internal Medicine/Pediatrics	OCC	Critical Care Medicine (Obstetrics & Gynecology)
MSR	Musculoskeletal Radiology	OFA	Foot and Ankle, Orthopedics
N	Neurology	OM	Occupational Medicine
NC	Nuclear Cardiology	OMF	Oral & Maxillofacial Surgery
NDN	Neurodevelopmental Disabilities (Psychiatry & Neurology)	OMM	Osteopathic Manipulative Medicine
NDP	Neurodevelopmental Disabilities (Pediatrics)	OMO	Musculoskeletal Oncology
NEP	Nephrology	ON	Medical Oncology
NM	Nuclear Medicine	OP	Pediatric Orthopedics
NMN	Neuromuscular Medicine	OPH	Ophthalmology
NO	Otology/Neurotology	ORS	Orthopedic Surgery
NP	Neuropathology	OS	Other (i.e., a specialty other than those appearing above)
NPM	Neonatal-Perinatal Medicine	OSM	Sports Medicine (Orthopedic Surgery)
NR	Nuclear Radiology	OSS	Orthopedic Surgery of the Spine
NRN	Neurology/Diagnostic Radiology/Neuroradiology	OTO	Otolaryngology
NS	Neurological Surgery	OTR	Orthopedic Trauma

Table 1.8

Physicians' Mean Age by Self-Designated Specialty and Activity (199 Specialties), 2006, continued

Specialty	Total Physicians	Patient Care				Other Professional Activity			
		Total Patient Care	Office Based	Hospital Based		Admin.	Med. Teach.	Research	Other
				Resid./ Fellows	Phys. Staff				
P	54.7	52.5	54.7	32.8	56.8	62.2	58.5	56.3	63.2
PA	56.7	57.2	56.7		59.0	67.8	64.3	62.3	69.5
PAN	40.9	39.2	40.9	33.9	40.3	55.3	47.6		
PCC	40.9	38.8	40.9	33.0	41.1	50.1	46.2	41.3	42.0
PCH	53.7	52.1	53.7	33.5	69.0	58.0	60.3	59.0	64.0
PCP	43.4	42.5	43.4	36.9	45.1	64.0	60.4	51.5	46.2
PCS	49.4	49.0	49.4		47.8	62.0		57.0	
PD	48.3	45.9	48.3	29.5	50.1	60.6	56.1	55.6	56.4
PDA	60.5	60.1	60.5		55.1	59.0	63.5	62.3	63.0
PDC	49.0	47.0	49.0	32.3	52.9	66.4	63.5	56.0	58.0
PDE	47.3	44.3	47.3	33.0	49.7	60.1	62.1	51.5	57.8
PDI	40.9	38.1	40.9	32.8	44.3	55.0	48.0	47.7	45.7
PDM	28.0	28.0		28.0					
PDO	46.4	45.6	46.4	35.2	50.7		65.4		
PDP	46.0	44.2	46.0	33.6	48.7	57.1	53.7	50.8	
PDR	48.6	48.5	48.6	34.3	54.5	64.7	57.2	64.8	57.6
PDS	51.9	50.9	51.9	34.9	53.3	67.3	64.5	59.6	56.0
PDT	59.0	59.0	59.0						
PE	40.7	37.5	40.7	32.8	39.7	55.0	42.0		
PEM	41.9	39.0	41.9	32.2	45.8	52.6	50.2	46.3	47.0
PFP	43.7	42.2	43.7	35.1	42.9	56.0	44.0		60.0
PG	45.0	41.7	45.0	32.4	46.2	55.9	55.2	47.9	61.3
PHL	50.2	49.8	50.2		41.3				
PHM	48.0	48.0	48.0			53.6	35.0	55.7	47.6
PHO	46.7	44.5	46.7	32.8	50.7	62.6	55.4	51.8	53.1
PHP	59.6	59.2	59.6	38.0	58.2	65.0	65.0	58.0	62.7
PLI	60.0	60.0	60.0					67.0	
PLM	51.6	52.6	51.6		56.6	54.8	54.4	45.3	57.0
PM	47.7	46.4	47.7	31.3	52.4	57.8	60.5	52.8	62.1
PMD	50.4	50.6	50.4		53.7	77.0	56.0	60.0	54.0
PMG	31.3	31.3		31.3					
PMM	46.0	45.1	46.0		40.7				
PMP	34.7	34.7		34.7					
PN	47.6	45.5	47.6	33.5	53.4	62.3	55.7	53.0	61.6
PO	50.1	50.3	50.1		55.4		57.0		
PP	48.4	47.1	48.4	37.3	49.8	59.0	56.5	64.0	56.5
PPM	29.3	29.3		29.3					
PPN	55.7	55.7	55.7			53.0			
PPR	43.5	39.3	43.5	32.8	46.7	64.0	58.0	46.9	57.5
PRD	33.9	32.7	33.9	32.0					

P	Psychiatry	PFP	Forensic Psychiatry
PA	Clinical Pharmacology	PG	Pediatric Gastroenterology
PAN	Pediatric Anesthesiology	PHL	Phlebology
PCC	Pulmonary Critical Care Medicine	PHM	Pharmaceutical Medicine
PCH	Chemical Pathology	PHO	Pediatric Hematology/Oncology
PCP	Cytopathology	PHP	Public Health and General Preventive Medicine
PCS	Pediatric Cardiothoracic Surgery	PLI	Clinical and Laboratory Immunology (Pediatrics)
PD	Pediatrics	PLM	Palliative Medicine
PDA	Pediatric Allergy	PM	Physical Medicine & Rehabilitation
PDC	Pediatric Cardiology	PMD	Pain Medicine
PDE	Pediatric Endocrinology	PMG	Pediatrics/Medical Genetics
PDI	Pediatric Infectious Disease	PMM	Sports Medicine (Physical Medicine & Rehabilitation)
PDM	Pediatrics/Dermatology	PMP	Pain Management (Physical Medicine & Rehabilitation)
PDO	Pediatric Otolaryngology	PN	Pediatric Nephrology
PDP	Pediatric Pulmonology	PO	Pediatric Ophthalmology
PDR	Pediatric Radiology	PP	Pediatric Pathology
PDS	Pediatric Surgery (Surgery)	PPM	Pediatrics/Physical Medicine & Rehabilitation
PDT	Medical Toxicology (Pediatrics)	PPN	Pain Medicine (Psychiatry)
PE	Pediatric Emergency Medicine (Emergency Medicine)	PPR	Pediatric Rheumatology
PEM	Pediatric Emergency Medicine (Pediatrics)	PRD	Procedural Dermatology

Table 1.8

Physicians' Mean Age by Self-Designated Specialty and Activity (199 Specialties), 2006, continued

| Specialty | Total Physicians | Patient Care | | | | Other Professional Activity | | | |
| | | Total Patient Care | Office Based | Hospital Based | | Admin. | Med. Teach. | Research | Other |
				Resid./ Fellows	Phys. Staff				
PRO	55.0	55.0	55.0						
PS	52.0	50.0	52.0	31.6	52.2	59.5	57.7	62.5	64.6
PSH	59.0	59.0	59.0						
PSM	39.6	38.0	39.6	31.6	43.2				
PTH	53.1	50.5	53.1	32.5	58.5	63.8	63.5	63.0	59.0
PTX	44.0	37.5	44.0	31.9				62.5	
PUD	53.8	53.6	53.8	33.3	54.9	61.1	60.6	57.4	61.5
PYA	70.6	70.5	70.6		67.3	73.0	71.8	79.8	68.0
PYG	45.1	44.9	45.1	39.2	47.8	61.3	49.4	49.7	60.5
PYM	42.7	37.9	42.7	35.8					
PYN	32.7	32.7		32.7					
R	61.7	61.8	61.7	34.0	62.3	65.6	63.2	61.3	63.7
REN	52.8	52.6	52.8		50.8	59.1	57.3	54.0	55.0
RHU	50.8	49.3	50.8	32.9	50.8	61.5	58.6	56.2	59.7
RNR	43.3	42.4	43.3	33.8	46.3	42.5	56.7	52.9	42.2
RO	49.8	48.0	49.8	31.6	53.5	60.4	55.3	57.5	53.8
RP	47.0	.						47.0	
RPM	47.5	47.3	47.5		47.0	54.0	36.0		
SCI	39.7	41.0	39.7	35.1	57.1	45.0		56.0	
SME	51.8	47.5	51.8	34.2	49.1	59.7	61.0	49.0	67.0
SO	49.7	49.2	49.7		47.4	63.3	55.6	56.6	54.5
SP	42.2	40.6	42.2	36.5	49.2		46.0		42.0
TRS	51.9	51.8	51.9		51.6	63.0	50.3	62.2	56.7
TS	53.7	52.8	53.7	35.3	54.4	66.7	65.1	61.8	69.7
TTS	48.5	48.4	48.5		47.9	60.0	57.0	50.6	64.0
U	52.8	51.1	52.8	30.9	53.5	63.7	57.8	56.4	66.8
UCM	53.8	53.7	53.8		53.0	44.3	57.5		
UM	53.9	52.8	53.9		49.5	55.5		50.0	72.0
UME	62.0	.					62.0		
UP	48.6	47.2	48.6	34.3	46.8	64.5	55.0	36.0	
US	47.3	40.6	47.3	29.0	50.2	60.3	58.4	56.7	53.3
VIR	42.5	42.0	42.5	34.5	44.3	51.5	55.7	56.3	
VM	51.4	51.5	51.4		55.0			61.0	
VN	33.3	34.7	33.3	34.9					
VS	50.2	49.1	50.2	35.1	49.9	61.4	59.4	58.2	61.8
Inactive	75.1								
Not Class	38.3								
Addr Unkn	77.9								

PRO	Proctology		SP	Selective Pathology
PS	Plastic Surgery		TRS	Trauma Surgery
PSH	Plastic Surgery Within the Head & Neck		TS	Thoracic Surgery
PSM	Sports Medicine (Pediatrics)		TTS	Transplant Surgery
PTH	Anatomic/Clinical Pathology		U	Urology
PTX	Medical Toxicology (Preventive Medicine)		UCM	Urgent Care Medicine
PUD	Pulmonary Disease		UM	Underseas Medicine (Preventive Medicine)
PYA	Psychoanalysis		UME	Underseas Medicine (Emergency Medicine)
PYG	Geriatric Psychiatry		UP	Pediatric Urology
PYM	Psychosomatic Medicine		US	Unspecified
PYN	Psychiatry/Neurology		VIR	Vascular and Interventional Radiology
R	Radiology		VM	Vascular Medicine
REN	Reproductive Endocrinology		VN	Vascular Neurology
RHU	Rheumatology		VS	Vascular Surgery
RNR	Neuroradiology			
RO	Radiation Oncology			
RP	Radiological Physics			
RPM	Pediatric Rehabilitation Medicine			
SCI	Spinal Cord Injury Medicine			
SME	Sleep Medicine			
SO	Surgical Oncology			

Table 1.9

Physicians Mean Age by Self-Designated Specialty and Activity (199 Specialties), 2006

Specialty	Total Physicians	Patient Care		Hospital Based		Other Professional Activity			
		Total Patient Care	Office Based	Resid./ Fellows	Phys. Staff	Admin.	Med. Teach.	Research	Other
Total Physicians	921,904	723,118	560,411	97,102	65,605	14,575	10,273	14,475	4,395
A	745	695	678		17	15	5	27	3
ADL	457	371	242	56	73	33	34	16	3
ADM	212	167	121		46	25	5	8	7
ADP	283	266	174	53	39	8	5	4	
AI	3,126	2,941	2,553	248	140	24	25	124	12
ALI	42	38	33		5	1	1	2	
AM	473	294	170	5	119	136	7	23	13
AMI	18	13	12		1	3	1	1	
AN	38,858	37,776	29,832	4,438	3,506	281	487	238	76
APM	1,904	1,883	1,594	182	107	7	8	4	2
AR	54	52	30	19	3	1	1		
AS	114	102	90		12	5	4	2	1
ATP	1,055	769	562	1	206	32	58	131	65
BBK	501	349	261	35	53	95	9	28	20
CBG	10	5	4		1			5	
CCA	431	414	320	41	53	4	9	2	2
CCG	7	5	2		3				2
CCM	1,303	1,200	875	109	216	31	43	26	3
CCP	1,232	1,177	734	301	142	12	19	22	2
CCS	573	556	384	102	70	4	5	7	1
CD	22,426	21,082	17,480	2,090	1,512	257	319	689	79
CFS	7	7	5	1	1				
CG	111	83	56		27	8	9	10	1
CHN	1,263	1,124	786	178	160	17	40	76	6
CHP	7,260	6,755	5,345	583	827	204	138	125	38
CLP	523	272	197		75	113	22	93	23
CMG	11	2	2				1	7	1
CN	648	637	474	137	26		3	5	3
CPP	82	82	0	82					
CRS	1,339	1,307	1,163	67	77	8	14	6	4
CS	67	67	66		1				
CTR	2	2	1	1					
D	10,707	10,452	8,905	1,079	468	49	78	112	16
DBP	52	50	10	39	1		2		
DDL	3	2	2						1
DIA	317	214	191		23	14	11	75	3
DMP	475	443	357	51	35	3	4	5	20
DR	24,622	23,884	17,576	3,969	2,339	144	240	117	237
DS	117	117	112		5				
EM	29,579	28,470	19,776	3,962	4,732	669	287	82	71

A	Allergy		CD	Cardiovascular Disease
ADL	Adolescent Medicine (Pediatrics)		CFS	Craniofacial Surgery
ADM	Addiction Medicine		CG	Clinical Genetics
ADP	Addiction Psychiatry		CHN	Child Neurology
AI	Allergy & Immunology		CHP	Child and Adolescent Psychiatry
ALI	Clinical Laboratory Immunology (Allergy & Immunology)		CLP	Clinical Pathology
AM	Aerospace Medicine		CMG	Clinical Molecular Genetics
AMI	Adolescent Medicine (Internal Medicine)		CN	Clinical Neurophysiology
AN	Anesthesiology		CPP	Pediatric Psychiatry/Child Psychiatry
APM	Pain Management		CRS	Colon & Rectal Surgery
AR	Abdominal Radiology		CS	Cosmetic Surgery
AS	Abdominal Surgery		CTR	Cardiothoracic Radiology
ATP	Anatomic Pathology		D	Dermatology
BBK	Blood Banking/Transfusion Medicine		DBP	Developmental-Behavioral Pediatrics
CBG	Clinical Biochemical Genetics		DDL	Clinical and Laboratory Dermatological Immunology
CCA	Critical Care Medicine (Anesthesiology)		DIA	Diabetes
CCG	Clinical Cytogenetics		DMP	Dermatopathology
CCM	Critical Care Medicine (Internal Medicine)		DR	Diagnostic Radiology
CCP	Pediatric Critical Care Medicine		DS	Dermatologic Surgery
CCS	Surgical Critical Care (Surgery)		EM	Emergency Medicine

Table 1.9

Physicians Mean Age by Self-Designated Specialty and Activity (199 Specialties), 2006, continued

Specialty	Total Physicians	Patient Care				Other Professional Activity			
		Total Patient Care	Office Based	Hospital Based		Admin.	Med. Teach.	Research	Other
				Resid./ Fellows	Phys. Staff				
EMP	23	23	0	23					
END	5,074	4,240	3,383	465	392	114	137	560	23
EP	37	2	2			4		20	11
ESM	16	15	10	4	1		1		
ESN	7	6	4	1	1		1		
ETX	66	60	32	24	4	1	2		3
FM	81,878	78,835	65,324	8,091	5,420	1,256	1,417	197	173
FOP	657	468	409	26	33	37	10	9	133
FPG	463	418	342	36	40	22	17	3	3
FPP	39	39	0	39					
FPS	387	383	364		19		3		1
FSM	475	472	362	89	21	1	2		
GE	12,268	11,634	9,881	1,058	695	115	164	332	23
GO	460	422	350		72	10	18	9	1
GP	10,493	10,099	8,872		1,227	214	32	42	106
GPM	2,093	1,622	1,177	219	226	221	42	148	60
GS	30,932	30,023	20,261	7,400	2,362	365	258	172	114
GYN	2,413	2,311	2,204		107	40	34	18	10
HEM	2,224	1,673	1,342	50	281	86	83	375	7
HEP	109	86	67		19	2	10	11	
HMP	497	475	344	84	47	3	5	10	4
HNS	236	216	193		23	6	8	5	1
HO	4,317	4,178	2,887	1,041	250	15	31	84	9
HOS	46	45	26		19		1		
HS	1,509	1,474	1,407		67	6	19	4	6
HSO	94	94	0	94					
HSP	15	15	0	15					
HSS	9	9	0	9					
IC	1,068	1,058	791	226	41	1	5	4	
ICE	910	893	697	144	52	3	6	7	1
ID	6,342	5,045	3,690	663	692	263	234	754	46
IFP	11	11	0	11					
IG	283	61	46		15	22	10	184	6
ILI	6	4	3		1		1	1	
IM	113,340	108,054	78,289	20,688	9,077	2,020	1,250	1,581	435
IMD	4	4	0	4					
IMG	2,973	2,655	2,013	242	400	126	73	110	9
IPM	19	19	0	19					
ISM	43	41	38	1	2		1	1	
LM	160	46	38		8	40	6	4	64
MDM	285	18	18			249	3	6	9
MEM	94	94	0	94					

EMP	Pediatrics/Emergency Medicine		HNS	Head & Neck Surgery
END	Endocrinology, Diabetes and Metabolism		HO	Hematology/Oncology
EP	Epidemiology		HOS	Hospitalist
ESM	Sports Medicine (Emergency Medicine)		HS	Hand Surgery
ESN	Endovascular Surgical Neuroradiology		HSO	Hand Surgery (Orthopedics)
ETX	Medical Toxicology (Emergency Medicine)		HSP	Hand Surgery (Plastic Surgery)
FM	Family Medicine		HSS	Hand Surgery (Surgery)
FOP	Forensic Pathology		IC	Interventional Cardiology
FPG	Geriatric Medicine (Family Practice)		ICE	Clinical Cardiac Electrophysiology
FPP	Family Practice/Psychiatry		ID	Infectious Disease
FPS	Facial Plastic Surgery		IFP	Internal Medicine/Family Practice
FSM	Sports Medicine (Family Practice)		IG	Immunology
GE	Gastroenterology		ILI	Clinical and Laboratory Immunology (Internal Medicine)
GO	Gynecological Oncology		IM	Internal Medicine
GP	General Practice		IMD	Internal Medicine/Dermatology
GPM	General Preventive Medicine		IMG	Geriatric Medicine (Internal Medicine)
GS	General Surgery		IPM	Internal Medicine (Preventive Medicine)
GYN	Gynecology		ISM	Sports Medicine (Internal Medicine)
HEM	Hematology (Internal Medicine)		LM	Legal Medicine
HEP	Hepatology		MDM	Medical Management
HMP	Hematology (Pathology)		MEM	Internal Medicine/Emergency Medicine

Table 1.9

Physicians Mean Age by Self-Designated Specialty and Activity (198 Specialties), 2006, continued

Specialty	Total Physicians	Patient Care		Hospital Based		Other Professional Activity			
		Total Patient Care	Office Based	Resid./ Fellows	Phys. Staff	Admin.	Med. Teach.	Research	Other
MFM	596	503	359		144	25	46	19	3
MG	394	290	169	77	44	16	14	73	1
MGP	13	13	2	11					
MM	65	44	29	8	7	7	3	9	2
MN	10	10	0	10					
MP	91	91	0	91					
MPD	3,904	3,841	2,300	1,340	201	8	35	15	5
MSR	59	58	40	17	1	1			
N	12,621	11,462	9,160	1,288	1,014	172	214	703	70
NC	3	2	1		1				1
NDN	6	6	1	4	1				
NDP	2	2	2						
NEP	7,410	6,761	5,571	730	460	125	126	380	18
NM	1,477	1,323	953	121	249	44	28	60	22
NMN	5	5	0	5					
NO	135	132	109	12	11	1	2		
NP	351	234	169	33	32	8	30	67	12
NPM	4,071	3,653	2,587	462	604	89	106	207	16
NR	137	132	117	5	10		1	4	
NRN	29	26	15	7	4	1		1	1
NS	5,358	5,212	4,060	793	359	34	48	39	25
NSP	31	30	24		6			1	
NTR	160	92	84		8	9	7	42	10
NUP	8	7	6		1				1
OAR	223	220	185	26	9		2	1	
OBG	37,996	37,022	30,626	4,205	2,191	324	414	176	60
OBS	228	205	173		32	6	12	5	
OCC	5	2	2			1		2	
OFA	78	78	59	13	6				
OM	2,641	1,891	1,550	32	309	520	39	82	109
OMF	102	97	86	3	8	1	4		
OMM	5	5	5						
OMO	61	58	48	6	4		3		
ON	5,386	4,639	4,021	146	472	152	57	520	18
OP	335	324	255	15	54	3	7	1	
OPH	17,873	17,480	15,588	1,125	767	98	122	140	33
ORS	21,785	21,341	17,164	3,058	1,119	107	126	77	134
OS	4,617	3,014	1,572	1,131	311	624	124	715	140
OSM	1,052	1,048	914	91	43	1	2	1	
OSS	573	564	516	20	28	1	5	1	2

MFM   Maternal & Fetal Medicine
MG   Medical Genetics
MGP   Molecular Genetic Pathology (Pathology)
MM   Medical Microbiology
MN   Internal Medicine/Neurology
MP   Internal Medicine/Psychiatry
MPD   Internal Medicine/Pediatrics
MSR   Musculoskeletal Radiology
N   Neurology
NC   Nuclear Cardiology
NDN   Neurodevelopmental Disabilities (Psychiatry & Neurology)
NDP   Neurodevelopmental Disabilities (Pediatrics)
NEP   Nephrology
NM   Nuclear Medicine
NMN   Neuromuscular Medicine
NO   Otology/Neurotology
NP   Neuropathology
NPM   Neonatal-Perinatal Medicine
NR   Nuclear Radiology
NRN   Neurology/Diagnostic Radiology/Neuroradiology

NS   Neurological Surgery
NSP   Pediatric Surgery (Neurology)
NTR   Nutrition
NUP   Neuropsychiatry
OAR   Adult Reconstructive Orthopedics
OBG   Obstetrics & Gynecology
OBS   Obstetrics
OCC   Critical Care Medicine (Obstetrics & Gynecology)
OFA   Foot and Ankle, Orthopedics
OM   Occupational Medicine
OMF   Oral & Maxillofacial Surgery
OMM   Osteopathic Manipulative Medicine
OMO   Musculoskeletal Oncology
ON   Medical Oncology
OP   Pediatric Orthopedics
OPH   Ophthalmology
ORS   Orthopedic Surgery
OS   Other (i.e., a specialty other than those appearing above)
OSM   Sports Medicine (Orthopedic Surgery)
OSS   Orthopedic Surgery of the Spine

Table 1.9

Physicians Mean Age by Self-Designated Specialty and Activity (197 Specialties), 2005, continued

Specialty	Total Physicians	Patient Care				Other Professional Activity			
		Total Patient Care	Office Based	Hospital Based		Admin.	Med. Teach.	Research	Other
				Resid./ Fellows	Phys. Staff				
OTO	9,701	9,513	7,979	1,057	477	65	82	28	13
OTR	90	86	74	4	8		4		
P	39,423	36,354	25,986	4,180	6,188	1,397	558	832	282
PA	330	55	43		12	54	11	202	8
PAN	438	427	298	101	28	3	8		
PCC	3,884	3,785	2,564	1,003	218	9	26	59	5
PCH	35	16	13	2	1	6	4	3	6
PCP	641	625	478	102	45	2	7	2	5
PCS	43	41	30		11	1		1	
PD	57,200	54,326	42,509	7,301	4,516	1,025	845	752	252
PDA	168	146	135		11	4	4	11	3
PDC	1,877	1,739	1,243	260	236	26	30	78	4
PDE	889	761	471	179	111	9	17	97	5
PDI	385	322	167	126	29	14	14	32	3
PDM	1	1	0	1					
PDO	138	133	111	13	9		5		
PDP	651	595	420	104	71	11	9	36	
PDR	685	650	504	46	100	3	21	6	5
PDS	810	756	596	56	104	12	26	15	1
PDT	2	2	2						
PE	104	102	48	39	15	1	1		
PEM	611	577	245	216	116	7	18	8	1
PFP	317	290	199	47	44	7	1		19
PG	644	608	377	162	69	8	9	16	3
PHL	62	62	59		3				
PHM	73	6	6			9	1	38	19
PHO	1,739	1,482	942	304	236	30	26	194	7
PHP	1,434	297	218	1	78	679	68	299	91
PLI	2	1	1					1	
PLM	121	84	67		17	22	5	3	7
PM	7,649	7,361	5,582	873	906	160	45	47	36
PMD	222	215	201		14	1	4	1	1
PMG	9	9	0	9					
PMM	17	17	14		3				
PMP	13	13	0	13					
PN	518	430	287	87	56	13	26	44	5
PO	185	184	177		7		1		
PP	116	106	74	15	17	2	2	2	4
PPM	11	11	0	11					
PPN	4	3	3			1			

OTO	Otolaryngology	PE	Pediatric Emergency Medicine (Emergency Medicine)
OTR	Orthopedic Trauma	PEM	Pediatric Emergency Medicine (Pediatrics)
P	Psychiatry	PFP	Forensic Psychiatry
PA	Clinical Pharmacology	PG	Pediatric Gastroenterology
PAN	Pediatric Anesthesiology	PHL	Phlebology
PCC	Pulmonary Critical Care Medicine	PHM	Pharmaceutical Medicine
PCH	Chemical Pathology	PHO	Pediatric Hematology/Oncology
PCP	Cytopathology	PHP	Public Health and General Preventive Medicine
PCS	Pediatric Cardiothoracic Surgery	PLI	Clinical and Laboratory Immunology (Pediatrics)
PD	Pediatrics	PLM	Palliative Medicine
PDA	Pediatric Allergy	PM	Physical Medicine & Rehabilitation
PDC	Pediatric Cardiology	PMD	Pain Medicine
PDE	Pediatric Endocrinology	PMG	Pediatrics/Medical Genetics
PDI	Pediatric Infectious Disease	PMM	Sports Medicine (Physical Medicine & Rehabilitation)
PDM	Pediatrics/Dermatology	PMP	Pain Management (Physical Medicine & Rehabilitation)
PDO	Pediatric Otolaryngology	PN	Pediatric Nephrology
PDP	Pediatric Pulmonology	PO	Pediatric Ophthalmology
PDR	Pediatric Radiology	PP	Pediatric Pathology
PDS	Pediatric Surgery (Surgery)	PPM	Pediatrics/Physical Medicine & Rehabilitation
PDT	Medical Toxicology (Pediatrics)	PPN	Pain Medicine (Psychiatry)

Table 1.9

Physicians Mean Age by Self-Designated Specialty and Activity (199 Specialties), 2006, continued

Specialty	Total Physicians	Patient Care		Hospital Based		Other Professional Activity			
		Total Patient Care	Office Based	Resid./ Fellows	Phys. Staff	Admin.	Med. Teach.	Research	Other
PPR	137	112	57	46	9	1	5	17	2
PRD	34	34	13	21					
PRO	1	1	1						
PS	6,592	6,480	5,584	636	260	25	45	21	21
PSH	2	2	2						
PSM	43	43	27	11	5				
PTH	14,659	12,879	8,828	2,097	1,954	443	252	449	636
PTX	15	13	6	7				2	
PUD	6,348	5,565	4,813	88	664	187	193	378	25
PYA	512	497	490		7	5	5	4	1
PYG	711	681	521	64	96	8	10	10	2
PYM	23	23	7	16					
PYN	16	16	0	16					
R	4,749	4,358	3,668	5	685	77	118	73	123
REN	635	571	511		60	14	23	25	2
RHU	4,438	3,936	3,303	336	297	85	109	283	25
RNR	1,675	1,642	1,290	211	141	2	19	7	5
RO	4,424	4,314	3,419	506	389	39	27	39	5
RP	1	0	0					1	
RPM	6	4	2		2	1	1		
SCI	65	63	38	16	9	1		1	
SME	178	162	108	37	17	6	1	8	1
SO	303	274	218		56	6	8	13	2
SP	240	238	151	78	9		1		1
TRS	252	221	143		78	13	10	5	3
TS	4,807	4,624	3,984	250	390	57	49	65	12
TTS	151	137	114		23	2	3	8	1
U	10,325	10,086	8,692	834	560	83	79	54	23
UCM	221	216	189		27	3	2		
UM	53	47	36		11	4		1	1
UME	1	0	0			1			
UP	193	188	158	16	14	2	2	1	
US	6,383	6,108	3,955	1,613	540	66	36	115	58
VIR	1,526	1,514	1,305	112	97	2	6	4	
VM	24	23	22		1			1	
VN	22	22	3	19					
VS	2,549	2,451	2,067	181	203	38	36	19	5
Inactive	108344								
Not Class	46,252								
Addr Unkn	472								

PPR	Pediatric Rheumatology	SME	Sleep Medicine
PRD	Procedural Dermatology	SO	Surgical Oncology
PRO	Proctology	SP	Selective Pathology
PS	Plastic Surgery	TRS	Trauma Surgery
PSH	Plastic Surgery Within the Head & Neck	TS	Thoracic Surgery
PSM	Sports Medicine (Pediatrics)	TTS	Transplant Surgery
PTH	Anatomic/Clinical Pathology	U	Urology
PTX	Medical Toxicology (Preventive Medicine)	UCM	Urgent Care Medicine
PUD	Pulmonary Disease	UM	Underseas Medicine (Preventive Medicine)
PYA	Psychoanalysis	UME	Underseas Medicine (Emergency Medicine)
PYG	Geriatric Psychiatry	UP	Pediatric Urology
PYM	Psychosomatic Medicine	US	Unspecified
PYN	Psychiatry/Neurology	VIR	Vascular and Interventional Radiology
R	Radiology	VM	Vascular Medicine
REN	Reproductive Endocrinology	VN	Vascular Neurology
RHU	Rheumatology	VS	Vascular Surgery
RNR	Neuroradiology		
RO	Radiation Oncology		
RP	Radiological Physics		
RPM	Pediatric Rehabilitation Medicine		
SCI	Spinal Cord Injury Medicine		

Table 1.10

International Medical Graduates by Self-Designated Specialty and Activity, 2006

Specialty	Total Physicians	Patient Care		Hospital Based		Other Professional Activity			
		Total Patient Care	Office Based	Resid./ Fellows	Phys. Staff	Admin.	Med. Teach.	Research	Other
Total Physicans	236,669	185,045	137,115	27,579	20,351	1,958	1,714	2,829	945
GP/FM Prac	22,250	21,839	16,333	3,770	1,736	192	114	31	74
FM	17,268	17,000	12,277	3,770	953	118	103	18	29
GP	4,982	4,839	4,056		783	74	11	13	45
Med. Spec.	92,987	89,997	66,113	15,871	8,013	627	719	1,460	184
AI	1,033	944	861	39	44	9	14	63	3
CD	6,822	6,563	5,384	683	496	27	60	158	14
D	645	615	535	36	44	3	10	16	1
GE	3,298	3,158	2,648	290	220	21	40	75	4
IM	57,029	55,446	39,073	11,533	4,840	345	355	778	105
PD	20,318	19,584	14,826	2,723	2,035	199	204	276	55
PDC	466	443	320	60	63	5	7	11	
PUD	3,376	3,244	2,466	507	271	18	29	83	2
Sur. Spec.	23,336	22,681	17,821	2,846	2,014	160	196	228	71
CRS	263	259	233	9	17		2	2	
GS	7,419	7,216	4,950	1,464	802	57	50	63	33
NS	752	731	573	86	72	2	7	11	1
OBG	7,446	7,252	5,741	925	586	59	70	54	11
OPH	1,423	1,376	1,205	91	80	5	13	27	2
ORS	1,610	1,565	1,339	99	127	11	13	13	8
OTO	932	900	808	35	57	7	8	15	2
PS	851	832	738	45	49	2	2	9	6
TS	1,052	1,011	867	55	89	4	10	25	2
U	1,588	1,539	1,367	37	135	13	21	9	6
Oth. Spec.	53,918	50,528	36,848	5,092	8,588	979	685	1,110	616
AM	37	26	16		10	5	1	4	1
AN	11,712	11,391	9,182	799	1,410	62	152	82	25
CHP	2,139	2,039	1,506	205	328	31	24	32	13
DR	2,858	2,727	2,028	257	442	15	43	29	44
EM	2,664	2,589	1,674	247	668	44	22	4	5
FOP	152	100	84	9	7	9	3	4	36
GPM	309	262	203	35	24	20	7	14	6
MG	131	110	61	33	16	3	1	17	
N	4,644	4,421	3,398	613	410	17	56	130	20
NM	536	499	336	56	107	7	8	14	8
OM	384	322	258	12	52	42	5	5	10
P	12,999	12,368	7,997	1,484	2,887	304	103	167	57
PHP	168	54	40		14	75	9	20	10
PM	2,374	2,292	1,714	191	387	38	20	8	16
PTH	6,361	5,566	3,703	856	1,007	166	134	244	251
R	1,670	1,538	1,145	88	305	17	33	41	41
RO	791	764	624	15	125	5	8	13	1
TTS	38	36	27		9			2	
OTH	977	584	441	20	123	88	37	228	40
UNSP	2,969	2,835	2,406	172	257	31	19	52	32
VM	5	5	5						
Inactive	22,838								
Not Class	21,255								
Addr Unkn	85								

Subspecialties in this table are condensed into major specialties. See Appendix A.

Table 1.11

International Medical Graduates by Age, Activity, and Sex, 2006

Activity	Total Physicians	< 35	35-44	45-54	55-64	≥ 65
Both Sexes						
Total Physicians	236,669	31,451	55,767	52,657	47,656	49,138
Patient Care	185,045	25,334	45,849	46,639	41,028	26,195
Office-Based Practice	137,115	5,979	34,999	40,372	34,611	21,154
Hospital-Based Practice	47,930	19,355	10,850	6,267	6,417	5,041
Residents	27,579	18,875	7,543	1,088	70	3
Full-Time Staff	20,351	480	3,307	5,179	6,347	5,038
Other Professional Activity	7,446	76	584	1,522	2,536	2,728
Administration	1,958	5	68	350	661	874
Medical Teaching	1,714	42	194	392	529	557
Research	2,829	20	265	599	1,039	906
Other	945	9	57	181	307	391
Inactive	22,838	19	211	850	2,517	19,241
Not Classified	21,255	6,020	9,123	3,646	1,565	901
Address Unknown	85	2			10	73
Male						
Total Physicians	165,377	17,695	34,391	37,589	35,650	40,052
Patient Care	128,486	14,330	28,309	33,439	31,036	21,372
Office-Based Practice	98,385	3,280	21,686	29,189	26,674	17,556
Hospital-Based Practice	30,101	11,050	6,623	4,250	4,362	3,816
Residents	16,021	10,763	4,550	665	40	3
Full-Time Staff	14,080	287	2,073	3,585	4,322	3,813
Other Professional Activity	5,559	43	356	1,083	1,851	2,226
Administration	1,468	4	36	251	476	701
Medical Teaching	1,241	23	117	272	365	464
Research	2,201	11	173	441	816	760
Other	649	5	30	119	194	301
Inactive	18,086	11	112	561	1,672	15,730
Not Classified	13,183	3,309	5,614	2,506	1,084	670
Address Unknown	63	2			7	54
Female						
Total Physicians	71,292	13,756	21,376	15,068	12,006	9,086
Patient Care	56,559	11,004	17,540	13,200	9,992	4,823
Office-Based Practice	38,730	2,699	13,313	11,183	7,937	3,598
Hospital-Based Practice	17,829	8,305	4,227	2,017	2,055	1,225
Residents	11,558	8,112	2,993	423	30	
Full-Time Staff	6,271	193	1,234	1,594	2,025	1,225
Other Professional Activity	1,887	33	228	439	685	502
Administration	490	1	32	99	185	173
Medical Teaching	473	19	77	120	164	93
Research	628	9	92	158	223	146
Other	296	4	27	62	113	90
Inactive	4,752	8	99	289	845	3,511
Not Classified	8,072	2,711	3,509	1,140	481	231
Address Unknown	22				3	19

Table 1.12

Male Physicians by Self-Designated Specialty and Activity, 2006

Specialty	Total Physicians	Total Patient Care	Office Based	Resid./ Fellows	Phys. Staff	Admin.	Med. Teach.	Research	Other
				Patient Care		Other Professional Activity			
				Hospital Based					
Total Physicians	665,647	509,474	407,907	55,078	46,489	11,817	7,618	11,394	3,188
GP/FM Prac	62,888	60,283	51,747	3,927	4,609	1,189	1,053	167	196
FM	54,450	52,134	44,483	3,927	3,724	1,030	1,032	133	121
GP	8,438	8,149	7,264		885	159	21	34	75
Med. Spec.	190,502	176,489	139,797	21,934	14,758	3,922	2,970	6,405	716
AI	3,042	2,674	2,434	124	116	54	28	273	13
CD	20,234	19,005	15,920	1,734	1,351	236	298	622	73
D	6,482	6,290	5,607	408	275	41	56	84	11
GE	10,833	10,267	8,907	760	600	112	141	293	20
IM	106,164	97,907	75,055	14,280	8,572	2,452	1,586	3,792	427
PD	33,740	31,214	24,609	3,664	2,941	824	644	914	144
PDC	1,336	1,224	894	157	173	24	22	63	3
PUD	8,671	7,908	6,371	807	730	179	195	364	25
Sur. Spec.	129,230	125,467	104,419	13,046	8,002	1,233	1,297	806	427
CRS	1,155	1,126	1,012	46	68	5	14	6	4
GS	31,853	30,747	22,666	5,458	2,623	430	339	214	123
NS	5,094	4,946	3,905	707	334	34	48	40	26
OBG	23,813	22,838	20,211	1,006	1,621	341	394	191	49
OPH	14,678	14,348	13,058	693	597	88	101	116	25
ORS	23,133	22,664	18,525	2,950	1,189	109	147	79	134
OTO	8,758	8,570	7,353	802	415	65	85	26	12
PS	6,191	6,086	5,346	496	244	23	43	19	20
TS	4,620	4,443	3,851	221	371	54	49	63	11
U	9,935	9,699	8,492	667	540	84	77	52	23
Oth. Spec.	160,871	147,235	111,944	16,171	19,120	5,473	2,298	4,016	1,849
AM	435	272	158	4	110	125	7	20	11
AN	31,824	30,983	25,148	3,099	2,736	240	359	186	56
CHP	3,934	3,604	2,892	238	474	146	86	75	23
DR	19,100	18,493	13,775	2,902	1,816	129	186	100	192
EM	23,157	22,176	15,769	2,515	3,892	615	235	70	61
FOP	437	305	266	18	21	28	7	7	90
GPM	1,344	1,025	730	124	171	168	22	91	38
MG	280	187	116	34	37	15	13	63	2
N	10,856	9,769	7,956	925	888	154	214	654	65
NM	1,179	1,055	767	86	202	37	25	49	13
OM	2,099	1,499	1,232	20	247	428	29	61	82
P	27,319	24,815	18,399	2,078	4,338	1,171	429	669	235
PHP	1,004	181	129	1	51	481	52	227	63
PM	5,061	4,865	3,763	546	556	112	28	36	20
PTH	12,551	10,536	7,605	1,225	1,706	550	283	643	539
R	7,500	7,095	5,921	317	857	77	134	78	116
RO	3,356	3,267	2,625	347	295	35	21	31	2
TTS	136	125	104		21	2	3	6	
OTH	4,220	2,119	1,754	30	335	909	138	855	199
UNSP	5,060	4,846	2,818	1,662	366	51	27	94	42
VM	19	18	17		1			1	
Inactive	94,469								
Not Class	27,358								
Addr Unkn	329								

Subspecialties in this table are condensed into major specialties. See Appendix A.

Table 1.13

Female Physicians by Self-Designated Specialty and Activity, 2006

Specialty	Total Physicians	Patient Care		Hospital Based		Other Professional Activity			
		Total Patient Care	Office Based	Resid./ Fellows	Phys. Staff	Admin.	Med. Teach.	Research	Other
Total Physicians	256,257	213,644	152,504	42,024	19,116	2,758	2,655	3,081	1,207
GP/FM Prac	30,471	29,591	23,153	4,339	2,099	304	415	75	86
FM	28,416	27,641	21,545	4,339	1,757	249	404	67	55
GP	2,055	1,950	1,608		342	55	11	8	31
Med. Spec.	100,154	95,573	67,513	19,864	8,196	1,100	1,245	1,863	373
AI	1,154	1,061	876	124	61	8	13	64	8
CD	2,192	2,077	1,560	356	161	21	21	67	6
D	4,262	4,198	3,313	692	193	8	22	28	6
GE	1,435	1,367	974	298	95	3	23	39	3
IM	49,541	47,140	32,229	10,779	4,132	597	600	1,023	181
PD	39,468	37,773	27,206	7,228	3,339	444	534	554	163
PDC	541	515	349	103	63	2	8	15	1
PUD	1,561	1,442	1,006	284	152	17	24	73	5
Sur. Spec.	32,140	31,600	22,699	7,064	1,837	130	230	128	52
CRS	185	182	152	21	9	3			
GS	5,703	5,597	2,926	2,294	377	27	39	29	11
NS	331	328	198	94	36	1	1	1	
OBG	18,520	18,198	14,014	3,199	985	79	153	63	27
OPH	3,380	3,316	2,707	432	177	10	22	24	8
ORS	1,163	1,154	695	377	82	3	2	2	2
OTO	1,216	1,208	846	280	82	1	4	2	1
PS	872	861	670	155	36	2	5	2	2
TS	187	181	133	29	19	3		2	1
U	583	575	358	183	34	1	4	3	
Oth. Spec.	60,580	56,880	39,139	10,757	6,984	1,224	765	1,015	696
AM	38	22	12	1	9	11		3	2
AN	9,369	9,090	6,598	1,562	930	52	145	58	24
CHP	3,326	3,151	2,453	345	353	58	52	50	15
DR	5,524	5,393	3,802	1,068	523	15	54	17	45
EM	6,830	6,687	4,286	1,514	887	60	58	12	13
FOP	220	163	143	8	12	9	3	2	43
GPM	817	657	489	102	66	57	20	60	23
MG	253	198	117	43	38	9	11	32	3
N	3,698	3,476	2,467	697	312	35	43	130	14
NM	298	268	186	35	47	7	3	11	9
OM	542	392	318	12	62	92	10	21	27
P	14,066	13,410	8,988	2,384	2,038	255	150	181	70
PHP	430	116	89		27	198	16	72	28
PM	2,675	2,581	1,871	348	362	49	17	12	16
PTH	6,620	5,927	3,860	1,292	775	164	114	156	259
R	1,386	1,311	1,033	98	180	9	32	17	17
RO	1,068	1,047	794	159	94	4	6	8	3
TTS	15	12	10		2			2	1
OTH	948	583	481	9	93	125	22	150	68
UNSP	2,452	2,391	1,137	1,080	174	15	9	21	16
VM	5	5	5						
Inactive	13,875								
Not Class	18,894								
Addr Unkn	143								

Subspecialties in this table are condensed into major specialties. See Appendix A.

Table 1.14

Total Physicians by Self-Designated Specialty and Corresponding Board Certification, 2006

Primary Specialty	Total Physicians	Total Certified	By Corresponding Board Only	By Corresponding Board and Other Boards	By Non-Corresponding Board	Not Board Certified
Total Physicians	921,904	638,987	496,475	23,588	118,924	282,917
Aerospace Medicine	473	327	204	46	77	146
Allergy/Immunology	4,196	3,697	471	2,002	1,224	499
Anesthesiology	41,193	29,709	26,762	1,251	1,696	11,484
Cardiovascular Disease	22,426	19,998	19,619	124	255	2,428
Child Psychiatry	7,260	5,041	4,735	218	88	2,219
Colon/Rectal Surgery	1,340	1,216	235	854	127	124
Dermatology	10,744	9,062	8,027	846	189	1,682
Diagnostic Radiology	24,624	19,620	18,371	1,057	192	5,004
Emergency Medicine	29,987	20,664	16,445	1,846	2,373	9,323
Family Medicine	82,866	60,649	58,869	698	1,082	22,217
Forensic Pathology	657	521	503	12	6	136
Gastroenterology	12,268	11,142	10,949	46	147	1,126
General Practice	10,493	1,080			1,080	9,413
General Preventive Medicine	2,161	1,547	841	344	362	614
General Surgery	37,556	23,894	20,278	677	2,939	13,662
Internal Medicine	155,705	109,520	100,602	2,452	6,466	46,185
Medical Genetics	533	477	102	292	83	56
Neurological Surgery	5,425	3,696	3,565	33	98	1,729
Neurology	14,554	10,672	8,491	1,499	682	3,882
Nuclear Medicine	1,477	1,214	502	568	144	263
Obstetrics/Gynecology	42,333	31,316	28,558	293	2,465	11,017
Occupational Medicine	2,641	1,833	997	461	375	808
Ophthalmology	18,058	15,212	14,755	227	230	2,846
Orthopedic Surgery	24,296	18,294	17,074	55	1,165	6,002
Otolaryngology	9,974	8,053	7,988	40	25	1,921
Pathology-Anatomic/Clinical	19,171	15,330	14,443	410	477	3,841
Pediatric Cardiology	1,877	1,728	1,684	35	9	149
Pediatrics	73,208	55,316	51,005	1,131	3,180	17,892
Physical Medicine & Rehabilitation	7,736	5,826	5,532	204	90	1,910
Plastic Surgery	7,063	5,653	3,815	1,201	637	1,410
Psychiatry	41,385	26,141	24,370	1,066	705	15,244
Public Health & General Preventive Medicine	1,434	943	457	136	350	491
Pulmonary Diseases	10,232	9,377	5,654	87	3,636	855
Radiation Oncology	4,424	3,594	3,322	242	30	830
Radiology	8,886	8,222	7,372	678	172	664
Thoracic Surgery	4,807	4,276	1,325	2,404	547	531
Transplant Surgery	151	119			119	32
Urological Surgery	10,518	8,517	8,450	46	21	2,001
Vascular Medicine	24	19			19	5
Other Specialty	5,168	2,853	103	7	2,743	2,315
Unspecified	7,512	688			688	6,824
Inactive	108,344	64,186			64,186	44,158
Not Classified	46,252	17,709			17,709	28,543
Address Unknown	472	36			36	436

Table 1.15

Male Physicians by Self-Designated Specialty and Corresponding Board Certification, 2006

Primary Specialty	Total Physicians	Total Certified	By Corresponding Board Only	By Corresponding Board and Other Boards	By Non-Corresponding Board	Not Board Certified
Total Physicians	665,647	473,134	358,886	18,873	95,375	192,513
Aerospace Medicine	435	303	189	42	72	132
Allergy/Immunology	3,042	2,673	327	1,430	916	369
Anesthesiology	31,824	23,673	21,284	996	1,393	8,151
Cardiovascular Disease	20,234	18,097	17,750	110	237	2,137
Child Psychiatry	3,934	2,819	2,649	130	40	1,115
Colon/Rectal Surgery	1,155	1,062	224	732	106	93
Dermatology	6,482	5,651	4,961	571	119	831
Diagnostic Radiology	19,100	15,414	14,348	919	147	3,686
Emergency Medicine	23,157	16,345	12,813	1,602	1,930	6,812
Family Medicine	54,450	39,778	38,354	563	861	14,672
Forensic Pathology	437	343	330	9	4	94
Gastroenterology	10,833	9,868	9,713	41	114	965
General Practice	8,438	873			873	7,565
General Preventive Medicine	1,344	967	528	227	212	377
General Surgery	31,853	21,171	17,918	640	2,613	10,682
Internal Medicine	106,164	76,162	69,840	1,797	4,525	30,002
Medical Genetics	280	252	61	150	41	28
Neurological Surgery	5,094	3,535	3,415	32	88	1,559
Neurology	10,856	8,296	6,626	1,201	469	2,560
Nuclear Medicine	1,179	996	389	497	110	183
Obstetrics/Gynecology	23,813	19,261	17,367	197	1,697	4,552
Occupational Medicine	2,099	1,443	778	358	307	656
Ophthalmology	14,678	12,657	12,301	199	157	2,021
Orthopedic Surgery	23,133	17,675	16,545	55	1,075	5,458
Otolaryngology	8,758	7,226	7,165	38	23	1,532
Pathology-Anatomic/Clinical	12,551	10,435	9,837	304	294	2,116
Pediatric Cardiology	1,336	1,238	1,203	28	7	98
Pediatrics	33,740	26,735	24,265	702	1,768	7,005
Physical Medicine & Rehabilitation	5,061	3,870	3,674	127	69	1,191
Plastic Surgery	6,191	5,049	3,376	1,100	573	1,142
Psychiatry	27,319	18,106	16,894	713	499	9,213
Public Health & General Preventive Medicine	1,004	675	338	97	240	329
Pulmonary Diseases	8,671	7,989	5,095	80	2,814	682
Radiation Oncology	3,356	2,779	2,553	207	19	577
Radiology	7,500	6,985	6,240	607	138	515
Thoracic Surgery	4,620	4,115	1,288	2,322	505	505
Transplant Surgery	136	107			107	29
Urological Surgery	9,935	8,216	8,154	46	16	1,719
Vascular Medicine	19	14			14	5
Other Specialty	4,220	2,307	94	4	2,209	1,913
Unspecified	5,060	443			443	4,617
Inactive	94,469	57,543			57,543	36,926
Not Classified	27,358	9,965			9,965	17,393
Address Unknown	329	23			23	306

Table 1.16

Female Physicians by Self-Designated Specialty and Corresponding Board Certification, 2006

Primary Specialty	Total Physicians	Total Certified	By Corresponding Board Only	By Corresponding Board and Other Boards	By Non-Corresponding Board	Not Board Certified
Total Physicians	256,257	165,853	137,589	4,715	23,549	90,404
Aerospace Medicine	38	24	15	4	5	14
Allergy/Immunology	1,154	1,024	144	572	308	130
Anesthesiology	9,369	6,036	5,478	255	303	3,333
Cardiovascular Disease	2,192	1,901	1,869	14	18	291
Child Psychiatry	3,326	2,222	2,086	88	48	1,104
Colon/Rectal Surgery	185	154	11	122	21	31
Dermatology	4,262	3,411	3,066	275	70	851
Diagnostic Radiology	5,524	4,206	4,023	138	45	1,318
Emergency Medicine	6,830	4,319	3,632	244	443	2,511
Family Medicine	28,416	20,871	20,515	135	221	7,545
Forensic Pathology	220	178	173	3	2	42
Gastroenterology	1,435	1,274	1,236	5	33	161
General Practice	2,055	207			207	1,848
General Preventive Medicine	817	580	313	117	150	237
General Surgery	5,703	2,723	2,360	37	326	2,980
Internal Medicine	49,541	33,358	30,762	655	1,941	16,183
Medical Genetics	253	225	41	142	42	28
Neurological Surgery	331	161	150	1	10	170
Neurology	3,698	2,376	1,865	298	213	1,322
Nuclear Medicine	298	218	113	71	34	80
Obstetrics/Gynecology	18,520	12,055	11,191	96	768	6,465
Occupational Medicine	542	390	219	103	68	152
Ophthalmology	3,380	2,555	2,454	28	73	825
Orthopedic Surgery	1,163	619	529		90	544
Otolaryngology	1,216	827	823	2	2	389
Pathology-Anatomic/Clinical	6,620	4,895	4,606	106	183	1,725
Pediatric Cardiology	541	490	481	7	2	51
Pediatrics	39,468	28,581	26,740	429	1,412	10,887
Physical Medicine & Rehabilitation	2,675	1,956	1,858	77	21	719
Plastic Surgery	872	604	439	101	64	268
Psychiatry	14,066	8,035	7,476	353	206	6,031
Public Health & General Preventive Medicine	430	268	119	39	110	162
Pulmonary Diseases	1,561	1,388	559	7	822	173
Radiation Oncology	1,068	815	769	35	11	253
Radiology	1,386	1,237	1,132	71	34	149
Thoracic Surgery	187	161	37	82	42	26
Transplant Surgery	15	12			12	3
Urological Surgery	583	301	296		5	282
Vascular Medicine	5	5			5	
Other Specialty	948	546	9	3	534	402
Unspecified	2,452	245			245	2,207
Inactive	13,875	6,643			6,643	7,232
Not Classified	18,894	7,744			7,744	11,150
Address Unknown	143	13			13	130

Table 1.17

Country and School of Graduation of Total Physicians by Year of Graduation, 2006

State School	Total Physicians	Prior 1950	1950-1959	1960-1969	1970-1979	1980-1989	1990-1999	2000-Present
Total Physicians	921,904	30,253	62,466	105547	161,230	219,789	208,039	134,580
US Active Schools	671,554	24,577	44,024	67,120	113691	155,954	156,158	110,030
AL-U Of Alabama	6,334	41	321	625	1,122	1,556	1,558	1,111
" -U Of So Alabama	1,833				189	607	615	422
AZ-U Of Arizona	2,973				605	822	879	667
AR-U Of Arkansas	5,823	208	433	685	1,029	1,255	1,287	926
CA-Loma Linda U	6,834	393	632	757	1,231	1,282	1,477	1,062
" -Stanford U	4,120	257	446	436	788	760	841	592
" -U Of Cal (Davis)	3,038				600	898	900	640
" -U Of Cal (Irvine)	4,659	2	5	1,628	663	862	882	617
" -U Of Cal (La)	6,540		137	552	1,309	1,710	1,697	1,135
" -U Of Cal (San Diego)	3,612				482	1,116	1,176	838
" -U Of Cal (Sf)	7,071	357	531	911	1,313	1,451	1,476	1,032
" -U Of So Cal (La)	6,286	198	457	604	1,015	1,502	1,434	1,076
CO-U Of Colorado	5,814	214	460	696	1,115	1,221	1,247	861
CT-U Of Connecticut	2,558				401	824	804	529
" -Yale U	4,972	295	486	679	882	971	973	686
DC-George Wash U	6,928	310	557	825	1,233	1,464	1,500	1,039
" -Georgetown U	8,539	329	674	902	1,573	2,021	1,922	1,118
" -Howard U	4,845	198	412	686	951	1,031	898	669
FL-U Of Florida	4,238			422	788	1,120	1,123	785
" -U Of Miami	6,164		129	588	1,278	1,714	1,452	1,003
" -U Of So Florida	2,702				291	820	918	673
GA-Emory U	5,171	245	450	593	914	1,151	1,070	748
" -Med Coll Of Georgia	7,429	206	483	755	1,310	1,737	1,735	1,203
" -Morehouse U	678					118	307	253
" -Mercer U	858					86	417	355
HI-U Of Hawaii	1,850				290	622	539	399
IL-Chgo Med School	6,440	162	490	590	909	1,409	1,616	1,264
" -Loyola U/Stritch	6,120	285	533	689	1,248	1,206	1,266	893
" -Northwestern U	8,803	568	965	1,189	1,549	1,713	1,676	1,143
" -Rush Med Coll	3,831	131			524	1,192	1,175	809
" -Southern Illinois U	2,040				234	634	680	492
" -U Of Chgo/Pritzker	4,950	260	464	606	859	1,037	1,017	707
" -U Of Illinois	13,768	823	1,053	1,609	2,378	3,068	2,857	1,980
IN-Indiana U	12,241	447	819	1,433	2,409	2,769	2,536	1,828
IA-U Of Iowa	7,762	358	660	972	1,427	1,631	1,647	1,067
KS-U Of Kansas	7,946	330	634	884	1,534	1,709	1,695	1,160
KY-U Of Kentucky	3,660			301	866	968	878	647
" -U Of Louisville	6,197	374	522	716	1,094	1,307	1,235	949
LA-Lsu (New Orleans)	7,782	306	638	964	1,351	1,678	1,650	1,195
" -Lsu (Shreveport)	2,863				306	931	946	680
" -Tulane U	7,696	520	824	1,053	1,342	1,464	1,440	1,053
MD-Johns Hopkins	5,767	385	507	720	1,051	1,157	1,152	795
" -U Of Maryland	7,491	493	643	882	1,415	1,630	1,459	969
" -Uniformed Services U	3,897					1,184	1,588	1,125
MA-Boston U	6,287	243	449	613	1,036	1,446	1,460	1,040
" -Harvard U	8,995	774	1,068	1,250	1,571	1,562	1,652	1,118
" -Tufts U	7,733	467	738	964	1,414	1,465	1,535	1,150
" -U Of Massachusetts	2,866				258	965	968	675
MI-Michigan State U	3,316				581	995	1,037	703
" -U Of Michigan	10,468	551	1,109	1,595	2,104	2,105	1,865	1,139
" -Wayne State U	10,009	286	417	867	1,816	2,487	2,464	1,672
MN-Mayo Medical School	1,211				156	378	391	286
" -U Of Minnesota	10,748	603	878	1,235	2,243	2,656	1,977	1,156
" -U Of Minnesota-Duluth	644						283	361
MS-U Of Mississippi	4,515		86	538	981	1,315	931	664
MO-St Louis U	7,171	412	721	876	1,267	1,455	1,420	1,020
" -U Of Mo (Columbia)	4,351		65	625	956	1,075	995	635
" -U Of Mo (Kansas City)	2,516				214	811	871	620
" -Washington U	6,147	409	671	751	1,122	1,257	1,173	764
NE-Creighton U	5,155	217	457	574	912	1,085	1,137	773

Table 1.17

Country and School of Graduation of Total Physicians by Year of Graduation, 2006, continued

State School	Total Physicians	Prior 1950	1950-1959	1960-1969	1970-1979	1980-1989	1990-1999	2000-Present
" -U Of Nebraska	6,151	300	551	691	1,306	1,306	1,175	822
NV-U Of Nevada	1,282					450	477	355
NH-Dartmouth Med School	2,110				274	564	758	514
NJ-N Jersey Med Sch (Newark)	5,931			617	1,024	1,471	1,666	1,153
" -N Jersey Med Sch (Rutgers)	3,960				296	1,200	1,433	1,031
NM-U Of New Mexico	2,391			32	496	700	685	478
NY-Albany Med Coll	5,374	159	336	526	923	1,245	1,304	881
" -Albert Einstein Coll Of Med	6,863		42	802	1,469	1,699	1,658	1,193
" -Columbia U	7,735	575	830	1,056	1,317	1,461	1,469	1,027
" -Cornell U	5,463	387	624	759	946	1,066	988	693
" -Mt Sinai School Of Med	3,950				640	1,254	1,296	760
" -New York Med Coll	9,191	437	780	1,061	1,668	1,942	1,944	1,359
" -New York U	8,562	727	946	1,140	1,471	1,687	1,481	1,110
" -Suny (Brooklyn)	10,300	466	943	1,365	1,966	2,159	2,043	1,358
" -Suny (Buffalo)	6,523	314	476	737	1,204	1,389	1,443	960
" -Suny (Stony Brook)	2,809				181	797	1,072	759
" -Suny (Syracuse)	6,506	210	447	728	1,086	1,471	1,475	1,089
" -U Of Rochester	4,822	276	491	610	836	968	959	682
NC-Bowman Gray	4,377	117	338	437	733	1,020	1,021	711
" -Duke University	5,296	312	524	733	994	1,086	1,009	638
" -East Carolina U	1,617					444	680	493
" -U Of No Carolina	5,910		253	560	1,002	1,521	1,530	1,044
ND-U Of No Dakota	1,518				153	443	533	389
OH-Case Western Res	6,593	352	531	722	1,139	1,460	1,408	981
" -Med Coll Of Ohio	3,872				470	1,181	1,272	949
" -Northeastern Ohio U	2,351					668	973	710
" -Ohio State U	9,866	290	772	1,222	2,012	2,106	2,052	1,412
" -U Of Cincinnati	7,278	355	566	775	1,229	1,824	1,481	1,048
" -Wright State U	2,217					768	850	599
OK-U Of Oklahoma	6,611	212	459	763	1,222	1,631	1,362	962
OR-U Of Oregon	4,882	287	438	633	961	1,021	897	645
PA-Med Coll Of Penn	10,373	673	885	1,209	2,061	2,882	2,595	68
" -Jefferson Med Coll	12,688	636	1,093	1,387	1,917	2,142	2,365	3,148
" -Pennsylvania State U	3,246				590	913	976	767
" -Temple U	8,815	549	814	1,142	1,552	1,743	1,701	1,314
" -U Of Pennsylvania	8,199	671	907	1,180	1,438	1,521	1,449	1,033
" -U Of Pittsburgh	6,386	358	578	790	1,116	1,285	1,285	974
PR-Ponce Med Sch	1,317					325	570	422
" -U Central Del Caribe	1,903					886	631	386
" -U Of Puerto Rico	4,762		208	414	954	1,407	1,061	718
RI-Brown U	2,126				294	710	686	436
SC-Med Coll Of So Carolina	6,135	164	412	615	1,208	1,483	1,308	945
" -U Of So Carolina	1,518					392	630	496
SD-U Of So Dakota	1,414				114	479	474	347
TN-East Tennessee State U	1,322					365	562	395
" -Meharry Med Coll	3,742	169	306	436	774	836	690	531
" -U Of Tennessee	8,933	426	1,087	1,426	1,742	1,681	1,490	1,081
" -Vanderbilt U	4,350	218	328	440	699	997	959	709
TX-Baylor Coll Of Med	7,013	199	478	704	1,353	1,553	1,602	1,124
" -Texas A&M U	1,267					327	467	473
" -Texas Tech U	2,779				184	771	994	830
" -U Of Tx (Dallas)	8,031	148	527	795	1,275	1,946	1,946	1,394
" -U Of Tx (Galveston)	8,834	306	793	1,051	1,639	1,880	1,860	1,305
" -U Of Tx (Houston)	5,153				351	1,568	1,857	1,377
" -U Of Tx (San Antonio)	5,919				873	1,738	1,954	1,354
UT-U Of Utah	4,277	109	285	436	799	990	973	685
VT-U Of Vermont	3,925	173	281	392	673	840	918	648
VA-Eastern Virginia Med Sch	2,584				156	794	938	696
" -Med Coll Of Va	7,425	402	623	696	1,288	1,612	1,613	1,191
" -U Of Virginia	5,956	274	471	614	1,016	1,314	1,325	942
WA-U Of Washington	6,679		448	693	1,120	1,673	1,566	1,179
WV-Marshall U	1,091					309	458	324

Table 1.17

Country and School of Graduation of Total Physicians by Year of Graduation, 2006, continued

State School	Total Physicians	Prior 1950	1950-1959	1960-1969	1970-1979	1980-1989	1990-1999	2000-Present
" -West Virginia U	3,264			333	727	827	784	593
WI-Med Coll Of Wisconsin	7,893	370	597	794	1,068	1,779	1,910	1,375
" -U Of Wisconsin	6,669	299	532	764	1,193	1,519	1,368	994
INA-Inactive Schools	1,527	285	2	94	2	608	323	213
CAN-Canadian Schools	12,154	560	1,386	1,851	2,566	2,649	2,539	603
IMG-Internat"L Schools	236,669	4,831	17,054	36,482	44,971	60,578	49,019	23,734

Note: Data for 1990 are as of January 1; data for all other years, December 31.

*Data were not available for Emergency Medicine prior to 1980 and Nuclear Medicine prior to 1985.

**Data on Medical Genetics were not available prior to 1994.

Table 1.18

Country and School of Graduation of Male Physicians by Year of Graduation, 2006

State School	Total Physicians	Prior 1950	1950-1959	1960-1969	1970-1979	1980-1989	1990-1999	2000-Present
Total Physicians	665,647	27,254	56,682	92,603	132,215	155,688	126,418	74,787
US Active Schools	489,635	22,584	41,159	62,694	96,569	110,885	95,516	60,228
AL-U Of Alabama	4,877	37	309	592	989	1,203	1,058	689
" -U Of So Alabama	1,258				160	472	384	242
AZ-U Of Arizona	1,830				476	549	453	352
AR-U Of Arkansas	4,608	199	406	651	919	977	855	601
CA-Loma Linda U	5,257	356	579	687	1,054	982	969	630
" -Stanford U	2,959	237	410	391	642	489	505	285
" -U Of Cal (Davis)	1,889				471	544	547	327
" -U Of Cal (Irvine)	3,549	2	3	1,541	569	582	518	334
" -U Of Cal (La)	4,516		126	512	1,150	1,183	962	583
" -U Of Cal (San Diego)	2,402				390	816	719	477
" -U Of Cal (Sf)	4,741	311	489	816	1,026	876	773	450
" -U Of So Cal (La)	4,632	189	431	566	840	1,131	869	606
CO-U Of Colorado	4,139	194	421	647	939	773	727	438
CT-U Of Connecticut	1,567				324	566	422	255
" -Yale U	3,647	258	446	626	729	660	581	347
DC-George Wash U	4,931	271	526	767	1,031	998	823	515
" -Georgetown U	6,609	328	633	869	1,356	1,534	1,291	598
" -Howard U	3,179	173	355	585	718	579	449	320
FL-U Of Florida	2,933			396	677	814	660	386
" -U Of Miami	4,511		118	552	1,138	1,314	902	487
" -U Of So Florida	1,845				244	612	607	382
GA-Emory U	3,984	242	442	572	818	830	666	414
" -Med Coll Of Georgia	5,898	189	460	728	1,179	1,380	1,178	784
" -Morehouse U	284					58	140	86
" -Mercer U	517					52	256	209
HI-U Of Hawaii	1,185				235	422	314	214
IL-Chgo Med School	4,924	157	479	585	829	1,057	1,053	764
" -Loyola U/Stritch	4,578	267	512	661	1,065	842	752	479
" -Northwestern U	6,657	546	914	1,131	1,312	1,158	958	638
" -Rush Med Coll	2,363	120			423	788	629	403
" -Southern Illinois U	1,302				194	442	395	271
" -U Of Chgo/Pritzker	3,729	237	428	551	737	786	631	359
" -U Of Illinois	10,693	756	990	1,508	2,074	2,301	1,886	1,178
IN-Indiana U	9,378	420	785	1,355	2,105	1,998	1,655	1,060
IA-U Of Iowa	5,976	329	637	924	1,254	1,166	1,040	626
KS-U Of Kansas	6,072	304	609	853	1,319	1,235	1,103	649
KY-U Of Kentucky	2,681			275	738	703	591	374
" -U Of Louisville	4,641	361	491	682	950	938	735	484
LA-Lsu (New Orleans)	5,988	278	595	895	1,206	1,261	1,068	685
" -Lsu (Shreveport)	2,080				281	729	665	405
" -Tulane U	5,981	481	791	1,019	1,188	1,033	884	585
MD-Johns Hopkins	4,316	331	464	671	887	840	677	446
" -U Of Maryland	5,541	453	615	824	1,192	1,174	823	460
" -Uniformed Services U	3,006					943	1,225	838
MA-Boston U	4,423	219	410	534	819	959	867	615
" -Harvard U	6,799	768	1,009	1,169	1,267	1,035	972	579
" -Tufts U	5,671	427	706	914	1,115	980	875	654
" -U Of Massachusetts	1,633				199	600	508	326
MI-Michigan State U	1,815				413	573	531	298
" -U Of Michigan	8,135	487	1,039	1,497	1,763	1,545	1,166	638
" -Wayne State U	7,300	265	396	806	1,563	1,828	1,497	945
MN-Mayo Medical School	754				125	262	227	140
" -U Of Minnesota	8,013	549	827	1,163	1,953	1,809	1,119	593
" -U Of Minnesota-Duluth	348						158	190
MS-U Of Mississippi	3,599		82	516	865	1,027	675	434
MO-St Louis U	5,816	412	709	841	1,148	1,147	1,006	553
" -U Of Mo (Columbia)	3,235		64	594	837	789	604	347
" -U Of Mo (Kansas City)	1,308				159	479	410	260
" -Washington U	4,729	383	629	706	941	936	755	379

Table 1.18

Country and School of Graduation of Male Physicians by Year of Graduation, 2006, continued

State School	Total Physicians	Prior 1950	1950-1959	1960-1969	1970-1979	1980-1989	1990-1999	2000-Present
NE-Creighton U	4,163	201	438	565	852	878	796	433
" -U Of Nebraska	4,752	279	527	663	1,162	930	711	480
NV-U Of Nevada	823					318	302	203
NH-Dartmouth Med School	1,239				208	341	423	267
NJ-N Jersey Med Sch (Newark)	4,210			570	885	1,011	1,058	686
" -N Jersey Med Sch (Rutgers)	2,529				219	861	887	562
NM-U Of New Mexico	1,444			29	402	452	350	211
NY-Albany Med Coll	3,788	138	318	495	783	877	746	431
" -Albert Einstein Coll Of Med	4,574		40	739	1,154	1,099	933	609
" -Columbia U	5,784	510	738	957	1,068	1,035	913	563
" -Cornell U	4,039	346	576	717	806	702	556	336
" -Mt Sinai School Of Med	2,404				500	830	690	384
" -New York Med Coll	6,844	377	709	987	1,421	1,393	1,256	701
" -New York U	6,443	650	859	1,016	1,193	1,168	941	616
" -Suny (Brooklyn)	7,768	439	869	1,228	1,656	1,584	1,284	708
" -Suny (Buffalo)	4,683	291	451	692	1,015	918	843	473
" -Suny (Stony Brook)	1,593				102	476	622	393
" -Suny (Syracuse)	4,747	187	418	677	936	1,044	869	616
" -U Of Rochester	3,562	250	460	578	723	677	531	343
NC-Bowman Gray	3,363	112	319	413	652	761	681	425
" -Duke University	4,066	296	495	705	819	744	655	352
" -East Carolina U	964					332	379	253
" -U Of No Carolina	4,059		245	540	852	1,016	876	530
ND-U Of No Dakota	1,000				135	333	331	201
OH-Case Western Res	4,689	332	483	651	935	930	773	585
" -Med Coll Of Ohio	2,549				380	801	790	578
" -Northeastern Ohio U	1,386					456	562	368
" -Ohio State U	7,617	272	745	1,146	1,760	1,529	1,324	841
" -U Of Cincinnati	5,579	325	543	747	1,098	1,298	922	646
" -Wright State U	1,279					565	445	269
OK-U Of Oklahoma	5,170	199	439	721	1,103	1,245	886	577
OR-U Of Oregon	3,732	266	413	603	851	737	521	341
PA-Med Coll Of Penn	6,468	471	555	800	1,333	1,815	1,463	31
" -Jefferson Med Coll	9,537	635	1,093	1,350	1,656	1,650	1,490	1,663
" -Pennsylvania State U	2,084				502	637	556	389
" -Temple U	6,692	499	751	1,040	1,339	1,236	1,064	763
" -U Of Pennsylvania	6,306	632	854	1,132	1,212	1,021	885	570
" -U Of Pittsburgh	4,826	333	556	746	941	923	825	502
PR-Ponce Med Sch	848					240	360	248
" -U Central Del Caribe	1,222					628	381	213
" -U Of Puerto Rico	3,061		176	339	712	911	575	348
RI-Brown U	1,224				219	447	369	189
SC-Med Coll Of So Carolina	4,766	157	401	590	1,100	1,135	847	536
" -U Of So Carolina	987					288	411	288
SD-U Of So Dakota	934				94	359	286	195
TN-East Tennessee State U	804					252	340	212
" -Meharry Med Coll	2,584	148	289	392	612	540	349	254
" -U Of Tennessee	7,363	401	1,027	1,351	1,578	1,358	1,000	648
" -Vanderbilt U	3,412	209	311	417	629	774	651	421
TX-Baylor Coll Of Med	5,194	184	452	677	1,188	1,111	989	593
" -Texas A&M U	748					238	282	228
" -Texas Tech U	1,976				150	570	720	536
" -U Of Tx (Dallas)	6,161	131	490	753	1,126	1,512	1,282	867
" -U Of Tx (Galveston)	6,764	276	749	997	1,422	1,393	1,210	717
" -U Of Tx (Houston)	3,194				297	1,063	1,064	770
" -U Of Tx (San Antonio)	3,875				746	1,217	1,235	677
UT-U Of Utah	3,586	105	277	429	742	824	754	455
VT-U Of Vermont	2,727	160	259	372	590	577	479	290
VA-Eastern Virginia Med Sch	1,523				112	526	516	369
" -Med Coll Of Va	5,558	359	569	662	1,124	1,168	1,035	641
" -U Of Virginia	4,557	259	457	591	910	1,023	807	510

Table 1.18

Country and School of Graduation of Male Physicians by Year of Graduation, 2006, continued

State School	Total Physicians	Prior 1950	1950-1959	1960-1969	1970-1979	1980-1989	1990-1999	2000-Present
WA-U Of Washington	4,604		418	658	948	1,126	874	580
WV-Marshall U	700					219	299	182
" -West Virginia U	2,424			306	647	629	486	356
WI-Med Coll Of Wisconsin	5,990	347	566	766	965	1,283	1,200	863
" -U Of Wisconsin	4,863	272	489	715	1,010	1,092	808	477
INA-Inactive Schools	1,134	274	2	91	1	441	204	121
CAN-Canadian Schools	9,501	500	1,308	1,665	2,154	1,878	1,653	343
IMG-Internat"L Schools	165,377	3,896	14,213	28,153	33,491	42,484	29,045	14,095

Note: Data for 1990 are as of January 1; data for all other years, December 31.

*Data were not available for Emergency Medicine prior to 1980 and Nuclear Medicine prior to 1985.

**Data on Medical Genetics were not available prior to 1994.

Table 1.19

Country and School of Graduation of Female Physicians by Year of Graduation, 2006

State / School	Total Physicians	Prior 1950	1950-1959	1960-1969	1970-1979	1980-1989	1990-1999	2000-Present
Total Physicians	256,257	2,999	5,784	12,944	29,015	64,101	81,621	59,793
US Active Schools	181,919	1,993	2,865	4,426	17,122	45,069	60,642	49,802
AL-U Of Alabama	1,457	4	12	33	133	353	500	422
" -U Of So Alabama	575				29	135	231	180
AZ-U Of Arizona	1,143				129	273	426	315
AR-U Of Arkansas	1,215	9	27	34	110	278	432	325
CA-Loma Linda U	1,577	37	53	70	177	300	508	432
" -Stanford U	1,161	20	36	45	146	271	336	307
" -U Of Cal (Davis)	1,149				129	354	353	313
" -U Of Cal (Irvine)	1,110		2	87	94	280	364	283
" -U Of Cal (La)	2,024		11	40	159	527	735	552
" -U Of Cal (San Diego)	1,210				92	300	457	361
" -U Of Cal (Sf)	2,330	46	42	95	287	575	703	582
" -U Of So Cal (La)	1,654	9	26	38	175	371	565	470
CO-U Of Colorado	1,675	20	39	49	176	448	520	423
CT-U Of Connecticut	991				77	258	382	274
" -Yale U	1,325	37	40	53	153	311	392	339
DC-George Wash U	1,997	39	31	58	202	466	677	524
" -Georgetown U	1,930	1	41	33	217	487	631	520
" -Howard U	1,666	25	57	101	233	452	449	349
FL-U Of Florida	1,305			26	111	306	463	399
" -U Of Miami	1,653		11	36	140	400	550	516
" -U Of So Florida	857				47	208	311	291
GA-Emory U	1,187	3	8	21	96	321	404	334
" -Med Coll Of Georgia	1,531	17	23	27	131	357	557	419
" -Morehouse U	394					60	167	167
" -Mercer U	341					34	161	146
HI-U Of Hawaii	665				55	200	225	185
IL-Chgo Med School	1,516	5	11	5	80	352	563	500
" -Loyola U/Stritch	1,542	18	21	28	183	364	514	414
" -Northwestern U	2,146	22	51	58	237	555	718	505
" -Rush Med Coll	1,468	11			101	404	546	406
" -Southern Illinois U	738				40	192	285	221
" -U Of Chgo/Pritzker	1,221	23	36	55	122	251	386	348
" -U Of Illinois	3,075	67	63	101	304	767	971	802
IN-Indiana U	2,863	27	34	78	304	771	881	768
IA-U Of Iowa	1,786	29	23	48	173	465	607	441
KS-U Of Kansas	1,874	26	25	31	215	474	592	511
KY-U Of Kentucky	979			26	128	265	287	273
" -U Of Louisville	1,556	13	31	34	144	369	500	465
LA-Lsu (New Orleans)	1,794	28	43	69	145	417	582	510
" -Lsu (Shreveport)	783				25	202	281	275
" -Tulane U	1,715	39	33	34	154	431	556	468
MD-Johns Hopkins	1,451	54	43	49	164	317	475	349
" -U Of Maryland	1,950	40	28	58	223	456	636	509
" -Uniformed Services U	891					241	363	287
MA-Boston U	1,864	24	39	79	217	487	593	425
" -Harvard U	2,196	6	59	81	304	527	680	539
" -Tufts U	2,062	40	32	50	299	485	660	496
" -U Of Massachusetts	1,233				59	365	460	349
MI-Michigan State U	1,501				168	422	506	405
" -U Of Michigan	2,333	64	70	98	341	560	699	501
" -Wayne State U	2,709	21	21	61	253	659	967	727
MN-Mayo Medical School	457				31	116	164	146
" -U Of Minnesota	2,735	54	51	72	290	847	858	563
" -U Of Minnesota-Duluth	296						125	171
MS-U Of Mississippi	916		4	22	116	288	256	230
MO-St Louis U	1,355		12	35	119	308	414	467
" -U Of Mo (Columbia)	1,116		1	31	119	286	391	288
" -U Of Mo (Kansas City)	1,208				55	332	461	360
" -Washington U	1,418	26	42	45	181	321	418	385

Table 1.19

Country and School of Graduation of Female Physicians by Year of Graduation, 2006, continued

State School	Total Physicians	Prior 1950	1950-1959	1960-1969	1970-1979	1980-1989	1990-1999	2000-Present
NE-Creighton U	992	16	19	9	60	207	341	340
" -U Of Nebraska	1,399	21	24	28	144	376	464	342
NV-U Of Nevada	459					132	175	152
NH-Dartmouth Med School	871				66	223	335	247
NJ-N Jersey Med Sch (Newark)	1,721			47	139	460	608	467
" -N Jersey Med Sch (Rutgers)	1,431				77	339	546	469
NM-U Of New Mexico	947			3	94	248	335	267
NY-Albany Med Coll	1,586	21	18	31	140	368	558	450
" -Albert Einstein Coll Of Med	2,289		2	63	315	600	725	584
" -Columbia U	1,951	65	92	99	249	426	556	464
" -Cornell U	1,424	41	48	42	140	364	432	357
" -Mt Sinai School Of Med	1,546				140	424	606	376
" -New York Med Coll	2,347	60	71	74	247	549	688	658
" -New York U	2,119	77	87	124	278	519	540	494
" -Suny (Brooklyn)	2,532	27	74	137	310	575	759	650
" -Suny (Buffalo)	1,840	23	25	45	189	471	600	487
" -Suny (Stony Brook)	1,216				79	321	450	366
" -Suny (Syracuse)	1,759	23	29	51	150	427	606	473
" -U Of Rochester	1,260	26	31	32	113	291	428	339
NC-Bowman Gray	1,014	5	19	24	81	259	340	286
" -Duke University	1,230	16	29	28	175	342	354	286
" -East Carolina U	653					112	301	240
" -U Of No Carolina	1,851		8	20	150	505	654	514
ND-U Of No Dakota	518				18	110	202	188
OH-Case Western Res	1,904	20	48	71	204	530	635	396
" -Med Coll Of Ohio	1,323				90	380	482	371
" -Northeastern Ohio U	965					212	411	342
" -Ohio State U	2,249	18	27	76	252	577	728	571
" -U Of Cincinnati	1,699	30	23	28	131	526	559	402
" -Wright State U	938					203	405	330
OK-U Of Oklahoma	1,441	13	20	42	119	386	476	385
OR-U Of Oregon	1,150	21	25	30	110	284	376	304
PA-Med Coll Of Penn	3,905	202	330	409	728	1,067	1,132	37
" -Jefferson Med Coll	3,151	1		37	261	492	875	1,485
" -Pennsylvania State U	1,162				88	276	420	378
" -Temple U	2,123	50	63	102	213	507	637	551
" -U Of Pennsylvania	1,893	39	53	48	226	500	564	463
" -U Of Pittsburgh	1,560	25	22	44	175	362	460	472
PR-Ponce Med Sch	469					85	210	174
" -U Central Del Caribe	681					258	250	173
" -U Of Puerto Rico	1,701		32	75	242	496	486	370
RI-Brown U	902				75	263	317	247
SC-Med Coll Of So Carolina	1,369	7	11	25	108	348	461	409
" -U Of So Carolina	531					104	219	208
SD-U Of So Dakota	480				20	120	188	152
TN-East Tennessee State U	518					113	222	183
" -Meharry Med Coll	1,158	21	17	44	162	296	341	277
" -U Of Tennessee	1,570	25	60	75	164	323	490	433
" -Vanderbilt U	938	9	17	23	70	223	308	288
TX-Baylor Coll Of Med	1,819	15	26	27	165	442	613	531
" -Texas A&M U	519					89	185	245
" -Texas Tech U	803				34	201	274	294
" -U Of Tx (Dallas)	1,870	17	37	42	149	434	664	527
" -U Of Tx (Galveston)	2,070	30	44	54	217	487	650	588
" -U Of Tx (Houston)	1,959				54	505	793	607
" -U Of Tx (San Antonio)	2,044				127	521	719	677
UT-U Of Utah	691	4	8	7	57	166	219	230
VT-U Of Vermont	1,198	13	22	20	83	263	439	358
VA-Eastern Virginia Med Sch	1,061				44	268	422	327
" -Med Coll Of Va	1,867	43	54	34	164	444	578	550
" -U Of Virginia	1,399	15	14	23	106	291	518	432

Table 1.19

Country and School of Graduation of Female Physicians by Year of Graduation, 2006, continued

State School	Total Physicians	Prior 1950	1950-1959	1960-1969	1970-1979	1980-1989	1990-1999	2000-Present
WA-U Of Washington	2,075		30	35	172	547	692	599
WV-Marshall U	391					90	159	142
" -West Virginia U	840			27	80	198	298	237
WI-Med Coll Of Wisconsin	1,903	23	31	28	103	496	710	512
" -U Of Wisconsin	1,806	27	43	49	183	427	560	517
INA-Inactive Schools	393	11		3	1	167	119	92
CAN-Canadian Schools	2,653	60	78	186	412	771	886	260
IMG-Internat"L Schools	71,292	935	2,841	8,329	11,480	18,094	19,974	9,639

Note: Data for 1990 are as of January 1; data for all other years, December 31.

*Data were not available for Emergency Medicine prior to 1980 and Nuclear Medicine prior to 1985.

**Data on Medical Genetics were not available prior to 1994.

Table 1.20

Physicians by Race/Ethnicity, 2006

Specialty	Total	White	Black	Hispanic	Asian	Other	American Indian/ Alaskan Native	Unknown
Total Physicians	921,904	514,254	32,452	46,214	113,585	12,572	1,444	201,383
Aerospace Medicine	473	299	9	12	12	5		136
Allergy/Immunology	4,196	2,548	84	163	613	82	5	701
Anesthesiology	41,193	22,269	1,430	1,898	6,103	650	83	8,760
Cardiovascular Disease	22,426	12,032	555	1,062	3,688	522	40	4,527
Child Psychiatry	7,260	4,158	382	484	979	103	21	1,133
Colon/Rectal Surgery	1,340	898	40	77	149	17		159
Dermatology	10,744	7,660	293	446	771	80	14	1,480
Diagnostic Radiology	24,624	15,458	463	1,101	2,880	171	29	4,522
Emergency Medicine	29,987	19,731	1,202	1,454	2,136	263	86	5,115
Family Medicine	82,866	48,022	3,572	4,571	7,618	954	284	17,845
Forensic Pathology	657	459	30	26	50	3	2	87
Gastroenterology	12,268	6,792	369	619	2,028	280	6	2,174
General Practice	10,493	3,530	178	736	1,479	65	4	4,501
General Preventive Medicine	2,161	1,229	198	101	192	6	4	431
General Surgery	37,556	22,235	1,413	1,986	4,130	384	76	7,332
Internal Medicine	155,705	71,866	6,316	8,247	28,402	3,571	166	37,137
Medical Genetics	533	384	8	24	40	4		73
Neurological Surgery	5,425	3,543	155	245	490	59	9	924
Neurology	14,554	8,116	283	767	2,160	370	17	2,841
Nuclear Medicine	1,477	708	32	82	273	28		354
Obstetrics/Gynecology	42,333	24,678	2,964	2,297	3,694	467	73	8,160
Occupational Medicine	2,641	1,753	96	72	150	21		549
Ophthalmology	18,058	11,978	425	705	1,748	241	24	2,937
Orthopedic Surgery	24,296	17,015	611	691	1,294	174	41	4,470
Otolaryngology	9,974	6,772	210	382	988	68	9	1,545
Pathology-Anatomic/Clinical	19,171	10,498	373	851	2,661	247	15	4,526
Pediatric Cardiology	1,877	1,157	36	106	253	32	2	291
Pediatrics	73,208	38,451	3,525	4,949	10,211	1,275	135	14,662
Physical Medicine & Rehabilitation	7,736	3,976	379	503	1,546	111	14	1,207
Plastic Surgery	7,063	4,879	158	307	624	72	6	1,017
Psychiatry	41,385	22,920	1,405	2,173	5,337	648	52	8,850
Public Health & General Preventive Medicine	1,434	898	67	32	63	10		364
Pulmonary Diseases	10,232	5,659	266	538	1,656	221	12	1,880
Radiation Oncology	4,424	2,590	128	185	774	58	8	681
Radiology	8,886	5,050	151	268	990	73	7	2,347
Thoracic Surgery	4,807	2,974	147	180	486	67	7	946
Transplant Surgery	151	87	3	4	15	2		40
Urological Surgery	10,518	6,829	291	400	959	108	13	1,918
Vascular Medicine	24	18	1		1	1		3
Other Specialty	5,168	2,969	110	155	276	36	5	1,617
Unspecified	7,512	2,244	258	295	638	84	21	3,972
Inactive	108,344	70,862	1,282	2,957	6,259	587	15	26,382
Not Classified	46,252	18,058	2,554	4,063	8,769	352	139	12,317
Address Unknown	472	2						470

Table 1.21

Male Physicians by Race/Ethnicity, 2006

Specialty	Total	White	Black	Hispanic	Asian	Other	American Indian/ Alaskan Native	Unknown
Total Physicians	665,647	383,473	17,313	31,205	72,121	8,831	834	151,870
Aerospace Medicine	435	276	8	10	11	5		125
Allergy/Immunology	3,042	1,951	35	106	336	58	4	552
Anesthesiology	31,824	17,675	878	1,441	4,355	509	68	6,898
Cardiovascular Disease	20,234	10,865	454	947	3,248	481	30	4,209
Child Psychiatry	3,934	2,380	123	242	451	57	11	670
Colon/Rectal Surgery	1,155	774	29	66	123	15		148
Dermatology	6,482	4,736	104	209	327	47	8	1,051
Diagnostic Radiology	19,100	12,209	281	793	2,038	120	19	3,640
Emergency Medicine	23,157	15,325	707	1,073	1,558	209	56	4,229
Family Medicine	54,450	32,636	1,561	2,860	4,151	578	143	12,521
Forensic Pathology	437	299	20	23	31	2		62
Gastroenterology	10,833	6,109	276	498	1,693	254	6	1,997
General Practice	8,438	2,981	138	614	1,057	47	2	3,599
General Preventive Medicine	1,344	798	71	59	109	2	2	303
General Surgery	31,853	18,677	1,043	1,627	3,435	335	59	6,677
Internal Medicine	106,164	50,217	3,672	5,558	17,562	2,450	97	26,608
Medical Genetics	280	205	5	14	16	3		37
Neurological Surgery	5,094	3,323	140	224	448	58	9	892
Neurology	10,856	6,079	164	541	1,486	283	13	2,290
Nuclear Medicine	1,179	600	22	64	202	16		275
Obstetrics/Gynecology	23,813	13,980	1,050	1,362	1,646	257	19	5,499
Occupational Medicine	2,099	1,428	49	59	109	16		438
Ophthalmology	14,678	10,011	261	496	1,172	183	15	2,540
Orthopedic Surgery	23,133	16,180	557	634	1,210	165	33	4,354
Otolaryngology	8,758	5,991	158	315	801	56	7	1,430
Pathology-Anatomic/Clinical	12,551	7,143	175	518	1,472	146	8	3,089
Pediatric Cardiology	1,336	842	19	66	162	22		225
Pediatrics	33,740	18,406	1,047	2,220	4,080	626	48	7,313
Physical Medicine & Rehabilitation	5,061	2,712	200	336	949	71	8	785
Plastic Surgery	6,191	4,285	114	264	525	66	5	932
Psychiatry	27,319	15,360	712	1,412	3,191	413	32	6,199
Public Health & General Preventive Medicine	1,004	642	31	27	40	7		257
Pulmonary Diseases	8,671	4,824	208	454	1,313	199	9	1,664
Radiation Oncology	3,356	2,039	72	138	539	38	7	523
Radiology	7,500	4,299	117	207	816	63	5	1,993
Thoracic Surgery	4,620	2,852	138	175	462	66	7	920
Transplant Surgery	136	75	2	4	15	2		38
Urological Surgery	9,935	6,445	248	351	893	104	11	1,883
Vascular Medicine	19	14	1		1			3
Other Specialty	4,220	2,438	71	120	198	28	4	1,361
Unspecified	5,060	1,517	116	193	379	41	13	2,801
Inactive	94,469	63,345	1,006	2,532	4,632	489	11	22,454
Not Classified	27,358	10,530	1,230	2,353	4,879	244	65	8,057
Address Unknown	329							329

Table 1.22

Female Physicians by Race/Ethnicity, 2006

Specialty	Total	White	Black	Hispanic	Asian	Other	American Indian/ Alaskan Native	Unknown
Total Physicians	256,257	130,781	15,139	15,009	41,464	3,741	610	49,513
Aerospace Medicine	38	23	1	2	1			11
Allergy/Immunology	1,154	597	49	57	277	24	1	149
Anesthesiology	9,369	4,594	552	457	1,748	141	15	1,862
Cardiovascular Disease	2,192	1,167	101	115	440	41	10	318
Child Psychiatry	3,326	1,778	259	242	528	46	10	463
Colon/Rectal Surgery	185	124	11	11	26	2		11
Dermatology	4,262	2,924	189	237	444	33	6	429
Diagnostic Radiology	5,524	3,249	182	308	842	51	10	882
Emergency Medicine	6,830	4,406	495	381	578	54	30	886
Family Medicine	28,416	15,386	2,011	1,711	3,467	376	141	5,324
Forensic Pathology	220	160	10	3	19	1	2	25
Gastroenterology	1,435	683	93	121	335	26		177
General Practice	2,055	549	40	122	422	18	2	902
General Preventive Medicine	817	431	127	42	83	4	2	128
General Surgery	5,703	3,558	370	359	695	49	17	655
Internal Medicine	49,541	21,649	2,644	2,689	10,840	1,121	69	10,529
Medical Genetics	253	179	3	10	24	1		36
Neurological Surgery	331	220	15	21	42	1		32
Neurology	3,698	2,037	119	226	674	87	4	551
Nuclear Medicine	298	108	10	18	71	12		79
Obstetrics/Gynecology	18,520	10,698	1,914	935	2,048	210	54	2,661
Occupational Medicine	542	325	47	13	41	5		111
Ophthalmology	3,380	1,967	164	209	576	58	9	397
Orthopedic Surgery	1,163	835	54	57	84	9	8	116
Otolaryngology	1,216	781	52	67	187	12	2	115
Pathology-Anatomic/Clinical	6,620	3,355	198	333	1,189	101	7	1,437
Pediatric Cardiology	541	315	17	40	91	10	2	66
Pediatrics	39,468	20,045	2,478	2,729	6,131	649	87	7,349
Physical Medicine & Rehabilitation	2,675	1,264	179	167	597	40	6	422
Plastic Surgery	872	594	44	43	99	6	1	85
Psychiatry	14,066	7,560	693	761	2,146	235	20	2,651
Public Health & General Preventive Medicine	430	256	36	5	23	3		107
Pulmonary Diseases	1,561	835	58	84	343	22	3	216
Radiation Oncology	1,068	551	56	47	235	20	1	158
Radiology	1,386	751	34	61	174	10	2	354
Thoracic Surgery	187	122	9	5	24	1		26
Transplant Surgery	15	12				1		2
Urological Surgery	583	384	43	49	66	4	2	35
Vascular Medicine	5	4	1					
Other Specialty	948	531	39	35	78	8	1	256
Unspecified	2,452	727	142	102	259	43	8	1,171
Inactive	13,875	7,517	276	425	1,627	98	4	3,928
Not Classified	18,894	7,528	1,324	1,710	3,890	108	74	4,260
Address Unknown	143	2						141

Chapter 2
Physician Distribution

This chapter provides information on the geographic distribution of physicians in the US and Possessions. The tabulations consist of summary tables by state of location, age, and sex, and summary tables by state of location, Major Professional Activity, and sex. These tables provide this information for the physician population as a whole and for International Medical Graduates (IMGs).

State of Location, Age, and Activity by Sex

Total US Physicians

Table 2.1 demonstrates that of the total 2006 US physician population (921,904), more than half (55.2%) were located in 10 states, each having more than 25,000 physicians. These 10 leading states were California (110,406), New York (83,826), Texas (54,971), Florida (53,566), Pennsylvania (42,204), Illinois (39,240), Ohio (34,091), Massachusetts (32,575), New Jersey (30,183), and Michigan (27,877).

Physicians younger than 45 years comprised 35% or more of the total physicians in each of these states except Florida (29.9%) and California (34.9%). The

state having the highest percentage of physicians in this age group was Massachusetts (44.0%).

Table 2.3 indicates that there were more female physicians in California in 2006 than in any other state (31,083, or 12.1% of total female physicians). New York followed with 26,763 female physicians and Texas with 14,675. These three states, in addition to Illinois (12,505), Pennsylvania (11,840), Florida (11,601), Massachusetts (11,055), and New Jersey (9,441), accounted for more than half (50.5%) of all female physicians in 2006.

The distribution of physicians by age categories reveals a higher proportion of female physicians than male physicians younger than 35 years. Table 3 demonstrates the percentage distributions by age groups and sex.

Male physicians younger than 35 (Table 2.2) showed the highest concentrations in New York (8,562), California (7,704), Texas (4,991), Pennsylvania (4,237), and Illinois (4,103). Nearly two fifths (38.4%) of all male physicians younger than 35 years were located in these states. Table 2.3 reveals that female physicians younger than 35 years accounted for the highest counts in New York (7,595), California (6,883), Texas (4,015), Illinois (3,727), and Pennsylvania (3,295). Cumulatively,

Mini-Table 3
Percent Distribution of Physicians by Age and Sex, 2006

Sex	Total	< 35	35–44	45–54	55–64	≥ 65
Both	100.0	15.3	23.1	24.3	18.0	19.2
Male	100.0	11.6	20.1	24.1	20.4	23.9
Female	100.0	25.1	31.1	24.8	11.8	7.1

Source: Tables 2.1, 2.2, and 2.3.

these five states accounted for 39.7% of all female physicians younger than 35 years.

State of Location and Activity

Tables 2.7 through 2.9 show the distribution of total physicians, male physicians, and female physicians among the states and major professional activity. Patient-Care physicians were in largest numbers in California (84,907), followed by New York (65,224), Texas (44,813), Florida (40,211), and Pennsylvania (32,324). Together, these states represented almost two fifths (37.0%) of all Patient-Care physicians. Residents/Fellows had the highest representation in New York, where they accounted for more than one fifth (20.9%) of Patient-Care physicians in that state.

For male physicians, Table 2.8 shows that Patient Care had the highest percentage representation in Alaska (83.2%), followed by Alabama (81.6%), Louisiana (81.2%), and Indiana (80.8%). Lowest representation among male physicians in Patient Care was in the District of Columbia (71.1%) and Maryland (71.6%).

Among female physicians (Table 2.9), Patient Care had the highest proportional representation in North Dakota (91.5%) and Idaho (89.8%). Lowest was the District of Columbia (78.5%). Female Residents/Fellows were found in highest numbers in New York (6,033), California (3,908), and Illinois (2,533).

International Medical Graduates (IMGs)

The states of New York (35,180), California (25,408), Florida (19,536), New Jersey (13,617), Illinois (13,439), and Texas (13,250) comprised half (50.9%) of all IMGs (Table 2.4). Of total IMGs, 36.9% were younger than 45 years. More than three fifths (59.7%) of IMGs in Arkansas were in the younger than 45-year age group, the highest proportion among the states.

The largest counts of male IMGs (Table 2.5) were found in New York (23,732), California (17,202), and Florida (14,995). Largest counts of female IMGs (Table 2.6) were found in New York (11,448), California (8,206), and New Jersey (4,772). The three highest-ranking states in each case accounted for approximately one third of the IMG population: 33.8% for male and 34.3% for female.

Table 4 indicates that the percentage distribution of female IMGs (Table 2.6) compared with the distribution of male IMGs (Table 2.5) varied widely in the younger and older age groups.

Of the five states with the largest counts of female IMGs—New York, California, New Jersey, Florida, and Illinois—proportionately the highest percentages of female IMGs younger than 35 years were found in New York (23.4%) and Illinois (22.7%).

More IMGs were in Office-Based practice in 2006 (57.9%) than in any other major professional activity (Table 2.10). Of the five states with the most IMGs (New York, California, Florida, New Jersey, and Illinois), California had the highest percentages of IMGs in Office-Based practice (67.1%), whereas New York had the lowest (48.0%).

New York (10,304), Pennsylvania (3,005), New Jersey (2,876), California (2,836), and Illinois (2,762) had the largest numbers of Hospital-Based IMGs. Of these states, New York had the largest percentage of its IMG population (29.3%) as Hospital-Based.

Mini-Table 4

Percentage Distribution of International Medical Graduates by Age and Sex, 2006

Sex	Total	< 35	35–44	45–54	55–64	≥ 65
Both	100.0	13.3	23.6	22.2	20.1	20.8
Male	100.0	10.7	20.8	22.7	21.6	24.2
Female	100.0	19.3	30.0	21.1	16.8	12.7

Source: Tables 2.4, 2.5, and 2.6.

Table 2.1

Total Physicians by Age and State of Location, 2006

State	Total Physicians	< 35	35-44	45-54	55-64	≥ 65
Total Physicians	921,904	141,492	213,311	223,864	166,005	177,232
Alabama	10,994	1,701	2,525	3,019	1,971	1,778
Alaska	1,697	135	460	487	362	253
Arizona	15,127	1,733	3,709	3,694	2,754	3,237
Arkansas	6,464	942	1,502	1,702	1,168	1,150
California	110,406	14,587	23,924	24,372	22,538	24,985
Colorado	14,175	1,765	3,532	3,555	2,679	2,644
Connecticut	14,488	2,289	3,198	3,589	2,595	2,817
Delaware	2,414	366	583	595	390	480
District Of Columbia	5,023	1,251	1,019	892	876	985
Florida	53,566	4,919	11,104	13,681	9,716	14,146
Georgia	22,805	3,186	5,879	6,120	3,893	3,727
Hawaii	4,599	537	995	1,190	928	949
Idaho	2,934	198	762	781	579	614
Illinois	39,240	7,830	9,123	8,952	6,794	6,541
Indiana	15,229	2,152	3,725	4,122	2,704	2,526
Iowa	6,428	981	1,488	1,696	1,127	1,136
Kansas	7,079	1,009	1,599	1,758	1,288	1,425
Kentucky	10,828	1,602	2,707	2,799	1,941	1,779
Louisiana	12,643	2,167	2,998	2,950	2,310	2,218
Maine	4,197	355	914	1,111	874	943
Maryland	25,969	3,942	6,003	6,307	4,749	4,968
Massachusetts	32,575	6,308	8,022	7,338	5,462	5,445
Michigan	27,877	5,222	6,450	6,350	4,813	5,042
Minnesota	16,756	2,800	4,149	4,316	2,803	2,688
Mississippi	5,890	718	1,426	1,551	1,092	1,103
Missouri	15,586	3,045	3,605	3,805	2,622	2,509
Montana	2,548	118	533	723	574	600
Nebraska	4,852	874	1,167	1,224	778	809
Nevada	5,384	514	1,479	1,333	933	1,125
New Hampshire	4,079	402	941	1,108	782	846
New Jersey	30,183	3,907	6,892	7,713	5,833	5,838
New Mexico	5,424	652	1,183	1,332	1,212	1,045
New York	83,826	16,157	17,990	18,742	14,312	16,625
North Carolina	25,385	3,987	6,585	6,616	3,987	4,210
North Dakota	1,745	186	440	463	355	301
Ohio	34,091	6,451	8,180	7,946	5,516	5,998
Oklahoma	7,111	972	1,482	1,825	1,424	1,408
Oregon	11,741	1,273	2,829	2,898	2,359	2,382
Pennsylvania	42,204	7,532	8,763	10,498	7,399	8,012
Rhode Island	4,368	876	1,054	985	633	820
South Carolina	11,241	1,736	2,834	2,684	1,951	2,036
South Dakota	1,975	199	468	584	393	331
Tennessee	17,791	2,686	4,273	4,789	3,123	2,920
Texas	54,971	9,006	14,236	13,231	9,407	9,091
Utah	6,093	912	1,582	1,496	1,103	1,000
Vermont	2,659	372	557	681	499	550
Virginia	23,545	3,475	5,552	5,842	4,195	4,481
Washington	19,864	2,172	4,562	5,081	4,067	3,982
West Virginia	4,710	731	1,043	1,047	957	932
Wisconsin	16,154	2,246	4,138	4,369	2,679	2,722
Wyoming	1,132	63	258	306	242	263
Possessions	12,338	2,011	2,460	3,447	2,066	2,354
APO's and FPO's	1,029	239	428	168	97	97
Address Unknown	472	3	1	1	101	366

Table 2.2

Male Physicians by Age and State of Location, 2006

State	Total Physicians	< 35	35-44	45-54	55-64	≥ 65
Total Physicians	665,647	77,168	133,515	160,253	135,790	158,921
Alabama	8,563	1,011	1,815	2,359	1,717	1,661
Alaska	1,187	63	284	321	292	227
Arizona	11,331	997	2,354	2,675	2,317	2,988
Arkansas	5,073	562	1,052	1,355	1,023	1,081
California	79,323	7,704	14,334	16,670	18,234	22,381
Colorado	10,079	901	2,103	2,389	2,246	2,440
Connecticut	10,252	1,214	1,851	2,511	2,131	2,545
Delaware	1,690	174	349	448	301	418
District Of Columbia	3,177	597	558	553	660	809
Florida	41,965	2,719	7,533	10,573	8,242	12,898
Georgia	16,699	1,700	3,736	4,527	3,271	3,465
Hawaii	3,338	316	578	857	766	821
Idaho	2,387	109	552	609	528	589
Illinois	26,735	4,103	5,527	6,200	5,248	5,657
Indiana	11,417	1,198	2,524	3,084	2,290	2,321
Iowa	4,957	596	1,021	1,280	989	1,071
Kansas	5,318	574	1,032	1,310	1,083	1,319
Kentucky	8,145	933	1,850	2,081	1,675	1,606
Louisiana	9,586	1,270	2,083	2,249	1,962	2,022
Maine	3,069	180	539	767	727	856
Maryland	17,589	2,015	3,454	4,121	3,673	4,326
Massachusetts	21,520	3,199	4,557	4,699	4,251	4,814
Michigan	19,780	2,942	3,932	4,543	3,855	4,508
Minnesota	12,003	1,529	2,575	3,061	2,344	2,494
Mississippi	4,732	468	1,067	1,216	951	1,030
Missouri	11,427	1,733	2,353	2,838	2,207	2,296
Montana	2,017	65	351	534	493	574
Nebraska	3,659	491	782	921	690	775
Nevada	4,179	296	1,053	1,037	792	1,001
New Hampshire	3,010	217	550	790	680	773
New Jersey	20,742	2,069	4,002	5,365	4,382	4,924
New Mexico	3,742	344	682	839	928	949
New York	57,063	8,562	10,731	12,871	10,959	13,940
North Carolina	18,612	2,173	4,180	4,894	3,440	3,925
North Dakota	1,379	116	291	363	317	292
Ohio	24,675	3,800	5,195	5,854	4,479	5,347
Oklahoma	5,527	605	1,018	1,373	1,228	1,303
Oregon	8,471	642	1,681	1,955	1,976	2,217
Pennsylvania	30,364	4,237	5,476	7,583	5,974	7,094
Rhode Island	2,968	432	611	675	523	727
South Carolina	8,669	995	1,962	2,060	1,716	1,936
South Dakota	1,546	108	303	461	358	316
Tennessee	13,666	1,598	2,897	3,716	2,734	2,721
Texas	40,296	4,991	9,297	9,691	7,922	8,395
Utah	4,870	584	1,151	1,176	1,003	956
Vermont	1,856	198	316	437	404	501
Virginia	16,756	1,821	3,361	4,128	3,429	4,017
Washington	14,285	1,089	2,741	3,431	3,376	3,648
West Virginia	3,659	474	713	822	803	847
Wisconsin	11,914	1,286	2,598	3,220	2,283	2,527
Wyoming	915	38	179	233	212	253
Possessions	8,374	983	1,452	2,399	1,546	1,994
APO's and FPO's	762	144	329	128	80	81
Address Unknown	329	3		1	80	245

Table 2.3

Female Physicians by Age and State of Location, 2006

State	Total Physicians	< 35	35-44	45-54	55-64	≥ 65
Total Physicians	256,257	64,324	79,796	63,611	30,215	18,311
Alabama	2,431	690	710	660	254	117
Alaska	510	72	176	166	70	26
Arizona	3,796	736	1,355	1,019	437	249
Arkansas	1,391	380	450	347	145	69
California	31,083	6,883	9,590	7,702	4,304	2,604
Colorado	4,096	864	1,429	1,166	433	204
Connecticut	4,236	1,075	1,347	1,078	464	272
Delaware	724	192	234	147	89	62
District Of Columbia	1,846	654	461	339	216	176
Florida	11,601	2,200	3,571	3,108	1,474	1,248
Georgia	6,106	1,486	2,143	1,593	622	262
Hawaii	1,261	221	417	333	162	128
Idaho	547	89	210	172	51	25
Illinois	12,505	3,727	3,596	2,752	1,546	884
Indiana	3,812	954	1,201	1,038	414	205
Iowa	1,471	385	467	416	138	65
Kansas	1,761	435	567	448	205	106
Kentucky	2,683	669	857	718	266	173
Louisiana	3,057	897	915	701	348	196
Maine	1,128	175	375	344	147	87
Maryland	8,380	1,927	2,549	2,186	1,076	642
Massachusetts	11,055	3,109	3,465	2,639	1,211	631
Michigan	8,097	2,280	2,518	1,807	958	534
Minnesota	4,753	1,271	1,574	1,255	459	194
Mississippi	1,158	250	359	335	141	73
Missouri	4,159	1,312	1,252	967	415	213
Montana	531	53	182	189	81	26
Nebraska	1,193	383	385	303	88	34
Nevada	1,205	218	426	296	141	124
New Hampshire	1,069	185	391	318	102	73
New Jersey	9,441	1,838	2,890	2,348	1,451	914
New Mexico	1,682	308	501	493	284	96
New York	26,763	7,595	7,259	5,871	3,353	2,685
North Carolina	6,773	1,814	2,405	1,722	547	285
North Dakota	366	70	149	100	38	9
Ohio	9,416	2,651	2,985	2,092	1,037	651
Oklahoma	1,584	367	464	452	196	105
Oregon	3,270	631	1,148	943	383	165
Pennsylvania	11,840	3,295	3,287	2,915	1,425	918
Rhode Island	1,400	444	443	310	110	93
South Carolina	2,572	741	872	624	235	100
South Dakota	429	91	165	123	35	15
Tennessee	4,125	1,088	1,376	1,073	389	199
Texas	14,675	4,015	4,939	3,540	1,485	696
Utah	1,223	328	431	320	100	44
Vermont	803	174	241	244	95	49
Virginia	6,789	1,654	2,191	1,714	766	464
Washington	5,579	1,083	1,821	1,650	691	334
West Virginia	1,051	257	330	225	154	85
Wisconsin	4,240	960	1,540	1,149	396	195
Wyoming	217	25	79	73	30	10
Possessions	3,964	1,028	1,008	1,048	520	360
APO's and FPO's	267	95	99	40	17	16
Address Unknown	143		1		21	121

Table 2.4

IMGs by Age and State of Location, 2006

State	Total Physicians	< 35	35-44	45-54	55-64	≥ 65
Total Physicians	236,669	31,451	55,767	52,657	47,656	49,138
Alabama	1,754	278	520	422	329	205
Alaska	118	6	38	28	27	19
Arizona	3,215	348	947	745	573	602
Arkansas	1,017	230	377	216	129	65
California	25,408	1,683	5,108	6,343	6,801	5,473
Colorado	1,053	120	317	209	202	205
Connecticut	4,192	836	1,050	863	674	769
Delaware	753	75	217	132	121	208
District Of Columbia	1,075	225	254	182	184	230
Florida	19,536	1,133	3,834	5,044	3,918	5,607
Georgia	4,438	557	1,215	1,111	821	734
Hawaii	708	51	102	140	174	241
Idaho	105	7	33	25	21	19
Illinois	13,439	2,117	2,828	2,514	3,031	2,949
Indiana	3,157	323	866	745	640	583
Iowa	1,252	193	377	270	206	206
Kansas	1,314	185	324	247	284	274
Kentucky	2,272	245	747	525	405	350
Louisiana	2,285	417	614	490	476	288
Maine	592	72	182	99	97	142
Maryland	7,106	672	1,575	1,587	1,537	1,735
Massachusetts	7,106	1,046	2,156	1,528	1,182	1,194
Michigan	9,459	1,840	2,298	1,774	1,878	1,669
Minnesota	2,482	477	907	508	253	337
Mississippi	780	104	281	188	117	90
Missouri	3,431	566	959	606	670	630
Montana	116	3	24	33	26	30
Nebraska	678	156	230	131	89	72
Nevada	1,580	186	452	335	256	351
New Hampshire	577	67	145	100	105	160
New Jersey	13,617	1,622	2,785	3,413	3,041	2,756
New Mexico	936	125	276	193	187	155
New York	35,180	6,072	7,246	7,390	6,739	7,733
North Carolina	3,221	356	986	848	515	516
North Dakota	459	94	144	88	70	63
Ohio	9,911	1,757	2,475	1,675	1,874	2,130
Oklahoma	1,351	235	332	300	288	196
Oregon	1,034	134	294	212	165	229
Pennsylvania	10,920	2,061	2,410	2,339	2,142	1,968
Rhode Island	1,177	180	280	221	170	326
South Carolina	1,427	203	444	348	186	246
South Dakota	270	46	85	65	33	41
Tennessee	2,930	457	887	700	508	378
Texas	13,250	1,468	3,725	3,074	2,681	2,302
Utah	510	78	172	123	83	54
Vermont	244	41	66	49	31	57
Virginia	4,981	481	1,192	1,074	979	1,255
Washington	2,448	258	716	494	426	554
West Virginia	1,711	223	369	295	391	433
Wisconsin	2,948	413	939	633	436	527
Wyoming	109	11	44	20	16	18
Possessions	6,833	916	912	1,945	1,424	1,636
APO's and FPO's	119		11	18	35	55
Address Unknown	85	2			10	73

Table 2.5

Male IMGs by Age and State of Location, 2006

State	Total Physicians	< 35	35-44	45-54	55-64	≥ 65
Total Physicians	165,377	17,695	34,391	37,589	35,650	40,052
Alabama	1,319	180	376	331	262	170
Alaska	75	1	23	18	20	13
Arizona	2,357	208	619	571	463	496
Arkansas	735	135	270	168	103	59
California	17,202	799	2,781	4,182	5,064	4,376
Colorado	699	64	174	146	152	163
Connecticut	2,845	445	603	631	522	644
Delaware	529	39	131	101	88	170
District Of Columbia	678	109	142	121	129	177
Florida	14,995	655	2,599	3,873	3,103	4,765
Georgia	3,184	305	785	817	638	639
Hawaii	491	32	51	94	133	181
Idaho	80	5	19	22	19	15
Illinois	8,977	1,105	1,694	1,694	2,131	2,353
Indiana	2,293	181	565	564	491	492
Iowa	953	134	264	208	167	180
Kansas	958	112	211	189	214	232
Kentucky	1,677	159	528	396	316	278
Louisiana	1,676	267	424	375	371	239
Maine	435	44	120	67	80	124
Maryland	4,878	369	939	1,079	1,088	1,403
Massachusetts	4,639	555	1,279	1,009	865	931
Michigan	6,430	1,045	1,353	1,270	1,399	1,363
Minnesota	1,716	291	586	384	186	269
Mississippi	573	75	196	143	88	71
Missouri	2,451	345	631	447	500	528
Montana	92	2	15	24	24	27
Nebraska	494	109	160	94	69	62
Nevada	1,129	103	304	258	192	272
New Hampshire	416	38	84	75	83	136
New Jersey	8,845	832	1,471	2,342	2,089	2,111
New Mexico	693	79	189	142	148	135
New York	23,732	3,395	4,285	5,130	4,889	6,033
North Carolina	2,324	199	628	648	403	446
North Dakota	350	64	102	66	60	58
Ohio	7,174	1,096	1,636	1,275	1,421	1,746
Oklahoma	992	147	226	237	221	161
Oregon	720	82	183	150	126	179
Pennsylvania	7,674	1,208	1,524	1,697	1,632	1,613
Rhode Island	856	105	170	167	143	271
South Carolina	1,028	116	305	263	133	211
South Dakota	203	32	52	51	30	38
Tennessee	2,142	303	587	532	408	312
Texas	9,486	802	2,330	2,257	2,096	2,001
Utah	379	54	122	92	68	43
Vermont	182	27	41	37	26	51
Virginia	3,460	248	733	737	707	1,035
Washington	1,653	123	433	330	320	447
West Virginia	1,350	151	258	234	322	385
Wisconsin	2,083	258	583	460	336	446
Wyoming	80	7	32	14	14	13
Possessions	4,844	454	571	1,365	1,061	1,393
APO's and FPO's	88		4	12	30	42
Address Unknown	63	2			7	54

Table 2.6

Female IMGs by Age and State of Location, 2006

State	Total Physicians	< 35	35-44	45-54	55-64	≥ 65
Total Physicians	71,292	13,756	21,376	15,068	12,006	9,086
Alabama	435	98	144	91	67	35
Alaska	43	5	15	10	7	6
Arizona	858	140	328	174	110	106
Arkansas	282	95	107	48	26	6
California	8,206	884	2,327	2,161	1,737	1,097
Colorado	354	56	143	63	50	42
Connecticut	1,347	391	447	232	152	125
Delaware	224	36	86	31	33	38
District Of Columbia	397	116	112	61	55	53
Florida	4,541	478	1,235	1,171	815	842
Georgia	1,254	252	430	294	183	95
Hawaii	217	19	51	46	41	60
Idaho	25	2	14	3	2	4
Illinois	4,462	1,012	1,134	820	900	596
Indiana	864	142	301	181	149	91
Iowa	299	59	113	62	39	26
Kansas	356	73	113	58	70	42
Kentucky	595	86	219	129	89	72
Louisiana	609	150	190	115	105	49
Maine	157	28	62	32	17	18
Maryland	2,228	303	636	508	449	332
Massachusetts	2,467	491	877	519	317	263
Michigan	3,029	795	945	504	479	306
Minnesota	766	186	321	124	67	68
Mississippi	207	29	85	45	29	19
Missouri	980	221	328	159	170	102
Montana	24	1	9	9	2	3
Nebraska	184	47	70	37	20	10
Nevada	451	83	148	77	64	79
New Hampshire	161	29	61	25	22	24
New Jersey	4,772	790	1,314	1,071	952	645
New Mexico	243	46	87	51	39	20
New York	11,448	2,677	2,961	2,260	1,850	1,700
North Carolina	897	157	358	200	112	70
North Dakota	109	30	42	22	10	5
Ohio	2,737	661	839	400	453	384
Oklahoma	359	88	106	63	67	35
Oregon	314	52	111	62	39	50
Pennsylvania	3,246	853	886	642	510	355
Rhode Island	321	75	110	54	27	55
South Carolina	399	87	139	85	53	35
South Dakota	67	14	33	14	3	3
Tennessee	788	154	300	168	100	66
Texas	3,764	666	1,395	817	585	301
Utah	131	24	50	31	15	11
Vermont	62	14	25	12	5	6
Virginia	1,521	233	459	337	272	220
Washington	795	135	283	164	106	107
West Virginia	361	72	111	61	69	48
Wisconsin	865	155	356	173	100	81
Wyoming	29	4	12	6	2	5
Possessions	1,989	462	341	580	363	243
APO's and FPO's	31		7	6	5	13
Address Unknown	22				3	19

Table 2.7

Total Physicians by State of Location and Major Professional Activity, 2006

State	Total Physicians	Patient Care				Other Professional Activity			
		Total Patient Care	Office Based	Hospital Based		Admin.	Med. Teach.	Research	Other*
				Resid./ Fellows	Phys. Staff				
Total Physicians	921,904	723,118	560,411	97,102	65,605	14,575	10,273	14,475	158,991
Alabama	10,994	9,091	7,250	1,194	647	129	92	133	1,549
Alaska	1,697	1,437	1,165	43	229	36	13	14	197
Arizona	15,127	11,622	9,667	998	957	231	154	134	2,986
Arkansas	6,464	5,316	4,216	651	449	57	97	48	946
California	110,406	84,907	70,083	8,465	6,359	1,764	1,036	1,856	20,843
Colorado	14,175	11,180	9,225	1,066	889	246	153	211	2,385
Connecticut	14,488	11,224	8,339	1,809	1,076	296	186	334	2,448
Delaware	2,414	1,927	1,521	212	194	38	20	25	404
District Of Columbia	5,023	3,710	2,196	968	546	201	115	159	838
Florida	53,566	40,211	33,863	2,884	3,464	717	453	397	11,788
Georgia	22,805	18,418	15,024	1,837	1,557	357	257	319	3,454
Hawaii	4,599	3,628	2,889	340	399	78	60	47	786
Idaho	2,934	2,373	2,087	66	220	35	12	7	507
Illinois	39,240	31,367	23,395	5,505	2,467	620	426	475	6,352
Indiana	15,229	12,560	10,206	1,312	1,042	198	130	182	2,159
Iowa	6,428	4,957	3,886	668	403	62	99	124	1,186
Kansas	7,079	5,602	4,474	637	491	95	87	50	1,245
Kentucky	10,828	8,825	7,199	1,018	608	128	116	84	1,675
Louisiana	12,643	10,393	8,087	1,540	766	130	196	97	1,827
Maine	4,197	3,250	2,606	229	415	94	53	28	772
Maryland	25,969	19,205	14,055	2,733	2,417	736	303	1,246	4,479
Massachusetts	32,575	24,657	17,291	4,587	2,779	597	328	1,214	5,779
Michigan	27,877	22,003	16,111	4,062	1,830	434	339	363	4,738
Minnesota	16,756	13,318	10,347	1,963	1,008	242	177	273	2,746
Mississippi	5,890	4,782	3,821	451	510	63	60	31	954
Missouri	15,586	12,590	9,301	2,126	1,163	202	212	274	2,308
Montana	2,548	1,991	1,728	37	226	29	13	14	501
Nebraska	4,852	3,874	2,992	589	293	70	71	51	786
Nevada	5,384	4,307	3,760	214	333	61	32	17	967
New Hampshire	4,079	3,176	2,561	260	355	50	33	56	764
New Jersey	30,183	24,128	18,874	2,855	2,399	507	306	513	4,729
New Mexico	5,424	4,162	3,210	478	474	93	66	74	1,029
New York	83,826	65,224	43,989	13,621	7,614	1,534	1,034	1,562	14,472
North Carolina	25,385	20,015	15,876	2,465	1,674	371	320	463	4,216
North Dakota	1,745	1,437	1,143	115	179	25	21	6	256
Ohio	34,091	26,844	19,866	4,610	2,368	452	385	424	5,986
Oklahoma	7,111	5,667	4,542	655	470	99	97	46	1,202
Oregon	11,741	9,036	7,538	736	762	182	122	146	2,255
Pennsylvania	42,204	32,324	23,343	5,881	3,100	727	493	908	7,752
Rhode Island	4,368	3,458	2,419	675	364	72	49	65	724
South Carolina	11,241	9,155	7,267	1,083	805	124	163	85	1,714
South Dakota	1,975	1,627	1,342	104	181	24	17	6	301
Tennessee	17,791	14,557	11,673	1,898	986	251	196	228	2,559
Texas	54,971	44,813	35,693	5,923	3,197	714	708	615	8,121
Utah	6,093	4,862	3,883	643	336	87	66	102	976
Vermont	2,659	1,980	1,418	313	249	47	41	56	535
Virginia	23,545	18,538	14,306	2,262	1,970	391	241	239	4,136
Washington	19,864	15,168	12,460	1,354	1,354	340	204	402	3,750
West Virginia	4,710	3,762	2,802	555	405	58	77	32	781
Wisconsin	16,154	13,126	10,611	1,529	986	221	196	182	2,429
Wyoming	1,132	903	780	33	90	18	8	4	199
Possessions	12,338	9,533	7,585	814	1,134	206	136	48	2,415
APO's and FPO's	1,029	898	446	36	416	36	4	6	85
Address Unknown	472								

* Includes Other, Inactive and Not Classified Physicians

Table 2.8

Male Physicians by State of Location and Major Professional Activity, 2006

State	Total Physicians	Patient Care				Other Professional Activity			
		Total Patient Care	Office Based	Hospital Based		Admin.	Med. Teach.	Research	Other*
				Resid./ Fellows	Phys. Staff				
Total Physicians	665,647	509,474	407,907	55,078	46,489	11,817	7,618	11,394	125,015
Alabama	8,563	6,987	5,754	757	476	110	77	111	1,278
Alaska	1,187	988	792	22	174	27	10	7	155
Arizona	11,331	8,445	7,173	572	700	194	108	105	2,479
Arkansas	5,073	4,100	3,370	391	339	44	72	43	814
California	79,323	59,179	50,120	4,557	4,502	1,439	786	1,469	16,450
Colorado	10,079	7,657	6,449	561	647	205	115	171	1,931
Connecticut	10,252	7,707	5,982	978	747	248	148	267	1,882
Delaware	1,690	1,311	1,082	103	126	30	14	18	317
District Of Columbia	3,177	2,260	1,413	481	366	157	87	116	557
Florida	41,965	30,616	26,371	1,622	2,623	609	346	319	10,075
Georgia	16,699	13,191	11,017	1,028	1,146	282	198	233	2,795
Hawaii	3,338	2,596	2,107	194	295	62	38	39	603
Idaho	2,387	1,882	1,678	30	174	33	8	6	458
Illinois	26,735	20,850	16,255	2,972	1,623	492	294	369	4,730
Indiana	11,417	9,230	7,730	746	754	172	99	141	1,775
Iowa	4,957	3,725	2,996	414	315	48	80	106	998
Kansas	5,318	4,076	3,367	367	342	84	64	44	1,050
Kentucky	8,145	6,543	5,515	602	426	108	85	68	1,341
Louisiana	9,586	7,788	6,248	952	588	108	148	84	1,458
Maine	3,069	2,279	1,856	117	306	80	45	24	641
Maryland	17,589	12,594	9,469	1,490	1,635	557	217	975	3,246
Massachusetts	21,520	15,691	11,337	2,502	1,852	503	236	926	4,164
Michigan	19,780	15,216	11,540	2,383	1,293	351	244	279	3,690
Minnesota	12,003	9,212	7,307	1,162	743	200	141	223	2,227
Mississippi	4,732	3,814	3,124	314	376	46	45	23	804
Missouri	11,427	9,043	6,922	1,270	851	168	168	229	1,819
Montana	2,017	1,520	1,344	23	153	27	6	13	451
Nebraska	3,659	2,840	2,252	366	222	61	55	44	659
Nevada	4,179	3,289	2,939	113	237	50	23	13	804
New Hampshire	3,010	2,263	1,862	152	249	44	27	48	628
New Jersey	20,742	16,305	13,188	1,598	1,519	390	204	389	3,454
New Mexico	3,742	2,779	2,176	271	332	71	42	53	797
New York	57,063	43,562	30,950	7,588	5,024	1,187	733	1,193	10,388
North Carolina	18,612	14,342	11,707	1,402	1,233	299	230	364	3,377
North Dakota	1,379	1,102	893	69	140	19	18	6	234
Ohio	24,675	18,920	14,472	2,778	1,670	380	281	341	4,753
Oklahoma	5,527	4,331	3,577	400	354	82	67	37	1,010
Oregon	8,471	6,205	5,308	364	533	150	98	119	1,899
Pennsylvania	30,364	22,703	17,078	3,420	2,205	579	348	731	6,003
Rhode Island	2,968	2,294	1,702	342	250	58	39	43	534
South Carolina	8,669	6,882	5,662	628	592	100	126	65	1,496
South Dakota	1,546	1,244	1,039	61	144	21	16	6	259
Tennessee	13,666	10,990	9,090	1,148	752	212	159	186	2,119
Texas	40,296	32,287	26,536	3,398	2,353	578	549	500	6,382
Utah	4,870	3,814	3,117	424	273	75	56	85	840
Vermont	1,856	1,313	959	182	172	39	30	46	428
Virginia	16,756	12,799	10,100	1,260	1,439	331	173	188	3,265
Washington	14,285	10,483	8,750	729	1,004	286	158	321	3,037
West Virginia	3,659	2,890	2,195	369	326	46	63	27	633
Wisconsin	11,914	9,426	7,778	924	724	195	142	141	2,010
Wyoming	915	711	622	20	69	18	6	1	179
Possessions	8,374	6,537	5,330	434	773	132	93	33	1,579
APO's and FPO's	762	663	307	28	328	30	3	6	60
Address Unknown	329								

* Includes Other, Inactive and Not Classified Physicians

Table 2.9

Female Physicians by State of Location and Major Professional Activity, 2006

State	Total Physicians	Patient Care				Other Professional Activity			
		Total Patient Care	Office Based	Hospital Based		Admin.	Med. Teach.	Research	Other*
				Resid./ Fellows	Phys. Staff				
Total Physicians	256,257	213,644	152,504	42,024	19,116	2,758	2,655	3,081	33,976
Alabama	2,431	2,104	1,496	437	171	19	15	22	271
Alaska	510	449	373	21	55	9	3	7	42
Arizona	3,796	3,177	2,494	426	257	37	46	29	507
Arkansas	1,391	1,216	846	260	110	13	25	5	132
California	31,083	25,728	19,963	3,908	1,857	325	250	387	4,393
Colorado	4,096	3,523	2,776	505	242	41	38	40	454
Connecticut	4,236	3,517	2,357	831	329	48	38	67	566
Delaware	724	616	439	109	68	8	6	7	87
District Of Columbia	1,846	1,450	783	487	180	44	28	43	281
Florida	11,601	9,595	7,492	1,262	841	108	107	78	1,713
Georgia	6,106	5,227	4,007	809	411	75	59	86	659
Hawaii	1,261	1,032	782	146	104	16	22	8	183
Idaho	547	491	409	36	46	2	4	1	49
Illinois	12,505	10,517	7,140	2,533	844	128	132	106	1,622
Indiana	3,812	3,330	2,476	566	288	26	31	41	384
Iowa	1,471	1,232	890	254	88	14	19	18	188
Kansas	1,761	1,526	1,107	270	149	11	23	6	195
Kentucky	2,683	2,282	1,684	416	182	20	31	16	334
Louisiana	3,057	2,605	1,839	588	178	22	48	13	369
Maine	1,128	971	750	112	109	14	8	4	131
Maryland	8,380	6,611	4,586	1,243	782	179	86	271	1,233
Massachusetts	11,055	8,966	5,954	2,085	927	94	92	288	1,615
Michigan	8,097	6,787	4,571	1,679	537	83	95	84	1,048
Minnesota	4,753	4,106	3,040	801	265	42	36	50	519
Mississippi	1,158	968	697	137	134	17	15	8	150
Missouri	4,159	3,547	2,379	856	312	34	44	45	489
Montana	531	471	384	14	73	2	7	1	50
Nebraska	1,193	1,034	740	223	71	9	16	7	127
Nevada	1,205	1,018	821	101	96	11	9	4	163
New Hampshire	1,069	913	699	108	106	6	6	8	136
New Jersey	9,441	7,823	5,686	1,257	880	117	102	124	1,275
New Mexico	1,682	1,383	1,034	207	142	22	24	21	232
New York	26,763	21,662	13,039	6,033	2,590	347	301	369	4,084
North Carolina	6,773	5,673	4,169	1,063	441	72	90	99	839
North Dakota	366	335	250	46	39	6	3		22
Ohio	9,416	7,924	5,394	1,832	698	72	104	83	1,233
Oklahoma	1,584	1,336	965	255	116	17	30	9	192
Oregon	3,270	2,831	2,230	372	229	32	24	27	356
Pennsylvania	11,840	9,621	6,265	2,461	895	148	145	177	1,749
Rhode Island	1,400	1,164	717	333	114	14	10	22	190
South Carolina	2,572	2,273	1,605	455	213	24	37	20	218
South Dakota	429	383	303	43	37	3	1		42
Tennessee	4,125	3,567	2,583	750	234	39	37	42	440
Texas	14,675	12,526	9,157	2,525	844	136	159	115	1,739
Utah	1,223	1,048	766	219	63	12	10	17	136
Vermont	803	667	459	131	77	8	11	10	107
Virginia	6,789	5,739	4,206	1,002	531	60	68	51	871
Washington	5,579	4,685	3,710	625	350	54	46	81	713
West Virginia	1,051	872	607	186	79	12	14	5	148
Wisconsin	4,240	3,700	2,833	605	262	26	54	41	419
Wyoming	217	192	158	13	21		2	3	20
Possessions	3,964	2,996	2,255	380	361	74	43	15	836
APO's and FPO's	267	235	139	8	88	6	1		25
Address Unknown	143								

* Includes Other, Inactive and Not Classified Physicians

Table 2.10

IMGs by State of Location and Major Professional Activity, 2006

State	Total Physicians	Patient Care		Hospital Based		Other Professional Activity			
		Total Patient Care	Office Based	Resid./ Fellows	Phys. Staff	Admin.	Med. Teach.	Research	Other*
Total Physicians	236,669	185,045	137,115	27,579	20,351	1,958	1,714	2,829	45,038
Alabama	1,754	1,471	1,063	251	157	9	9	19	246
Alaska	118	92	80	2	10	1	1	2	22
Arizona	3,215	2,552	2,083	233	236	14	29	28	592
Arkansas	1,017	881	581	214	86	3	7	9	117
California	25,408	19,884	17,048	1,097	1,739	227	179	337	4,781
Colorado	1,053	796	636	86	74	5	9	15	228
Connecticut	4,192	3,277	2,180	763	334	33	34	52	796
Delaware	753	590	474	46	70	6	1	4	152
District Of Columbia	1,075	740	397	238	105	26	17	32	260
Florida	19,536	14,786	12,541	824	1,421	162	104	138	4,346
Georgia	4,438	3,661	2,844	446	371	28	31	37	681
Hawaii	708	538	432	45	61	6	11	11	142
Idaho	105	85	63	4	18		1	1	18
Illinois	13,439	10,571	7,809	1,762	1,000	110	116	128	2,514
Indiana	3,157	2,670	2,123	254	293	16	9	15	447
Iowa	1,252	945	697	143	105	9	12	26	260
Kansas	1,314	1,065	769	142	154	10	7	17	215
Kentucky	2,272	1,849	1,455	200	194	12	16	15	380
Louisiana	2,285	1,884	1,254	422	208	16	35	24	326
Maine	592	454	331	53	70	5	3	3	127
Maryland	7,106	5,308	4,030	604	674	81	54	196	1,467
Massachusetts	7,106	5,106	3,550	887	669	60	35	204	1,701
Michigan	9,459	7,640	5,294	1,664	682	71	66	90	1,592
Minnesota	2,482	1,897	1,305	412	180	6	13	49	517
Mississippi	780	666	470	76	120	3	2	9	100
Missouri	3,431	2,741	1,877	538	326	18	37	48	587
Montana	116	93	77	1	15	1		1	21
Nebraska	678	555	347	152	56	5	5	7	106
Nevada	1,580	1,258	1,055	92	111	8	6	5	303
New Hampshire	577	441	342	40	59	1		7	128
New Jersey	13,617	11,099	8,223	1,548	1,328	136	86	153	2,143
New Mexico	936	743	552	106	85	5	4	8	176
New York	35,180	27,197	16,893	6,571	3,733	355	285	471	6,872
North Carolina	3,221	2,501	1,949	253	299	30	35	48	607
North Dakota	459	391	259	69	63	2	1		65
Ohio	9,911	7,534	5,240	1,478	816	63	59	88	2,167
Oklahoma	1,351	1,138	791	205	142	4	8	5	196
Oregon	1,034	731	596	67	68	10	8	14	271
Pennsylvania	10,920	8,582	5,577	2,042	963	86	83	157	2,012
Rhode Island	1,177	893	644	132	117	5	6	8	265
South Carolina	1,427	1,171	886	132	153	11	11	18	216
South Dakota	270	231	157	41	33			2	37
Tennessee	2,930	2,433	1,765	448	220	12	21	43	421
Texas	13,250	10,735	8,552	1,285	898	71	118	143	2,183
Utah	510	409	308	63	38	6	5	13	77
Vermont	244	146	92	40	14	3	3	5	87
Virginia	4,981	3,783	2,894	414	475	52	33	29	1,084
Washington	2,448	1,808	1,476	151	181	22	19	39	560
West Virginia	1,711	1,401	966	233	202	8	10	5	287
Wisconsin	2,948	2,427	1,875	363	189	13	28	28	452
Wyoming	109	93	66	22	5	1		1	14
Possessions	6,833	5,000	4,103	225	672	107	41	22	1,663
APO's and FPO's	119	103	44		59	4	1		11
Address Unknown	85								

* Includes Other, Inactive and Not Classified Physicians

Table 2.11

Male IMGs by State of Location and Major Professional Activity, 2006

State	Total Physicians	Patient Care				Other Professional Activity			
		Total Patient Care	Office Based	Hospital Based		Admin.	Med. Teach.	Research	Other*
				Resid./ Fellows	Phys. Staff				
Total Physicians	165,377	128,486	98,385	16,021	14,080	1,468	1,241	2,201	31,918
Alabama	1,319	1,106	825	166	115	9	9	17	178
Alaska	75	58	51	1	6	1	1	1	14
Arizona	2,357	1,869	1,552	138	179	9	20	22	437
Arkansas	735	634	447	125	62	3	7	9	82
California	17,202	13,425	11,734	541	1,150	167	129	255	3,226
Colorado	699	511	410	46	55	5	6	12	165
Connecticut	2,845	2,185	1,522	426	237	24	30	43	563
Delaware	529	409	333	23	53	3	1	3	113
District Of Columbia	678	461	271	121	69	19	11	24	163
Florida	14,995	11,221	9,687	464	1,070	128	82	110	3,454
Georgia	3,184	2,621	2,102	252	267	16	25	27	495
Hawaii	491	381	312	24	45	5	7	10	88
Idaho	80	63	46	2	15		1	1	15
Illinois	8,977	6,952	5,339	962	651	80	81	100	1,764
Indiana	2,293	1,916	1,576	140	200	15	8	12	342
Iowa	953	716	550	87	79	6	9	20	202
Kansas	958	776	598	74	104	8	5	14	155
Kentucky	1,677	1,386	1,124	130	132	8	13	12	258
Louisiana	1,676	1,397	964	277	156	14	23	21	221
Maine	435	323	248	28	47	5	3	3	101
Maryland	4,878	3,613	2,811	348	454	56	39	150	1,020
Massachusetts	4,639	3,259	2,294	506	459	47	24	161	1,148
Michigan	6,430	5,153	3,713	962	478	48	50	70	1,109
Minnesota	1,716	1,281	888	259	134	5	9	36	385
Mississippi	573	493	358	49	86	2	2	7	69
Missouri	2,451	1,943	1,370	331	242	14	27	40	427
Montana	92	69	55		14	1		1	21
Nebraska	494	407	256	108	43	4	4	7	72
Nevada	1,129	905	779	54	72	6	3	4	211
New Hampshire	416	318	248	25	45	1		5	92
New Jersey	8,845	7,172	5,506	852	814	94	59	112	1,408
New Mexico	693	548	412	69	67	4	2	7	132
New York	23,732	18,166	11,916	3,790	2,460	279	193	359	4,735
North Carolina	2,324	1,802	1,444	144	214	24	24	36	438
North Dakota	350	295	206	41	48	1	1		53
Ohio	7,174	5,421	3,903	932	586	47	44	61	1,601
Oklahoma	992	836	602	126	108	3	5	5	143
Oregon	720	489	404	38	47	7	8	12	204
Pennsylvania	7,674	6,003	4,117	1,224	662	66	56	127	1,422
Rhode Island	856	647	478	84	85	5	4	5	195
South Carolina	1,028	832	654	78	100	8	7	13	168
South Dakota	203	172	121	24	27			2	29
Tennessee	2,142	1,770	1,321	291	158	11	19	37	305
Texas	9,486	7,704	6,327	729	648	54	83	113	1,532
Utah	379	297	228	41	28	4	5	11	62
Vermont	182	106	66	29	11	3	2	5	66
Virginia	3,460	2,575	1,994	247	334	42	25	22	796
Washington	1,653	1,200	996	75	129	16	14	32	391
West Virginia	1,350	1,109	785	162	162	5	9	5	222
Wisconsin	2,083	1,705	1,329	231	145	13	22	21	322
Wyoming	80	69	50	15	4	1		1	9
Possessions	4,844	3,642	3,032	130	480	68	29	18	1,087
APO's and FPO's	88	75	31		44	4	1		8
Address Unknown	63								

* Includes Other, Inactive and Not Classified Physicians

Table 2.12

Female IMGs by State of Location and Major Professional Activity, 2006

State	Total Physicians	Patient Care		Hospital Based		Other Professional Activity			
		Total Patient Care	Office Based	Resid./ Fellows	Phys. Staff	Admin.	Med. Teach.	Research	Other*
Total Physicians	71,292	56,559	38,730	11,558	6,271	490	473	628	13,120
Alabama	435	365	238	85	42			2	68
Alaska	43	34	29	1	4			1	8
Arizona	858	683	531	95	57	5	9	6	155
Arkansas	282	247	134	89	24				35
California	8,206	6,459	5,314	556	589	60	50	82	1,555
Colorado	354	285	226	40	19		3	3	63
Connecticut	1,347	1,092	658	337	97	9	4	9	233
Delaware	224	181	141	23	17	3		1	39
District Of Columbia	397	279	126	117	36	7	6	8	97
Florida	4,541	3,565	2,854	360	351	34	22	28	892
Georgia	1,254	1,040	742	194	104	12	6	10	186
Hawaii	217	157	120	21	16	1	4	1	54
Idaho	25	22	17	2	3				3
Illinois	4,462	3,619	2,470	800	349	30	35	28	750
Indiana	864	754	547	114	93	1	1	3	105
Iowa	299	229	147	56	26	3	3	6	58
Kansas	356	289	171	68	50	2	2	3	60
Kentucky	595	463	331	70	62	4	3	3	122
Louisiana	609	487	290	145	52	2	12	3	105
Maine	157	131	83	25	23				26
Maryland	2,228	1,695	1,219	256	220	25	15	46	447
Massachusetts	2,467	1,847	1,256	381	210	13	11	43	553
Michigan	3,029	2,487	1,581	702	204	23	16	20	483
Minnesota	766	616	417	153	46	1	4	13	132
Mississippi	207	173	112	27	34	1		2	31
Missouri	980	798	507	207	84	4	10	8	160
Montana	24	24	22	1	1				
Nebraska	184	148	91	44	13	1	1		34
Nevada	451	353	276	38	39	2	3	1	92
New Hampshire	161	123	94	15	14			2	36
New Jersey	4,772	3,927	2,717	696	514	42	27	41	735
New Mexico	243	195	140	37	18	1	2	1	44
New York	11,448	9,031	4,977	2,781	1,273	76	92	112	2,137
North Carolina	897	699	505	109	85	6	11	12	169
North Dakota	109	96	53	28	15	1			12
Ohio	2,737	2,113	1,337	546	230	16	15	27	566
Oklahoma	359	302	189	79	34	1	3		53
Oregon	314	242	192	29	21	3		2	67
Pennsylvania	3,246	2,579	1,460	818	301	20	27	30	590
Rhode Island	321	246	166	48	32		2	3	70
South Carolina	399	339	232	54	53	3	4	5	48
South Dakota	67	59	36	17	6				8
Tennessee	788	663	444	157	62	1	2	6	116
Texas	3,764	3,031	2,225	556	250	17	35	30	651
Utah	131	112	80	22	10	2		2	15
Vermont	62	40	26	11	3		1		21
Virginia	1,521	1,208	900	167	141	10	8	7	288
Washington	795	608	480	76	52	6	5	7	169
West Virginia	361	292	181	71	40	3	1		65
Wisconsin	865	722	546	132	44		6	7	130
Wyoming	29	24	16	7	1				5
Possessions	1,989	1,358	1,071	95	192	39	12	4	576
APO's and FPO's	31	28	13		15				3
Address Unknown	22								

Includes Other, Inactive and Not Classified Physicians

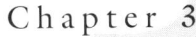

Chapter 3

Analysis of Professional Activity by Self-Designated Specialty and Geographic Region

This chapter includes detailed tables of physicians by specialty and major professional activity for census regions and divisions, metropolitan areas, states, and counties. These data are useful for determining health program options and strategies to complement policy-related research. It is recognized, however, that important influences not reflected in these data have an impact on the distribution patterns of physicians. These determinants of physician location include community of origin, medical education experience, hospital facilities, population size (as well as composition and change), urbanization, licensure requirements, and cultural, social, and environmental conditions.

Total US Physicians

Table 3.1

The geographic distribution for the 921,904 physicians in the US and Possessions is presented in Tables 3.1 through 3.14. Although no interpretation is presented or intended for the complex issue of physician diffusion, the data are useful to study the composition of the physician supply by specialty and major professional activity at the national, state, county, and metropolitan levels. In Table 3.1, total physician count includes the categories of Not Classified (46,252), Inactive (108,344), and Address Unknown (472).

In 2006, four fifths (78.4%) of the 921,904 physicians were in Patient Care (Table 3.1). Of the 723,118 physicians in Patient Care, 77.5% were in Office-Based practice, 13.4% were in residency/fellowship training, and 9.1% comprised full-time

Hospital Staff. Patient Care physicians in the primary care specialties of Family Medicine, General Practice, Internal Medicine, Pediatrics, and Obstetrics/Gynecology accounted for 344,944 physicians or nearly one half (47.7%) of all physicians in active Patient Care. The five highest specialties ranked by size for total physicians included Internal Medicine, Family Medicine, Pediatrics, Obstetrics/Gynecology, and Psychiatry. Table 5 illustrates the percentage distribution of physicians in these specialties by Patient Care, Office-Based practice, residency/fellowship training, full-time Hospital Staff, and other activities as of 2006.

International Medical Graduates (IMGs)

Tables 3.2 through 3.4

Nearly all (96.1%) IMGs who were not categorized as Inactive, Not Classified, or Address Unknown in 2006 were in Patient Care (Table 3.2). Internal Medicine comprised three fifths (61.3%) of all IMGs in the medical specialties, whereas 31.8% of all physicians in surgical specialties were in General Surgery.

Of the 192,491 IMGs who were not categorized as Inactive, Not Classified, or Address Unknown, 60.7% were located in the South and Northeast census regions (Table 3.3). These regions consisted of nearly two thirds of all IMGs in Administration (62.2%) and in Research (64.8%). More than half (60.4%) of all IMGs in Medical Teaching were concentrated in the Middle Atlantic (454), South Atlantic (296), and East North Central (278) cen-

Mini-Table 5

Percent Distribution of Five Highest Ranking Self-Designated Specialties by Selected Major Professional Activity, 2006

Specialty	Total	Patient Care*	Office-Based	Residents/ Fellows	Hosp. Staff	Other Prof. Activity**
Internal Medicine	100.0	93.2	68.9	16.1	8.2	6.8
Family Medicine	100.0	96.3	79.7	10.0	6.6	3.7
Pediatrics	100.0	94.2	70.8	14.9	8.6	5.8
Obstetrics/Gynecology	100.0	96.9	80.8	9.9	6.2	3.1
Psychiatry	100.0	92.4	66.2	10.8	15.4	7.6

Source: Table 3.1
* Includes Office-Based practice, Residents/Fellows, and Hospital Staff.
** Includes Medical Teaching, Administration, Research, and Other.

sus divisions (Table 3.4). IMGs in Administration also represented the highest frequencies in these census divisions, or 64.0% of all IMGs in Administration.

US Physicians by Geographic Region

Tables 3.5 through 3.11

Patient Care accounted for 78.4% of all physicians in 2006 (Table 3.1). Of the total number of physicians in Patient Care (723,118), more than three fourths (77.5%) were in Office-Based practice. Of a total of 97,102 Residents/Fellows, more than half (58.3%) were specialists in the disciplines of Internal Medicine, Pediatrics, Family Medicine, General Surgery, and Anesthesiology. Percentages of total physicians in residency/fellowship training in these specialties are as follows: Internal Medicine, 25.8%; Pediatrics, 11.2%; Family Medicine, 8.5%; General Surgery, 8.0%; and Anesthesiology, 4.8%.

Regarding physicians in census regions, the South (32.7%) and the Northeast (23.7%) accounted for the largest percentages (Table 3.5). The North Central region had proportionately more physicians in Patient Care (79.8%) than any other region, whereas the Northeast had the greatest proportion of physicians in residency/fellowship training (13.8%).

Table 3.6 presents physician data by census division (see Appendix D). The South Atlantic census division had the highest number of physicians in 2006

with 174,658. The Middle Atlantic census division ranked second with 156,213, followed by the Pacific census division with 148,307 and the East North Central division with 132,591 physicians.

Population and physician/population ratios for the divisions are provided in Table 6. These ratios are presented as general guidelines to compare the distribution of physicians among the divisions and not as definitive measures of physician supply. It is recognized that the quality and quantity of health care are predicated on a variety of factors such as medical need for services, demographic composition, geographical location, and socioeconomic variables, among others.

As Table 6 indicates, the New England and Middle Atlantic divisions had the largest numbers of physicians per 100,000 civilian population, with 437 and 386, respectively. The fewest numbers of physicians per 100,000 civilian population were located in the Mountain (253) and West South Central (237) divisions. The ratios for the divisions are illustrated in Figure 4.

Table 3.7 represents the distribution of physicians by state, specialty, and major professional activity. One third of all physicians (32.8%) were concentrated in California (12.0%), New York (9.1%), Texas (6.0%), and Florida (5.8%).

In Table 3.9, the specialty and activity distributions of physicians are displayed by census division and county group. County group classifies a physician's county of location by its population size (see Appendix E). Table 3.10 reports the specialty and activity distributions of physicians by census division,

Mini-Table 6

Physicians, Population, and Physician/Population Ratios by Census Division, 2006

Census Division	Physicians	Population (in millions)**	Physician Pop./Ratio
Total*	921,904	299,398	308
New England	62,366	14,270	437
Middle Atlantic	156,213	40,471	386
East North Central	132,591	46,276	287
West North Central	54,421	19,942	273
South Atlantic	174,658	57,144	306
East South Central	45,503	17,754	256
West South Central	81,189	34,186	237
Mountain	52,817	20,846	253
Pacific	148,307	48,510	306

Includes the 50 states and DC but excludes Possessions.

** Population estimates as of July 1, 2006.*

Source: Tables 3.6 and 3.8, US Census Bureau, Population Division, Table 1: Annual Estimates of the Population for the United States, Regions, and States and for Puerto Rico: April 1, 2000 to July 1, 2006

Figure 4

Physicians per 100,000 Civilian Population by Census Division, 2006*

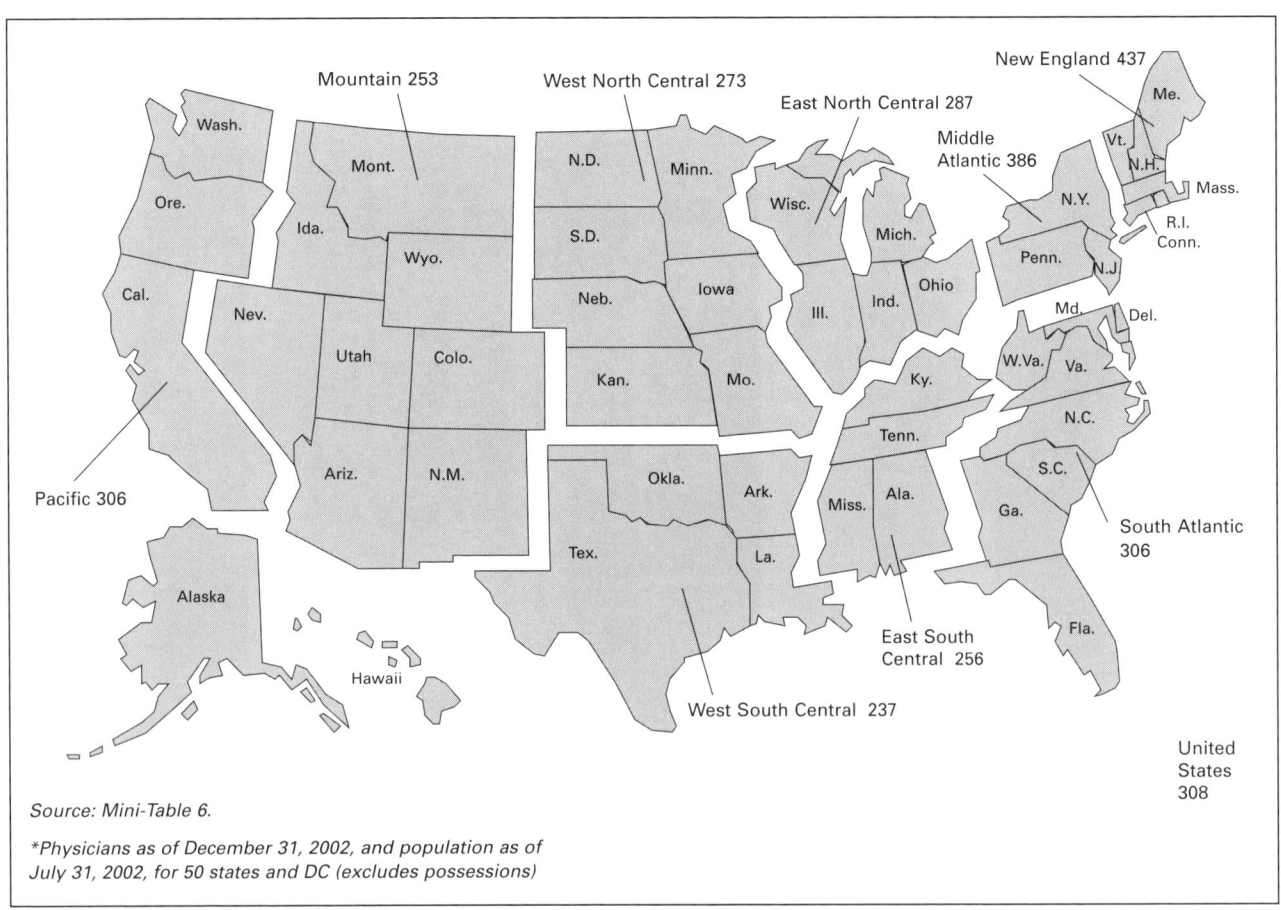

Source: Mini-Table 6.

Physicians as of December 31, 2002, and population as of July 31, 2002, for 50 states and DC (excludes possessions)

state, and county group. Table 3.11 reports the specialty and activity distributions of physicians by state and county. The top 10 counties with the largest numbers of physicians are Los Angeles, CA (31,094), Cook, IL (21,969), New York, NY (20,593), Harris, TX (11,973), San Diego, CA (10,747), Orange, CA (10,088), Miami-Dade, FL (9,495), Maricopa, AZ (9,460), King, WA (9,378), and Suffolk, MA (9,211). Taken together, these 10 counties make up 15.6% of the physicians in the US.

Metropolitan Data

Tables 3.12 through 3.14

Table 3.12 illustrates that of the total number of physicians in metropolitan areas, 78.9% were in Patient Care. Office-Based practice accounted for more than three fourths (76.5%) of these Patient Care physicians in 2006. The specialties showing the largest numbers of physicians in Office-Based practice were Internal Medicine, General/Family Medicine, Pediatrics, Obstetrics/Gynecology, and Anesthesiology. These disciplines represented more than half (52.7%) of all Office-Based physicians in metropolitan areas.

Physicians in metropolitan areas comprised 80.0% of all physicians in Hospital-Based practice. This significant distribution reflects the clustering of interns, residents, fellows, and full-time staff in large metropolitan and university-affiliated teaching hospitals.

In 2006, the 280 metropolitan statistical areas (MSAs) listed in Table 3.14 contained 76.9% of the total physician population of 921,904. In those metropolitan areas, Office-Based medical specialties represented 75.3% of metropolitan medical specialties physicians in Patient Care, whereas the Surgical Specialties were 80.2%, Other Specialties were 73.3%, and Family/General Practice were 81.7% (Table 3.12).

Table 3.1

Total Physicians in the United States and Possessions by Self-Designated Specialty and Activity, 2006

Specialty	Total Physicians	Patient Care				Other Professional Activity			
		Total Patient Care	Office Based	Hospital Based		Admin.	Med. Teach.	Research	Other
				Resid./ Fellows	Phys. Staff				
Total Physicians	921,904	723,118	560,411	97,102	65,605	14,575	10,273	14,475	4,395
GP/FM Prac	93,359	89,874	74,900	8,266	6,708	1,493	1,468	242	282
FM	82,866	79,775	66,028	8,266	5,481	1,279	1,436	200	176
GP	10,493	10,099	8,872		1,227	214	32	42	106
Med. Spec.	290,656	272,062	207,310	41,798	22,954	5,022	4,215	8,268	1,089
AI	4,196	3,735	3,310	248	177	62	41	337	21
CD	22,426	21,082	17,480	2,090	1,512	257	319	689	79
D	10,744	10,488	8,920	1,100	468	49	78	112	17
GE	12,268	11,634	9,881	1,058	695	115	164	332	23
IM	155,705	145,047	107,284	25,059	12,704	3,049	2,186	4,815	608
PD	73,208	68,987	51,815	10,892	6,280	1,268	1,178	1,468	307
PDC	1,877	1,739	1,243	260	236	26	30	78	4
PUD	10,232	9,350	7,377	1,091	882	196	219	437	30
Sur. Spec.	161,370	157,067	127,118	20,110	9,839	1,363	1,527	934	479
CRS	1,340	1,308	1,164	67	77	8	14	6	4
GS	37,556	36,344	25,592	7,752	3,000	457	378	243	134
NS	5,425	5,274	4,103	801	370	35	49	41	26
OBG	42,333	41,036	34,225	4,205	2,606	420	547	254	76
OPH	18,058	17,664	15,765	1,125	774	98	123	140	33
ORS	24,296	23,818	19,220	3,327	1,271	112	149	81	136
OTO	9,974	9,778	8,199	1,082	497	66	89	28	13
PS	7,063	6,947	6,016	651	280	25	48	21	22
TS	4,807	4,624	3,984	250	390	57	49	65	12
U	10,518	10,274	8,850	850	574	85	81	55	23
Oth. Spec.	221,451	204,115	151,083	26,928	26,104	6,697	3,063	5,031	2,545
AM	473	294	170	5	119	136	7	23	13
AN	41,193	40,073	31,746	4,661	3,666	292	504	244	80
CHP	7,260	6,755	5,345	583	827	204	138	125	38
DR	24,624	23,886	17,577	3,970	2,339	144	240	117	237
EM	29,987	28,863	20,055	4,029	4,779	675	293	82	74
FOP	657	468	409	26	33	37	10	9	133
GPM	2,161	1,682	1,219	226	237	225	42	151	61
MG	533	385	233	77	75	24	24	95	5
N	14,554	13,245	10,423	1,622	1,200	189	257	784	79
NM	1,477	1,323	953	121	249	44	28	60	22
OM	2,641	1,891	1,550	32	309	520	39	82	109
P	41,385	38,225	27,387	4,462	6,376	1,426	579	850	305
PHP	1,434	297	218	1	78	679	68	299	91
PM	7,736	7,446	5,634	894	918	161	45	48	36
PTH	19,171	16,463	11,465	2,517	2,481	714	397	799	798
R	8,886	8,406	6,954	415	1,037	86	166	95	133
RO	4,424	4,314	3,419	506	389	39	27	39	5
TTS	151	137	114		23	2	3	8	1
OTH	5,168	2,702	2,235	39	428	1,034	160	1,005	267
UNSP	7,512	7,237	3,955	2,742	540	66	36	115	58
VM	24	23	22		1			1	
Inactive	108,344								
Not Class	46,252								
Address Unknown	472								

Subspecialties in this table are condensed into major specialties. See Appendix A.

Table 3.2

International Medical Graduates in the United States and Possessions by Self-Designated Specialty and Activity, 2006

Specialty	Total Physicians	Patient Care				Other Professional Activity			
		Total Patient Care	Office Based	Hospital Based		Admin.	Med. Teach.	Research	Other
				Resid./ Fellows	Phys. Staff				
Total Physicians	192,491	185,045	137,115	27,579	20,351	1,958	1,714	2,829	945
GP/FM Prac	22,250	21,839	16,333	3,770	1,736	192	114	31	74
FM	17,268	17,000	12,277	3,770	953	118	103	18	29
GP	4,982	4,839	4,056		783	74	11	13	45
Med. Spec.	92,987	89,997	66,113	15,871	8,013	627	719	1,460	184
AI	1,033	944	861	39	44	9	14	63	3
CD	6,822	6,563	5,384	683	496	27	60	158	14
D	645	615	535	36	44	3	10	16	1
GE	3,298	3,158	2,648	290	220	21	40	75	4
IM	57,029	55,446	39,073	11,533	4,840	345	355	778	105
PD	20,318	19,584	14,826	2,723	2,035	199	204	276	55
PDC	466	443	320	60	63	5	7	11	
PUD	3,376	3,244	2,466	507	271	18	29	83	2
Sur. Spec.	23,336	22,681	17,821	2,846	2,014	160	196	228	71
CRS	263	259	233	9	17		2	2	
GS	7,419	7,216	4,950	1,464	802	57	50	63	33
NS	752	731	573	86	72	2	7	11	1
OBG	7,446	7,252	5,741	925	586	59	70	54	11
OPH	1,423	1,376	1,205	91	80	5	13	27	2
ORS	1,610	1,565	1,339	99	127	11	13	13	8
OTO	932	900	808	35	57	7	8	15	2
PS	851	832	738	45	49	2	2	9	6
TS	1,052	1,011	867	55	89	4	10	25	2
U	1,588	1,539	1,367	37	135	13	21	9	6
Oth. Spec.	53,918	50,528	36,848	5,092	8,588	979	685	1,110	616
AM	37	26	16		10	5	1	4	1
AN	11,712	11,391	9,182	799	1,410	62	152	82	25
CHP	2,139	2,039	1,506	205	328	31	24	32	13
DR	2,858	2,727	2,028	257	442	15	43	29	44
EM	2,664	2,589	1,674	247	668	44	22	4	5
FOP	152	100	84	9	7	9	3	4	36
GPM	309	262	203	35	24	20	7	14	6
MG	131	110	61	33	16	3	1	17	
N	4,644	4,421	3,398	613	410	17	56	130	20
NM	536	499	336	56	107	7	8	14	8
OM	384	322	258	12	52	42	5	5	10
P	12,999	12,368	7,997	1,484	2,887	304	103	167	57
PHP	168	54	40		14	75	9	20	10
PM	2,374	2,292	1,714	191	387	38	20	8	16
PTH	6,361	5,566	3,703	856	1,007	166	134	244	251
R	1,670	1,538	1,145	88	305	17	33	41	41
RO	791	764	624	15	125	5	8	13	1
TTS	38	36	27		9			2	
OTH	977	584	441	20	123	88	37	228	40
UNSP	2,969	2,835	2,406	172	257	31	19	52	32
VM	5	5	5						

Note: Above excludes Inactive, Not Classified and Address Unknown Physicians.

Subspecialties in this table are condensed into major specialties. See Appendix A.

Table 3.3

International Medical Graduates by Census Region, Self-Designated Specialty, and Activity, 2006
Northeast

Specialty	Total Physicians	Total Patient Care	Office Based	Resid./ Fellows	Phys. Staff	Admin.	Med. Teach.	Research	Other
			Patient Care	Hospital Based		Other Professional Activity			
Total Physicians	59,773	57,195	37,832	12,076	7,287	684	535	1,060	299
GP/FM Prac.	4,003	3,923	2,699	900	324	38	20	7	15
FM	3,342	3,287	2,193	900	194	27	20	3	5
GP	661	636	506		130	11		4	10
Med. Spec.	30,057	28,997	18,567	7,588	2,842	236	228	525	71
AI	293	257	224	17	16	5	5	25	1
CD	1,818	1,736	1,323	259	154	14	15	49	4
D	191	179	158	7	14	1	2	9	
GE	893	844	646	124	74	7	11	28	3
IM	19,151	18,583	11,210	5,716	1,657	133	108	282	45
PD	6,607	6,352	4,288	1,252	812	67	71	99	18
PDC	124	120	81	13	26	1	1	2	
PUD	980	926	637	200	89	8	15	31	
Sur. Spec.	7,819	7,571	5,415	1,423	733	51	72	104	21
CRS	71	69	63	1	5			2	
GS	2,673	2,590	1,510	783	297	25	17	34	7
NS	199	187	137	27	23		3	9	
OBG	2,604	2,542	1,835	478	229	13	24	19	6
OPH	443	426	366	36	24	2	4	10	1
ORS	475	460	385	42	33	2	6	6	1
OTO	317	299	265	8	26	3	6	8	1
PS	256	251	216	15	20			3	2
TS	298	281	228	21	32	2	4	10	1
U	483	466	410	12	44	4	8	3	2
Oth. Spec.	17,894	16,704	11,151	2,165	3,388	359	215	424	192
AM	4	4	3		1				
AN	3,912	3,798	2,992	337	469	29	45	30	10
CHP	777	734	501	87	146	16	6	13	8
DR	920	881	619	111	151	6	8	11	14
EM	866	838	438	103	297	16	7	2	3
FOP	44	25	21		4	3		3	13
GPM	75	67	48	10	9	2	2	2	2
MG	36	28	14	9	5			8	
N	1,419	1,340	930	234	176	7	18	46	8
NM	182	167	105	28	34	4	3	5	3
OM	81	61	48	3	10	15	2	2	1
P	4,782	4,524	2,609	705	1,210	125	44	73	16
PHP	43	12	10		2	21	3	4	3
PM	962	920	660	93	167	20	11	2	9
PTH	2,215	1,958	1,155	365	438	56	42	87	72
R	533	497	346	30	121	4	6	14	12
RO	249	236	178	6	52	1	4	7	1
TTS	11	11	7		4				
OTH	296	155	102	9	44	26	11	93	11
UNSP	486	447	364	35	48	8	3	22	6
VM	1	1	1						

Note: Above excludes Inactive, Not Classified and Address Unknown Physicians.

Subspecialties in this table are condensed into major specialties. See Appendix A.

Table 3.3

International Medical Graduates by Census Region, Self-Designated Specialty, and Activity, 2006, continued
North Central

Specialty	Total Physicians	Patient Care		Hospital Based		Other Professional Activity			
		Total Patient Care	Office Based	Resid./ Fellows	Phys. Staff	Admin.	Med. Teach.	Research	Other
Total Physicians	40,036	38,667	27,752	7,018	3,897	323	353	498	195
GP/FM Prac.	4,984	4,910	3,396	1,148	366	30	24	7	13
FM	4,246	4,198	2,802	1,148	248	18	23	2	5
GP	738	712	594		118	12	1	5	8
Med. Spec.	19,338	18,815	13,301	3,985	1,529	90	145	263	25
AI	235	226	205	13	8	3	1	5	
CD	1,578	1,529	1,233	189	107	2	10	35	2
D	131	128	106	14	8		2	1	
GE	664	639	539	72	28	1	8	16	
IM	12,256	11,957	8,115	2,872	970	56	80	150	13
PD	3,668	3,555	2,551	658	346	21	39	44	9
PDC	108	104	59	25	20	3	1		
PUD	698	677	493	142	42	4	4	12	1
Sur. Spec.	4,594	4,487	3,489	626	372	25	30	41	11
CRS	67	67	63	2	2				
GS	1,477	1,446	1,008	289	149	3	12	11	5
NS	193	187	148	23	16	2	2	1	1
OBG	1,396	1,364	1,036	219	109	11	8	11	2
OPH	264	257	220	18	19	2	1	4	
ORS	282	275	235	16	24	2	1	2	2
OTO	178	175	150	17	8			3	
PS	158	153	134	14	5	1	1	3	
TS	249	240	201	18	21	1	2	6	
U	330	323	294	10	19	3	3		1
Oth. Spec.	11,120	10,455	7,566	1,259	1,630	178	154	187	146
AM	6	5	3		2	1			
AN	2,481	2,422	1,887	235	300	9	34	10	6
CHP	395	377	277	43	57	5	5	5	3
DR	654	628	474	73	81	1	9	3	13
EM	490	473	296	61	116	9	8		
FOP	31	21	18	2	1	1	2	1	6
GPM	48	44	37	4	3	1	1	2	
MG	18	15	9	4	2		1	2	
N	1,070	1,019	770	161	88	5	15	26	5
NM	122	109	74	12	23	1	4	5	3
OM	93	78	63	2	13	8	1	2	4
P	2,446	2,344	1,559	300	485	62	11	21	8
PHP	11	2	2			6		1	2
PM	455	444	314	50	80	4	3	1	3
PTH	1,476	1,281	861	205	215	35	40	53	67
R	407	378	297	14	67	6	7	5	11
RO	213	208	175	5	28	3	1	1	
TTS	7	6	5		1			1	
OTH	195	118	85	9	24	16	8	42	11
UNSP	500	481	358	79	44	5	4	6	4
VM	2	2	2						

Note: Above excludes Inactive, Not Classified and Address Unknown Physicians.

Subspecialties in this table are condensed into major specialties. See Appendix A.

Table 3.3

International Medical Graduates by Census Region, Self-Designated Specialty, and Activity, 2006, continued
South

Specialty	Total Physicians	Patient Care		Hospital Based		Other Professional Activity			
		Total Patient Care	Office Based	Resid./ Fellows	Phys. Staff	Admin.	Med. Teach.	Research	Other
Total Physicians	57,080	54,998	42,912	6,291	5,795	534	512	774	262
GP/FM Prac.	7,272	7,150	5,349	1,228	573	59	34	9	20
FM	5,829	5,745	4,182	1,228	335	41	29	6	8
GP	1,443	1,405	1,167		238	18	5	3	12
Med. Spec.	28,006	27,156	21,555	3,182	2,419	178	218	410	44
AI	317	289	273	6	10	1	7	20	
CD	2,376	2,298	1,950	187	161	9	20	42	7
D	180	173	150	14	9	1	3	2	1
GE	1,139	1,104	956	71	77	5	14	16	
IM	16,512	16,067	12,400	2,168	1,499	102	105	216	22
PD	6,183	5,966	4,809	604	553	54	62	88	13
PDC	153	146	120	14	12	1	2	4	
PUD	1,146	1,113	897	118	98	5	5	22	1
Sur. Spec.	6,624	6,448	5,303	596	549	42	59	49	26
CRS	88	86	76	4	6		2		
GS	2,096	2,038	1,534	269	235	18	13	11	16
NS	231	228	184	24	20		2	1	
OBG	1,892	1,844	1,523	186	135	14	25	8	1
OPH	446	428	380	31	17	1	6	11	
ORS	513	499	420	34	45	5	4	3	2
OTO	255	251	231	8	12		1	3	
PS	270	264	237	13	14		1	2	3
TS	314	303	270	13	20	1	3	6	1
U	519	507	448	14	45	3	2	4	3
Oth. Spec.	15,178	14,244	10,705	1,285	2,254	255	201	306	172
AM	14	8	5		3	3		3	
AN	3,211	3,127	2,569	174	384	15	42	24	3
CHP	624	601	457	61	83	6	9	7	1
DR	809	770	579	61	130	3	14	9	13
EM	833	818	597	59	162	7	5	1	2
FOP	54	38	31	6	1	4			12
GPM	115	92	66	18	8	12	3	6	2
MG	44	39	20	14	5	3		2	
N	1,488	1,433	1,149	189	95	3	15	32	5
NM	132	127	88	7	32	1	1	2	1
OM	94	80	64	4	12	9	1		4
P	3,593	3,431	2,296	372	763	63	31	47	21
PHP	68	21	17		4	31	3	11	2
PM	573	558	438	34	86	7	1	5	2
PTH	1,784	1,557	1,093	215	249	45	34	76	72
R	485	433	315	33	85	3	19	16	14
RO	220	216	184	3	29	1	2	1	
TTS	16	15	11		4			1	
OTH	278	177	137	1	39	27	13	50	11
UNSP	742	702	588	34	80	12	8	13	7
VM	1	1	1						

Note: Above excludes Inactive, Not Classified and Address Unknown Physicians.

Subspecialties in this table are condensed into major specialties. See Appendix A.

Table 3.3

International Medical Graduates by Census Region, Self-Designated Specialty, and Activity, 2006, continued
West

Specialty	Total Physicians	Patient Care				Other Professional Activity			
		Total Patient Care	Office Based	Resid./ Fellows	Phys. Staff	Admin.	Med. Teach.	Research	Other
Total Physicians	30,293	29,082	24,472	1,969	2,641	306	272	475	158
GP/FM Prac.	4,338	4,251	3,546	468	237	34	29	6	18
FM	3,388	3,323	2,717	468	138	22	28	6	9
GP	950	928	829		99	12	1		9
Med. Spec.	14,062	13,562	11,560	972	1,030	96	111	253	40
AI	183	167	154	3	10		1	13	2
CD	973	928	814	43	71	2	12	30	1
D	131	123	113	1	9	1	3	4	
GE	589	559	497	23	39	8	7	14	1
IM	8,304	8,056	6,782	659	615	46	54	125	23
PD	3,288	3,166	2,733	188	245	38	26	45	13
PDC	74	66	55	8	3		3	5	
PUD	520	497	412	47	38	1	5	17	
Sur. Spec.	3,724	3,622	3,166	189	267	32	26	34	10
CRS	32	32	28	2	2				
GS	1,011	985	780	120	85	10	5	7	4
NS	118	118	95	11	12				
OBG	1,294	1,253	1,140	35	78	13	11	16	1
OPH	244	239	216	6	17		2	2	1
ORS	313	308	280	6	22	1		2	2
OTO	145	139	131	2	6	4		1	1
PS	160	157	145	3	9	1		1	1
TS	185	181	164	3	14		1	3	
U	222	210	187	1	22	3	7	2	
Oth. Spec.	8,169	7,647	6,200	340	1,107	144	106	182	90
AM	13	9	5		4	1	1	1	1
AN	2,013	1,952	1,664	51	237	7	31	17	6
CHP	318	305	254	14	37	4	2	7	
DR	452	426	339	12	75	5	12	6	3
EM	386	381	294	20	67	3	1	1	
FOP	20	13	11	1	1	1	1		5
GPM	57	47	42	3	2	4	1	4	1
MG	32	28	18	6	4			4	
N	628	592	522	27	43	2	7	26	1
NM	97	93	67	9	17	1		2	1
OM	84	77	63	3	11	5	1	1	
P	1,946	1,849	1,367	100	382	48	17	22	10
PHP	30	12	7		5	10	2	4	2
PM	347	335	276	10	49	6	4		2
PTH	836	728	567	68	93	28	16	28	36
R	229	214	174	11	29	4	1	6	4
RO	103	99	84	1	14		1	3	
TTS	4	4	4						
OTH	163	99	87		12	12	4	41	7
UNSP	410	383	354	4	25	3	4	9	11
VM	1	1	1						

Note: Above excludes Inactive, Not Classified and Address Unknown Physicians.

Subspecialties in this table are condensed into major specialties. See Appendix A.

Table 3.3

International Medical Graduates by Census Region, Self-Designated Specialty, and Activity, 2006, continued
Possessions

Specialty	Total Physicians	Patient Care				Other Professional Activity			
		Total Patient Care	Office Based	Hospital Based		Admin.	Med. Teach.	Research	Other
				Resid./ Fellows	Phys. Staff				
Total Physicians	5,309	5,103	4,147	225	731	111	42	22	31
GP/FM Prac.	1,653	1,605	1,343	26	236	31	7	2	8
FM	463	447	383	26	38	10	3	1	2
GP	1,190	1,158	960		198	21	4	1	6
Med. Spec.	1,524	1,467	1,130	144	193	27	17	9	4
AI	5	5	5						
CD	77	72	64	5	3		3	2	
D	12	12	8		4				
GE	13	12	10		2			1	
IM	806	783	566	118	99	8	8	5	2
PD	572	545	445	21	79	19	6		2
PDC	7	7	5		2				
PUD	32	31	27		4			1	
Sur. Spec.	575	553	448	12	93	10	9		3
CRS	5	5	3		2				
GS	162	157	118	3	36	1	3		1
NS	11	11	9	1	1				
OBG	260	249	207	7	35	8	2		1
OPH	26	26	23		3				
ORS	27	23	19	1	3	1	2		1
OTO	37	36	31		5		1		
PS	7	7	6		1				
TS	6	6	4		2				
U	34	33	28		5		1		
Oth. Spec.	1,557	1,478	1,226	43	209	43	9	11	16
AN	95	92	70	2	20	2		1	
CHP	25	22	17		5		2		1
DR	23	22	17		5				1
EM	89	79	49	4	26	9	1		
FOP	3	3	3						
GPM	14	12	10		2	1			1
MG	1							1	
N	39	37	27	2	8		1		1
NM	3	3	2		1				
OM	32	26	20		6	5			1
P	232	220	166	7	47	6		4	2
PHP	16	7	4		3	7	1		1
PM	37	35	26	4	5	1	1		
PTH	50	42	27	3	12	2	2		4
R	16	16	13		3				
RO	6	5	3		2			1	
OTH	45	35	30	1	4	7	1	2	
UNSP	831	822	742	20	60	3		2	4

Note: Above excludes Inactive, Not Classified and Address Unknown Physicians.

Subspecialties in this table are condensed into major specialties. See Appendix A.

Table 3.4

International Medical Graduates by Census Division, Self-Designated Specialty, and Activity, 2006
New England

Specialty	Total Physicians	Patient Care				Other Professional Activity			
		Total Patient Care	Office Based	Hospital Based		Admin.	Med. Teach.	Research	Other
				Resid./ Fellows	Phys. Staff				
Total Physicians	10,833	10,317	7,139	1,915	1,263	107	81	279	49
GP/FM Prac.	622	612	457	110	45	6	1		3
FM	511	504	363	110	31	4	1		2
GP	111	108	94		14	2			1
Med. Spec.	5,215	4,989	3,367	1,145	477	37	32	148	9
AI	56	46	37	5	4		1	8	1
CD	338	318	230	51	37	2	3	14	1
D	51	45	38	4	3	1		5	
GE	185	177	136	23	18			8	
IM	3,557	3,436	2,207	927	302	20	16	78	7
PD	786	746	569	88	89	11	6	23	
PDC	26	25	18	4	3		1		
PUD	216	196	132	43	21	3	5	12	
Sur. Spec.	1,283	1,232	919	198	115	9	7	31	4
CRS	10	9	7		2			1	
GS	420	399	240	118	41	5	3	11	2
NS	55	51	38	7	6		1	3	
OBG	377	371	299	42	30			4	2
OPH	79	75	59	10	6	1	1	2	
ORS	86	83	67	6	10		1	2	
OTO	68	62	54	1	7	2		4	
PS	46	46	39	6	1				
TS	64	60	52	5	3			4	
U	78	76	64	3	9	1	1		
Oth. Spec.	3,713	3,484	2,396	462	626	55	41	100	33
AN	861	834	610	95	129	5	12	8	2
CHP	157	152	111	21	20	2	2	1	
DR	218	214	151	32	31		1	1	2
EM	169	166	81	18	67	3			
FOP	7	5	3		2				2
GPM	35	34	24	5	5	1			
MG	13	9	5	3	1			4	
N	303	290	206	41	43		2	10	1
NM	34	31	22	8	1		1	2	
OM	19	15	12	1	2	4			
P	860	817	511	121	185	19	5	14	5
PHP	9	1	1			4	1	2	1
PM	103	98	74	4	20	2	1		2
PTH	541	486	316	93	77	7	9	25	14
R	119	112	87	9	16		1	5	1
RO	41	38	31		7			2	1
TTS	3	3	2		1				
OTH	53	18	12	2	4	8	5	20	2
UNSP	167	160	136	9	15		1	6	
VM	1	1	1						

Note: Above excludes Inactive, Not Classified and Address Unknown Physicians.

Subspecialties in this table are condensed into major specialties. See Appendix A.

Table 3.4

International Medical Graduates by Census Division, Self-Designated Specialty, and Activity, 2006, continued
Middle Atlantic

Specialty	Total Physicians	Patient Care				Other Professional Activity			
		Total Patient Care	Office Based	Hospital Based		Admin.	Med. Teach.	Research	Other
				Resid./ Fellows	Phys. Staff				
Total Physicians	48,940	46,878	30,693	10,161	6,024	577	454	781	250
GP/FM Prac.	3,381	3,311	2,242	790	279	32	19	7	12
FM	2,831	2,783	1,830	790	163	23	19	3	3
GP	550	528	412		116	9		4	9
Med. Spec.	24,842	24,008	15,200	6,443	2,365	199	196	377	62
AI	237	211	187	12	12	5	4	17	
CD	1,480	1,418	1,093	208	117	12	12	35	3
D	140	134	120	3	11		2	4	
GE	708	667	510	101	56	7	11	20	3
IM	15,594	15,147	9,003	4,789	1,355	113	92	204	38
PD	5,821	5,606	3,719	1,164	723	56	65	76	18
PDC	98	95	63	9	23	1		2	
PUD	764	730	505	157	68	5	10	19	
Sur. Spec.	6,536	6,339	4,496	1,225	618	42	65	73	17
CRS	61	60	56	1	3			1	
GS	2,253	2,191	1,270	665	256	20	14	23	5
NS	144	136	99	20	17		2	6	
OBG	2,227	2,171	1,536	436	199	13	24	15	4
OPH	364	351	307	26	18	1	3	8	1
ORS	389	377	318	36	23	2	5	4	1
OTO	249	237	211	7	19	1	6	4	1
PS	210	205	177	9	19			3	2
TS	234	221	176	16	29	2	4	6	1
U	405	390	346	9	35	3	7	3	2
Oth. Spec.	14,181	13,220	8,755	1,703	2,762	304	174	324	159
AM	4	4	3		1				
AN	3,051	2,964	2,382	242	340	24	33	22	8
CHP	620	582	390	66	126	14	4	12	8
DR	702	667	468	79	120	6	7	10	12
EM	697	672	357	85	230	13	7	2	3
FOP	37	20	18		2	3		3	11
GPM	40	33	24	5	4	1	2	2	2
MG	23	19	9	6	4			4	
N	1,116	1,050	724	193	133	7	16	36	7
NM	148	136	83	20	33	4	2	3	3
OM	62	46	36	2	8	11	2	2	1
P	3,922	3,707	2,098	584	1,025	106	39	59	11
PHP	34	11	9		2	17	2	2	2
PM	859	822	586	89	147	18	10	2	7
PTH	1,674	1,472	839	272	361	49	33	62	58
R	414	385	259	21	105	4	5	9	11
RO	208	198	147	6	45	1	4	5	
TTS	8	8	5		3				
OTH	243	137	90	7	40	18	6	73	9
UNSP	319	287	228	26	33	8	2	16	6

Note: Above excludes Inactive, Not Classified and Address Unknown Physicians.

Subspecialties in this table are condensed into major specialties. See Appendix A.

Table 3.4

International Medical Graduates by Census Division, Self-Designated Specialty, and Activity, 2006, continued
East North Central

Specialty	Total Physicians	Patient Care				Other Professional Activity			
		Total Patient Care	Office Based	Hospital Based		Admin.	Med. Teach.	Research	Other
				Resid./ Fellows	Phys. Staff				
Total Physicians	31,903	30,842	22,341	5,521	2,980	273	278	349	161
GP/FM Prac.	4,056	3,994	2,816	894	284	23	22	6	11
FM	3,427	3,385	2,303	894	188	14	22	2	4
GP	629	609	513		96	9		4	7
Med. Spec.	15,541	15,141	10,767	3,200	1,174	78	117	184	21
AI	179	174	161	6	7	2		3	
CD	1,223	1,188	966	142	80	2	7	25	1
D	109	106	89	12	5		2	1	
GE	490	473	401	50	22	1	7	9	
IM	9,810	9,582	6,570	2,289	723	50	64	102	12
PD	3,105	3,012	2,146	574	292	18	32	35	8
PDC	77	74	39	19	16	2	1		
PUD	548	532	395	108	29	3	4	9	
Sur. Spec.	3,726	3,644	2,862	506	276	21	23	28	10
CRS	56	56	53	1	2				
GS	1,177	1,151	834	213	104	2	12	7	5
NS	150	146	116	16	14	2	1		1
OBG	1,208	1,184	895	203	86	10	5	8	1
OPH	202	198	170	14	14	1	1	2	
ORS	217	211	180	13	18	2		2	2
OTO	148	147	129	13	5			1	
PS	135	131	114	14	3	1	1	2	
TS	190	181	156	11	14	1	2	6	
U	243	239	215	8	16	2	1		1
Oth. Spec.	8,580	8,063	5,896	921	1,246	151	116	131	119
AM	4	4	2		2				
AN	2,073	2,023	1,574	198	251	9	28	7	6
CHP	271	258	190	30	38	4	4	3	2
DR	508	487	369	57	61	1	5	3	12
EM	396	385	246	52	87	7	4		
FOP	29	19	16	2	1	1	2	1	6
GPM	30	28	25	1	2	1		1	
MG	10	8	4	2	2			2	
N	780	752	572	115	65	2	8	14	4
NM	96	85	60	10	15	1	3	4	3
OM	77	64	51	2	11	6	1	2	4
P	1,780	1,699	1,169	180	350	53	10	12	6
PHP	8	1	1			6			1
PM	337	327	234	38	55	3	3	1	3
PTH	1,179	1,019	693	143	183	32	35	41	52
R	328	304	237	11	56	5	4	5	10
RO	165	161	135	4	22	3	1		
TTS	4	3	3					1	
OTH	140	86	64	5	17	13	6	29	6
UNSP	363	348	249	71	28	4	2	5	4
VM	2	2	2						

Note: Above excludes Inactive, Not Classified and Address Unknown Physicians.

Subspecialties in this table are condensed into major specialties. See Appendix A.

Table 3.4

International Medical Graduates by Census Division, Self-Designated Specialty, and Activity, 2006, continued
West North Central

| Specialty | Total Physicians | Patient Care | | | | Other Professional Activity | | | |
		Total Patient Care	Office Based	Resid./ Fellows	Phys. Staff	Admin.	Med. Teach.	Research	Other
Total Physicians	8,133	7,825	5,411	1,497	917	50	75	149	34
GP/FM Prac.	928	916	580	254	82	7	2	1	2
FM	819	813	499	254	60	4	1		1
GP	109	103	81		22	3	1	1	1
Med. Spec.	3,797	3,674	2,534	785	355	12	28	79	4
AI	56	52	44	7	1	1	1	2	
CD	355	341	267	47	27		3	10	1
D	22	22	17	2	3				
GE	174	166	138	22	6		1	7	
IM	2,446	2,375	1,545	583	247	6	16	48	1
PD	563	543	405	84	54	3	7	9	1
PDC	31	30	20	6	4	1			
PUD	150	145	98	34	13	1		3	1
Sur. Spec.	868	843	627	120	96	4	7	13	1
CRS	11	11	10	1					
GS	300	295	174	76	45	1		4	
NS	43	41	32	7	2		1	1	
OBG	188	180	141	16	23	1	3	3	1
OPH	62	59	50	4	5	1		2	
ORS	65	64	55	3	6		1		
OTO	30	28	21	4	3			2	
PS	23	22	20		2			1	
TS	59	59	45	7	7				
U	87	84	79	2	3	1	2		
Oth. Spec.	2,540	2,392	1,670	338	384	27	38	56	27
AM	2	1	1			1			
AN	408	399	313	37	49		6	3	
CHP	124	119	87	13	19	1	1	2	1
DR	146	141	105	16	20		4		1
EM	94	88	50	9	29	2	4		
FOP	2	2	2						
GPM	18	16	12	3	1		1	1	
MG	8	7	5	2			1		
N	290	267	198	46	23	3	7	12	1
NM	26	24	14	2	8		1	1	
OM	16	14	12		2	2			
P	666	645	390	120	135	9	1	9	2
PHP	3	1	1					1	1
PM	118	117	80	12	25	1			
PTH	297	262	168	62	32	3	5	12	15
R	79	74	60	3	11	1	3		1
RO	48	47	40	1	6			1	
TTS	3	3	2		1				
OTH	55	32	21	4	7	3	2	13	5
UNSP	137	133	109	8	16	1	2	1	

Note: Above excludes Inactive, Not Classified and Address Unknown Physicians.

Subspecialties in this table are condensed into major specialties. See Appendix A.

Table 3.4

International Medical Graduates by Census Division, Self-Designated Specialty, and Activity, 2006, continued
South Atlantic

| Specialty | Total Physicians | Patient Care | | | | Other Professional Activity | | | |
| | | Total Patient Care | Office Based | Hospital Based | | Admin. | Med. Teach. | Research | Other |
				Resid./ Fellows	Phys. Staff				
Total Physicians	35,336	33,941	26,981	3,190	3,770	404	296	507	188
GP/FM Prac.	4,292	4,203	3,333	511	359	46	19	5	19
FM	3,241	3,186	2,479	511	196	28	15	4	8
GP	1,051	1,017	854		163	18	4	1	11
Med. Spec.	17,141	16,599	13,424	1,643	1,532	136	129	247	30
AI	187	165	157	3	5	1	4	17	
CD	1,337	1,295	1,121	76	98	5	12	22	3
D	128	123	109	9	5		3	1	1
GE	686	664	578	38	48	4	9	9	
IM	10,288	9,997	7,887	1,170	940	82	64	130	15
PD	3,770	3,638	2,990	275	373	40	32	50	10
PDC	84	78	59	12	7	1	2	3	
PUD	661	639	523	60	56	3	3	15	1
Sur. Spec.	4,320	4,213	3,487	347	379	29	29	34	15
CRS	57	57	50	2	5				
GS	1,353	1,316	985	166	165	13	6	9	9
NS	137	135	114	8	13		1	1	
OBG	1,275	1,246	1,035	115	96	10	12	6	1
OPH	280	269	249	11	9		2	9	
ORS	337	329	279	18	32	3	4	1	
OTO	166	163	154	4	5		1	2	
PS	177	173	156	7	10		1	1	2
TS	179	175	155	8	12	1	1	2	
U	359	350	310	8	32	2	1	3	3
Oth. Spec.	9,583	8,926	6,737	689	1,500	193	119	221	124
AM	7	4	3		1	1		2	
AN	1,974	1,921	1,561	116	244	9	25	17	2
CHP	395	382	298	24	60	3	7	2	1
DR	489	463	364	24	75	3	4	9	10
EM	599	587	430	33	124	7	3	1	1
FOP	34	25	21	3	1	4			5
GPM	87	66	54	9	3	11	2	6	2
MG	23	21	11	8	2			2	
N	856	817	674	83	60	3	8	25	3
NM	79	75	51	3	21	1	1	1	1
OM	57	44	33	2	9	9			4
P	2,380	2,261	1,516	216	529	47	23	35	14
PHP	52	14	11		3	27	2	8	1
PM	367	357	275	22	60	5	1	4	
PTH	1,058	892	641	97	154	34	19	58	55
R	316	282	206	20	56	1	10	12	11
RO	128	126	111	3	12		1	1	
TTS	8	7	4		3			1	
OTH	178	115	88	1	26	17	9	28	9
UNSP	495	466	384	25	57	11	4	9	5
VM	1	1	1						

Note: Above excludes Inactive, Not Classified and Address Unknown Physicians.

Subspecialties in this table are condensed into major specialties. See Appendix A.

Table 3.4

International Medical Graduates by Census Division, Self-Designated Specialty, and Activity, 2006, continued
East South Central

Specialty	Total Physicians	Patient Care		Hospital Based		Other Professional Activity			
		Total Patient Care	Office Based	Resid./ Fellows	Phys. Staff	Admin.	Med. Teach.	Research	Other
Total Physicians	6,616	6,419	4,753	975	691	36	48	86	27
GP/FM Prac.	820	813	541	201	71	5	1	1	
FM	719	713	470	201	42	5	1		
GP	101	100	71		29			1	
Med. Spec.	3,337	3,249	2,448	500	301	15	19	52	2
AI	31	30	27	1	2			1	
CD	288	283	233	32	18	1	1	3	
D	8	7	5	1	1			1	
GE	127	125	109	9	7		1	1	
IM	2,082	2,033	1,480	362	191	8	11	28	2
PD	607	582	449	73	60	5	6	14	
PDC	17	16	14		2			1	
PUD	177	173	131	22	20	1		3	
Sur. Spec.	643	626	501	72	53	2	5	4	6
CRS	7	7	7						
GS	251	244	177	42	25		1	1	5
NS	25	24	19	3	2		1		
OBG	139	135	112	13	10	2	2		
OPH	46	43	38	4	1		1	2	
ORS	43	42	31	4	7				1
OTO	26	26	23		3				
PS	26	26	22	3	1				
TS	41	40	35	2	3			1	
U	39	39	37	1	1				
Oth. Spec.	1,816	1,731	1,263	202	266	14	23	29	19
AM	1	1	1						
AN	380	372	308	17	47	1	4	3	
CHP	63	61	43	10	8		1	1	
DR	82	79	57	9	13		2		1
EM	84	84	59	3	22				
FOP	4	2	2						2
GPM	13	12	5	7			1		
MG	4	3	2	1		1			
N	233	225	184	31	10		4	3	1
NM	20	20	14	2	4				
OM	10	10	8	1	1				
P	467	449	281	71	97	6	1	7	4
PHP	3	2	2				1		
PM	47	46	37	2	7				1
PTH	205	187	121	39	27	1	4	7	6
R	47	43	25	6	12	1	1	1	1
RO	22	22	17		5				
TTS	2	2	2						
OTH	37	23	17		6	4	1	7	2
UNSP	92	88	78	3	7		3		1

Note: Above excludes Inactive, Not Classified and Address Unknown Physicians.

Subspecialties in this table are condensed into major specialties. See Appendix A.

Table 3.4

International Medical Graduates by Census Division, Self-Designated Specialty, and Activity, 2006, continued
West South Central

Specialty	Total Physicians	Patient Care				Other Professional Activity			
		Total Patient Care	Office Based	Resid./ Fellows	Phys. Staff	Admin.	Med. Teach.	Research	Other
Total Physicians	15,128	14,638	11,178	2,126	1,334	94	168	181	47
GP/FM Prac.	2,160	2,134	1,475	516	143	8	14	3	1
FM	1,869	1,846	1,233	516	97	8	13	2	
GP	291	288	242		46		1	1	1
Med. Spec.	7,528	7,308	5,683	1,039	586	27	70	111	12
AI	99	94	89	2	3		3	2	
CD	751	720	596	79	45	3	7	17	4
D	44	43	36	4	3	1			
GE	326	315	269	24	22	1	4	6	
IM	4,142	4,037	3,033	636	368	12	30	58	5
PD	1,806	1,746	1,370	256	120	9	24	24	3
PDC	52	52	47	2	3				
PUD	308	301	243	36	22	1	2	4	
Sur. Spec.	1,661	1,609	1,315	177	117	11	25	11	5
CRS	24	22	19	2	1		2		
GS	492	478	372	61	45	5	6	1	2
NS	69	69	51	13	5				
OBG	478	463	376	58	29	2	11	2	
OPH	120	116	93	16	7	1	3		
ORS	133	128	110	12	6	2		2	1
OTO	63	62	54	4	4			1	
PS	67	65	59	3	3			1	1
TS	94	88	80	3	5		2	3	1
U	121	118	101	5	12	1	1	1	
Oth. Spec.	3,779	3,587	2,705	394	488	48	59	56	29
AM	6	3	1		2	2		1	
AN	857	834	700	41	93	5	13	4	1
CHP	166	158	116	27	15	3	1	4	
DR	238	228	158	28	42		8		2
EM	150	147	108	23	16		2		1
FOP	16	11	8	3					5
GPM	15	14	7	2	5	1			
MG	17	15	7	5	3	2			
N	399	391	291	75	25		3	4	1
NM	33	32	23	2	7			1	
OM	27	26	23	1	2		1		
P	746	721	499	85	137	10	7	5	3
PHP	13	5	4		1	4		3	1
PM	159	155	126	10	19	2		1	1
PTH	521	478	331	79	68	10	11	11	11
R	122	108	84	7	17	1	8	3	2
RO	70	68	56		12	1	1		
TTS	6	6	5		1				
OTH	63	39	32		7	6	3	15	
UNSP	155	148	126	6	16	1	1	4	1

Note: Above excludes Inactive, Not Classified and Address Unknown Physicians.

Subspecialties in this table are condensed into major specialties. See Appendix A.

Table 3.4

International Medical Graduates by Census Division, Self-Designated Specialty, and Activity, 2006, continued
Mountain

| Specialty | Total Physicians | Patient Care | | Hospital Based | | Other Professional Activity | | | |
		Total Patient Care	Office Based	Resid./ Fellows	Phys. Staff	Admin.	Med. Teach.	Research	Other
Total Physicians	6,222	6,029	4,840	607	582	40	54	72	27
GP/FM Prac.	818	806	629	131	46	4	6	1	1
FM	718	708	547	131	30	3	6	1	
GP	100	98	82		16	1			1
Med. Spec.	3,185	3,103	2,536	322	245	14	22	39	7
AI	49	49	46	3					
CD	231	224	191	21	12		1	6	
D	18	17	15	1	1			1	
GE	156	150	135	5	10	2	1	2	1
IM	1,981	1,937	1,562	212	163	9	12	19	4
PD	597	581	473	60	48	3	4	7	2
PDC	17	15	12	3			2		
PUD	136	130	102	17	11		2	4	
Sur. Spec.	590	576	465	62	49	4	4	5	1
CRS	6	6	5		1				
GS	187	184	129	36	19		1	1	1
NS	27	27	19	7	1				
OBG	181	175	150	14	11	3		3	
OPH	32	31	26	1	4			1	
ORS	48	48	40	3	5				
OTO	16	16	14		2				
PS	17	16	14	1	1	1			
TS	39	38	37		1		1		
U	37	35	31		4		2		
Oth. Spec.	1,629	1,544	1,210	92	242	18	22	27	18
AM	6	3	2		1	1	1		1
AN	430	418	355	11	52	2	7	2	1
CHP	67	64	49	5	10	1		2	
DR	105	97	74	4	19	1	4	1	2
EM	91	90	68	5	17		1		
FOP	6	6	6						
GPM	12	11	8	1	2	1			
MG	8	7	4	1	2			1	
N	144	138	110	15	13		1	5	
NM	5	5	4	1					
OM	16	16	13	1	2				
P	352	341	237	29	75	4	4	3	
PHP	4	1			1	2		1	
PM	87	85	70	5	10	1			1
PTH	146	129	98	11	20	3	2	5	7
R	41	37	30	2	5	1		1	2
RO	21	20	17		3			1	
TTS	1	1	1						
OTH	27	19	16		3	1	1	4	2
UNSP	60	56	48	1	7			1	2

Note: Above excludes Inactive, Not Classified and Address Unknown Physicians.

Subspecialties in this table are condensed into major specialties. See Appendix A.

Table 3.4

International Medical Graduates by Census Division, Self-Designated Specialty, and Activity, 2006, continued
Pacific

Specialty	Total Physicians	Patient Care		Hospital Based		Other Professional Activity			
		Total Patient Care	Office Based	Resid./ Fellows	Phys. Staff	Admin.	Med. Teach.	Research	Other
Total Physicians	24,071	23,053	19,632	1,362	2,059	266	218	403	131
GP/FM Prac.	3,520	3,445	2,917	337	191	30	23	5	17
FM	2,670	2,615	2,170	337	108	19	22	5	9
GP	850	830	747		83	11	1		8
Med. Spec.	10,877	10,459	9,024	650	785	82	89	214	33
AI	134	118	108		10		1	13	2
CD	742	704	623	22	59	2	11	24	1
D	113	106	98		8	1	3	3	
GE	433	409	362	18	29	6	6	12	
IM	6,323	6,119	5,220	447	452	37	42	106	19
PD	2,691	2,585	2,260	128	197	35	22	38	11
PDC	57	51	43	5	3		1	5	
PUD	384	367	310	30	27	1	3	13	
Sur. Spec.	3,134	3,046	2,701	127	218	28	22	29	9
CRS	26	26	23	2	1				
GS	824	801	651	84	66	10	4	6	3
NS	91	91	76	4	11				
OBG	1,113	1,078	990	21	67	10	11	13	1
OPH	212	208	190	5	13		2	1	1
ORS	265	260	240	3	17	1		2	2
OTO	129	123	117	2	4	4		1	1
PS	143	141	131	2	8			1	1
TS	146	143	127	3	13			3	
U	185	175	156	1	18	3	5	2	
Oth. Spec.	6,540	6,103	4,990	248	865	126	84	155	72
AM	7	6	3		3			1	
AN	1,583	1,534	1,309	40	185	5	24	15	5
CHP	251	241	205	9	27	3	2	5	
DR	347	329	265	8	56	4	8	5	1
EM	295	291	226	15	50	3		1	
FOP	14	7	5	1	1	1	1		5
GPM	45	36	34	2		3	1	4	1
MG	24	21	14	5	2			3	
N	484	454	412	12	30	2	6	21	1
NM	92	88	63	8	17	1		2	1
OM	68	61	50	2	9	5	1	1	
P	1,594	1,508	1,130	71	307	44	13	19	10
PHP	26	11	7		4	8	2	3	2
PM	260	250	206	5	39	5	4		1
PTH	690	599	469	57	73	25	14	23	29
R	188	177	144	9	24	3	1	5	2
RO	82	79	67	1	11		1	2	
TTS	3	3	3						
OTH	136	80	71		9	11	3	37	5
UNSP	350	327	306	3	18	3	3	8	9
VM	1	1	1						

Note: Above excludes Inactive, Not Classified and Address Unknown Physicians.

Subspecialties in this table are condensed into major specialties. See Appendix A.

Table 3.4

International Medical Graduates by Census Division, Self-Designated Specialty, and Activity, 2006, continued
Possessions

| Specialty | Total Physicians | Patient Care | | | | Other Professional Activity | | | |
		Total Patient Care	Office Based	Resid./ Fellows	Phys. Staff	Admin.	Med. Teach.	Research	Other
Total Physicians	5,309	5,103	4,147	225	731	111	42	22	31
GP/FM Prac.	1,653	1,605	1,343	26	236	31	7	2	8
FM	463	447	383	26	38	10	3	1	2
GP	1,190	1,158	960		198	21	4	1	6
Med. Spec.	1,524	1,467	1,130	144	193	27	17	9	4
AI	5	5	5						
CD	77	72	64	5	3		3	2	
D	12	12	8		4				
GE	13	12	10		2			1	
IM	806	783	566	118	99	8	8	5	2
PD	572	545	445	21	79	19	6		2
PDC	7	7	5		2				
PUD	32	31	27		4			1	
Sur. Spec.	575	553	448	12	93	10	9		3
CRS	5	5	3		2				
GS	162	157	118	3	36	1	3		1
NS	11	11	9	1	1				
OBG	260	249	207	7	35	8	2		1
OPH	26	26	23		3				
ORS	27	23	19	1	3	1	2		1
OTO	37	36	31		5		1		
PS	7	7	6		1				
TS	6	6	4		2				
U	34	33	28		5		1		
Oth. Spec.	1,557	1,478	1,226	43	209	43	9	11	16
AN	95	92	70	2	20	2		1	
CHP	25	22	17		5		2		1
DR	23	22	17		5				1
EM	89	79	49	4	26	9	1		
FOP	3	3	3						
GPM	14	12	10		2	1			1
MG	1							1	
N	39	37	27	2	8		1		1
NM	3	3	2		1				
OM	32	26	20		6	5			1
P	232	220	166	7	47	6		4	2
PHP	16	7	4		3	7	1		1
PM	37	35	26	4	5	1	1		
PTH	50	42	27	3	12	2	2		4
R	16	16	13		3				
RO	6	5	3		2			1	
OTH	45	35	30	1	4	7	1	2	
UNSP	831	822	742	20	60	3		2	4

Note: Above excludes Inactive, Not Classified and Address Unknown Physicians.

Subspecialties in this table are condensed into major specialties. See Appendix A.

Table 3.5

Physicians by Census Region, Self-Designated Specialty, and Activity, 2006
Northeast

Specialty	Total Physicians	Patient Care				Other Professional Activity			
		Total Patient Care	Office Based	Hospital Based		Admin.	Med. Teach.	Research	Other
				Resid./ Fellows	Phys. Staff				
Total Physicians	218,579	169,421	120,840	30,230	18,351	3,924	2,523	4,736	1,128
GP/FM Prac.	12,771	12,208	9,747	1,489	972	238	235	47	43
FM	11,533	11,039	8,746	1,489	804	205	231	33	25
GP	1,238	1,169	1,001		168	33	4	14	18
Med. Spec.	78,156	72,376	50,632	14,755	6,989	1,513	1,170	2,737	360
AI	971	843	738	62	43	20	9	94	5
CD	6,006	5,581	4,408	707	466	90	84	219	32
D	2,485	2,402	2,026	267	109	12	23	45	3
GE	3,217	3,017	2,445	349	223	34	47	107	12
IM	44,047	40,552	27,007	9,676	3,869	977	637	1,672	209
PD	18,325	17,179	12,012	3,249	1,918	319	290	446	91
PDC	444	408	250	70	88	5	8	21	2
PUD	2,661	2,394	1,746	375	273	56	72	133	6
Sur. Spec.	36,379	35,307	26,985	5,838	2,484	340	307	299	126
CRS	364	355	316	20	19	1	4	3	1
GS	8,928	8,597	5,415	2,414	768	134	78	82	37
NS	1,090	1,052	759	190	103	5	11	18	4
OBG	9,515	9,212	7,255	1,219	738	103	106	73	21
OPH	4,311	4,211	3,735	301	175	16	28	42	14
ORS	5,211	5,100	3,889	982	229	23	27	27	34
OTO	2,024	1,982	1,617	239	126	11	19	10	2
PS	1,487	1,467	1,230	159	78	4	5	5	6
TS	1,075	1,014	816	80	118	23	12	24	2
U	2,374	2,317	1,953	234	130	20	17	15	5
Oth. Spec.	54,426	49,530	33,476	8,148	7,906	1,833	811	1,653	599
AM	29	19	13		6	8		1	1
AN	9,159	8,852	6,653	1,285	914	80	124	84	19
CHP	2,148	1,969	1,469	196	304	72	34	53	20
DR	5,720	5,519	3,694	1,190	635	40	59	49	53
EM	6,025	5,754	3,248	1,254	1,252	170	62	26	13
FOP	128	81	70	5	6	13	1	4	29
GPM	387	308	207	70	31	35	14	19	11
MG	121	91	41	29	21	5	3	21	1
N	3,909	3,476	2,537	520	419	59	80	270	24
NM	384	338	228	43	67	13	9	18	6
OM	475	287	219	10	58	130	8	20	30
P	13,032	11,903	7,941	1,629	2,333	503	191	351	84
PHP	282	62	49		13	131	16	51	22
PM	2,144	2,047	1,453	275	319	53	17	12	15
PTH	4,657	3,950	2,360	754	836	199	101	245	162
R	2,180	2,055	1,581	125	349	27	32	36	30
RO	993	961	686	135	140	8	7	15	2
TTS	40	37	29		8	1		2	
OTH	1,271	553	421	13	119	269	43	339	67
UNSP	1,337	1,263	572	615	76	17	10	37	10
VM	5	5	5						
Inactive	22,926								
Not Class	13,921								

Note: Above excludes Address Unknown.

Subspecialties in this table are condensed into major specialties. See Appendix A.

Table 3.5

Physicians by Census Region, Self-Designated Specialty, and Activity, 2006, continued
North Central

Specialty	Total Physicians	Patient Care				Other Professional Activity			
		Total Patient Care	Office Based	Hospital Based		Admin.	Med. Teach.	Research	Other
				Resid./ Fellows	Phys. Staff				
Total Physicians	187,012	149,305	113,674	23,220	12,411	2,645	2,160	2,410	755
GP/FM Prac.	23,102	22,215	18,334	2,347	1,534	354	421	56	56
FM	21,501	20,683	16,990	2,347	1,346	321	415	47	35
GP	1,601	1,532	1,344		188	33	6	9	21
Med. Spec.	57,446	54,104	40,232	9,621	4,251	942	838	1,402	160
AI	884	819	720	79	20	10	9	42	4
CD	4,568	4,307	3,519	515	273	42	63	139	17
D	1,982	1,949	1,578	292	79	3	14	13	3
GE	2,274	2,152	1,807	233	112	16	32	72	2
IM	30,984	29,063	21,119	5,586	2,358	603	456	774	88
PD	14,401	13,647	9,844	2,581	1,222	215	223	277	39
PDC	426	401	266	80	55	5	5	14	1
PUD	1,927	1,766	1,379	255	132	48	36	71	6
Sur. Spec.	32,656	31,880	25,170	4,891	1,819	235	291	184	66
CRS	305	301	267	18	16	1	3		
GS	7,865	7,640	5,311	1,776	553	68	73	63	21
NS	1,178	1,146	840	219	87	12	13	3	4
OBG	8,214	7,982	6,516	951	515	75	100	49	8
OPH	3,637	3,566	3,152	291	123	21	20	23	7
ORS	5,032	4,956	3,884	843	229	18	27	14	17
OTO	2,053	2,014	1,623	308	83	11	19	6	3
PS	1,239	1,213	985	188	40	7	12	6	1
TS	1,048	1,012	868	59	85	9	10	13	4
U	2,085	2,050	1,724	238	88	13	14	7	1
Oth. Spec.	44,071	41,106	29,938	6,361	4,807	1,114	610	768	473
AM	48	31	19	1	11	12	1	4	
AN	8,386	8,197	6,264	1,205	728	45	92	38	14
CHP	1,271	1,190	927	117	146	30	29	17	5
DR	5,355	5,224	3,806	980	438	23	53	10	45
EM	6,356	6,114	4,102	1,049	963	142	68	21	11
FOP	122	89	79	6	4	6	3	1	23
GPM	244	191	156	19	16	24	5	19	5
MG	100	75	49	13	13		6	17	2
N	3,012	2,785	2,148	418	219	32	48	131	16
NM	287	257	187	21	49	8	8	9	5
OM	651	512	420	6	86	93	6	15	25
P	6,886	6,432	4,647	786	999	214	95	108	37
PHP	148	32	21		11	72	10	25	9
PM	1,692	1,637	1,195	229	213	30	8	10	7
PTH	4,276	3,690	2,627	571	492	165	96	143	182
R	1,845	1,766	1,494	91	181	14	24	12	29
RO	976	959	739	136	84	8	6	3	
TTS	37	30	26		4		2	4	1
OTH	960	519	424	22	73	186	43	165	47
UNSP	1,410	1,367	599	691	77	10	7	16	10
VM	9	9	9						
Inactive	20,676								
Not Class	9,061								

Note: Above excludes Address Unknown.

Subspecialties in this table are condensed into major specialties. See Appendix A.

Table 3.5

Physicians by Census Region, Self-Designated Specialty, and Activity, 2006, continued
South

Specialty	Total Physicians	Patient Care				Other Professional Activity			
		Total Patient Care	Office Based	Hospital Based		Admin.	Med. Teach.	Research	Other
				Resid./ Fellows	Phys. Staff				
Total Physicians	301,350	238,385	189,391	28,329	20,665	4,564	3,511	4,247	1,347
GP/FM Prac.	32,317	31,134	25,996	2,789	2,349	502	518	73	90
FM	28,707	27,644	22,931	2,789	1,924	433	508	65	57
GP	3,610	3,490	3,065		425	69	10	8	33
Med. Spec.	92,957	87,374	68,972	11,315	7,087	1,456	1,405	2,402	320
AI	1,431	1,268	1,136	71	61	18	17	121	7
CD	7,633	7,265	6,167	620	478	81	95	174	18
D	3,568	3,501	2,980	370	151	19	23	19	6
GE	4,237	4,060	3,541	300	219	33	53	86	5
IM	47,711	44,618	34,391	6,302	3,925	846	709	1,376	162
PD	24,284	22,866	17,692	3,283	1,891	400	433	477	108
PDC	612	564	441	66	57	10	9	28	1
PUD	3,481	3,232	2,624	303	305	49	66	121	13
Sur. Spec.	56,223	54,747	45,171	6,263	3,313	471	599	255	151
CRS	452	440	394	20	26	2	5	3	2
GS	12,715	12,298	8,966	2,311	1,021	152	152	66	47
NS	1,968	1,921	1,557	248	116	12	15	10	10
OBG	14,957	14,495	12,313	1,379	803	137	234	62	29
OPH	6,093	5,949	5,286	394	269	37	49	48	10
ORS	8,287	8,150	6,650	1,016	484	43	53	17	24
OTO	3,632	3,567	3,037	359	171	22	28	9	6
PS	2,549	2,506	2,209	204	93	9	21	6	7
TS	1,730	1,674	1,478	77	119	21	15	15	5
U	3,840	3,747	3,281	255	211	36	27	19	11
Oth. Spec.	70,557	65,130	49,252	7,962	7,916	2,135	989	1,517	786
AM	245	148	84	4	60	75	4	11	7
AN	13,687	13,344	10,650	1,473	1,221	103	156	63	21
CHP	2,221	2,075	1,660	176	239	58	49	32	7
DR	8,242	8,029	6,076	1,217	736	39	72	30	72
EM	9,773	9,450	6,955	1,049	1,446	182	92	23	26
FOP	257	190	162	14	14	12	3	2	50
GPM	900	675	460	94	121	103	17	79	26
MG	178	133	83	24	26	12	13	20	
N	4,689	4,323	3,507	473	343	60	75	215	16
NM	428	385	273	35	77	13	7	20	3
OM	790	539	437	8	94	182	15	23	31
P	11,676	10,815	7,830	1,256	1,729	385	180	209	87
PHP	642	112	76	1	35	316	26	161	27
PM	2,102	2,031	1,572	242	217	39	10	17	5
PTH	6,440	5,596	4,013	822	761	202	128	253	261
R	2,961	2,786	2,340	123	323	22	70	30	53
RO	1,497	1,463	1,217	143	103	16	8	8	2
TTS	52	48	38		10	1	1	2	
OTH	1,611	904	743	2	159	293	50	285	79
UNSP	2,159	2,077	1,070	806	201	22	13	34	13
VM	7	7	6		1				
Inactive	36,242								
Not Class	13,054								

Note: Above excludes Address Unknown.

Subspecialties in this table are condensed into major specialties. See Appendix A.

Table 3.5

Physicians by Census Region, Self-Designated Specialty, and Activity, 2006, continued
West

| | | Patient Care | | | | Other Professional Activity | | | |
| | | | | Hospital Based | | | | | |
Specialty	Total Physicians	Total Patient Care	Office Based	Resid./ Fellows	Phys. Staff	Admin.	Med. Teach.	Research	Other
Total Physicians	201,124	155,576	128,475	14,473	12,628	3,200	1,939	3,028	1,108
GP/FM Prac.	22,732	21,961	18,906	1,596	1,459	351	274	63	83
FM	20,048	19,374	16,541	1,596	1,237	295	268	54	57
GP	2,684	2,587	2,365		222	56	6	9	26
Med. Spec.	58,584	54,865	45,002	5,708	4,155	1,041	737	1,703	238
AI	893	788	701	35	52	14	6	80	5
CD	3,990	3,712	3,203	233	276	43	70	154	11
D	2,607	2,537	2,258	163	116	14	17	34	5
GE	2,423	2,292	1,995	166	131	32	30	65	4
IM	31,227	29,147	23,613	3,210	2,324	594	359	983	144
PD	14,998	14,167	11,403	1,700	1,064	295	209	263	64
PDC	376	347	272	44	31	6	8	15	
PUD	2,070	1,875	1,557	157	161	43	38	109	5
Sur. Spec.	34,345	33,419	28,430	2,989	2,000	294	308	193	131
CRS	210	203	181	9	13	4	2		1
GS	7,588	7,366	5,590	1,195	581	96	67	32	27
NS	1,162	1,129	928	138	63	6	9	10	8
OBG	9,014	8,738	7,639	623	476	93	99	68	16
OPH	3,834	3,758	3,428	136	194	22	26	26	2
ORS	5,595	5,446	4,674	462	310	27	39	23	60
OTO	2,169	2,122	1,841	173	108	21	21	3	2
PS	1,753	1,724	1,559	98	67	6	11	4	8
TS	930	900	804	33	63	4	12	13	1
U	2,090	2,033	1,786	122	125	15	22	14	6
Oth. Spec.	49,190	45,331	36,137	4,180	5,014	1,514	620	1,069	656
AM	128	81	50		31	36	2	5	4
AN	9,720	9,448	7,999	681	768	60	129	58	25
CHP	1,538	1,444	1,235	89	120	43	23	23	5
DR	5,106	4,927	3,870	561	496	37	52	27	63
EM	7,603	7,331	5,633	648	1,050	167	69	12	24
FOP	144	102	95	1	6	6	3	2	31
GPM	578	464	372	35	57	58	5	33	18
MG	132	85	59	11	15	7	2	36	2
N	2,800	2,525	2,136	191	198	37	51	165	22
NM	344	313	241	20	52	8	3	13	7
OM	684	520	450	8	62	108	10	24	22
P	9,286	8,600	6,635	740	1,225	311	106	177	92
PHP	332	82	67		15	147	15	60	28
PM	1,587	1,523	1,253	120	150	37	9	9	9
PTH	3,668	3,116	2,389	360	367	139	69	157	187
R	1,831	1,732	1,486	73	173	23	39	16	21
RO	934	910	760	92	58	5	6	12	1
TTS	22	22	21		1				
OTH	1,253	674	605	1	68	271	21	213	74
UNSP	1,497	1,430	779	549	102	14	6	26	21
VM	3	2	2					1	
Inactive	27,635								
Not Class	8,638								

Note: Above excludes Address Unknown.

Subspecialties in this table are condensed into major specialties. See Appendix A.

Table 3.5

Physicians by Census Region, Self-Designated Specialty, and Activity, 2006, continued
Possessions

Specialty	Total Physicians	Patient Care				Other Professional Activity			
		Total Patient Care	Office Based	Hospital Based		Admin.	Med. Teach.	Research	Other
				Resid./ Fellows	Phys. Staff				
Total Physicians	13,367	10,431	8,031	850	1,550	242	140	54	57
GP/FM Prac.	2,437	2,356	1,917	45	394	48	20	3	10
FM	1,077	1,035	820	45	170	25	14	1	2
GP	1,360	1,321	1,097	224	23	6	2	8	
Med. Spec.	3,507	3,339	2,470	399	470	69	64	24	11
AI	17	17	15	1	1				
CD	229	217	183	15	19	1	7	3	1
D	102	99	78	8	13	1	1	1	
GE	117	113	93	10	10	2	2		
IM	1,736	1,667	1,154	285	228	29	25	10	5
PD	1,194	1,124	862	79	183	38	22	5	5
PDC	19	19	14	5					
PUD	93	83	71	1	11	7	3		
Sur. Spec.	1,773	1,718	1,364	129	225	24	23	3	5
CRS	9	9	6	3					
GS	460	443	310	56	77	7	8	2	
NS	27	26	19	6	1	1			
OBG	633	609	502	33	74	12	8	2	2
OPH	183	180	164	3	13	2	1		
ORS	171	166	123	24	19	1	3	1	
OTO	96	93	81	3	9	1	2		
PS	41	41	35	2	4				
TS	24	24	18	1	5				
U	129	127	106	1	20	1	1		
Oth. Spec.	3,207	3,018	2,280	277	461	101	33	24	31
AM	23	15	4	11	5	2	1		
AN	241	232	180	17	35	4	3	1	1
CHP	82	77	54	5	18	1	3	1	
DR	201	187	131	22	34	5	4	1	4
EM	230	214	117	29	68	14	2		
FOP	6	6	3	3					
GPM	52	44	24	8	12	5	1	1	1
MG	2	1	1	1					
N	144	136	95	20	21	1	3	3	1
NM	34	30	24	2	4	2	1	1	
OM	41	33	24	9	7	1			
P	505	475	334	51	90	13	7	5	5
PHP	30	9	5	4	13	1	2	5	
PM	211	208	161	28	19	2	1		
PTH	130	111	76	10	25	9	3	1	6
R	69	67	53	3	11	1	1		
RO	24	21	17	4	2	1			
OTH	73	52	42	1	9	15	3	3	
UNSP	1,109	1,100	935	81	84	3	2	4	
Inactive	865								
Not Class	1,578								

Note: Above excludes Address Unknown.

Subspecialties in this table are condensed into major specialties. See Appendix A.

Table 3.6

Physicians by Census Division, Self-Designated Specialty, and Activity, 2006
New England

Specialty	Total Physicians	Patient Care		Hospital Based		Other Professional Activity			
		Total Patient Care	Office Based	Resid./ Fellows	Phys. Staff	Admin.	Med. Teach.	Research	Other
Total Physicians	62,366	47,745	34,634	7,873	5,238	1,156	690	1,753	342
GP/FM Prac.	3,555	3,414	2,842	283	289	66	50	13	12
FM	3,282	3,157	2,608	283	266	58	49	9	9
GP	273	257	234		23	8	1	4	3
Med. Spec.	22,154	20,249	14,559	3,682	2,008	431	316	1,054	104
AI	262	215	177	22	16	7	2	36	2
CD	1,606	1,469	1,121	203	145	24	24	75	14
D	717	687	566	81	40	5	5	19	1
GE	905	841	662	111	68	7	12	44	1
IM	12,748	11,557	8,051	2,343	1,163	288	188	660	55
PD	4,986	4,654	3,403	781	470	80	62	160	30
PDC	137	133	82	33	18		2	2	
PUD	793	693	497	108	88	20	21	58	1
Sur. Spec.	9,802	9,507	7,391	1,453	663	93	71	99	32
CRS	72	70	61	4	5		1	1	
GS	2,443	2,341	1,526	628	187	34	18	37	13
NS	329	318	239	48	31		3	7	1
OBG	2,528	2,450	1,987	273	190	32	24	19	3
OPH	1,074	1,051	942	52	57	3	6	10	4
ORS	1,573	1,538	1,208	249	81	5	10	11	9
OTO	551	540	453	50	37	4	3	4	
PS	365	361	288	58	15	1	2		1
TS	278	261	207	25	29	8	2	7	
U	589	577	480	66	31	6	2	3	1
Oth. Spec.	16,175	14,575	9,842	2,455	2,278	566	253	587	194
AM	10	5	5			4		1	
AN	2,539	2,441	1,724	444	273	24	45	25	4
CHP	679	627	479	65	83	19	12	18	3
DR	1,702	1,641	1,095	364	182	13	19	14	15
EM	1,950	1,863	1,078	339	446	62	16	7	2
FOP	29	16	14		2	2	1		10
GPM	132	107	65	29	13	9	4	8	4
MG	52	37	16	14	7	4		11	
N	1,124	989	729	124	136	7	22	95	11
NM	88	74	56	12	6	1	4	9	
OM	166	101	78	5	18	36	2	10	17
P	3,940	3,566	2,479	461	626	169	59	116	30
PHP	95	12	10		2	35	6	28	14
PM	369	345	251	31	63	14	3	3	4
PTH	1,511	1,287	784	266	237	61	32	90	41
R	618	579	440	55	84	5	7	18	9
RO	289	277	193	44	40	3	1	7	1
TTS	13	11	9		2	1		1	
OTH	401	151	117	3	31	95	15	113	27
UNSP	466	444	218	199	27	2	5	13	2
VM	2	2	2						
Inactive	6,503								
Not Class	4,177								

Note: Above excludes Address Unknown.

Subspecialties in this table are condensed into major specialties. See Appendix A.

Table 3.6

Physicians by Census Division, Self-Designated Specialty, and Activity, 2006, continued
Middle Atlantic

Specialty	Total Physicians	Patient Care				Other Professional Activity			
		Total Patient Care	Office Based	Hospital Based		Admin.	Med. Teach.	Research	Other
				Resid./ Fellows	Phys. Staff				
Total Physicians	156,213	121,676	86,206	22,357	13,113	2,768	1,833	2,983	786
GP/FM Prac.	9,216	8,794	6,905	1,206	683	172	185	34	31
FM	8,251	7,882	6,138	1,206	538	147	182	24	16
GP	965	912	767		145	25	3	10	15
Med. Spec.	56,002	52,127	36,073	11,073	4,981	1,082	854	1,683	256
AI	709	628	561	40	27	13	7	58	3
CD	4,400	4,112	3,287	504	321	66	60	144	18
D	1,768	1,715	1,460	186	69	7	18	26	2
GE	2,312	2,176	1,783	238	155	27	35	63	11
IM	31,299	28,995	18,956	7,333	2,706	689	449	1,012	154
PD	13,339	12,525	8,609	2,468	1,448	239	228	286	61
PDC	307	275	168	37	70	5	6	19	2
PUD	1,868	1,701	1,249	267	185	36	51	75	5
Sur. Spec.	26,577	25,800	19,594	4,385	1,821	247	236	200	94
CRS	292	285	255	16	14	1	3	2	1
GS	6,485	6,256	3,889	1,786	581	100	60	45	24
NS	761	734	520	142	72	5	8	11	3
OBG	6,987	6,762	5,268	946	548	71	82	54	18
OPH	3,237	3,160	2,793	249	118	13	22	32	10
ORS	3,638	3,562	2,681	733	148	18	17	16	25
OTO	1,473	1,442	1,164	189	89	7	16	6	2
PS	1,122	1,106	942	101	63	3	3	5	5
TS	797	753	609	55	89	15	10	17	2
U	1,785	1,740	1,473	168	99	14	15	12	4
Oth. Spec.	38,251	34,955	23,634	5,693	5,628	1,267	558	1,066	405
AM	19	14	8		6	4			1
AN	6,620	6,411	4,929	841	641	56	79	59	15
CHP	1,469	1,342	990	131	221	53	22	35	17
DR	4,018	3,878	2,599	826	453	27	40	35	38
EM	4,075	3,891	2,170	915	806	108	46	19	11
FOP	99	65	56	5	4	11		4	19
GPM	255	201	142	41	18	26	10	11	7
MG	69	54	25	15	14	1	3	10	1
N	2,785	2,487	1,808	396	283	52	58	175	13
NM	296	264	172	31	61	12	5	9	6
OM	309	186	141	5	40	94	6	10	13
P	9,092	8,337	5,462	1,168	1,707	334	132	235	54
PHP	187	50	39		11	96	10	23	8
PM	1,775	1,702	1,202	244	256	39	14	9	11
PTH	3,146	2,663	1,576	488	599	138	69	155	121
R	1,562	1,476	1,141	70	265	22	25	18	21
RO	704	684	493	91	100	5	6	8	1
TTS	27	26	20		6			1	
OTH	870	402	304	10	88	174	28	226	40
UNSP	871	819	354	416	49	15	5	24	8
VM	3	3	3						
Inactive	16,423								
Not Class	9,744								

Note: Above excludes Address Unknown.

Subspecialties in this table are condensed into major specialties. See Appendix A.

Table 3.6

Physicians by Census Division, Self-Designated Specialty, and Activity, 2006, continued
East North Central

| Specialty | Total Physicians | Patient Care | | | | Other Professional Activity | | | |
		Total Patient Care	Office Based	Resid./ Fellows	Phys. Staff	Admin.	Med. Teach.	Research	Other
Total Physicians	132,591	105,900	80,189	17,018	8,693	1,925	1,476	1,626	556
GP/FM Prac.	15,030	14,463	11,839	1,632	992	228	260	36	43
FM	13,840	13,322	10,838	1,632	852	207	257	29	25
GP	1,190	1,141	1,001		140	21	3	7	18
Med. Spec.	41,860	39,523	29,278	7,208	3,037	696	577	952	112
AI	624	581	520	46	15	8	4	29	2
CD	3,189	3,015	2,465	360	190	31	41	90	12
D	1,384	1,357	1,112	197	48	3	12	9	3
GE	1,583	1,507	1,261	165	81	11	20	43	2
IM	22,812	21,466	15,587	4,207	1,672	450	310	525	61
PD	10,610	10,068	7,181	1,995	892	154	164	198	26
PDC	306	290	185	62	43	4	4	7	1
PUD	1,352	1,239	967	176	96	35	22	51	5
Sur. Spec.	23,016	22,467	17,657	3,546	1,264	176	197	125	51
CRS	217	213	192	10	11	1	3		
GS	5,536	5,381	3,716	1,296	369	48	50	41	16
NS	836	815	598	153	64	8	8	1	4
OBG	6,057	5,883	4,754	735	394	63	70	35	6
OPH	2,533	2,481	2,195	202	84	13	14	18	7
ORS	3,375	3,324	2,585	596	143	12	20	9	10
OTO	1,400	1,375	1,117	206	52	9	12	1	3
PS	858	839	671	138	30	5	8	5	1
TS	730	704	615	38	51	7	5	11	3
U	1,474	1,452	1,214	172	66	10	7	4	1
Oth. Spec.	31,577	29,447	21,415	4,632	3,400	825	442	513	350
AM	33	20	14		6	9	1	3	
AN	6,102	5,966	4,534	881	551	30	67	27	12
CHP	878	819	643	77	99	21	25	9	4
DR	3,666	3,574	2,597	669	308	16	35	7	34
EM	4,818	4,636	3,142	845	649	107	47	18	10
FOP	88	64	59	4	1	5	2	1	16
GPM	155	125	107	11	7	15	3	9	3
MG	69	52	35	9	8		2	14	1
N	2,058	1,905	1,475	282	148	21	31	87	14
NM	206	186	137	16	33	5	5	6	4
OM	490	384	311	3	70	67	5	13	21
P	4,926	4,588	3,362	526	700	168	71	70	29
PHP	100	18	11		7	56	7	13	6
PM	1,249	1,202	880	177	145	25	6	10	6
PTH	2,976	2,549	1,784	389	376	131	79	88	129
R	1,335	1,280	1,080	66	134	13	13	8	21
RO	685	671	505	104	62	8	4	2	
TTS	25	19	17		2		2	3	1
OTH	670	370	311	14	45	122	32	115	31
UNSP	1,039	1,010	402	559	49	6	5	10	8
VM	9	9	9						
Inactive	14,393								
Not Class	6,715								

Note: Above excludes Address Unknown.

Subspecialties in this table are condensed into major specialties. See Appendix A.

Table 3.6

Physicians by Census Division, Self-Designated Specialty, and Activity, 2006, continued
West North Central

| Specialty | Total Physicians | Patient Care | | | | Other Professional Activity | | | |
| | | Total Patient Care | Office Based | Hospital Based | | Admin. | Med. Teach. | Research | Other |
				Resid./ Fellows	Phys. Staff				
Total Physicians	54,421	43,405	33,485	6,202	3,718	720	684	784	199
GP/FM Prac.	8,072	7,752	6,495	715	542	126	161	20	13
FM	7,661	7,361	6,152	715	494	114	158	18	10
GP	411	391	343		48	12	3	2	3
Med. Spec.	15,586	14,581	10,954	2,413	1,214	246	261	450	48
AI	260	238	200	33	5	2	5	13	2
CD	1,379	1,292	1,054	155	83	11	22	49	5
D	598	592	466	95	31		2	4	
GE	691	645	546	68	31	5	12	29	
IM	8,172	7,597	5,532	1,379	686	153	146	249	27
PD	3,791	3,579	2,663	586	330	61	59	79	13
PDC	120	111	81	18	12	1	1	7	
PUD	575	527	412	79	36	13	14	20	1
Sur. Spec.	9,640	9,413	7,513	1,345	555	59	94	59	15
CRS	88	88	75	8	5				
GS	2,329	2,259	1,595	480	184	20	23	22	5
NS	342	331	242	66	23	4	5	2	
OBG	2,157	2,099	1,762	216	121	12	30	14	2
OPH	1,104	1,085	957	89	39	8	6	5	
ORS	1,657	1,632	1,299	247	86	6	7	5	7
OTO	653	639	506	102	31	2	7	5	
PS	381	374	314	50	10	2	4	1	
TS	318	308	253	21	34	2	5	2	1
U	611	598	510	66	22	3	7	3	
Oth. Spec.	12,494	11,659	8,523	1,729	1,407	289	168	255	123
AM	15	11	5	1	5	3		1	
AN	2,284	2,231	1,730	324	177	15	25	11	2
CHP	393	371	284	40	47	9	4	8	1
DR	1,689	1,650	1,209	311	130	7	18	3	11
EM	1,538	1,478	960	204	314	35	21	3	1
FOP	34	25	20	2	3	1	1		7
GPM	89	66	49	8	9	9	2	10	2
MG	31	23	14	4	5		4	3	1
N	954	880	673	136	71	11	17	44	2
NM	81	71	50	5	16	3	3	3	1
OM	161	128	109	3	16	26	1	2	4
P	1,960	1,844	1,285	260	299	46	24	38	8
PHP	48	14	10		4	16	3	12	3
PM	443	435	315	52	68	5	2		1
PTH	1,300	1,141	843	182	116	34	17	55	53
R	510	486	414	25	47	1	11	4	8
RO	291	288	234	32	22		2	1	
TTS	12	11	9		2			1	
OTH	290	149	113	8	28	64	11	50	16
UNSP	371	357	197	132	28	4	2	6	2
Inactive	6,283								
Not Class	2,346								

Note: Above excludes Address Unknown.

Subspecialties in this table are condensed into major specialties. See Appendix A.

Table 3.6

Physicians by Census Division, Self-Designated Specialty, and Activity, 2006, continued
South Atlantic

Specialty	Total Physicians	Patient Care				Other Professional Activity			
		Total Patient Care	Office Based	Hospital Based		Admin.	Med. Teach.	Research	Other
				Resid./ Fellows	Phys. Staff				
Total Physicians	174,658	134,941	106,910	14,999	13,032	2,993	1,949	2,965	887
GP/FM Prac.	16,897	16,212	13,440	1,331	1,441	299	280	48	58
FM	14,877	14,284	11,781	1,331	1,172	244	272	44	33
GP	2,020	1,928	1,659		269	55	8	4	25
Med. Spec.	54,554	50,961	40,280	6,142	4,539	969	784	1,607	233
AI	793	680	604	37	39	11	11	87	4
CD	4,396	4,172	3,557	309	306	54	53	107	10
D	2,139	2,089	1,796	196	97	13	16	15	6
GE	2,496	2,393	2,109	152	132	19	27	52	5
IM	28,538	26,513	20,495	3,515	2,503	577	399	930	119
PD	13,858	12,964	10,004	1,715	1,245	263	238	311	82
PDC	352	319	233	45	41	7	9	17	
PUD	1,982	1,831	1,482	173	176	25	31	88	7
Sur. Spec.	31,166	30,303	24,993	3,241	2,069	285	304	177	97
CRS	249	246	219	12	15	2			1
GS	6,963	6,709	4,870	1,195	644	92	82	49	31
NS	1,063	1,030	816	139	75	8	8	9	8
OBG	8,386	8,123	6,873	726	524	85	118	37	23
OPH	3,522	3,434	3,064	208	162	17	22	40	9
ORS	4,508	4,428	3,641	506	281	29	33	11	7
OTO	1,945	1,910	1,620	188	102	12	14	5	4
PS	1,470	1,443	1,284	101	58	7	11	5	4
TS	910	886	761	49	76	12	4	7	1
U	2,150	2,094	1,845	117	132	21	12	14	9
Oth. Spec.	41,118	37,465	28,197	4,285	4,983	1,440	581	1,133	499
AM	119	70	31	2	37	40	2	4	3
AN	7,376	7,180	5,713	727	740	56	85	43	12
CHP	1,352	1,263	1,012	97	154	40	29	17	3
DR	4,588	4,459	3,407	608	444	27	40	22	40
EM	5,921	5,709	4,182	619	908	124	57	15	16
FOP	151	112	93	9	10	10	3	2	24
GPM	676	487	325	63	99	79	12	74	24
MG	99	76	47	14	15	4	7	12	
N	2,757	2,510	2,031	261	218	43	36	159	9
NM	248	220	147	17	56	8	4	13	3
OM	432	275	213	4	58	108	8	17	24
P	7,271	6,688	4,877	693	1,118	262	114	155	52
PHP	505	74	49		25	250	19	141	21
PM	1,148	1,106	851	122	133	21	7	13	1
PTH	3,556	2,989	2,120	410	459	137	79	183	168
R	1,697	1,593	1,306	86	201	14	38	23	29
RO	866	843	706	83	54	12	5	4	2
TTS	28	24	16		8	1	1	2	
OTH	982	500	394	1	105	186	28	209	59
UNSP	1,342	1,283	674	469	140	18	7	25	9
VM	4	4	3		1				
Inactive	23,224								
Not Class	7,699								

Note: Above excludes Address Unknown.

Subspecialties in this table are condensed into major specialties. See Appendix A.

Table 3.6

Physicians by Census Division, Self-Designated Specialty, and Activity, 2006, continued
East South Central

Specialty	Total Physicians	Patient Care				Other Professional Activity			
		Total Patient Care	Office Based	Resid./ Fellows	Phys. Staff	Admin.	Med. Teach.	Research	Other
Total Physicians	45,503	37,255	29,943	4,561	2,751	571	464	476	180
GP/FM Prac.	5,433	5,259	4,502	414	343	84	76	5	9
FM	4,865	4,701	4,000	414	287	77	76	4	7
GP	568	558	502		56	7		1	2
Med. Spec.	14,059	13,363	10,620	1,819	924	175	181	307	33
AI	209	192	175	11	6	2	2	10	3
CD	1,141	1,093	945	97	51	9	15	21	3
D	451	446	400	34	12	1	1	3	
GE	623	601	526	45	30	3	7	12	
IM	7,299	6,923	5,346	1,031	546	95	92	170	19
PD	3,626	3,446	2,687	537	222	54	54	66	6
PDC	85	76	64	6	6	1		8	
PUD	625	586	477	58	51	10	10	17	2
Sur. Spec.	9,186	8,997	7,494	1,084	419	60	79	25	25
CRS	50	48	45		3		1	1	
GS	2,241	2,188	1,628	430	130	17	24	4	8
NS	353	350	297	42	11		2		1
OBG	2,310	2,249	1,932	219	98	20	28	11	2
OPH	893	879	798	58	23	5	5	4	
ORS	1,403	1,385	1,118	186	81	4	4	2	8
OTO	630	623	546	54	23		3	2	2
PS	367	364	323	33	8		3		
TS	315	301	269	13	19	6	4	1	3
U	624	610	538	49	23	8	5		1
Oth. Spec.	10,268	9,636	7,327	1,244	1,065	252	128	139	113
AM	23	18	14		4	4		1	
AN	2,065	2,011	1,605	242	164	19	26	6	3
CHP	279	260	213	18	29	4	8	5	2
DR	1,325	1,294	985	222	87	8	7	4	12
EM	1,384	1,348	989	135	224	20	8	5	3
FOP	40	26	22		4				14
GPM	72	58	46	8	4	9	3	1	1
MG	25	18	10	3	5	3		4	
N	709	654	539	74	41	9	17	26	3
NM	57	53	40	8	5	1		3	
OM	130	92	80	1	11	28	2	4	4
P	1,558	1,473	1,039	199	235	40	18	18	9
PHP	54	15	13		2	28	2	5	4
PM	267	257	205	25	27	8			2
PTH	1,022	916	667	143	106	22	17	28	39
R	458	435	384	9	42	4	8	1	10
RO	232	228	184	23	21		1	3	
TTS	7	7	6		1				
OTH	241	163	135	1	27	43	7	23	5
UNSP	320	310	151	133	26	2	4	2	2
Inactive	4,865								
Not Class	1,692								

Note: Above excludes Address Unknown.

Subspecialties in this table are condensed into major specialties. See Appendix A.

Table 3.6

Physicians by Census Division, Self-Designated Specialty, and Activity, 2006, continued
West South Central

Specialty	Total Physicians	Patient Care				Other Professional Activity			
		Total Patient Care	Office Based	Hospital Based		Admin.	Med. Teach.	Research	Other
				Resid./ Fellows	Phys. Staff				
Total Physicians	81,189	66,189	52,538	8,769	4,882	1,000	1,098	806	280
GP/FM Prac.	9,987	9,663	8,054	1,044	565	119	162	20	23
FM	8,965	8,659	7,150	1,044	465	112	160	17	17
GP	1,022	1,004	904		100	7	2	3	6
Med. Spec.	24,344	23,050	18,072	3,354	1,624	312	440	488	54
AI	429	396	357	23	16	5	4	24	
CD	2,096	2,000	1,665	214	121	18	27	46	5
D	978	966	784	140	42	5	6	1	
GE	1,118	1,066	906	103	57	11	19	22	
IM	11,874	11,182	8,550	1,756	876	174	218	276	24
PD	6,800	6,456	5,001	1,031	424	83	141	100	20
PDC	175	169	144	15	10	2		3	1
PUD	874	815	665	72	78	14	25	16	4
Sur. Spec.	15,871	15,447	12,684	1,938	825	126	216	53	29
CRS	153	146	130	8	8		4	2	1
GS	3,511	3,401	2,468	686	247	43	46	13	8
NS	552	541	444	67	30	4	5	1	1
OBG	4,261	4,123	3,508	434	181	32	88	14	4
OPH	1,678	1,636	1,424	128	84	15	22	4	1
ORS	2,376	2,337	1,891	324	122	10	16	4	9
OTO	1,057	1,034	871	117	46	10	11	2	
PS	712	699	602	70	27	2	7	1	3
TS	505	487	448	15	24	3	7	7	1
U	1,066	1,043	898	89	56	7	10	5	1
Oth. Spec.	19,171	18,029	13,728	2,433	1,868	443	280	245	174
AM	103	60	39	2	19	31	2	6	4
AN	4,246	4,153	3,332	504	317	28	45	14	6
CHP	590	552	435	61	56	14	12	10	2
DR	2,329	2,276	1,684	387	205	4	25	4	20
EM	2,468	2,393	1,784	295	314	38	27	3	7
FOP	66	52	47	5		2			12
GPM	152	130	89	23	18	15	2	4	1
MG	54	39	26	7	6	5	6	4	
N	1,223	1,159	937	138	84	8	22	30	4
NM	123	112	86	10	16	4	3	4	
OM	228	172	144	3	25	46	5	2	3
P	2,847	2,654	1,914	364	376	83	48	36	26
PHP	83	23	14	1	8	38	5	15	2
PM	687	668	516	95	57	10	3	4	2
PTH	1,862	1,691	1,226	269	196	43	32	42	54
R	806	758	650	28	80	4	24	6	14
RO	399	392	327	37	28	4	2	1	
TTS	17	17	16		1				
OTH	388	241	214		27	64	15	53	15
UNSP	497	484	245	204	35	2	2	7	2
VM	3	3	3						
Inactive	8,153								
Not Class	3,663								

Note: Above excludes Address Unknown.

Subspecialties in this table are condensed into major specialties. See Appendix A.

Table 3.6

Physicians by Census Division, Self-Designated Specialty, and Activity, 2006, continued
Mountain

Specialty	Total Physicians	Patient Care		Hospital Based		Other Professional Activity			
		Total Patient Care	Office Based	Resid./ Fellows	Phys. Staff	Admin.	Med. Teach.	Research	Other
Total Physicians	52,817	41,400	34,340	3,535	3,525	800	504	563	262
GP/FM Prac.	6,679	6,463	5,495	471	497	93	93	11	19
FM	6,191	5,996	5,072	471	453	79	91	11	14
GP	488	467	423		44	14	2		5
Med. Spec.	14,543	13,706	11,150	1,395	1,161	265	198	319	55
AI	230	212	188	13	11	2	1	14	1
CD	1,078	1,022	888	65	69	10	14	29	3
D	614	593	534	39	20	2	6	11	2
GE	652	628	550	45	33	7	7	9	1
IM	7,531	7,092	5,646	770	676	150	95	161	33
PD	3,716	3,510	2,803	407	300	78	59	54	15
PDC	95	85	70	11	4	2	5	3	
PUD	627	564	471	45	48	14	11	38	
Sur. Spec.	9,344	9,139	7,884	727	528	66	72	35	32
CRS	57	56	50	2	4				1
GS	2,124	2,074	1,601	302	171	25	13	5	7
NS	333	329	276	42	11	1	1	2	
OBG	2,414	2,349	2,053	167	129	21	20	18	6
OPH	969	956	872	31	53	5	5	3	
ORS	1,610	1,578	1,380	106	92	4	11	5	12
OTO	553	539	488	29	22	3	10	1	
PS	435	431	405	11	15	1	2		1
TS	257	250	233	6	11	1	4	1	1
U	592	577	526	31	20	5	6		4
Oth. Spec.	12,963	12,092	9,811	942	1,339	376	141	198	156
AM	49	28	19		9	15	2	2	2
AN	2,825	2,771	2,428	151	192	10	30	9	5
CHP	421	395	328	24	43	12	5	8	1
DR	1,432	1,388	1,106	124	158	9	10	5	20
EM	2,220	2,148	1,660	172	316	46	16	2	8
FOP	42	37	36		1				5
GPM	116	93	79	5	9	13		7	3
MG	25	20	12	3	5			5	
N	723	664	565	57	42	9	16	32	2
NM	44	41	33	2	6	1		1	1
OM	189	141	123	1	17	34	3	4	7
P	2,027	1,881	1,406	162	313	72	24	30	20
PHP	70	14	12		2	34		18	4
PM	467	451	392	26	33	8	2	3	3
PTH	969	844	662	88	94	28	16	30	51
R	525	498	437	18	43	9	10	3	5
RO	250	247	216	18	13	1		1	1
TTS	3	3	3						
OTH	315	184	162	1	21	74	5	36	16
UNSP	250	243	131	90	22	1	2	2	2
VM	1	1	1						
Inactive	7,516								
Not Class	1,772								

Note: Above excludes Address Unknown.

Subspecialties in this table are condensed into major specialties. See Appendix A.

Table 3.6

Physicians by Census Division, Self-Designated Specialty, and Activity, 2006, continued
Pacific

Specialty	Total Physicians	Patient Care				Other Professional Activity			
		Total Patient Care	Office Based	Hospital Based		Admin.	Med. Teach.	Research	Other
				Resid./ Fellows	Phys. Staff				
Total Physicians	148,307	114,176	94,135	10,938	9,103	2,400	1,435	2,465	846
GP/FM Prac.	16,053	15,498	13,411	1,125	962	258	181	52	64
FM	13,857	13,378	11,469	1,125	784	216	177	43	43
GP	2,196	2,120	1,942		178	42	4	9	21
Med. Spec.	44,041	41,159	33,852	4,313	2,994	776	539	1,384	183
AI	663	576	513	22	41	12	5	66	4
CD	2,912	2,690	2,315	168	207	33	56	125	8
D	1,993	1,944	1,724	124	96	12	11	23	3
GE	1,771	1,664	1,445	121	98	25	23	56	3
IM	23,696	22,055	17,967	2,440	1,648	444	264	822	111
PD	11,282	10,657	8,600	1,293	764	217	150	209	49
PDC	281	262	202	33	27	4	3	12	
PUD	1,443	1,311	1,086	112	113	29	27	71	5
Sur. Spec.	25,001	24,280	20,546	2,262	1,472	228	236	158	99
CRS	153	147	131	7	9	4	2		
GS	5,464	5,292	3,989	893	410	71	54	27	20
NS	829	800	652	96	52	5	8	8	8
OBG	6,600	6,389	5,586	456	347	72	79	50	10
OPH	2,865	2,802	2,556	105	141	17	21	23	2
ORS	3,985	3,868	3,294	356	218	23	28	18	48
OTO	1,616	1,583	1,353	144	86	18	11	2	2
PS	1,318	1,293	1,154	87	52	5	9	4	7
TS	673	650	571	27	52	3	8	12	
U	1,498	1,456	1,260	91	105	10	16	14	2
Oth. Spec.	36,227	33,239	26,326	3,238	3,675	1,138	479	871	500
AM	79	53	31		22	21		3	2
AN	6,895	6,677	5,571	530	576	50	99	49	20
CHP	1,117	1,049	907	65	77	31	18	15	4
DR	3,674	3,539	2,764	437	338	28	42	22	43
EM	5,383	5,183	3,973	476	734	121	53	10	16
FOP	102	65	59	1	5	6	3	2	26
GPM	462	371	293	30	48	45	5	26	15
MG	107	65	47	8	10	7	2	31	2
N	2,077	1,861	1,571	134	156	28	35	133	20
NM	300	272	208	18	46	7	3	12	6
OM	495	379	327	7	45	74	7	20	15
P	7,259	6,719	5,229	578	912	239	82	147	72
PHP	262	68	55		13	113	15	42	24
PM	1,120	1,072	861	94	117	29	7	6	6
PTH	2,699	2,272	1,727	272	273	111	53	127	136
R	1,306	1,234	1,049	55	130	14	29	13	16
RO	684	663	544	74	45	4	6	11	
TTS	19	19	18		1				
OTH	938	490	443		47	197	16	177	58
UNSP	1,247	1,187	648	459	80	13	4	24	19
VM	2	1	1					1	
Inactive	20,119								
Not Class	6,866								

Note: Above excludes Address Unknown.

Subspecialties in this table are condensed into major specialties. See Appendix A.

Table 3.6

Physicians by Census Division, Self-Designated Specialty, and Activity, 2006, continued
Possessions

Specialty	Total Physicians	Patient Care				Other Professional Activity			
		Total Patient Care	Office Based	Hospital Based		Admin.	Med. Teach.	Research	Other
				Resid./ Fellows	Phys. Staff				
Total Physicians	13,367	10,431	8,031	850	1,550	242	140	54	57
GP/FM Prac.	2,437	2,356	1,917	45	394	48	20	3	10
FM	1,077	1,035	820	45	170	25	14	1	2
GP	1,360	1,321	1,097		224	23	6	2	8
Med. Spec.	3,507	3,339	2,470	399	470	69	64	24	11
AI	17	17	15	1	1				
CD	229	217	183	15	19	1	7	3	1
D	102	99	78	8	13	1	1	1	
GE	117	113	93	10	10		2	2	
IM	1,736	1,667	1,154	285	228	29	25	10	5
PD	1,194	1,124	862	79	183	38	22	5	5
PDC	19	19	14		5				
PUD	93	83	71	1	11		7	3	
Sur. Spec.	1,773	1,718	1,364	129	225	24	23	3	5
CRS	9	9	6		3				
GS	460	443	310	56	77	7	8		2
NS	27	26	19	6	1		1		
OBG	633	609	502	33	74	12	8	2	2
OPH	183	180	164	3	13	2		1	
ORS	171	166	123	24	19	1	3		1
OTO	96	93	81	3	9	1	2		
PS	41	41	35	2	4				
TS	24	24	18	1	5				
U	129	127	106	1	20	1	1		
Oth. Spec.	3,207	3,018	2,280	277	461	101	33	24	31
AM	23	15	4		11	5		2	1
AN	241	232	180	17	35	4	3	1	1
CHP	82	77	54	5	18	1	3		1
DR	201	187	131	22	34	5	4	1	4
EM	230	214	117	29	68	14	2		
FOP	6	6	3		3				
GPM	52	44	24	8	12	5	1	1	1
MG	2	1	1					1	
N	144	136	95	20	21	1	3	3	1
NM	34	30	24	2	4	2	1		1
OM	41	33	24		9	7			1
P	505	475	334	51	90	13	7	5	5
PHP	30	9	5		4	13	1	2	5
PM	211	208	161	28	19	2	1		
PTH	130	111	76	10	25	9	3	1	6
R	69	67	53	3	11		1	1	
RO	24	21	17		4	2		1	
OTH	73	52	42	1	9	15	3	3	
UNSP	1,109	1,100	935	81	84	3		2	4
Inactive	865								
Not Class	1,578								

Note: Above excludes Address Unknown.

Subspecialties in this table are condensed into major specialties. See Appendix A.

Table 3.7

Physicians by State, Self-Designated Specialty, and Activity, 2006
Alabama

| Specialty | Total Physicians | Patient Care | | Hospital Based | | Other Professional Activity | | | |
		Total Patient Care	Office Based	Resid./ Fellows	Phys. Staff	Admin.	Med. Teach.	Research	Other
Total Physicians	10,994	9,091	7,250	1,194	647	129	92	133	43
GP/FM Prac.	1,335	1,308	1,073	148	87	15	12		
FM	1,207	1,182	959	148	75	13	12		
GP	128	126	114		12	2			
Med. Prac.	3,449	3,269	2,569	482	218	45	41	86	8
AI	46	38	36	2		1	1	6	
CD	295	283	247	20	16	1	1	10	
D	118	117	105	12				1	
GE	159	154	131	16	7		3	2	
IM	1,857	1,739	1,318	289	132	33	25	53	7
PD	820	790	609	127	54	8	9	12	1
PDC	14	14	13		1				
PUD	140	134	110	16	8	2	2	2	
Sur. Spec.	2,275	2,234	1,901	236	97	10	17	7	7
CRS	15	15	14		1				
GS	539	524	400	93	31	5	5		5
NS	74	74	67	5	2				
OBG	563	546	476	48	22	3	8	5	1
OPH	218	217	196	16	5			1	
ORS	367	367	295	52	20				
OTO	185	183	168	11	4			1	1
PS	81	80	76	3	1		1		
TS	81	79	69	3	7		2		
U	152	149	140	5	4	2	1		
Oth. Spec.	2,429	2,280	1,707	328	245	59	22	40	28
AM	8	5	4		1	2		1	
AN	474	462	376	51	35	7	3	1	1
CHP	70	67	53	5	9	1	1	1	
DR	326	318	235	63	20	1		2	5
EM	279	272	198	26	48	4	1	2	
FOP	15	8	7		1				7
GPM	19	15	12		3	3		1	
MG	6	3	1	2		1		2	
N	187	178	139	28	11		3	6	
NM	10	9	6	3				1	
OM	29	22	17		5	6	1		
P	350	330	238	37	55	10	4	4	2
PHP	11	1	1			6		2	2
PM	73	71	49	15	7	2			
PTH	235	218	154	42	22	3	3	7	4
R	119	108	95	5	8	3	3		5
RO	61	59	50	8	1			2	
OTH	68	47	37		10	10	2	7	2
UNSP	89	87	35	43	9		1	1	
Not Class	405								
Inactive	1,101								

Note: Excludes Address Unknown.

Subspecialties in this table are condensed into major specialties. See Appendix A.

Table 3.7

Physicians by State, Self-Designated Specialty, and Activity, 2006, continued
Alaska

| Specialty | Total Physicians | Patient Care | | | | Other Professional Activity | | | |
| | | Total Patient Care | Office Based | Hospital Based | | Admin. | Med. Teach. | Research | Other |
				Resid./ Fellows	Phys. Staff				
Total Physicians	1,697	1,437	1,165	43	229	36	13	14	10
GP/FM Prac.	394	381	295	25	61	7	4	2	
FM	364	352	268	25	59	6	4	2	
GP	30	29	27		2	1			
Med. Prac.	356	342	282	4	56	6	3	3	2
AI	6	6	2		4				
CD	23	23	21		2				
D	10	10	9		1				
GE	11	11	9		2				
IM	173	168	132	4	32		2	1	2
PD	122	113	101		12	6	1	2	
PDC	1	1	1						
PUD	10	10	7		3				
Sur. Spec.	340	332	276	5	51	1	2	3	2
CRS	1	1	1						
GS	77	74	56		18	1	1		1
NS	7	7	7						
OBG	84	83	77	2	4		1		
OPH	29	29	25	1	3				
ORS	77	74	56	1	17			2	1
OTO	32	32	25	1	6				
PS	7	6	6					1	
TS	4	4	3		1				
U	22	22	20		2				
Oth. Spec.	420	382	312	9	61	22	4	6	6
AM	6	4	2		2	2			
AN	85	82	70	2	10	1	2		
CHP	9	8	7		1			1	
DR	43	41	33	1	7	1			1
EM	91	88	68	3	17	3			
GPM	9	7	5		2	1		1	
N	13	13	12		1				
OM	5	3	3			1		1	
P	83	76	64		12	5		1	1
PHP	8	1	1			4		1	2
PM	13	13	12		1				
PTH	23	19	12		7		1	1	2
R	11	10	9		1		1		
RO	6	6	6						
OTH	6	2	2			4			
UNSP	9	9	6	3					
Not Class	37								
Inactive	150								

Note: Excludes Address Unknown.

Subspecialties in this table are condensed into major specialties. See Appendix A.

Table 3.7

Physicians by State, Self-Designated Specialty, and Activity, 2006, continued
Arizona

Specialty	Total Physicians	Patient Care				Other Professional Activity			
		Total Patient Care	Office Based	Hospital Based		Admin.	Med. Teach.	Research	Other
				Resid./ Fellows	Phys. Staff				
Total Physicians	15,127	11,622	9,667	998	957	231	154	134	61
GP/FM Prac.	1,525	1,468	1,269	100	99	28	23	4	2
FM	1,371	1,321	1,135	100	86	22	23	4	1
GP	154	147	134		13	6			1
Med. Prac.	4,442	4,222	3,428	422	372	77	63	67	13
AI	54	54	51	1	2				
CD	353	339	296	24	19	2	3	7	2
D	194	190	171	12	7		2	2	
GE	215	210	182	17	11	1	2	2	
IM	2,282	2,159	1,729	217	213	43	31	41	8
PD	1,116	1,058	816	138	104	25	20	10	3
PDC	30	28	25		3		2		
PUD	198	184	158	13	13	6	3	5	
Sur. Spec.	2,559	2,500	2,146	221	133	18	19	15	7
CRS	23	23	22		1				
GS	607	591	440	106	45	5	6	3	2
NS	94	94	71	19	4				
OBG	681	660	561	61	38	9	3	9	
OPH	276	272	254	6	12	2	1	1	
ORS	370	362	328	18	16	1	2	2	3
OTO	126	124	117	1	6		2		
PS	136	136	130	2	4				
TS	80	78	75	1	2		2		
U	166	160	148	7	5	1	3		2
Oth. Spec.	3,676	3,432	2,824	255	353	108	49	48	39
AM	6	3	3			1		2	
AN	865	849	763	29	57	4	10	1	1
CHP	103	98	86	5	7	1	1	2	1
DR	429	414	328	44	42	5	4	2	4
EM	559	536	414	56	66	11	8	1	3
FOP	11	10	10						1
GPM	27	21	21			2		3	1
MG	4	3	3					1	
N	241	224	188	21	15	2	7	8	
NM	18	16	14		2	1			1
OM	44	32	30		2	11		1	
P	574	535	394	43	98	20	9	6	4
PHP	17	3	3			8		5	1
PM	100	97	88	2	7	2		1	
PTH	249	220	175	19	26	7	4	5	13
R	178	168	144	10	14	5	3		2
RO	74	74	64	5	5				
TTS	1	1	1						
OTH	107	62	57		5	27	2	9	7
UNSP	68	65	37	21	7	1	1	1	
VM	1	1	1						
Not Class	595								
Inactive	2,330								

Note: Excludes Address Unknown.

Subspecialties in this table are condensed into major specialties. See Appendix A.

Table 3.7

Physicians by State, Self-Designated Specialty, and Activity, 2006, continued
Arkansas

| Specialty | Total Physicians | Patient Care | | | | Other Professional Activity | | | |
		Total Patient Care	Office Based	Resid./ Fellows	Phys. Staff	Admin.	Med. Teach.	Research	Other
Total Physicians	6,464	5,316	4,216	651	449	57	97	48	22
GP/FM Prac.	1,237	1,197	983	140	74	6	30	1	3
FM	1,128	1,089	887	140	62	6	30	1	2
GP	109	108	96		12				1
Med. Prac.	1,678	1,594	1,251	209	134	21	35	24	4
AI	26	25	25					1	
CD	162	155	125	13	17	2	1	4	
D	71	70	56	12	2	1			
GE	79	75	65	2	8	1	2	1	
IM	766	731	564	101	66	10	14	9	2
PD	496	468	359	75	34	4	15	8	1
PDC	11	11	10		1				
PUD	67	59	47	6	6	3	3	1	1
Sur. Spec.	1,170	1,153	983	107	63	4	9	3	1
CRS	6	6	6						
GS	279	270	207	39	24	3	3	2	1
NS	48	48	40	6	2				
OBG	267	264	238	17	9		3		
OPH	134	132	113	8	11		2		
ORS	185	184	159	23	2		1		
OTO	89	89	70	11	8				
PS	34	33	32		1			1	
TS	40	40	38		2				
U	88	87	80	3	4	1			
Oth. Spec.	1,455	1,372	999	195	178	26	23	20	14
AM	1					1			
AN	300	294	203	58	33	2	2	2	
CHP	41	37	27	3	7	1	2	1	
DR	192	186	135	32	19		5		1
EM	186	181	123	23	35	1	3		1
FOP	4	4	4						
GPM	8	7	4	1	2	1			
MG	3	2	1		1	1			
N	89	83	66	11	6		3	2	1
NM	13	13	10	1	2				
OM	10	10	8	1	1				
P	227	211	146	27	38	5	4	6	1
PHP	6	1	1			4		1	
PM	55	52	36	9	7		1	2	
PTH	150	136	98	24	14	2	2	4	6
R	83	80	73	3	4	1	1		1
RO	26	26	26						
OTH	35	24	19		5	7		1	3
UNSP	26	25	19	2	4			1	
Not Class	163								
Inactive	761								

Note: Excludes Address Unknown.

Subspecialties in this table are condensed into major specialties. See Appendix A.

Table 3.7

Physicians by State, Self-Designated Specialty, and Activity, 2006, continued
California

| Specialty | Total Physicians | Patient Care | | | | Other Professional Activity | | | |
| | | Total Patient Care | Office Based | Hospital Based | | Admin. | Med. Teach. | Research | Other |
				Resid./ Fellows	Phys. Staff				
Total Physicians	110,406	84,907	70,083	8,465	6,359	1,764	1,036	1,856	625
GP/FM Prac.	10,873	10,524	9,139	810	575	161	107	32	49
FM	9,110	8,822	7,579	810	433	131	104	24	29
GP	1,763	1,702	1,560		142	30	3	8	20
Med. Prac.	33,679	31,476	25,991	3,394	2,091	594	408	1,054	147
AI	524	453	405	20	28	7	5	56	3
CD	2,286	2,103	1,821	139	143	28	44	104	7
D	1,567	1,532	1,359	103	70	10	8	16	1
GE	1,334	1,250	1,069	104	77	19	19	44	2
IM	17,928	16,684	13,697	1,866	1,121	335	199	621	89
PD	8,723	8,251	6,645	1,050	556	171	113	148	40
PDC	223	207	157	29	21	4	1	11	
PUD	1,094	996	838	83	75	20	19	54	5
Sur. Spec.	18,664	18,124	15,367	1,713	1,044	177	177	119	67
CRS	116	111	97	5	9	4	1		
GS	4,013	3,888	2,962	649	277	49	40	21	15
NS	596	578	463	79	36	4	6	4	4
OBG	4,977	4,818	4,196	361	261	60	54	36	9
OPH	2,177	2,122	1,930	80	112	14	18	21	2
ORS	2,918	2,839	2,433	269	137	16	22	13	28
OTO	1,157	1,131	976	104	51	15	7	2	2
PS	1,085	1,064	951	73	40	5	8	3	5
TS	536	517	454	22	41	2	8	9	
U	1,089	1,056	905	71	80	8	13	10	2
Oth. Spec.	26,972	24,783	19,586	2,548	2,649	832	344	651	362
AM	45	29	17		12	12		2	2
AN	5,114	4,957	4,121	413	423	36	66	38	17
CHP	840	790	687	49	54	23	12	14	1
DR	2,643	2,543	1,957	339	247	19	32	17	32
EM	3,879	3,738	2,822	415	501	83	38	7	13
FOP	78	51	46		5	4	2		21
GPM	314	253	204	22	27	31	5	12	13
MG	80	52	37	7	8	6	1	20	1
N	1,565	1,396	1,186	97	113	24	25	109	11
NM	237	216	164	13	39	6	2	8	5
OM	349	269	238	5	26	50	5	16	9
P	5,626	5,223	4,113	440	670	181	57	113	52
PHP	177	42	33		9	90	9	22	14
PM	798	769	612	73	84	17	4	4	4
PTH	2,029	1,708	1,299	208	201	90	42	96	93
R	996	935	796	35	104	13	24	9	15
RO	507	491	394	63	34	3	4	9	
TTS	15	15	15						
OTH	686	362	327		35	134	12	132	46
UNSP	992	943	517	369	57	10	4	22	13
VM	2	1	1					1	
Not Class	5,488								
Inactive	14,730								

Note: Excludes Address Unknown.

Subspecialties in this table are condensed into major specialties. See Appendix A.

Table 3.7

Physicians by State, Self-Designated Specialty, and Activity, 2006, continued
Colorado

Specialty	Total Physicians	Patient Care				Other Professional Activity			
		Total Patient Care	Office Based	Hospital Based		Admin.	Med. Teach.	Research	Other
				Resid./ Fellows	Phys. Staff				
Total Physicians	14,175	11,180	9,225	1,066	889	246	153	211	70
GP/FM Prac.	1,796	1,729	1,470	143	116	32	26	3	6
FM	1,701	1,636	1,383	143	110	30	26	3	6
GP	95	93	87		6	2			
Med. Prac.	3,930	3,648	2,956	428	264	72	60	132	18
AI	105	92	73	12	7	1	1	10	1
CD	248	235	204	17	14	3	4	6	
D	159	153	131	15	7	1		4	1
GE	160	155	132	13	10	1	1	3	
IM	2,018	1,874	1,498	226	150	36	29	67	12
PD	1,027	956	773	121	62	27	17	23	4
PDC	28	23	15	8		1	3	1	
PUD	185	160	130	16	14	2	5	18	
Sur. Spec.	2,544	2,477	2,107	218	152	22	27	10	8
CRS	14	13	12	1					1
GS	580	564	428	99	37	10	4		2
NS	84	81	74	4	3	1	1	1	
OBG	660	646	553	49	44	5	5	4	
OPH	272	266	237	12	17	2	2	2	
ORS	451	440	381	29	30	1	6	2	2
OTO	166	159	139	11	9		7		
PS	109	108	103	1	4				1
TS	53	51	46	2	3	1		1	
U	155	149	134	10	5	2	2		2
Oth. Spec.	3,590	3,326	2,692	277	357	120	40	66	38
AM	23	12	10		2	9	2		
AN	728	710	620	37	53	3	11	3	1
CHP	146	138	111	9	18	3	2	3	
DR	345	336	258	32	46	3	2	1	3
EM	646	627	483	55	89	13	3	1	2
FOP	8	6	6						2
GPM	50	37	32	2	3	9		3	1
MG	10	8	5	2	1			2	
N	159	144	125	13	6	2	3	9	1
NM	12	12	7	1	4				
OM	68	54	49		5	8	1	2	3
P	599	556	449	41	66	21	2	13	7
PHP	26	4	3		1	15		6	1
PM	156	147	126	13	8	4	2	1	2
PTH	270	238	181	28	29	9	5	8	10
R	128	121	104	4	13		4	2	1
RO	58	57	48	7	2	1			
TTS	1	1	1						
OTH	77	39	35		4	20	2	12	4
UNSP	80	79	39	33	7		1		
Not Class	436								
Inactive	1,879								

Note: Excludes Address Unknown.

Subspecialties in this table are condensed into major specialties. See Appendix A.

Table 3.7

Physicians by State, Self-Designated Specialty, and Activity, 2006, continued
Connecticut

Specialty	Total Physicians	Patient Care				Other Professional Activity			
		Total Patient Care	Office Based	Hospital Based		Admin.	Med. Teach.	Research	Other
				Resid./ Fellows	Phys. Staff				
Total Physicians	14,488	11,224	8,339	1,809	1,076	296	186	334	78
GP/FM Prac.	602	577	492	51	34	12	9	3	1
FM	545	521	439	51	31	11	9	3	1
GP	57	56	53		3	1			
Med. Prac.	5,370	4,965	3,621	909	435	110	95	181	19
AI	76	64	56	5	3	1	1	8	2
CD	374	356	292	36	28	8	4	5	1
D	189	184	162	14	8			5	
GE	232	219	184	22	13	1	5	7	
IM	3,131	2,870	1,980	631	259	73	62	115	11
PD	1,137	1,069	793	171	105	21	13	29	5
PDC	24	23	17	6			1		
PUD	207	180	137	24	19	6	9	12	
Sur. Spec.	2,512	2,443	1,978	352	113	26	16	19	8
CRS	25	24	23	1				1	
GS	568	544	355	154	35	8	7	5	4
NS	82	80	64	10	6		1	1	
OBG	710	691	567	85	39	10	3	6	
OPH	306	298	277	11	10	2	1	3	2
ORS	372	367	312	47	8	1	2	1	1
OTO	144	142	119	14	9	1		1	
PS	94	93	81	10	2	1			
TS	65	61	56	3	2	3	1		
U	146	143	124	17	2		1	1	1
Oth. Spec.	3,634	3,239	2,248	497	494	148	66	131	50
AM	4	2	2			2			
AN	568	548	423	75	50	5	12	2	1
CHP	169	157	124	14	19	4	3	5	
DR	401	383	290	67	26	5	6	1	6
EM	408	387	182	83	122	17	3	1	
FOP	5	2	1		1	1			2
GPM	30	26	20	6		1	1	2	
MG	12	6	5	1		2		4	
N	210	191	152	24	15		3	14	2
NM	28	22	17	5			3	3	
OM	56	33	24	2	7	12	2	3	6
P	937	833	573	104	156	48	12	39	5
PHP	15	2	2			4	1	5	3
PM	83	76	65	2	9	3	1		3
PTH	341	284	168	59	57	18	11	17	11
R	124	116	98	6	12	1	4	2	1
RO	67	62	48	9	5	1		4	
TTS	4	3	3					1	
OTH	98	39	28		11	22	3	24	10
UNSP	74	67	23	40	4	2	1	4	
Not Class	783								
Inactive	1,587								

Note: Excludes Address Unknown.

Subspecialties in this table are condensed into major specialties. See Appendix A.

Table 3.7

Physicians by State, Self-Designated Specialty, and Activity, 2006, continued
Delaware

Specialty	Total Physicians	Patient Care		Hospital Based		Other Professional Activity			
		Total Patient Care	Office Based	Resid./ Fellows	Phys. Staff	Admin.	Med. Teach.	Research	Other
Total Physicians	2,414	1,927	1,521	212	194	38	20	25	12
GP/FM Prac.	250	237	187	25	25	7	5	1	
FM	234	222	177	25	20	7	4	1	
GP	16	15	10		5		1		
Med. Prac.	770	739	581	88	70	9	6	12	4
AI	8	7	7					1	
CD	61	60	55	1	4		1		
D	18	18	16	1	1				
GE	30	29	27		2			1	
IM	362	347	275	44	28	5	2	6	2
PD	256	246	175	39	32	3	3	2	2
PDC	7	6	2	3	1			1	
PUD	28	26	24		2	1		1	
Sur. Spec.	439	428	363	35	30	6	3	2	
CRS	4	4	4						
GS	114	109	85	17	7	4		1	
NS	15	14	11	2	1		1		
OBG	102	98	75	11	12	2	2		
OPH	43	43	41	1	1				
ORS	70	69	66		3			1	
OTO	23	23	17	3	3				
PS	24	24	24						
TS	14	14	13		1				
U	30	30	27	1	2				
Oth. Spec.	563	523	390	64	69	16	6	10	8
AN	90	87	71	4	12	2	1		
CHP	19	18	12	2	4	1			
DR	67	63	50	11	2	1		1	2
EM	92	89	55	23	11	3			
FOP	5	4	2		2		1		
GPM	4	2	1		1	1		1	
MG	3	2	1		1		1		
N	32	32	28		4				
NM	5	5	4	1					
OM	13	9	6		3	4			
P	92	90	65	10	15		1	1	
PHP	3	1	1			1		1	
PM	29	29	27		2				
PTH	38	35	29	1	5	1	1		1
R	26	22	17	1	4		1	1	2
RO	12	12	11		1				
OTH	14	5	5			2		4	3
UNSP	19	18	5	11	2			1	
Not Class	111								
Inactive	281								

Note: Excludes Address Unknown.

Subspecialties in this table are condensed into major specialties. See Appendix A.

Table 3.7

Physicians by State, Self-Designated Specialty, and Activity, 2006, continued
District of Columbia

| Specialty | Total Physicians | Patient Care | | Hospital Based | | Other Professional Activity | | | |
		Total Patient Care	Office Based	Resid./ Fellows	Phys. Staff	Admin.	Med. Teach.	Research	Other
Total Physicians	5,023	3,710	2,196	968	546	201	115	159	38
GP/FM Prac.	216	198	132	23	43	11	5	1	1
FM	183	168	112	23	33	9	5	1	
GP	33	30	20		10	2			1
Med. Prac.	1,805	1,592	923	439	230	65	47	91	10
AI	30	21	18	1	2	1	1	7	
CD	122	102	66	17	19	7	3	10	
D	61	58	41	14	3	1	1		1
GE	66	62	52	5	5		2	2	
IM	995	875	489	267	119	38	24	51	7
PD	461	416	226	121	69	15	12	16	2
PDC	20	18	10	7	1	2			
PUD	50	40	21	7	12	1	4	5	
Sur. Spec.	890	839	473	277	89	19	21	8	3
CRS	7	7	5	1	1				
GS	240	221	100	96	25	7	7	4	1
NS	37	35	16	14	5		2		
OBG	231	214	120	69	25	8	5	2	2
OPH	107	105	72	25	8		1	1	
ORS	106	103	59	36	8	1	2		
OTO	43	42	27	12	3	1			
PS	38	36	19	12	5		2		
TS	30	27	23	2	2	2	1		
U	51	49	32	10	7		1	1	
Oth. Spec.	1,312	1,081	668	229	184	106	42	59	24
AM	6	3	1		2	3			
AN	138	127	87	18	22	4	7		
CHP	52	45	36	4	5	3	2	2	
DR	132	128	71	44	13		2	2	
EM	109	104	60	29	15	2	1	2	
FOP	3	2	1	1					1
GPM	27	11	7	2	2	7	1	4	4
MG	6	5	1	2	2		1		
N	87	74	40	18	16	3	2	6	2
NM	16	11	7		4	3	1		1
OM	18	7	4		3	6	1	2	2
P	340	296	218	42	36	22	7	11	4
PHP	36	2	2			22	2	8	2
PM	34	31	17	8	6		1	2	
PTH	139	104	47	23	34	10	9	12	4
R	48	45	34	5	6		2		1
RO	19	19	11	4	4				
TTS	2	2	1		1				
OTH	56	23	14		9	20	3	7	3
UNSP	44	42	9	29	4	1		1	
Not Class	423								
Inactive	377								

Note: Excludes Address Unknown.

Subspecialties in this table are condensed into major specialties. See Appendix A.

Table 3.7

Physicians by State, Self-Designated Specialty, and Activity, 2006, continued
Florida

| Specialty | Total Physicians | Patient Care | | | | Other Professional Activity | | | |
| | | Total Patient Care | Office Based | Hospital Based | | Admin. | Med. Teach. | Research | Other |
				Resid./ Fellows	Phys. Staff				
Total Physicians	53,566	40,211	33,863	2,884	3,464	717	453	397	241
GP/FM Prac.	4,911	4,723	4,043	290	390	98	66	5	19
FM	3,947	3,794	3,213	290	291	75	64	4	10
GP	964	929	830		99	23	2	1	9
Med. Prac.	16,108	15,443	13,121	1,142	1,180	226	181	211	47
AI	197	191	177	5	9	2	2	2	
CD	1,581	1,529	1,367	67	95	17	13	16	6
D	749	739	670	47	22	1	3	4	2
GE	844	828	742	44	42	5	5	6	
IM	8,157	7,795	6,584	558	653	126	100	114	22
PD	3,820	3,637	2,958	384	295	68	53	49	13
PDC	103	97	82	6	9	2	2	2	
PUD	657	627	541	31	55	5	3	18	4
Sur. Spec.	9,178	8,979	7,850	582	547	58	72	38	31
CRS	107	105	89	8	8	1			1
GS	1,848	1,804	1,425	192	187	14	14	8	8
NS	330	321	267	28	26	4	1	2	2
OBG	2,238	2,182	1,926	137	119	12	30	10	4
OPH	1,158	1,138	1,055	43	40	4	5	6	5
ORS	1,312	1,285	1,120	82	83	11	10	4	2
OTO	573	566	503	38	25	1	5		1
PS	577	567	538	20	9	3	3	1	3
TS	323	314	290	6	18	6		3	
U	712	697	637	28	32	2	4	4	5
Oth. Spec.	11,822	11,066	8,849	870	1,347	335	134	143	144
AM	40	24	6	2	16	12	2	2	
AN	2,577	2,521	2,075	220	226	22	18	15	1
CHP	306	290	245	18	27	10	4	1	1
DR	1,428	1,395	1,116	135	144	7	12	3	11
EM	1,622	1,562	1,189	102	271	42	13	1	4
FOP	59	45	42	2	1	6			8
GPM	111	87	63	13	11	17	1	3	3
MG	16	11	7	3	1		2	3	
N	849	804	695	59	50	11	9	22	3
NM	64	60	42	5	13		2		2
OM	97	72	57		15	18	1	1	5
P	1,761	1,649	1,240	114	295	55	22	23	12
PHP	57	14	11		3	34	1	7	1
PM	306	299	262	14	23	6		1	
PTH	1,009	866	674	74	118	35	20	25	63
R	542	516	438	18	60	3	9	3	11
RO	295	290	256	17	17	2	2	1	
TTS	12	9	7		2	1	1	1	
OTH	251	151	127		24	46	12	25	17
UNSP	419	400	296	74	30	8	3	6	2
VM	1	1	1						
Not Class	1,865								
Inactive	9,682								

Note: Excludes Address Unknown.

Subspecialties in this table are condensed into major specialties. See Appendix A.

Table 3.7

Physicians by State, Self-Designated Specialty, and Activity, 2006, continued
Georgia

| Specialty | Total Physicians | Patient Care | | Hospital Based | | Other Professional Activity | | | |
		Total Patient Care	Office Based	Resid./ Fellows	Phys. Staff	Admin.	Med. Teach.	Research	Other
Total Physicians	22,805	18,418	15,024	1,837	1,557	357	257	319	122
GP/FM Prac.	2,344	2,246	1,858	194	194	40	46	7	5
FM	2,112	2,027	1,672	194	161	32	45	6	2
GP	232	219	186		33	8	1	1	3
Med. Prac.	7,271	6,888	5,607	720	561	110	103	141	29
AI	88	82	75	4	3		2	4	
CD	521	507	422	51	34	3	8	3	
D	276	271	233	27	11	2	2	1	
GE	310	303	272	19	12	2	2	3	
IM	3,841	3,611	2,858	436	317	72	62	82	14
PD	1,940	1,841	1,528	157	156	28	20	36	15
PDC	47	43	32	6	5		1	3	
PUD	248	230	187	20	23	3	6	9	
Sur. Spec.	4,437	4,345	3,711	411	223	35	33	11	13
CRS	33	33	30	2	1				
GS	1,024	993	759	168	66	9	10	5	7
NS	143	141	114	17	10	1			1
OBG	1,382	1,346	1,198	91	57	15	14	4	3
OPH	419	414	364	28	22	3	1	1	
ORS	596	588	506	52	30	3	4		1
OTO	278	274	250	14	10	1	1	1	1
PS	187	185	163	13	9		2		
TS	108	107	89	11	7	1			
U	267	264	238	15	11	2	1		
Oth. Spec.	5,421	4,939	3,848	512	579	172	75	160	75
AM	13	3	2		1	9		1	
AN	941	924	777	81	66	4	10		3
CHP	157	149	124	11	14	1	7		
DR	597	585	449	85	51	1	5	1	5
EM	848	816	622	80	114	21	8	2	1
FOP	24	16	13	1	2	1		1	6
GPM	155	119	70	6	43	10	1	19	6
MG	11	8	5	1	2		2	1	
N	330	308	271	23	14	5	3	13	1
NM	17	15	9		6		1	1	
OM	71	47	40		7	14	1	5	4
P	906	853	650	69	134	21	14	14	4
PHP	145	20	8		12	47	6	66	6
PM	141	136	110	11	15	1	2	2	
PTH	461	399	305	61	33	16	7	17	22
R	244	227	190	10	27	3	5	4	5
RO	116	113	97	10	6	2		1	
OTH	103	66	48		18	13	3	9	12
UNSP	140	134	58	63	13	3		3	
VM	1	1			1				
Not Class	877								
Inactive	2,455								

Note: Excludes Address Unknown.

Subspecialties in this table are condensed into major specialties. See Appendix A.

Table 3.7

Physicians by State, Self-Designated Specialty, and Activity, 2006, continued
Hawaii

| Specialty | Total Physicians | Patient Care | | | | Other Professional Activity | | | |
| | | Total Patient Care | Office Based | Hospital Based | | Admin. | Med. Teach. | Research | Other |
				Resid./ Fellows	Phys. Staff				
Total Physicians	4,599	3,628	2,889	340	399	78	60	47	31
GP/FM Prac.	417	403	337	22	44	4	8		2
FM	339	327	269	22	36	4	7		1
GP	78	76	68		8		1		1
Med. Prac.	1,439	1,364	1,104	123	137	27	20	21	7
AI	20	18	16		2			2	
CD	65	64	57	1	6			1	
D	53	51	42	1	8	1		1	
GE	42	42	40		2				
IM	799	758	609	80	69	18	12	8	3
PD	415	389	305	40	44	6	8	8	4
PDC	6	6	6						
PUD	39	36	29	1	6	2		1	
Sur. Spec.	809	781	617	100	64	6	13	5	4
CRS	3	3	3						
GS	174	166	117	33	16	4	3	1	
NS	24	22	18		4			1	1
OBG	247	231	188	31	12	2	10	3	1
OPH	96	96	92		4				
ORS	121	119	80	26	13				2
OTO	47	47	34	6	7				
PS	31	31	29	1	1				
TS	19	19	18		1				
U	47	47	38	3	6				
Oth. Spec.	1,179	1,080	831	95	154	41	19	21	18
AM	11	9	5		4	2			
AN	165	163	141	4	18	1	1		
CHP	71	65	52	6	7	3	3		
DR	119	118	85	17	16			1	
EM	171	162	140	3	19	7	1		1
FOP	4	2	1	1		1			1
GPM	31	26	19		7	2		3	
N	52	51	38		13			1	
NM	14	12	8		4		1	1	
OM	24	20	17		3	3			1
P	263	240	159	43	38	10	7	1	5
PHP	14	5	3		2		4	4	1
PM	38	36	32		4	1			1
PTH	85	71	52	12	7	4		3	7
R	47	44	36		8		2	1	
RO	16	16	16						
OTH	29	16	15		1	6		6	1
UNSP	25	24	12	9	3	1			
Not Class	152								
Inactive	603								

Note: Excludes Address Unknown.

Subspecialties in this table are condensed into major specialties. See Appendix A.

Table 3.7

Physicians by State, Self-Designated Specialty, and Activity, 2006, continued
Idaho

Specialty	Total Physicians	Patient Care		Hospital Based		Other Professional Activity			
		Total Patient Care	Office Based	Resid./ Fellows	Phys. Staff	Admin.	Med. Teach.	Research	Other
Total Physicians	2,934	2,373	2,087	66	220	35	12	7	14
GP/FM Prac.	566	552	483	36	33	6	7	1	
FM	528	514	449	36	29	6	7	1	
GP	38	38	34		4				
Med. Prac.	619	594	518	17	59	14	3	4	4
AI	12	12	12						
CD	52	51	48		3			1	
D	35	35	34		1				
GE	38	36	33		3	1		1	
IM	316	300	255	15	30	11	2	1	2
PD	131	126	108	2	16	2	1		2
PDC	3	3	3						
PUD	32	31	25		6			1	
Sur. Spec.	592	583	550	4	29	3	2	1	3
CRS	3	3	3						
GS	137	135	120	2	13	1			1
NS	25	25	24		1				
OBG	142	138	132		6	2	1	1	
OPH	55	55	53		2				
ORS	126	124	116	2	6				2
OTO	37	36	36				1		
PS	18	18	18						
TS	8	8	8						
U	41	41	40		1				
Oth. Spec.	664	644	536	9	99	12		1	7
AM	1								
AN	115	115	102	3	10				
CHP	20	20	18		2				
DR	129	127	108	1	18				2
EM	131	129	97	2	30	2			
FOP	2	2	2						
GPM	3	1	1			1			1
N	33	32	30		2				1
NM	1	1	1						
OM	8	6	3		3	1			1
P	77	75	56	1	18	2			
PHP	2	1	1			1			
PM	27	27	24		3				
PTH	43	40	33		7	1			2
R	36	35	33		2	1			
RO	16	16	15		1				
OTH	7	4	4			2		1	
UNSP	13	13	8	2	3				
Not Class	38								
Inactive	455								

Note: *Excludes Address Unknown.*

Subspecialties in this table are condensed into major specialties. See Appendix A.

Table 3.7

Physicians by State, Self-Designated Specialty, and Activity, 2006, continued
Illinois

Specialty	Total Physicians	Patient Care				Other Professional Activity			
		Total Patient Care	Office Based	Hospital Based		Admin.	Med. Teach.	Research	Other
				Resid./ Fellows	Phys. Staff				
Total Physicians	39,240	31,367	23,395	5,505	2,467	620	426	475	178
GP/FM Prac.	3,875	3,735	3,004	488	243	63	55	9	13
FM	3,474	3,354	2,663	488	203	53	55	5	7
GP	401	381	341		40	10		4	6
Med. Prac.	13,268	12,558	9,172	2,520	866	242	164	265	39
AI	195	176	157	13	6	4	2	12	1
CD	961	902	731	121	50	14	9	31	5
D	410	402	330	59	13	1	4	3	
GE	500	476	408	46	22	3	8	12	1
IM	7,601	7,185	5,045	1,618	522	156	87	153	20
PD	3,131	2,983	2,171	597	215	52	46	41	9
PDC	75	69	48	11	10	2	1	2	1
PUD	395	365	282	55	28	10	7	11	2
Sur. Spec.	6,561	6,384	5,014	1,024	346	57	58	45	17
CRS	55	52	44	3	5	1	2		
GS	1,521	1,476	1,001	376	99	13	12	14	6
NS	231	225	163	42	20	3	3		
OBG	1,859	1,803	1,492	202	109	21	17	15	3
OPH	736	723	629	68	26	2	6	3	2
ORS	925	907	698	180	29	4	8	3	3
OTO	376	369	293	59	17	3	3		1
PS	255	246	193	44	9	4	2	2	1
TS	188	179	160	8	11	1	2	6	
U	415	404	341	42	21	5	3	2	1
Oth. Spec.	9,362	8,690	6,205	1,473	1,012	258	149	156	109
AM	11	5	4		1	6			
AN	1,867	1,822	1,336	309	177	9	25	8	3
CHP	224	207	171	19	17	6	6	3	2
DR	1,003	973	694	203	76	7	10	2	11
EM	1,387	1,335	862	258	215	34	11	5	2
FOP	23	19	18	1			2		2
GPM	40	32	30	2		3	1	2	2
MG	14	12	11		1			2	
N	624	579	433	92	54	9	8	25	3
NM	56	51	36	5	10		2	1	2
OM	123	94	76	2	16	16	2	2	9
P	1,572	1,460	1,104	175	181	56	23	19	14
PHP	26	4	3		1	11	2	6	3
PM	387	368	237	69	62	9	5	2	3
PTH	917	783	534	134	115	38	32	33	31
R	363	344	280	22	42	5	4	3	7
RO	176	172	127	30	15	1	2	1	
TTS	7	5	4		1		1	1	
OTH	220	112	98		14	44	11	39	14
UNSP	320	311	145	152	14	4	2	2	1
VM	2	2	2						
Not Class	2,245								
Inactive	3,929								

Note: Excludes Address Unknown.

Subspecialties in this table are condensed into major specialties. See Appendix A.

Table 3.7

Physicians by State, Self-Designated Specialty, and Activity, 2006, continued
Indiana

Specialty	Total Physicians	Patient Care				Other Professional Activity			
		Total Patient Care	Office Based	Hospital Based		Admin.	Med. Teach.	Research	Other
				Resid./ Fellows	Phys. Staff				
Total Physicians	15,229	12,560	10,206	1,312	1,042	198	130	182	70
GP/FM Prac.	2,428	2,354	1,943	209	202	36	32	1	5
FM	2,251	2,181	1,789	209	183	35	32		3
GP	177	173	154		19	1		1	2
Med. Prac.	4,287	4,045	3,213	487	345	63	42	124	13
AI	56	53	53			1		2	
CD	399	386	342	22	22	2	4	5	2
D	147	144	128	13	3		1		2
GE	186	182	162	13	7	2		2	
IM	2,157	1,999	1,573	242	184	42	25	84	7
PD	1,136	1,089	796	180	113	11	10	25	1
PDC	27	27	23	3	1				
PUD	179	165	136	14	15	5	2	6	1
Sur. Spec.	2,714	2,672	2,301	256	115	13	20	8	1
CRS	28	28	27		1				
GS	588	578	463	85	30	2	3	4	1
NS	91	91	75	12	4				
OBG	702	680	585	54	41	8	12	2	
OPH	280	278	262	15	1	2			
ORS	451	448	383	47	18		2	1	
OTO	190	189	169	16	4		1		
PS	96	96	87	7	2				
TS	105	102	86	5	11	1	1	1	
U	183	182	164	15	3		1		
Oth. Spec.	3,711	3,489	2,749	360	380	86	36	49	51
AM	3	2	2			1			
AN	925	910	767	79	64	3	7	2	3
CHP	94	89	78	2	9	2	2		1
DR	442	431	343	61	27	2	3	1	5
EM	539	516	389	59	68	16	4	1	2
FOP	9	6	6						3
GPM	14	10	7	1	2	2		2	
MG	5	4	3	1				1	
N	243	229	202	17	10	2	3	7	2
NM	19	17	15	1	1	1			1
OM	63	52	41		11	8			3
P	462	434	303	28	103	9	4	12	3
PHP	9					7	1	1	
PM	112	109	91	9	9	2		1	
PTH	345	289	213	32	44	20	7	8	21
R	172	169	148	7	14	1			2
RO	95	94	80	7	7			1	
TTS	6	5	5					1	
OTH	69	42	35	1	6	10	4	10	3
UNSP	85	81	21	55	5		1	1	2
Not Class	427								
Inactive	1,662								

Note: Excludes Address Unknown.

Subspecialties in this table are condensed into major specialties. See Appendix A.

Table 3.7

Physicians by State, Self-Designated Specialty, and Activity, 2006, continued
Iowa

Specialty	Total Physicians	Patient Care				Other Professional Activity			
		Total Patient Care	Office Based	Hospital Based		Admin.	Med. Teach.	Research	Other
				Resid./ Fellows	Phys. Staff				
Total Physicians	6,428	4,957	3,886	668	403	62	99	124	24
GP/FM Prac.	1,152	1,093	896	119	78	13	36	4	6
FM	1,099	1,045	853	119	73	9	36	4	5
GP	53	48	43		5	4			1
Med. Prac.	1,516	1,390	1,086	201	103	20	28	75	3
AI	31	27	22	5		1		3	
CD	146	135	117	14	4	1	1	9	
D	78	77	55	15	7			1	
GE	71	68	60	1	7			3	
IM	721	654	511	94	49	10	16	39	2
PD	378	348	265	56	27	7	8	14	1
PDC	22	19	13	4	2	1	1	1	
PUD	69	62	43	12	7		2	5	
Sur. Spec.	1,167	1,143	913	157	73	4	13	7	
CRS	2	2	2						
GS	305	299	215	55	29	2	4		
NS	34	34	22	9	3				
OBG	216	209	177	17	15	2	3	2	
OPH	158	151	133	14	4		4	3	
ORS	198	195	154	32	9		1	2	
OTO	100	100	78	17	5				
PS	32	32	30	1	1				
TS	42	41	35	2	4		1		
U	80	80	67	10	3				
Oth. Spec.	1,431	1,331	991	191	149	25	22	38	15
AM	2	1	1			1			
AN	318	310	239	49	22		6	2	
CHP	40	39	29	4	6	1			
DR	193	188	142	30	16	1	2		2
EM	130	124	74	22	28	4	1		1
FOP	6	6	5		1				
GPM	15	11	8	2	1	1		3	
MG	4	4	3	1					
N	103	93	75	11	7	1	2	6	1
NM	17	16	13		3		1		
OM	19	18	14		4			1	
P	206	189	130	22	37	4	2	11	
PHP	9	3	3			1	1	3	1
PM	28	26	21	1	4	2			
PTH	171	148	117	21	10	3	3	9	8
R	46	44	40		4		2		
RO	40	39	33	4	2		1		
TTS	1	1	1						
OTH	28	19	15		4	6	1		2
UNSP	55	52	28	24				3	
Not Class	301								
Inactive	861								

Note: Excludes Address Unknown.

Subspecialties in this table are condensed into major specialties. See Appendix A.

Table 3.7

Physicians by State, Self-Designated Specialty, and Activity, 2006, continued
Kansas

Specialty	Total Physicians	Patient Care		Hospital Based		Other Professional Activity			
		Total Patient Care	Office Based	Resid./ Fellows	Phys. Staff	Admin.	Med. Teach.	Research	Other
Total Physicians	7,079	5,602	4,474	637	491	95	87	50	27
GP/FM Prac.	1,112	1,060	888	92	80	19	29	4	
FM	1,046	996	839	92	65	17	29	4	
GP	66	64	49		15	2			
Med. Prac.	1,805	1,723	1,371	205	147	24	30	20	8
AI	31	30	26	3	1			1	
CD	177	170	152	6	12		6	1	
D	69	69	58	5	6				
GE	75	73	69	3	1		1	1	
IM	897	853	656	122	75	14	14	13	3
PD	471	448	343	61	44	6	9	4	4
PDC	7	7	6		1				
PUD	78	73	61	5	7	4			1
Sur. Spec.	1,289	1,265	1,037	161	67	6	10	5	3
CRS	10	10	10						
GS	314	306	221	56	29	2	3	2	1
NS	31	29	25	4		1	1		
OBG	289	283	230	41	12	1	4	1	
OPH	154	151	137	8	6	2	1		
ORS	231	229	189	31	9				2
OTO	78	77	66	9	2			1	
PS	61	61	51	7	3				
TS	40	39	36		3			1	
U	81	80	72	5	3		1		
Oth. Spec.	1,655	1,554	1,178	179	197	46	18	21	16
AM	2	1	1			1			
AN	332	323	264	37	22	3	4	1	1
CHP	64	62	47	4	11	2			
DR	231	227	180	31	16	1	1		2
EM	191	187	135	13	39	3	1		
FOP	4	3	3						1
GPM	5	4	2		2			1	
MG	1	1			1				
N	110	106	89	9	8	2	2		
NM	6	6	3		3				
OM	18	15	13		2	1			2
P	288	266	179	43	44	10	6	6	
PHP	6	1	1			5			
PM	62	62	42	6	14				
PTH	161	146	111	16	19	5	1	4	5
R	59	55	44	2	9	1	1		2
RO	36	36	29	4	3				
OTH	42	20	15	1	4	9	2	8	3
UNSP	37	33	20	13		3		1	
Not Class	243								
Inactive	975								

Note: Excludes Address Unknown.

Subspecialties in this table are condensed into major specialties. See Appendix A.

Table 3.7

Physicians by State, Self-Designated Specialty, and Activity, 2006, continued
Kentucky

Specialty	Total Physicians	Patient Care				Other Professional Activity			
		Total Patient Care	Office Based	Hospital Based		Admin.	Med. Teach.	Research	Other
				Resid./ Fellows	Phys. Staff				
Total Physicians	10,828	8,825	7,199	1,018	608	128	116	84	45
GP/FM Prac.	1,346	1,303	1,141	87	75	25	15	2	1
FM	1,207	1,164	1,011	87	66	25	15	2	1
GP	139	139	130		9				
Med. Prac.	3,186	3,058	2,494	378	186	29	44	48	7
AI	58	57	55		2				1
CD	261	254	216	25	13	2	4	1	
D	113	113	104	7	2				
GE	124	117	107	7	3		3	4	
IM	1,601	1,540	1,231	196	113	9	19	29	4
PD	873	834	662	130	42	15	16	7	1
PDC	20	18	18					2	
PUD	136	125	101	13	11	3	2	5	1
Sur. Spec.	2,061	2,013	1,702	224	87	13	18	7	10
CRS	15	14	14					1	
GS	516	503	397	84	22	4	6	2	1
NS	76	74	61	12	1		1		1
OBG	520	509	436	50	23	5	4	2	
OPH	188	184	173	9	2	1	2	1	
ORS	310	302	246	37	19	1	1		6
OTO	124	123	107	10	6		1		
PS	94	92	80	10	2		2		
TS	81	77	70	4	3	1		1	2
U	137	135	118	8	9	1	1		
Oth. Spec.	2,605	2,451	1,862	329	260	61	39	27	27
AM	6	5	4		1	1			
AN	555	542	423	75	44	5	8		
CHP	86	79	64	8	7		4	2	1
DR	313	310	257	35	18	1	2		
EM	412	404	288	48	68	2	2	2	2
FOP	12	7	6		1				5
GPM	13	11	9	1	1	1	1		
MG	6	5	3	1	1	1			
N	156	139	118	14	7	6	3	7	1
NM	11	10	9		1			1	
OM	30	21	20		1	4	1	4	
P	403	380	270	57	53	9	5	4	5
PHP	9	3	2		1	5	1		
PM	73	71	57	9	5	2			
PTH	222	195	134	34	27	5	7	4	11
R	67	63	56		7		2		2
RO	57	55	40	8	7		1	1	
TTS	4	4	3		1				
OTH	65	44	41		3	18	1	2	
UNSP	105	103	58	39	6	1	1		
Not Class	473								
Inactive	1,157								

Note: Excludes Address Unknown.

Subspecialties in this table are condensed into major specialties. See Appendix A.

Table 3.7

Physicians by State, Self-Designated Specialty, and Activity, 2006, continued
Louisiana

Specialty	Total Physicians	Patient Care				Other Professional Activity			
		Total Patient Care	Office Based	Hospital Based		Admin.	Med. Teach.	Research	Other
				Resid./ Fellows	Phys. Staff				
Total Physicians	12,643	10,393	8,087	1,540	766	130	196	97	36
GP/FM Prac.	1,325	1,292	1,038	160	94	6	23	3	1
FM	1,138	1,107	877	160	70	5	23	3	
GP	187	185	161		24	1			1
Med. Prac.	3,988	3,788	2,910	622	256	41	90	62	7
AI	59	57	50	6	1		2		
CD	349	337	279	46	12	1	7	4	
D	171	169	134	30	5		2		
GE	170	163	134	22	7	3	2	2	
IM	1,970	1,862	1,374	349	139	21	45	39	3
PD	1,078	1,026	801	153	72	13	22	14	3
PDC	21	20	17		3	1			
PUD	170	154	121	16	17	2	10	3	1
Sur. Spec.	2,707	2,629	2,122	367	140	22	45	7	4
CRS	23	21	19	1	1		2		
GS	607	589	417	138	34	9	7	1	1
NS	104	101	76	17	8		2	1	
OBG	695	670	561	75	34	7	15	2	1
OPH	294	286	244	30	12	3	4	1	
ORS	398	393	309	53	31		4		1
OTO	214	211	180	25	6	1	2		
PS	88	85	77	6	2		3		
TS	85	81	75	2	4	1	2	1	
U	199	192	164	20	8	1	4	1	1
Oth. Spec.	2,832	2,684	2,017	391	276	61	38	25	24
AM	3	1			1	2			
AN	517	509	399	73	37	3	4	1	
CHP	72	65	50	10	5	3	2	2	
DR	347	341	252	63	26	1	3		2
EM	514	503	332	104	67	4	6		1
FOP	9	8	8						1
GPM	21	19	17	1	1	2			
MG	7	6	5	1			1		
N	184	177	142	19	16		4	2	1
NM	13	11	9		2	2			
OM	31	28	23		5	2	1		
P	470	440	330	60	50	19	7	1	3
PHP	15	5	1	1	3	5	1	4	
PM	107	104	85	11	8	2		1	
PTH	250	225	168	26	31	6	6	3	10
R	110	101	85	1	15	1	1	1	6
RO	44	44	41		3				
TTS	3	3	3						
OTH	53	34	31		3	8	2	9	
UNSP	61	59	35	21	3	1		1	
VM	1	1	1						
Not Class	577								
Inactive	1,214								

Note: Excludes Address Unknown.

Subspecialties in this table are condensed into major specialties. See Appendix A.

Table 3.7

Physicians by State, Self-Designated Specialty, and Activity, 2006, continued
Maine

| Specialty | Total Physicians | Patient Care | | | | Other Professional Activity | | | |
| | | Total Patient Care | Office Based | Resid./ Fellows | Phys. Staff | Admin. | Med. Teach. | Research | Other |
				Hospital Based					
Total Physicians	4,197	3,250	2,606	229	415	94	53	28	28
GP/FM Prac.	603	571	461	59	51	13	16	2	1
FM	582	551	442	59	50	12	16	2	1
GP	21	20	19		1	1			
Med. Prac.	1,109	1,042	855	69	118	28	18	11	10
AI	10	9	7		2			1	
CD	91	82	75	4	3	1	3	1	4
D	20	20	18		2				
GE	45	42	41		1	2		1	
IM	612	578	460	37	81	18	9	3	4
PD	266	250	205	25	20	7	3	4	2
PDC	8	8	6		2				
PUD	57	53	43	3	7		3	1	
Sur. Spec.	705	687	592	34	61	7	6	3	2
CRS	4	4	4						
GS	194	192	154	17	21	1	1		
NS	26	25	22	1	2			1	
OBG	166	160	130	13	17	3	2		1
OPH	70	67	66		1		3		
ORS	130	128	114	2	12			1	1
OTO	34	34	33		1				
PS	15	15	15						
TS	23	20	17		3	2		1	
U	43	42	37	1	4	1			
Oth. Spec.	1,036	950	698	67	185	46	13	12	15
AN	171	167	128	16	23	2		2	
CHP	56	50	38	1	11	3	2	1	
DR	101	101	74	13	14				
EM	174	166	94	17	55	6	1		1
FOP	4	1	1						3
GPM	7	4	1		3	2	1		
MG	3	2			2			1	
N	49	46	42		4	1	1		1
NM	2	2	2						
OM	18	15	13		2	1			2
P	236	221	157	15	49	10	2	1	2
PHP	12	1	1			6	1	2	2
PM	29	23	18		5	3	2		1
PTH	62	57	49		8	1	1	2	1
R	42	41	35	1	5		1		
RO	16	16	15		1				
OTH	27	10	9		1	11	1	3	2
UNSP	27	27	21	4	2				
Not Class	116								
Inactive	628								

Note: Excludes Address Unknown.

Subspecialties in this table are condensed into major specialties. See Appendix A.

Table 3.7

Physicians by State, Self-Designated Specialty, and Activity, 2006, continued
Maryland

Specialty	Total Physicians	Patient Care				Other Professional Activity			
		Total Patient Care	Office Based	Hospital Based		Admin.	Med. Teach.	Research	Other
				Resid./ Fellows	Phys. Staff				
Total Physicians	25,969	19,205	14,055	2,733	2,417	736	303	1,246	173
GP/FM Prac.	1,359	1,288	1,060	84	144	31	18	11	11
FM	1,197	1,139	940	84	115	26	17	10	5
GP	162	149	120		29	5	1	1	6
Med. Prac.	9,314	8,145	5,893	1,341	911	280	145	679	65
AI	210	143	113	13	17	5	3	56	3
CD	617	554	456	50	48	13	8	40	2
D	294	279	224	31	24	3	4	7	1
GE	341	316	260	35	21	4	3	17	1
IM	5,247	4,548	3,193	865	490	173	79	409	38
PD	2,267	2,006	1,443	293	270	76	39	126	20
PDC	35	30	18	5	7	1	1	3	
PUD	303	269	186	49	34	5	8	21	
Sur. Spec.	4,212	4,018	3,066	555	397	68	48	63	15
CRS	29	28	26	1	1	1			
GS	945	886	566	209	111	18	20	17	4
NS	156	149	107	28	14	2		3	2
OBG	1,132	1,080	883	92	105	25	13	9	5
OPH	537	505	427	41	37	5	4	22	1
ORS	605	591	444	96	51	7	3	2	2
OTO	269	261	195	41	25	3	3	2	
PS	184	178	144	17	17	2	1	2	1
TS	110	107	86	8	13		1	2	
U	245	233	188	22	23	5	3	4	
Oth. Spec.	6,778	5,754	4,036	753	965	357	92	493	82
AM	21	13	8		5	6			2
AN	1,062	1,023	784	94	145	8	12	17	2
CHP	270	248	203	13	32	12	4	4	2
DR	567	547	379	86	82	6	3	6	5
EM	721	690	492	89	109	21	5	3	2
FOP	24	19	14	2	3	1	1	1	2
GPM	213	143	93	28	22	25	7	33	5
MG	32	22	11	6	5	3		7	
N	510	406	281	63	62	15	7	80	2
NM	65	55	35	5	15	3		7	
OM	82	42	28	1	13	27		7	5
P	1,398	1,225	896	119	210	79	20	60	14
PHP	132	11	9		2	69	5	43	4
PM	192	180	117	28	35	5	3	4	
PTH	624	481	296	73	112	25	11	83	24
R	209	187	136	16	35	3	6	11	2
RO	117	110	83	14	13	3	2	2	
TTS	4	4	1		3				
OTH	254	84	59		25	44	3	114	9
UNSP	281	264	111	116	37	2	2	11	2
Not Class	1,668								
Inactive	2,638								

Note: Excludes Address Unknown.

Subspecialties in this table are condensed into major specialties. See Appendix A.

Table 3.7

Physicians by State, Self-Designated Specialty, and Activity, 2006, continued
Massachusetts

Specialty	Total Physicians	Patient Care		Hospital Based		Other Professional Activity			
		Total Patient Care	Office Based	Resid./ Fellows	Phys. Staff	Admin.	Med. Teach.	Research	Other
Total Physicians	32,575	24,657	17,291	4,587	2,779	597	328	1,214	180
GP/FM Prac.	1,320	1,271	1,065	112	94	24	16	2	7
FM	1,188	1,150	958	112	80	19	15		4
GP	132	121	107		14	5	1	2	3
Med. Prac.	12,093	10,887	7,636	2,136	1,115	237	147	763	59
AI	145	114	88	17	9	4	1	26	
CD	887	786	557	136	93	13	16	63	9
D	376	357	292	40	25	3	3	12	1
GE	485	439	321	74	44	3	6	36	1
IM	7,012	6,253	4,320	1,318	615	164	87	476	32
PD	2,698	2,507	1,779	460	268	39	26	111	15
PDC	90	88	50	26	12		1	1	
PUD	400	343	229	65	49	11	7	38	1
Sur. Spec.	4,702	4,537	3,363	819	355	47	31	68	19
CRS	32	31	25	2	4		1		
GS	1,211	1,150	688	365	97	21	5	27	8
NS	150	144	109	18	17			5	1
OBG	1,140	1,103	888	124	91	12	12	12	1
OPH	516	505	434	35	36	1	2	6	2
ORS	751	729	540	152	37	4	5	7	6
OTO	274	266	215	29	22	2	3	3	
PS	197	194	147	37	10		2		1
TS	157	147	104	22	21	3	1	6	
U	274	268	213	35	20	4		2	
Oth. Spec.	8,861	7,962	5,227	1,520	1,215	289	134	381	95
AM	4	2	2			1		1	
AN	1,400	1,334	871	308	155	14	28	21	3
CHP	351	323	244	37	42	11	7	9	1
DR	896	864	533	225	106	5	11	11	5
EM	983	940	563	198	179	30	9	4	
FOP	12	8	8				1		3
GPM	65	51	34	11	6	3	2	6	3
MG	35	27	11	12	4	2		6	
N	689	590	410	71	109	4	13	76	6
NM	52	44	31	7	6	1	1	6	
OM	70	38	29	3	6	18		7	7
P	2,163	1,955	1,372	250	333	93	34	60	21
PHP	57	6	4		2	21	4	19	7
PM	211	204	140	27	37	5		2	
PTH	846	725	441	168	116	31	10	60	20
R	359	333	233	44	56	4	2	14	6
RO	170	163	101	32	30	2	1	3	1
TTS	7	6	5		1	1			
OTH	196	66	49	3	14	43	8	69	10
UNSP	293	281	144	124	13		3	7	2
VM	2	2	2						
Not Class	2,780								
Inactive	2,819								

Note: Excludes Address Unknown.

Subspecialties in this table are condensed into major specialties. See Appendix A.

Table 3.7

Physicians by State, Self-Designated Specialty, and Activity, 2006, continued
Michigan

Specialty	Total Physicians	Patient Care				Other Professional Activity			
		Total Patient Care	Office Based	Hospital Based		Admin.	Med. Teach.	Research	Other
				Resid./ Fellows	Phys. Staff				
Total Physicians	27,877	22,003	16,111	4,062	1,830	434	339	363	99
GP/FM Prac.	2,815	2,705	2,156	351	198	42	54	10	4
FM	2,595	2,497	1,967	351	179	36	51	8	3
GP	220	208	189		19	6	3	2	1
Med. Prac.	8,904	8,381	6,129	1,619	633	155	142	213	13
AI	145	139	126	8	5	2	1	3	
CD	630	596	473	94	29	6	5	23	
D	295	288	231	49	8	1	2	4	
GE	278	258	209	31	18	2	3	15	
IM	5,036	4,722	3,413	968	341	106	77	124	7
PD	2,190	2,076	1,461	407	208	28	49	32	5
PDC	72	68	40	20	8	2		2	
PUD	258	234	176	42	16	8	5	10	1
Sur. Spec.	4,909	4,787	3,593	908	286	39	49	25	9
CRS	63	62	55	4	3		1		
GS	1,267	1,236	802	349	85	13	10	5	3
NS	171	168	126	30	12		1		2
OBG	1,367	1,317	976	226	115	16	24	9	1
OPH	556	544	479	47	18	2	5	4	1
ORS	614	604	448	135	21	5	4		1
OTO	248	244	199	36	9	1	1	1	1
PS	203	197	156	35	6	1	2	3	
TS	133	130	114	10	6	1		2	
U	287	285	238	36	11		1	1	
Oth. Spec.	6,610	6,130	4,233	1,184	713	198	94	115	73
AM	5	2	1		1	1		2	
AN	973	950	721	151	78	3	13	4	3
CHP	208	189	132	19	38	8	7	4	
DR	808	782	518	194	70	2	14	2	8
EM	1,157	1,125	686	304	135	22	10		
FOP	18	10	9		1	2			6
GPM	27	22	18	3	1	5			
MG	17	13	7	3	3		1	3	
N	411	375	285	61	29	2	9	22	3
NM	55	47	32	6	9	2	2	4	
OM	117	92	78		14	19		3	3
P	1,081	993	726	114	153	45	16	20	7
PHP	34	6	4		2	23		4	1
PM	289	278	218	38	22	5	1	3	2
PTH	587	504	336	80	88	24	13	16	30
R	275	263	219	14	30	2	3	3	4
RO	160	154	99	32	23	6			
TTS	5	4	3		1				1
OTH	119	61	51	4	6	27	5	21	5
UNSP	262	258	88	161	9			4	
VM	2	2	2						
Not Class	1,504								
Inactive	3,135								

Note: Excludes Address Unknown.

Subspecialties in this table are condensed into major specialties. See Appendix A.

Table 3.7

Physicians by State, Self-Designated Specialty, and Activity, 2006, continued
Minnesota

| Specialty | Total Physicians | Patient Care | | | | Other Professional Activity | | | |
| | | Total Patient Care | Office Based | Hospital Based | | Admin. | Med. Teach. | Research | Other |
				Resid./ Fellows	Phys. Staff				
Total Physicians	16,756	13,318	10,347	1,963	1,008	242	177	273	58
GP/FM Prac.	2,799	2,704	2,342	210	152	41	44	6	4
FM	2,719	2,628	2,274	210	144	38	43	6	4
GP	80	76	68		8	3	1		
Med. Prac.	4,810	4,479	3,377	777	325	81	64	171	15
AI	72	67	62	5		1	1	3	
CD	425	397	312	56	29	3	5	20	
D	197	195	149	39	7		1	1	
GE	229	209	168	30	11	1	4	15	
IM	2,577	2,379	1,733	445	201	56	36	94	12
PD	1,119	1,059	822	169	68	15	16	26	3
PDC	38	34	27	6	1			4	
PUD	153	139	104	27	8	5	1	8	
Sur. Spec.	2,687	2,625	2,049	443	133	17	22	20	3
CRS	43	43	36	5	2				
GS	633	613	401	175	37	4	4	10	2
NS	95	91	59	25	7	1	2	1	
OBG	605	594	524	50	20	2	6	3	
OPH	304	301	263	26	12	2		1	
ORS	500	494	380	90	24	3	2	1	
OTO	168	164	122	30	12	1	2	1	
PS	93	91	78	10	3	2			
TS	78	74	53	11	10		2	1	1
U	168	160	133	21	6	2	4	2	
Oth. Spec.	3,772	3,510	2,579	533	398	103	47	76	36
AM	2	2	1		1				
AN	561	546	422	85	39	4	5	5	1
CHP	103	99	82	9	8	2	1	1	
DR	536	525	391	92	42	2	6	1	2
EM	515	491	315	81	95	15	8	1	
FOP	11	7	4	1	2	1	1		2
GPM	37	30	22	5	3	3		4	
MG	15	11	7	2	2			3	1
N	330	306	240	47	19	3	6	14	1
NM	13	13	10		3				
OM	63	45	37	3	5	15	1		2
P	554	520	385	58	77	18	7	6	3
PHP	22	6	5		1	5	2	8	1
PM	169	164	118	29	17	2	2		1
PTH	373	328	233	60	35	12	2	16	15
R	163	158	135	7	16		2	1	2
RO	80	79	59	14	6		1		
TTS	3	3	3						
OTH	84	41	29	4	8	21	3	16	3
UNSP	138	136	81	36	19				2
Not Class	745								
Inactive	1,943								

Note: Excludes Address Unknown.

Subspecialties in this table are condensed into major specialties. See Appendix A.

Table 3.7

Physicians by State, Self-Designated Specialty, and Activity, 2006, continued
Mississippi

Specialty	Total Physicians	Patient Care		Hospital Based		Other Professional Activity			
		Total Patient Care	Office Based	Resid./ Fellows	Phys. Staff	Admin.	Med. Teach.	Research	Other
Total Physicians	5,890	4,782	3,821	451	510	63	60	31	37
GP/FM Prac.	806	775	659	37	79	12	15	1	3
FM	701	673	570	37	66	10	15	1	2
GP	105	102	89		13	2			1
Med. Prac.	1,625	1,560	1,252	155	153	23	17	19	6
AI	26	23	17	3	3		1		2
CD	139	132	116	9	7	2	3	1	1
D	44	43	41	1	1	1			
GE	102	101	87	6	8			1	
IM	833	800	612	89	99	11	7	13	2
PD	391	374	312	41	21	7	6	3	1
PDC	4	4	4						
PUD	86	83	63	6	14	2		1	
Sur. Spec.	1,267	1,241	1,024	125	92	8	11	3	4
CRS	2	2	2						
GS	277	272	210	35	27	1	2	1	1
NS	65	64	52	8	4		1		
OBG	333	325	276	25	24	1	4	2	1
OPH	138	135	124	8	3	2	1		
ORS	178	177	132	24	21	1			
OTO	101	99	83	10	6		1		1
PS	44	44	38	5	1				
TS	44	40	36	1	3	2	1		1
U	85	83	71	9	3	1	1		
Oth. Spec.	1,275	1,206	886	134	186	20	17	8	24
AM	5	4	3		1	1			
AN	250	245	187	27	31	1	4		
CHP	31	29	23	1	5			1	1
DR	148	145	109	24	12				3
EM	203	193	139	23	31	4	4	1	1
GPM	11	7	6	1		2	1		1
MG	6	5	3		2	1			
N	94	88	74	9	5		3	1	2
NM	8	8	5		3				
OM	5	5	4		1				
P	204	197	123	26	48	3	2	1	1
PHP	6	4	3		1	2			
PM	24	22	17		5	1			1
PTH	143	126	89	14	23	4	1	2	10
R	67	64	55		9		2		1
RO	23	23	19		4				
OTH	20	16	11	1	4	1		2	1
UNSP	27	25	16	8	1				2
Not Class	176								
Inactive	741								

Note: Excludes Address Unknown.

Subspecialties in this table are condensed into major specialties. See Appendix A.

Table 3.7

Physicians by State, Self-Designated Specialty, and Activity, 2006, continued
Missouri

Specialty	Total Physicians	Patient Care		Hospital Based		Other Professional Activity			
		Total Patient Care	Office Based	Resid./ Fellows	Phys. Staff	Admin.	Med. Teach.	Research	Other
Total Physicians	15,586	12,590	9,301	2,126	1,163	202	212	274	57
GP/FM Prac.	1,369	1,320	1,100	123	97	23	19	6	1
FM	1,247	1,202	993	123	86	22	18	4	1
GP	122	118	107		11	1	1	2	
Med. Prac.	5,281	4,933	3,523	954	456	78	100	155	15
AI	88	78	60	15	3		4	4	2
CD	444	404	318	60	26	6	10	19	5
D	181	179	135	36	8		1	1	
GE	229	213	175	28	10	2	5	9	
IM	2,793	2,606	1,833	530	243	43	54	84	6
PD	1,311	1,232	835	249	148	23	22	32	2
PDC	39	37	23	8	6			2	
PUD	196	184	144	28	12	4	4	4	
Sur. Spec.	2,909	2,825	2,206	437	182	20	37	20	7
CRS	23	23	18	2	3				
GS	646	622	445	124	53	6	9	7	2
NS	121	117	86	22	9	1	2	1	
OBG	729	702	564	84	54	7	11	7	2
OPH	318	315	269	34	12	2	1		
ORS	444	435	336	73	26	1	4	1	3
OTO	192	185	142	37	6		4	3	
PS	140	137	104	30	3		2	1	
TS	111	107	90	6	11	2	2		
U	185	182	152	25	5	1	2		
Oth. Spec.	3,776	3,512	2,472	612	428	81	56	93	34
AM	4	3	1	1	1			1	
AN	712	696	521	108	67	5	8	3	
CHP	116	106	82	13	11	2	2	6	
DR	486	474	309	129	36	2	6	2	2
EM	496	475	297	67	111	11	9	1	
FOP	12	8	7	1					4
GPM	23	14	11	1	2	4	2	1	2
MG	9	6	3	1	2		3		
N	298	267	177	64	26	5	4	22	
NM	32	24	14	5	5	3	2	3	
OM	47	38	36		2	8		1	
P	596	567	402	82	83	9	4	12	4
PHP	8	3	1		2	4			1
PM	127	126	94	14	18	1			
PTH	381	332	237	61	34	9	7	17	16
R	171	162	138	14	10		6	3	
RO	86	85	69	10	6			1	
TTS	3	3	1		2				
OTH	85	42	34	1	7	17	3	18	5
UNSP	84	81	38	40	3	1		2	
Not Class	783								
Inactive	1,468								

Note: Excludes Address Unknown.

Subspecialties in this table are condensed into major specialties. See Appendix A.

Table 3.7

Physicians by State, Self-Designated Specialty, and Activity, 2006, continued
Montana

| Specialty | Total Physicians | Patient Care | | | | Other Professional Activity | | | |
		Total Patient Care	Office Based	Resid./ Fellows	Phys. Staff	Admin.	Med. Teach.	Research	Other
Total Physicians	2,548	1,991	1,728	37	226	29	13	14	10
GP/FM Prac.	445	433	365	19	49	5	6		1
FM	424	413	347	19	47	4	6		1
GP	21	20	18		2	1			
Med. Prac.	554	534	460	8	66	10	2	7	1
AI	8	7	7					1	
CD	40	39	36		3			1	
D	32	32	31		1				
GE	26	26	25		1				
IM	307	294	238	7	49	8	1	3	1
PD	115	113	101	1	11	1	1		
PDC	1	1	1						
PUD	25	22	21		1	1		2	
Sur. Spec.	495	486	443	7	36	3	2	1	3
GS	109	107	91	4	12	1			1
NS	21	21	21						
OBG	113	110	100	1	9	1		1	1
OPH	47	47	44		3				
ORS	109	105	99	1	5	1	2		1
OTO	29	29	27	1	1				
PS	15	15	14		1				
TS	17	17	13		4				
U	35	35	34		1				
Oth. Spec.	563	538	460	3	75	11	3	6	5
AM	122	121	112		9		1		
AN	14	13	12		1	1			
CHP	65	65	60		5				
DR	103	99	75	2	22	3			1
EM	2	1	1						1
FOP	3	3	3						
GPM	3	3			3				
MG	36	35	33		2	1			
N	1	1	1						
OM	5	5	3		2				
P	85	78	65		13	3	1	1	2
PM	20	20	17		3				
PTH	44	40	33		7		1	2	1
R	22	22	20		2				
RO	13	13	12		1				
OTH	20	14	10		4	3		3	
UNSP	5	5	3	1	1				
Not Class	29								
Inactive	462								

Note: Excludes Address Unknown.

Subspecialties in this table are condensed into major specialties. See Appendix A.

Table 3.7

Physicians by State, Self-Designated Specialty, and Activity, 2006, continued
Nebraska

Specialty	Total Physicians	Patient Care				Other Professional Activity			
		Total Patient Care	Office Based	Resid./ Fellows	Phys. Staff	Admin.	Med. Teach.	Research	Other
Total Physicians	4,852	3,874	2,992	589	293	70	71	51	17
GP/FM Prac.	881	848	689	91	68	13	19		1
FM	848	818	661	91	66	12	18		
GP	33	30	28		2	1	1		1
Med. Prac.	1,247	1,170	873	217	80	23	27	23	4
AI	21	19	15	4				2	
CD	119	118	92	19	7	1			
D	33	32	32					1	
GE	52	48	42	6		2	1	1	
IM	636	590	411	133	46	12	17	15	2
PD	328	311	235	49	27	8	4	3	2
PDC	8	8	8						
PUD	50	44	38	6			5	1	
Sur. Spec.	899	877	714	128	35	9	8	5	
CRS	8	8	7	1					
GS	239	230	160	57	13	5	1	3	
NS	31	31	25	6					
OBG	190	184	154	22	8		5	1	
OPH	94	92	82	7	3	2			
ORS	161	160	132	20	8	1			
OTO	73	71	63	7	1	1	1		
PS	31	30	28	2			1		
TS	21	21	20	1					
U	51	50	43	5	2			1	
Oth. Spec.	1,056	979	716	153	110	25	17	23	12
AM	3	2			2	1			
AN	233	230	174	42	14	1	2		
CHP	35	34	26	3	5			1	
DR	145	141	104	29	8		3		1
EM	117	115	73	20	22	1	1		
GPM	5	3	3			1		1	
N	58	53	48	3	2		3	2	
NM	7	6	6						1
OM	6	4	3		1	2			
P	171	161	107	26	28	5	2	2	1
PHP	1					1			
PM	24	24	17	1	6				
PTH	127	110	79	20	11	4	2	8	3
R	38	35	28	2	5				3
RO	22	22	21		1				
TTS	3	2	2					1	
OTH	39	17	13	2	2	9	2	8	3
UNSP	22	20	12	5	3		2		
Not Class	190								
Inactive	579								

Note: Excludes Address Unknown.

Subspecialties in this table are condensed into major specialties. See Appendix A.

Table 3.7

Physicians by State, Self-Designated Specialty, and Activity, 2006, continued
Nevada

| Specialty | Total Physicians | Patient Care | | | | Other Professional Activity | | | |
| | | Total Patient Care | Office Based | Hospital Based | | Admin. | Med. Teach. | Research | Other |
				Resid./ Fellows	Phys. Staff				
Total Physicians	5,384	4,307	3,760	214	333	61	32	17	21
GP/FM Prac.	563	551	485	27	39	7	3		2
FM	507	498	436	27	35	4	3		2
GP	56	53	49		4	3			
Med. Prac.	1,637	1,588	1,359	111	118	23	17	7	2
AI	16	15	14		1			1	
CD	146	142	134	1	7	1	1	2	
D	49	49	48		1				
GE	60	59	59				1		
IM	945	914	756	80	78	17	10	2	2
PD	360	350	292	30	28	4	4	2	
PDC	10	10	10						
PUD	51	49	46		3	1	1		
Sur. Spec.	925	912	822	42	48	6	3	2	2
CRS	6	6	4	1	1				
GS	209	206	160	24	22	3			
NS	30	30	29	1					
OBG	258	250	230	11	9	2	3	1	2
OPH	92	92	83	2	7				
ORS	138	137	133		4	1			
OTO	49	48	47		1			1	
PS	47	47	43	3	1				
TS	34	34	33		1				
U	62	62	60		2				
Oth. Spec.	1,313	1,256	1,094	34	128	25	9	8	15
AM	3	3	1		2				
AN	361	358	328	7	23	2		1	
CHP	27	26	22	2	2			1	
DR	150	146	135	1	10				4
EM	217	216	185	7	24	1			
FOP	8	7	7						1
GPM	10	10	8		2				
MG	2	1	1					1	
N	67	62	57		5		3	2	
NM	3	3	3						
OM	13	9	8		1	3			1
P	173	165	113	14	38	3	3		2
PHP	5	2	2			1		2	
PM	59	57	54		3	2			
PTH	87	78	69		9	3	1		5
R	52	48	45		3	1	1	1	1
RO	29	28	28						1
OTH	31	21	16		5	9	1		
UNSP	16	16	12	3	1				
Not Class	173								
Inactive	773								

Note: Excludes Address Unknown.

Subspecialties in this table are condensed into major specialties. See Appendix A.

Table 3.7

Physicians by State, Self-Designated Specialty, and Activity, 2006, continued
New Hampshire

Specialty	Total Physicians	Patient Care				Other Professional Activity			
		Total Patient Care	Office Based	Hospital Based		Admin.	Med. Teach.	Research	Other
				Resid./ Fellows	Phys. Staff				
Total Physicians	4,079	3,176	2,561	260	355	50	33	56	22
GP/FM Prac.	484	468	392	18	58	9	1	4	2
FM	457	442	368	18	56	9	1	3	2
GP	27	26	24		2			1	
Med. Prac.	1,176	1,119	887	104	128	13	13	26	5
AI	10	10	9		1				
CD	91	90	77	8	5			1	
D	41	41	34	5	2				
GE	53	52	46	3	3		1		
IM	640	602	448	68	86	9	7	19	3
PD	295	281	236	18	27	3	5	4	2
PDC	4	3	3					1	
PUD	42	40	34	2	4	1		1	
Sur. Spec.	724	710	605	49	56	2	6	5	1
CRS	3	3	3						
GS	175	169	134	18	17	2	2	1	1
NS	24	23	17	4	2		1		
OBG	197	193	169	9	15		3	1	
OPH	68	67	65		2			1	
ORS	130	128	103	13	12			2	
OTO	40	40	38	1	1				
PS	22	22	18	1	3				
TS	17	17	15		2				
U	48	48	43	3	2				
Oth. Spec.	953	879	677	89	113	26	13	21	14
AM	2	1	1			1			
AN	174	169	135	17	17	1	4		
CHP	31	31	27	3	1				
DR	111	107	84	12	11	1			3
EM	153	149	105	4	40	3			1
FOP	1								1
GPM	15	12	2	10		2			1
N	59	57	49	7	1	1		1	
NM	2	2	2						
OM	12	6	5		1	4			2
P	185	170	134	17	19	4	5	6	
PHP	2	1	1					1	
PM	20	18	17		1	1		1	
PTH	80	71	54	8	9	2	2	2	3
R	36	35	30	1	4			1	
RO	10	10	8		2				
OTH	33	15	11		4	6	2	7	3
UNSP	27	25	12	10	3			2	
Not Class	126								
Inactive	616								

Note: Excludes Address Unknown.

Subspecialties in this table are condensed into major specialties. See Appendix A.

Table 3.7

Physicians by State, Self-Designated Specialty, and Activity, 2006, continued
New Jersey

| Specialty | Total Physicians | Patient Care | | | | Other Professional Activity | | | |
| | | Total Patient Care | Office Based | Hospital Based | | Admin. | Med. Teach. | Research | Other |
				Resid./ Fellows	Phys. Staff				
Total Physicians	30,183	24,128	18,874	2,855	2,399	507	306	513	194
GP/FM Prac.	1,609	1,537	1,222	198	117	21	30	11	10
FM	1,380	1,323	1,057	198	68	14	30	8	5
GP	229	214	165		49	7		3	5
Med. Prac.	11,648	10,915	8,441	1,444	1,030	207	159	300	67
AI	160	147	133	7	7	3		8	2
CD	959	902	785	55	62	13	9	30	5
D	340	329	301	16	12	2	2	6	1
GE	492	473	415	33	25	4	2	11	2
IM	6,234	5,797	4,321	969	507	126	83	185	43
PD	3,008	2,850	2,155	332	363	48	50	48	12
PDC	65	58	40		18	1	2	2	2
PUD	390	359	291	32	36	10	11	10	
Sur. Spec.	5,305	5,158	4,358	514	286	53	42	32	20
CRS	64	62	57	4	1			1	1
GS	1,204	1,165	844	210	111	18	10	6	5
NS	111	108	91	8	9		1	1	1
OBG	1,531	1,479	1,255	132	92	13	24	11	4
OPH	617	607	579	22	6	4	1	3	2
ORS	722	709	610	86	13	6	1	1	5
OTO	274	271	249	11	11	3			
PS	230	226	201	13	12	2	1	1	
TS	164	151	128	7	16	5		7	1
U	388	380	344	21	15	2	4	1	1
Oth. Spec.	7,086	6,518	4,853	699	966	226	75	170	97
AM	6	6	2		4				
AN	1,516	1,480	1,229	117	134	11	8	12	5
CHP	242	224	171	19	34	6	3	6	3
DR	748	722	536	115	71	4	4	5	13
EM	691	666	452	92	122	16	6	2	1
FOP	15	8	8			4		2	1
GPM	45	35	24	5	6	3	3	3	1
MG	10	7	3	1	3		1	2	
N	519	473	380	45	48	9	8	25	4
NM	47	40	33		7	1	1	2	3
OM	88	53	42	2	9	25	2	2	6
P	1,448	1,347	920	128	299	42	15	29	15
PHP	24	3	3			13	4	2	2
PM	375	359	255	43	61	10	3	2	1
PTH	542	458	307	59	92	27	7	24	26
R	305	291	254	5	32	3	2	3	6
RO	141	137	114	7	16	1		3	
TTS	7	6	5		1			1	
OTH	190	88	67	3	18	48	7	42	5
UNSP	127	115	48	58	9	3	1	3	5
Not Class	1,443								
Inactive	3,092								

Note: Excludes Address Unknown.

Subspecialties in this table are condensed into major specialties. See Appendix A.

Table 3.7

Physicians by State, Self-Designated Specialty, and Activity, 2006, continued
New Mexico

| Specialty | Total Physicians | Patient Care | | | | Other Professional Activity | | | |
| | | Total Patient Care | Office Based | Hospital Based | | Admin. | Med. Teach. | Research | Other |
				Resid./ Fellows	Phys. Staff				
Total Physicians	5,424	4,162	3,210	478	474	93	66	74	47
GP/FM Prac.	791	766	617	62	87	7	13	2	3
FM	728	705	566	62	77	6	13	2	2
GP	63	61	51		10	1			1
Med. Prac.	1,491	1,383	1,052	170	161	34	28	34	12
AI	12	12	12						
CD	107	101	76	11	14	1	2	2	1
D	52	47	41	5	1		3	1	1
GE	69	62	48	9	5	2	2	2	1
IM	814	756	563	102	91	20	11	22	5
PD	378	351	266	38	47	8	9	6	4
PDC	6	5	5			1			
PUD	53	49	41	5	3	2	1	1	
Sur. Spec.	825	804	646	90	68	7	10		4
CRS	4	4	3		1				
GS	202	197	147	24	26	2	3		
NS	21	21	17	3	1				
OBG	219	213	177	27	9	1	4		1
OPH	74	73	68		5	1			
ORS	147	144	104	25	15				3
OTO	53	52	44	5	3	1			
PS	31	28	23	1	4	1	2		
TS	27	27	27						
U	47	45	36	5	4	1	1		
Oth. Spec.	1,335	1,209	895	156	158	45	15	38	28
AM	10	5	3		2	3			2
AN	218	216	167	30	19		1	1	
CHP	60	53	41	4	8	4	2	1	
DR	118	109	67	25	17	1	1	2	5
EM	242	230	158	28	44	9	3		
FOP	10	10	9		1				
GPM	13	11	7	1	3	1		1	
MG	2	2	2						
N	69	61	48	8	5	1	2	5	
NM	5	5	5						
OM	23	18	16		2	4			1
P	280	252	180	35	37	12	4	8	4
PHP	12	3	2		1	4		3	2
PM	26	26	23		3				
PTH	120	100	74	20	6	1	1	8	10
R	41	40	35	1	4		1		
RO	22	21	18		3			1	
OTH	40	25	23	1	1	5		7	3
UNSP	24	22	17	3	2			1	1
Not Class	239								
Inactive	743								

Note: Excludes Address Unknown.

Subspecialties in this table are condensed into major specialties. See Appendix A.

Table 3.7

Physicians by State, Self-Designated Specialty, and Activity, 2006, continued
New York

| Specialty | Total Physicians | Patient Care | | Hospital Based | | Other Professional Activity | | | |
		Total Patient Care	Office Based	Resid./ Fellows	Phys. Staff	Admin.	Med. Teach.	Research	Other
Total Physicians	83,826	65,224	43,989	13,621	7,614	1,534	1,034	1,562	377
GP/FM Prac.	3,866	3,715	2,875	532	308	72	56	11	12
FM	3,434	3,307	2,522	532	253	62	54	6	5
GP	432	408	353		55	10	2	5	7
Med. Prac.	31,013	28,887	18,879	7,059	2,949	626	506	864	130
AI	372	324	282	24	18	8	4	36	
CD	2,180	2,034	1,554	299	181	35	38	67	6
D	969	942	801	102	39	5	12	9	1
GE	1,204	1,127	908	131	88	16	23	32	6
IM	17,820	16,542	10,142	4,749	1,651	412	268	520	78
PD	7,378	6,933	4,520	1,580	833	131	125	153	36
PDC	161	145	88	19	38	2	4	10	
PUD	929	840	584	155	101	17	32	37	3
Sur. Spec.	13,996	13,580	9,952	2,563	1,065	117	134	116	49
CRS	140	137	125	6	6	1	2		
GS	3,389	3,267	1,899	1,044	324	52	33	26	11
NS	394	380	263	80	37	1	5	7	1
OBG	3,778	3,660	2,776	564	320	37	39	33	9
OPH	1,756	1,717	1,482	159	76	3	14	17	5
ORS	1,838	1,798	1,295	409	94	5	10	11	14
OTO	789	768	591	117	60	3	13	4	1
PS	624	613	533	47	33	1	2	3	5
TS	362	340	260	28	52	6	7	8	1
U	926	900	728	109	63	8	9	7	2
Oth. Spec.	20,856	19,042	12,283	3,467	3,292	719	338	571	186
AM	7	5	3		2	1			1
AN	3,433	3,323	2,454	521	348	30	44	26	10
CHP	883	803	569	84	150	36	15	20	9
DR	2,023	1,952	1,218	475	259	16	20	18	17
EM	1,996	1,907	1,016	508	383	57	25	6	1
FOP	60	42	35	4	3	5		1	12
GPM	145	119	82	30	7	17	4	4	1
MG	37	27	13	7	7		2	7	1
N	1,568	1,393	951	264	178	31	42	95	7
NM	176	159	93	24	42	8	2	4	3
OM	125	75	58	2	15	40	1	6	3
P	5,650	5,175	3,263	811	1,101	223	88	136	28
PHP	129	41	31		10	62	4	18	4
PM	945	903	613	146	144	19	11	4	8
PTH	1,641	1,383	759	287	337	77	46	84	51
R	822	775	553	47	175	15	11	12	9
RO	339	327	221	52	54	2	5	4	1
TTS	13	13	9		4				
OTH	414	194	140	5	49	75	15	112	18
UNSP	449	425	201	200	24	5	3	14	2
VM	1	1	1						
Not Class	6,012								
Inactive	8,083								

Note: Excludes Address Unknown.

Subspecialties in this table are condensed into major specialties. See Appendix A.

Table 3.7

Physicians by State, Self-Designated Specialty, and Activity, 2006, continued
North Carolina

Specialty	Total Physicians	Patient Care — Total Patient Care	Office Based	Hospital Based — Resid./ Fellows	Phys. Staff	Other Professional Activity — Admin.	Med. Teach.	Research	Other
Total Physicians	25,385	20,015	15,876	2,465	1,674	371	320	463	102
GP/FM Prac.	2,880	2,788	2,334	217	237	37	40	10	5
FM	2,719	2,630	2,194	217	219	35	40	10	4
GP	161	158	140		18	2			1
Med. Prac.	7,777	7,216	5,679	989	548	130	124	282	25
AI	87	73	65	5	3	2	2	9	1
CD	631	593	497	58	38	5	7	26	
D	323	315	265	39	11	3	2	3	
GE	376	349	313	22	14	5	11	10	1
IM	4,021	3,727	2,877	533	317	77	51	155	11
PD	2,017	1,873	1,432	298	143	36	47	50	11
PDC	47	42	35	3	4		2	3	
PUD	275	244	195	31	18	2	2	26	1
Sur. Spec.	4,684	4,551	3,784	523	244	39	57	26	11
CRS	18	18	17		1				
GS	1,094	1,057	791	199	67	15	11	7	4
NS	158	152	127	19	6		3	1	2
OBG	1,286	1,241	1,051	117	73	10	28	5	2
OPH	461	448	413	18	17	3	4	6	
ORS	721	710	579	95	36	3	5	2	1
OTO	298	292	256	26	10	2	2	2	
PS	177	175	151	22	2	1	1		
TS	129	124	102	12	10	2	1	1	1
U	342	334	297	15	22	3	2	2	1
Oth. Spec.	5,930	5,460	4,079	736	645	165	99	145	61
AM	5	4	3		1	1			
AN	959	926	684	150	92	7	17	8	1
CHP	213	194	149	16	29	7	7	5	
DR	723	696	551	100	45	8	10	4	5
EM	1,018	987	706	133	148	11	15	2	3
FOP	12	9	7	2			1		2
GPM	73	55	42	7	6	4		12	2
MG	12	10	6	2	2	1	1		
N	396	369	301	38	30	1	6	20	
NM	36	34	24	4	6	1		1	
OM	49	29	24		5	16	1		3
P	1,051	967	711	103	153	30	19	27	8
PHP	43	9	7		2	21	2	9	2
PM	174	167	119	29	19	5	1	1	
PTH	495	423	300	76	47	19	9	23	21
R	276	260	213	19	28	2	7	2	5
RO	148	143	119	18	6	4			1
TTS	3	3	3						
OTH	116	55	48	1	6	25	2	28	6
UNSP	127	119	61	38	20	2	1	3	2
VM	1	1	1						
Not Class	1,135								
Inactive	2,979								

Note: Excludes Address Unknown.

Subspecialties in this table are condensed into major specialties. See Appendix A.

Table 3.7

Physicians by State, Self-Designated Specialty, and Activity, 2006, continued
North Dakota

| Specialty | Total Physicians | Patient Care | | Hospital Based | | Other Professional Activity | | | |
		Total Patient Care	Office Based	Resid./ Fellows	Phys. Staff	Admin.	Med. Teach.	Research	Other
Total Physicians	1,745	1,437	1,143	115	179	25	21	6	10
GP/FM Prac.	372	355	278	48	29	10	6		1
FM	345	330	255	48	27	9	6		
GP	27	25	23		2	1			1
Med. Prac.	438	420	342	27	51	8	6	3	1
AI	9	9	7	1	1				
CD	30	30	26		4				
D	17	17	16		1				
GE	15	15	14		1				
IM	269	255	194	26	35	6	5	2	1
PD	83	81	73		8	2			
PDC	1	1	1						
PUD	14	12	11		1		1	1	
Sur. Spec.	297	288	243	15	30	2	4	1	2
CRS	1	1	1						
GS	85	82	60	12	10	1	2		
NS	11	10	6		4	1			
OBG	50	49	46		3		1		
OPH	34	34	33		1				
ORS	51	48	42	1	5			1	2
OTO	18	18	16	1	1				
PS	11	10	10				1		
TS	17	17	11	1	5				
U	19	19	18		1				
Oth. Spec.	392	374	280	25	69	5	5	2	6
AM	2	2	1		1				
AN	64	64	54	2	8				
CHP	17	15	13	1	1	1			1
DR	43	41	37		4	1			1
EM	47	46	31		15		1		
FOP	1	1	1						
GPM	3	3	2		1				
MG	1						1		
N	22	22	13	2	7				
OM	3	3	2		1				
P	77	75	49	13	13		1	1	
PHP	2	1			1			1	
PM	15	15	11		4				
PTH	40	33	27	1	5	1	2		4
R	18	18	16		2				
RO	12	12	9		3				
TTS	1	1	1						
OTH	5	3	2		1	2			
UNSP	19	19	11	6	2				
Not Class	45								
Inactive	201								

Note: Excludes Address Unknown.

Subspecialties in this table are condensed into major specialties. See Appendix A.

Table 3.7

Physicians by State, Self-Designated Specialty, and Activity, 2006, continued
Ohio

Specialty	Total Physicians	Patient Care				Other Professional Activity			
		Total Patient Care	Office Based	Hospital Based		Admin.	Med. Teach.	Research	Other
				Resid./ Fellows	Phys. Staff				
Total Physicians	34,091	26,844	19,866	4,610	2,368	452	385	424	131
GP/FM Prac.	3,491	3,350	2,742	393	215	51	72	9	9
FM	3,215	3,081	2,526	393	162	47	72	9	6
GP	276	269	216		53	4			3
Med. Prac.	10,808	10,216	7,321	1,997	898	153	160	248	31
AI	127	119	102	14	3	1	1	6	
CD	883	831	671	94	66	7	18	23	4
D	346	337	271	53	13	1	5	2	1
GE	424	399	321	51	27	4	7	13	1
IM	5,540	5,233	3,718	1,067	448	96	85	109	17
PD	3,022	2,859	1,920	644	295	40	40	75	8
PDC	102	97	53	23	21			2	3
PUD	364	341	265	51	25	4	2	17	
Sur. Spec.	6,034	5,904	4,496	1,040	368	45	44	30	11
CRS	55	55	50	3	2				
GS	1,515	1,471	976	375	120	12	18	13	1
NS	228	220	150	52	18	4	3	1	
OBG	1,501	1,470	1,185	198	87	11	10	8	2
OPH	631	620	539	55	26	4	2	3	2
ORS	883	871	642	181	48	2	4	3	3
OTO	388	380	291	73	16	4	4		
PS	207	205	163	32	10		2		
TS	221	212	185	9	18	4		2	3
U	405	400	315	62	23	4	1		
Oth. Spec.	7,903	7,374	5,307	1,180	887	203	109	137	80
AM	13	10	6		4	1	1	1	
AN	1,501	1,472	1,087	235	150	8	11	7	3
CHP	230	214	165	27	22	5	8	2	1
DR	879	860	625	141	94	4	6	2	7
EM	1,214	1,156	803	198	155	24	19	10	5
FOP	26	19	17	2		2		1	4
GPM	52	45	38	5	2	3	1	3	
MG	23	15	8	4	3		1	6	1
N	522	484	355	86	43	7	7	20	4
NM	46	44	30	1	13	2			
OM	137	101	77	1	23	23		7	6
P	1,208	1,131	792	162	177	42	17	15	3
PHP	22	7	4		3	12	2	1	
PM	287	278	201	46	31	6		2	1
PTH	772	668	463	109	96	33	22	22	27
R	351	334	287	13	34	4	4	2	7
RO	165	163	130	21	12	1	1		
TTS	6	4	4				1	1	
OTH	179	110	90	7	13	24	6	32	7
UNSP	266	255	121	122	12	2	2	3	4
VM	4	4	4						
Not Class	2,085								
Inactive	3,770								

Note: Excludes Address Unknown.

Subspecialties in this table are condensed into major specialties. See Appendix A.

Table 3.7

Physicians by State, Self-Designated Specialty, and Activity, 2006, continued
Oklahoma

Specialty	Total Physicians	Patient Care				Other Professional Activity			
		Total Patient Care	Office Based	Hospital Based		Admin.	Med. Teach.	Research	Other
				Resid./ Fellows	Phys. Staff				
Total Physicians	7,111	5,667	4,542	655	470	99	97	46	30
GP/FM Prac.	1,064	1,035	800	142	93	13	12	1	3
FM	958	931	714	142	75	12	12	1	2
GP	106	104	86		18	1			1
Med. Prac.	1,927	1,807	1,455	222	130	39	45	31	5
AI	24	23	22		1			1	
CD	187	182	161	11	10	2	1	2	
D	72	69	61	7	1	1	1	1	
GE	96	93	83	8	2		3		
IM	990	921	720	117	84	28	22	17	2
PD	472	438	344	70	24	6	16	9	3
PDC	9	9	9						
PUD	77	72	55	9	8	2	2	1	
Sur. Spec.	1,358	1,324	1,101	146	77	12	17	3	2
CRS	15	15	12		3				
GS	317	308	222	59	27	5	3		1
NS	56	54	48	4	2	1	1		
OBG	331	318	266	30	22	2	9	2	
OPH	145	142	130	8	4	1	1	1	
ORS	227	226	185	29	12	1			
OTO	85	84	75	8	1	1			
PS	41	41	41						
TS	37	34	33		1		2		1
U	104	102	89	8	5	1	1		
Oth. Spec.	1,590	1,501	1,186	145	170	35	23	11	20
AM	10	5	4		1	3		2	
AN	358	355	304	27	24		1		2
CHP	36	31	22		9	2	2	1	
DR	221	212	164	32	16		3		6
EM	168	163	139	1	23	2	2	1	
FOP	4	2	2						2
GPM	12	11	6	2	3	1			
MG	4	2	2			1	1		
N	95	93	73	13	7		1	1	
NM	9	9	7	1	1				
OM	37	28	21		7	8			1
P	292	279	187	44	48	4	6	1	2
PHP	6	1	1			3	2		
PM	31	31	29		2				
PTH	144	130	102	17	11	6	4		4
R	57	55	49	2	4		1		1
RO	40	38	35		3	2			
TTS	4	4	3		1				
OTH	27	17	16		1	3		5	2
UNSP	34	34	19	6	9				
VM	1	1	1						
Not Class	225								
Inactive	947								

Note: Excludes Address Unknown.

Subspecialties in this table are condensed into major specialties. See Appendix A.

Table 3.7

Physicians by State, Self-Designated Specialty, and Activity, 2006, continued
Oregon

Specialty	Total Physicians	Patient Care				Other Professional Activity			
		Total Patient Care	Office Based	Hospital Based		Admin.	Med. Teach.	Research	Other
				Resid./ Fellows	Phys. Staff				
Total Physicians	11,741	9,036	7,538	736	762	182	122	146	60
GP/FM Prac.	1,399	1,352	1,192	71	89	26	12	5	4
FM	1,276	1,237	1,087	71	79	19	12	4	4
GP	123	115	105		10	7		1	
Med. Prac.	3,261	3,085	2,534	315	236	45	44	77	10
AI	35	32	32			2		1	
CD	186	177	147	10	20	2	3	3	1
D	135	131	114	11	6			4	
GE	131	124	114	6	4	2	2	3	
IM	1,955	1,841	1,463	221	157	27	26	53	8
PD	697	666	573	56	37	11	11	8	1
PDC	19	19	12	4	3				
PUD	103	95	79	7	9	1	2	5	
Sur. Spec.	2,048	1,999	1,728	170	101	18	14	9	8
CRS	12	12	11	1					
GS	486	473	345	87	41	7	3	2	1
NS	97	96	85	9	2		1		
OBG	525	512	463	26	23	3	5	5	
OPH	224	220	203	11	6	3		1	
ORS	326	314	284	14	16	3	2		7
OTO	139	135	120	11	4	2	2		
PS	65	65	55	5	5				
TS	43	42	40	1	1			1	
U	131	130	122	5	3		1		
Oth. Spec.	2,838	2,600	2,084	180	336	93	52	55	38
AM	1					1			
AN	564	548	470	27	51	2	12	2	
CHP	85	79	70	3	6	3			3
DR	303	294	247	20	27	4	3	1	1
EM	549	525	395	33	97	12	10	2	
FOP	8	6	6				1	1	
GPM	35	24	21	1	2	7		3	1
MG	8	4	3	1				4	
N	174	150	128	13	9	3	6	13	2
NM	13	13	11	2					
OM	29	20	16		4	6	2		1
P	477	441	330	32	79	17	10	4	5
PHP	18	9	7		2	6		2	1
PM	75	72	66	1	5	3			
PTH	200	162	117	17	28	9	3	11	15
R	78	75	68	3	4		1	1	1
RO	59	57	51	3	3	1	1		
OTH	90	50	42		8	19	3	10	8
UNSP	72	71	36	24	11			1	
Not Class	458								
Inactive	1,737								

Note: Excludes Address Unknown.

Subspecialties in this table are condensed into major specialties. See Appendix A.

Table 3.7

Physicians by State, Self-Designated Specialty, and Activity, 2006, continued
Pennsylvania

| Specialty | Total Physicians | Patient Care | | | | Other Professional Activity | | | |
| | | Total Patient Care | Office Based | Hospital Based | | Admin. | Med. Teach. | Research | Other |
				Resid./ Fellows	Phys. Staff				
Total Physicians	42,204	32,324	23,343	5,881	3,100	727	493	908	215
GP/FM Prac.	3,741	3,542	2,808	476	258	79	99	12	9
FM	3,437	3,252	2,559	476	217	71	98	10	6
GP	304	290	249		41	8	1	2	3
Med. Prac.	13,341	12,325	8,753	2,570	1,002	249	189	519	59
AI	177	157	146	9	2	2	3	14	1
CD	1,261	1,176	948	150	78	18	13	47	7
D	459	444	358	68	18		4	11	
GE	616	576	460	74	42	7	10	20	3
IM	7,245	6,656	4,493	1,615	548	151	98	307	33
PD	2,953	2,742	1,934	556	252	60	53	85	13
PDC	81	72	40	18	14	2		7	
PUD	549	502	374	80	48	9	8	28	2
Sur. Spec.	7,276	7,062	5,284	1,308	470	77	60	52	25
CRS	88	86	73	6	7		1	1	
GS	1,892	1,824	1,146	532	146	30	17	13	8
NS	256	246	166	54	26	4	2	3	1
OBG	1,678	1,623	1,237	250	136	21	19	10	5
OPH	864	836	732	68	36	6	7	12	3
ORS	1,078	1,055	776	238	41	7	6	4	6
OTO	410	403	324	61	18	1	3	2	1
PS	268	267	208	41	18			1	
TS	271	262	221	20	21	4	3	2	
U	471	460	401	38	21	4	2	4	1
Oth. Spec.	10,309	9,395	6,498	1,527	1,370	322	145	325	122
AM	6	3	3			3			
AN	1,671	1,608	1,246	203	159	15	27	21	
CHP	344	315	250	28	37	11	4	9	5
DR	1,247	1,204	845	236	123	7	16	12	8
EM	1,388	1,318	702	315	301	35	15	11	9
FOP	24	15	13	1	1	2		1	6
GPM	65	47	36	6	5	6	3	4	5
MG	22	20	9	7	4	1		1	
N	698	621	477	87	57	12	8	55	2
NM	73	65	46	7	12	3	2	3	
OM	96	58	41	1	16	29	3	2	4
P	1,994	1,815	1,279	229	307	69	29	70	11
PHP	34	6	5		1	21	2	3	2
PM	455	440	334	55	51	10		3	2
PTH	963	822	510	142	170	34	16	47	44
R	435	410	334	18	58	4	12	3	6
RO	224	220	158	32	30	2	1	1	
TTS	7	7	6		1				
OTH	266	120	97	2	21	51	6	72	17
UNSP	295	279	105	158	16	7	1	7	1
VM	2	2	2						
Not Class	2,289								
Inactive	5,248								

Note: Excludes Address Unknown.

Subspecialties in this table are condensed into major specialties. See Appendix A.

Table 3.7

Physicians by State, Self-Designated Specialty, and Activity, 2006, continued
Puerto Rico

Specialty	Total Physicians	Patient Care				Other Professional Activity			
		Total Patient Care	Office Based	Hospital Based		Admin.	Med. Teach.	Research	Other
				Resid./ Fellows	Phys. Staff				
Total Physicians	11,900	9,173	7,318	806	1,049	197	136	48	47
GP/FM Prac.	2,136	2,065	1,742	41	282	39	20	3	9
FM	805	772	661	41	70	16	14	1	2
GP	1,331	1,293	1,081		212	23	6	2	7
Med. Prac.	3,170	3,011	2,281	387	343	64	63	22	10
AI	12	12	12						
CD	219	207	178	14	15	1	7	3	1
D	88	86	72	8	6		1	1	
GE	111	107	89	10	8		2	2	
IM	1,567	1,505	1,058	278	169	26	24	8	4
PD	1,071	1,002	790	76	136	37	22	5	5
PDC	14	14	13		1				
PUD	88	78	69	1	8		7	3	
Sur. Spec.	1,480	1,432	1,180	122	130	19	22	3	4
CRS	7	7	6		1				
GS	373	358	257	53	48	6	8		1
NS	27	26	19	6	1		1		
OBG	538	517	434	33	50	10	7	2	2
OPH	167	165	154	3	8	1		1	
ORS	126	121	96	22	3	1	3		1
OTO	78	75	68	3	4	1	2		
PS	37	37	32	2	3				
TS	22	22	18		4				
U	105	104	96		8		1		
Oth. Spec.	2,815	2,665	2,115	256	294	75	31	20	24
AN	1	1	1						
AN	208	200	163	15	22	3	3	1	1
CHP	67	62	51	5	6	1	3		1
DR	169	157	116	18	23	3	4	1	4
EM	172	156	92	28	36	14	2		
FOP	3	3	3						
GPM	21	16	14		2	2	1	1	1
MG	2	1	1					1	
N	128	121	87	20	14		3	3	1
NM	32	28	24	2	2	2	1		1
OM	35	29	23		6	6			
P	454	428	310	51	67	11	6	5	4
PHP	19	7	4		3	9		1	2
PM	202	200	157	27	16	1	1		
PTH	104	89	71	10	8	6	3	1	5
R	63	61	51	2	8		1	1	
RO	22	20	17		3	1		1	
OTH	66	48	40	1	7	13	3	2	
UNSP	1,047	1,038	890	77	71	3		2	4
Not Class	1,494								
Inactive	805								

Note: Excludes Address Unknown.

Subspecialties in this table are condensed into major specialties. See Appendix A.

Table 3.7

Physicians by State, Self-Designated Specialty, and Activity, 2006, continued
Rhode Island

Specialty	Total Physicians	Patient Care		Hospital Based		Other Professional Activity			
		Total Patient Care	Office Based	Resid./ Fellows	Phys. Staff	Admin.	Med. Teach.	Research	Other
Total Physicians	4,368	3,458	2,419	675	364	72	49	65	23
GP/FM Prac.	229	220	173	26	21	2	6		1
FM	211	202	157	26	19	2	6		1
GP	18	18	16		2				
Med. Prac.	1,672	1,573	1,088	348	137	27	27	37	8
AI	12	11	10		1	1			
CD	111	109	92	9	8	1		1	
D	69	64	44	17	3	2	2	1	
GE	67	67	53	7	7				
IM	936	879	587	219	73	17	12	24	4
PD	411	381	259	87	35	5	12	9	4
PDC	7	7	4		3				
PUD	59	55	39	9	7	1	1	2	
Sur. Spec.	735	715	544	123	48	8	6	4	2
CRS	7	7	6	1					
GS	174	169	116	43	10	1		4	
NS	32	31	20	8	3		1		
OBG	203	195	153	27	15	5	2		1
OPH	78	78	65	6	7				
ORS	114	111	84	19	8		2		1
OTO	35	34	30	1	3	1			
PS	29	29	19	10					
TS	12	12	11		1				
U	51	49	40	8	1	1	1		
Oth. Spec.	1,031	950	614	178	158	35	10	24	12
AN	118	117	101	2	14	1			
CHP	45	39	24	8	7	1		3	2
DR	122	118	82	28	8	2		1	1
EM	162	155	97	36	22	4	1	2	
FOP	4	3	2		1	1			
GPM	4	4	2		2				
MG	2	2		1	1				
N	77	71	53	15	3	1	4		1
NM	4	4	4						
OM	8	7	5		2	1			
P	254	236	133	54	49	10	2	6	
PHP	4	1	1			2		1	
PM	13	12	5	1	6	1			
PTH	102	83	36	14	33	6	3	5	5
R	36	34	27	3	4			1	1
RO	18	18	15	2	1				
TTS	2	2	1		1				
OTH	28	16	15		1	5		5	2
UNSP	28	28	11	14	3				
Not Class	244								
Inactive	457								

Note: *Excludes Address Unknown.*

Subspecialties in this table are condensed into major specialties. See Appendix A.

Table 3.7

Physicians by State, Self-Designated Specialty, and Activity, 2006, continued
South Carolina

Specialty	Total Physicians	Patient Care		Hospital Based		Other Professional Activity			
		Total Patient Care	Office Based	Resid./ Fellows	Phys. Staff	Admin.	Med. Teach.	Research	Other
Total Physicians	11,241	9,155	7,267	1,083	805	124	163	85	29
GP/FM Prac.	1,575	1,518	1,224	184	110	14	35	6	2
FM	1,455	1,405	1,123	184	98	10	35	5	
GP	120	113	101		12	4		1	2
Med. Prac.	3,143	2,989	2,338	377	274	37	68	44	5
AI	50	48	46	1	1		1	1	
CD	268	256	225	15	16	3	7	2	
D	128	126	106	12	8	1	1		
GE	166	159	140	9	10	2	2	3	
IM	1,550	1,476	1,138	193	145	18	26	29	1
PD	850	802	583	132	87	10	28	7	3
PDC	31	29	17	8	4		1	1	
PUD	100	93	83	7	3	3	2	1	1
Sur. Spec.	2,233	2,175	1,798	251	126	15	27	10	6
CRS	16	16	15		1				
GS	536	515	377	91	47	8	8	2	3
NS	59	56	49	5	2		1	2	
OBG	594	583	487	59	37	1	8	1	1
OPH	241	237	217	15	5	1		3	
ORS	365	355	286	55	14	1	6	2	1
OTO	127	125	105	14	6		2		
PS	82	81	74	4	3	1			
TS	69	67	57	4	6	1	1		
U	144	140	131	4	5	2	1		1
Oth. Spec.	2,605	2,473	1,907	271	295	58	33	25	16
AM	7	7	3		4				
AN	462	453	389	35	29	4	3	2	
CHP	120	113	84	16	13	1	2	4	
DR	286	281	210	39	32	1	1	1	2
EM	467	455	353	32	70	7	5		
FOP	9	9	7	1	1				
GPM	15	13	7	3	3	1	1		
MG	11	10	10					1	
N	135	127	107	9	11	3	4	1	
NM	12	10	8	1	1			2	
OM	25	23	20		3	2			
P	475	448	304	66	78	12	8	4	3
PHP	25	6	5		1	15	1	1	2
PM	61	60	55	1	4				1
PTH	218	199	147	29	23	3	5	4	7
R	100	98	88	3	7		1	1	
RO	44	43	39	4					1
TTS	2	2	1		1				
OTH	45	30	24		6	9	2	4	
UNSP	85	85	45	32	8				
VM	1	1	1						
Not Class	331								
Inactive	1,354								

Note: Excludes Address Unknown.

Subspecialties in this table are condensed into major specialties. See Appendix A.

Table 3.7

Physicians by State, Self-Designated Specialty, and Activity, 2006, continued
South Dakota

Specialty	Total Physicians	Patient Care				Other Professional Activity			
		Total Patient Care	Office Based	Hospital Based		Admin.	Med. Teach.	Research	Other
				Resid./ Fellows	Phys. Staff				
Total Physicians	1,975	1,627	1,342	104	181	24	17	6	6
GP/FM Prac.	387	372	302	32	38	7	8		
FM	357	342	277	32	33	7	8		
GP	30	30	25		5				
Med. Prac.	489	466	382	32	52	12	6	3	2
AI	8	8	8						
CD	38	38	37		1				
D	23	23	21		2				
GE	20	19	18		1		1		
IM	279	260	194	29	37	12	4	2	1
PD	101	100	90	2	8				1
PDC	5	5	3		2				
PUD	15	13	11	1	1		1	1	
Sur. Spec.	392	390	351	4	35	1		1	
CRS	1	1	1						
GS	107	107	93	1	13				
NS	19	19	19						
OBG	78	78	67	2	9				
OPH	42	41	40		1			1	
ORS	72	71	66		5	1			
OTO	24	24	19	1	4				
PS	13	13	13						
TS	9	9	8		1				
U	27	27	25		2				
Oth. Spec.	412	399	307	36	56	4	3	2	4
AN	64	62	56	1	5	2			
CHP	18	16	5	6	5	1	1		
DR	55	54	46		8				1
EM	42	40	35	1	4	1		1	
GPM	1	1	1						
MG	1	1	1						
N	33	33	31		2				
NM	6	6	4		2				
OM	5	5	4		1				
P	68	66	33	16	17		2		
PM	18	18	12	1	5				
PTH	47	44	39	3	2			1	2
R	15	14	13		1				1
RO	15	15	14		1				
TTS	1	1	1						
OTH	7	7	5		2				
UNSP	16	16	7	8	1				
Not Class	39								
Inactive	256								

Note: Excludes Address Unknown.

Subspecialties in this table are condensed into major specialties. See Appendix A.

Table 3.7

Physicians by State, Self-Designated Specialty, and Activity, 2006, continued
Tennessee

Specialty	Total Physicians	Patient Care				Other Professional Activity			
		Total Patient Care	Office Based	Hospital Based		Admin.	Med. Teach.	Research	Other
				Resid./ Fellows	Phys. Staff				
Total Physicians	17,791	14,557	11,673	1,898	986	251	196	228	55
GP/FM Prac.	1,946	1,873	1,629	142	102	32	34	2	5
FM	1,750	1,682	1,460	142	80	29	34	1	4
GP	196	191	169		22	3		1	1
Med. Prac.	5,799	5,476	4,305	804	367	78	79	154	12
AI	79	74	67	6	1	1		4	
CD	446	424	366	43	15	4	7	9	2
D	176	173	150	14	9		1	2	
GE	238	229	201	16	12	3	1	5	
IM	3,008	2,844	2,185	457	202	42	41	75	6
PD	1,542	1,448	1,104	239	105	24	23	44	3
PDC	47	40	29	6	5	1		6	
PUD	263	244	203	23	18	3	6	9	1
Sur. Spec.	3,583	3,509	2,867	499	143	29	33	8	4
CRS	18	17	15		2		1		
GS	909	889	621	218	50	7	11	1	1
NS	138	138	117	17	4				
OBG	894	869	744	96	29	11	12	2	
OPH	349	343	305	25	13	2	2	2	
ORS	548	539	445	73	21	2	3	2	2
OTO	220	218	188	23	7		1	1	
PS	148	148	129	15	4				
TS	109	105	94	5	6	3	1		
U	250	243	209	27	7	4	2		1
Oth. Spec.	3,959	3,699	2,872	453	374	112	50	64	34
AM	4	4	3		1				
AN	786	762	619	89	54	6	11	5	2
CHP	92	85	73	4	8	3	3	1	
DR	538	521	384	100	37	6	5	2	4
EM	490	479	364	38	77	10	1		
FOP	13	11	9		2				2
GPM	29	25	19	6		3	1		
MG	7	5	3		2			2	
N	272	249	208	23	18	3	8	12	
NM	28	26	20	5	1	1		1	
OM	66	44	39	1	4	18			4
P	601	566	408	79	79	18	7	9	1
PHP	28	7	7			15	1	3	2
PM	97	93	82	1	10	3			1
PTH	422	377	290	53	34	10	6	15	14
R	205	200	178	4	18	1	1	1	2
RO	91	91	75	7	9				
TTS	3	3	3						
OTH	88	56	46		10	14	4	12	2
UNSP	99	95	42	43	10	1	2	1	
Not Class	638								
Inactive	1,866								

Note: Excludes Address Unknown.

Subspecialties in this table are condensed into major specialties. See Appendix A.

Table 3.7

Physicians by State, Self-Designated Specialty, and Activity, 2006, continued
Texas

Specialty	Total Physicians	Patient Care		Hospital Based		Other Professional Activity			
		Total Patient Care	Office Based	Resid./ Fellows	Phys. Staff	Admin.	Med. Teach.	Research	Other
Total Physicians	54,971	44,813	35,693	5,923	3,197	714	708	615	192
GP/FM Prac.	6,361	6,139	5,233	602	304	94	97	15	16
FM	5,741	5,532	4,672	602	258	89	95	12	13
GP	620	607	561		46	5	2	3	3
Med. Prac.	16,751	15,861	12,456	2,301	1,104	211	270	371	38
AI	320	291	260	17	14	5	2	22	
CD	1,398	1,326	1,100	144	82	13	18	36	5
D	664	658	533	91	34	3	3		
GE	773	735	624	71	40	7	12	19	
IM	8,148	7,668	5,892	1,189	587	115	137	211	17
PD	4,754	4,524	3,497	733	294	60	88	69	13
PDC	134	129	108	15	6	1		3	1
PUD	560	530	442	41	47	7	10	11	2
Sur. Spec.	10,636	10,341	8,478	1,318	545	88	145	40	22
CRS	109	104	93	7	4		2	2	1
GS	2,308	2,234	1,622	450	162	26	33	10	5
NS	344	338	280	40	18	3	2		1
OBG	2,968	2,871	2,443	312	116	23	61	10	3
OPH	1,105	1,076	937	82	57	11	15	2	1
ORS	1,566	1,534	1,238	219	77	9	11	4	8
OTO	669	650	546	73	31	8	9	2	
PS	549	540	452	64	24	2	4		3
TS	343	332	302	13	17	2	3	6	
U	675	662	565	58	39	4	5	4	
Oth. Spec.	13,294	12,472	9,526	1,702	1,244	321	196	189	116
AM	89	54	35	2	17	25	2	4	4
AN	3,071	2,995	2,426	346	223	23	38	11	4
CHP	441	419	336	48	35	8	6	6	2
DR	1,569	1,537	1,133	260	144	3	14	4	11
EM	1,600	1,546	1,190	167	189	31	16	2	5
FOP	49	38	33	5		2			9
GPM	111	93	62	19	12	11	2	4	1
MG	40	29	18	6	5	3	4	4	
N	855	806	656	95	55	8	14	25	2
NM	88	79	60	8	11	2	3	4	
OM	150	106	92	2	12	36	4	2	2
P	1,858	1,724	1,251	233	240	55	31	28	20
PHP	56	16	11		5	26	2	10	2
PM	494	481	366	75	40	8	2	1	2
PTH	1,318	1,200	858	202	140	29	20	35	34
R	556	522	443	22	57	2	21	5	6
RO	289	284	225	37	22	2	2	1	
TTS	10	10	10						
OTH	273	166	148		18	46	13	38	10
UNSP	376	366	172	175	19	1	2	5	2
VM	1	1	1						
Not Class	2,698								
Inactive	5,231								

Note: Excludes Address Unknown.

Subspecialties in this table are condensed into major specialties. See Appendix A.

Table 3.7

Physicians by State, Self-Designated Specialty, and Activity, 2006, continued
Utah

| Specialty | Total Physicians | Patient Care | | | | Other Professional Activity | | | |
		Total Patient Care	Office Based	Resid./ Fellows	Phys. Staff	Admin.	Med. Teach.	Research	Other
Total Physicians	6,093	4,862	3,883	643	336	87	66	102	31
GP/FM Prac.	742	722	621	56	45	6	11	1	2
FM	703	687	588	56	43	5	10	1	
GP	39	35	33		2	1	1		2
Med. Prac.	1,670	1,547	1,202	238	107	28	25	65	5
AI	21	18	17		1	1		2	
CD	117	102	82	12	8	2	4	9	
D	85	79	70	7	2	1	1	4	
GE	77	73	65	6	2	2	1	1	
IM	736	688	511	123	54	10	11	24	3
PD	542	511	403	77	31	10	7	12	2
PDC	17	15	11	3	1			2	
PUD	75	61	43	10	8	2	1	11	
Sur. Spec.	1,174	1,152	955	144	53	6	6	6	4
CRS	7	7	6		1				
GS	225	219	163	42	14	3		2	1
NS	49	48	31	15	2			1	
OBG	290	283	253	18	12		3	2	2
OPH	137	136	118	11	7		1		
ORS	206	204	159	31	14		1	1	
OTO	82	80	68	11	1	2			
PS	77	77	72	4	1				
TS	33	31	27	3	1		1		1
U	68	67	58	9		1			
Oth. Spec.	1,562	1,441	1,105	205	131	47	24	30	20
AM	3	2			2	1			
AN	364	350	286	45	19	1	7	3	3
CHP	47	43	35	4	4	3		1	
DR	163	158	123	20	15		3		2
EM	265	257	212	21	24	5	2		1
FOP	1	1	1						
GPM	8	8	5	2	1				
MG	4	3	1	1	1			1	
N	108	96	74	15	7	3	1	8	
NM	4	3	2	1				1	
OM	25	15	12	1	2	6	2	1	1
P	199	183	119	28	36	8	5	2	1
PHP	8	1	1			5		2	
PM	74	73	57	11	5			1	
PTH	129	105	77	21	7	6	3	6	9
R	58	55	47	3	5	2	1		
RO	31	31	25	6					
TTS	1	1	1						
OTH	31	18	16		2	7		4	2
UNSP	39	38	11	26	1				1
Not Class	253								
Inactive	692								

Note: Excludes Address Unknown.

Subspecialties in this table are condensed into major specialties. See Appendix A.

Table 3.7

Physicians by State, Self-Designated Specialty, and Activity, 2006, continued
Vermont

Specialty	Total Physicians	Patient Care				Other Professional Activity			
		Total Patient Care	Office Based	Hospital Based		Admin.	Med. Teach.	Research	Other
				Resid./ Fellows	Phys. Staff				
Total Physicians	2,659	1,980	1,418	313	249	47	41	56	11
GP/FM Prac.	317	307	259	17	31	6	2	2	
FM	299	291	244	17	30	5	2	1	
GP	18	16	15		1	1		1	
Med. Prac.	734	663	472	116	75	16	16	36	3
AI	9	7	7			1		1	
CD	52	46	28	10	8	1	1	4	
D	22	21	16	5				1	
GE	23	22	17	5		1			
IM	417	375	256	70	49	7	11	23	1
PD	179	166	131	20	15	5	3	3	2
PDC	4	4	2	1	1				
PUD	28	22	15	5	2	1	1	4	
Sur. Spec.	424	415	309	76	30	3	6		
CRS	1	1			1				
GS	121	117	79	31	7	1	3		
NS	15	15	7	7	1				
OBG	112	108	80	15	13	2	2		
OPH	36	36	35		1				
ORS	76	75	55	16	4		1		
OTO	24	24	18	5	1				
PS	8	8	8						
TS	4	4	4						
U	27	27	23	2	2				
Oth. Spec.	660	595	378	104	113	22	17	18	8
AN	108	106	66	26	14	1	1		
CHP	27	27	22	2	3				
DR	71	68	32	19	17		2	1	
EM	70	66	37	1	28	2	2		
FOP	3	2	2						1
GPM	11	10	6	2	2	1			
N	40	34	23	7	4		1	4	1
OM	2	2	2						
P	165	151	110	21	20	4	4	4	2
PHP	5	1	1			2			2
PM	13	12	6	1	5	1			
PTH	80	67	36	17	14	3	5	4	1
R	21	20	17		3				1
RO	8	8	6	1	1				
OTH	19	5	5			8	1	5	
UNSP	17	16	7	7	2		1		
Not Class	128								
Inactive	396								

Note: Excludes Address Unknown.

Subspecialties in this table are condensed into major specialties. See Appendix A.

Table 3.7

Physicians by State, Self-Designated Specialty, and Activity, 2006, continued
Virginia

| Specialty | Total Physicians | Patient Care | | Hospital Based | | Other Professional Activity | | | |
		Total Patient Care	Office Based	Resid./ Fellows	Phys. Staff	Admin.	Med. Teach.	Research	Other
Total Physicians	23,545	18,538	14,306	2,262	1,970	391	241	239	148
GP/FM Prac.	2,690	2,573	2,097	226	250	55	45	5	12
FM	2,444	2,344	1,919	226	199	44	42	5	9
GP	246	229	178		51	11	3		3
Med. Prac.	7,028	6,674	5,216	809	649	95	83	131	45
AI	106	98	86	8	4	1		7	
CD	472	454	380	34	40	5	4	8	1
D	254	249	210	23	16	2	1		2
GE	317	302	264	16	22	1	2	9	3
IM	3,660	3,460	2,614	481	365	57	43	77	23
PD	1,913	1,824	1,433	221	170	25	27	22	15
PDC	54	48	31	7	10	1	1	4	
PUD	252	239	198	19	22	3	5	4	1
Sur. Spec.	4,206	4,100	3,281	482	337	41	32	17	16
CRS	31	31	29		2				
GS	919	888	601	178	109	15	7	5	4
NS	133	130	99	21	10	1		1	1
OBG	1,211	1,179	988	115	76	10	12	4	6
OPH	461	451	392	28	31	1	7	1	1
ORS	621	615	496	74	45	3	3		
OTO	273	266	217	30	19	4	1		2
PS	171	167	144	12	11		2	2	
TS	93	92	75	5	12			1	
U	293	281	240	19	22	7		3	2
Oth. Spec.	5,633	5,191	3,712	745	734	200	81	86	75
AM	26	15	7		8	9		1	1
AN	990	964	721	114	129	5	15	1	5
CHP	193	185	141	16	28	4	3	1	
DR	639	619	470	91	58	3	4	4	9
EM	874	847	600	120	127	11	7	3	6
FOP	11	6	5		1	2			3
GPM	74	55	40	4	11	13	1	1	4
MG	7	7	5		2				
N	343	316	248	42	26	5	5	16	1
NM	30	27	17	1	9	1		2	
OM	58	35	25	1	9	16	2		5
P	1,081	1,007	693	141	173	39	15	14	6
PHP	56	11	6		5	37	2	4	2
PM	185	179	122	31	26	3		3	
PTH	441	366	245	60	61	23	17	16	19
R	208	198	158	14	26	1	5	1	3
RO	98	96	76	16	4	1	1		
TTS	5	4	3		1			1	
OTH	116	62	52		10	25	3	18	8
UNSP	198	192	78	94	20	2	1		3
Not Class	1,074								
Inactive	2,914								

Note: Excludes Address Unknown.

Subspecialties in this table are condensed into major specialties. See Appendix A.

Table 3.7

Physicians by State, Self-Designated Specialty, and Activity, 2006, continued
Virgin Islands

Specialty	Total Physicians	Patient Care				Other Professional Activity			
		Total Patient Care	Office Based	Hospital Based		Admin.	Med. Teach.	Research	Other
				Resid./ Fellows	Phys. Staff				
Total Physicians	200	167	124	5	38	2			
GP/FM Prac.	22	22	17	2	3				
FM	17	17	14	2	1				
GP	5	5	3		2				
Med. Prac.	50	50	35	2	13				
AI	1	1	1						
CD	4	4	3		1				
D	2	2	2						
GE	2	2	2						
IM	25	25	17	2	6				
PD	16	16	10		6				
Sur. Spec.	56	55	45	1	9	1			
GS	12	12	10		2				
OBG	24	23	19		4	1			
OPH	6	6	6						
ORS	6	6	5	1					
OTO	2	2	2						
PS	2	2	2						
TS	1	1			1				
U	3	3	1		2				
Oth. Spec.	41	40	27		13	1			
AN	7	7	6		1				
DR	3	3	2		1				
EM	6	6	2		4				
GPM	1	1	1						
N	3	3	3						
NM	1	1			1				
OM	1	1			1				
P	7	7	4		3				
PHP	1	1	1						
PM	4	3	2		1		1		
PTH	1	1			1				
R	1	1	1						
UNSP	5	5	5						
Not Class	8								
Inactive	23								

Note: Excludes Address Unknown.

Subspecialties in this table are condensed into major specialties. See Appendix A.

Table 3.7

Physicians by State, Self-Designated Specialty, and Activity, 2006, continued
Washington

Specialty	Total Physicians	Patient Care				Other Professional Activity			
		Total Patient Care	Office Based	Hospital Based		Admin.	Med. Teach.	Research	Other
				Resid./ Fellows	Phys. Staff				
Total Physicians	19,864	15,168	12,460	1,354	1,354	340	204	402	120
GP/FM Prac.	2,970	2,838	2,448	197	193	60	50	13	9
FM	2,768	2,640	2,266	197	177	56	50	13	9
GP	202	198	182		16	4			
Med. Prac.	5,306	4,892	3,941	477	474	104	64	229	17
AI	78	67	58	2	7	3		7	1
CD	352	323	269	18	36	3	9	17	
D	228	220	200	9	11	1	3	2	2
GE	253	237	213	11	13	4	2	9	1
IM	2,841	2,604	2,066	269	269	64	25	139	9
PD	1,325	1,238	976	147	115	23	17	43	4
PDC	32	29	26		3		2	1	
PUD	197	174	133	21	20	6	6	11	
Sur. Spec.	3,140	3,044	2,558	274	212	26	30	22	18
CRS	21	20	19	1			1		
GS	714	691	509	124	58	10	7	3	3
NS	105	97	79	8	10	1	1	3	3
OBG	767	745	662	36	47	7	9	6	
OPH	339	335	306	13	16		3	1	
ORS	543	522	441	46	35	4	4	3	10
OTO	241	238	198	22	18	1	2		
PS	130	127	113	8	6		1		2
TS	71	68	56	4	8	1		2	
U	209	201	175	12	14	2	2	4	
Oth. Spec.	4,818	4,394	3,513	406	475	150	60	138	76
AM	16	11	7		4	4		1	
AN	967	927	769	84	74	10	18	9	3
CHP	112	107	91	7	9	2	3		
DR	566	543	442	60	41	4	7	3	9
EM	693	670	548	22	100	16	4	1	2
FOP	12	6	6			1		1	4
GPM	73	61	44	7	10	4		7	1
MG	19	9	7		2	1	1	7	1
N	273	251	207	24	20	1	4	10	7
NM	36	31	25	3	3	1		3	1
OM	88	67	53	2	12	14		3	4
P	810	739	563	63	113	26	8	28	9
PHP	45	11	11			13	2	13	6
PM	196	182	139	20	23	8	3	2	1
PTH	362	312	247	35	30	8	7	16	19
R	174	170	140	17	13	1	1	2	
RO	96	93	77	8	8		1	2	
TTS	4	4	3		1				
OTH	127	60	57		3	34	1	29	3
UNSP	149	140	77	54	9	2		1	6
Not Class	731								
Inactive	2,899								

Note: Excludes Address Unknown.

Subspecialties in this table are condensed into major specialties. See Appendix A.

Table 3.7

Physicians by State, Self-Designated Specialty, and Activity, 2006, continued
West Virginia

Specialty	Total Physicians	Patient Care				Other Professional Activity			
		Total Patient Care	Office Based	Hospital Based		Admin.	Med. Teach.	Research	Other
				Resid./ Fellows	Phys. Staff				
Total Physicians	4,710	3,762	2,802	555	405	58	77	32	22
GP/FM Prac.	672	641	505	88	48	6	20	2	3
FM	586	555	431	88	36	6	20	2	3
GP	86	86	74		12				
Med. Prac.	1,338	1,275	922	237	116	17	27	16	3
AI	17	17	17						
CD	123	117	89	16	12	1	2	2	1
D	36	34	31	2	1		2		
GE	46	45	39	2	4			1	
IM	705	674	467	138	69	11	12	7	1
PD	334	319	226	70	23	2	9	3	1
PDC	8	6	6			1	1		
PUD	69	63	47	9	7	2	1	3	
Sur. Spec.	887	868	667	125	76	4	11	2	2
CRS	4	4	4						
GS	243	236	166	45	25	2	5		
NS	32	32	26	5	1				
OBG	210	200	145	35	20	2	6	2	
OPH	95	93	83	9	1				2
ORS	112	112	85	16	11				
OTO	61	61	50	10	1				
PS	30	30	27	1	2				
TS	34	34	26	1	7				
U	66	66	55	3	8				
Oth. Spec.	1,054	978	708	105	165	31	19	12	14
AM	1	1	1						
AN	157	155	125	11	19		2		
CHP	22	21	18	1	2	1			
DR	149	145	111	17	17		3		1
EM	170	159	105	11	43	6	3	2	
FOP	4	2	2						2
GPM	4	2	2			1		1	
MG	1	1	1						
N	75	74	60	9	5			1	
NM	3	3	1		2				
OM	19	11	9	2		5	1	2	
P	167	153	100	29	24	4	8	1	1
PHP	8					4		2	2
PM	26	25	22		3	1			
PTH	131	116	77	13	26	5		3	7
R	44	40	32		8	2	2		
RO	17	17	14		3				
OTH	27	24	17		7	2			1
UNSP	29	29	11	12	6				
Not Class	215								
Inactive	544								

Note: Excludes Address Unknown.

Subspecialties in this table are condensed into major specialties. See Appendix A.

Table 3.7

Physicians by State, Self-Designated Specialty, and Activity, 2006, continued
Wisconsin

| Specialty | Total Physicians | Patient Care | | | | Other Professional Activity | | | |
		Total Patient Care	Office Based	Resid./ Fellows	Phys. Staff	Admin.	Med. Teach.	Research	Other
Total Physicians	16,154	13,126	10,611	1,529	986	221	196	182	78
GP/FM Prac.	2,421	2,319	1,994	191	134	36	47	7	12
FM	2,305	2,209	1,893	191	125	36	47	7	6
GP	116	110	101		9				6
Med. Prac.	4,593	4,323	3,443	585	295	83	69	102	16
AI	101	94	82	11	1			6	1
CD	316	300	248	29	23	2	5	8	1
D	186	186	152	23	11				
GE	195	192	161	24	7		2	1	
IM	2,478	2,327	1,838	312	177	50	36	55	10
PD	1,131	1,061	833	167	61	23	19	25	3
PDC	30	29	21	5	3		1		
PUD	156	134	108	14	12	8	6	7	1
Sur. Spec.	2,798	2,720	2,253	318	149	22	26	17	13
CRS	16	16	16						
GS	645	620	474	111	35	8	7	5	5
NS	115	111	84	17	10	1	1		2
OBG	628	613	516	55	42	7	7	1	
OPH	330	316	286	17	13	3	1	8	2
ORS	502	494	414	53	27	1	2	2	3
OTO	198	193	165	22	6	1	3		1
PS	97	95	72	20	3		2		
TS	83	81	70	6	5		2		
U	184	181	156	17	8	1	1	1	
Oth. Spec.	3,991	3,764	2,921	435	408	80	54	56	37
AM	1	1	1						
AN	836	812	623	107	82	7	11	6	
CHP	122	120	97	10	13		2		
DR	534	528	417	70	41	1	2		3
EM	521	504	402	26	76	11	3	2	1
FOP	12	10	9	1		1			1
GPM	22	16	14		2	2	1	2	1
MG	10	8	6	1	1			2	
N	258	238	200	26	12	1	4	13	2
NM	30	27	24	3			1	1	1
OM	50	45	39		6	1	3	1	
P	603	570	437	47	86	16	11	4	2
PHP	9	1			1	3	2	1	2
PM	174	169	133	15	21	3		2	
PTH	355	305	238	34	33	16	5	9	20
R	174	170	146	10	14	1	2		1
RO	89	88	69	14	5		1		
TTS	1	1	1						
OTH	83	45	37	2	6	17	6	13	2
UNSP	106	105	27	69	9				1
VM	1	1	1						
Not Class	454								
Inactive	1,897								

Note: Excludes Address Unknown.

Subspecialties in this table are condensed into major specialties. See Appendix A.

Table 3.7

Physicians by State, Self-Designated Specialty, and Activity, 2006, continued
Wyoming

Specialty	Total Physicians	Patient Care				Other Professional Activity			
		Total Patient Care	Office Based	Hospital Based		Admin.	Med. Teach.	Research	Other
				Resid./ Fellows	Phys. Staff				
Total Physicians	1,132	903	780	33	90	18	8	4	8
GP/FM Prac.	251	242	185	28	29	2	4		3
FM	229	222	168	28	26	2	3		2
GP	22	20	17		3		1		1
Med. Prac.	200	190	175	1	14	7		3	
AI	2	2	2						
CD	15	13	12		1	1		1	
D	8	8	8						
GE	7	7	6		1				
IM	113	107	96		11	5		1	
PD	47	45	44		1	1		1	
PUD	8	8	7	1					
Sur. Spec.	230	225	215	1	9	1	3		1
GS	55	55	52	1	2				
NS	9	9	9						
OBG	51	49	47		2	1	1		
OPH	16	15	15				1		
ORS	63	62	60		2				
OTO	11	11	10		1				
PS	2	2	2						
TS	5	4	4				1		
U	18	18	16		2				
Oth. Spec.	260	246	205	3	38	8	1	1	4
AM	3	3	2		1				
AN	52	52	50		2				
CHP	4	4	3		1				
DR	33	33	27	1	5				
EM	57	54	36	1	17	2			1
GPM	2	2	2						
N	10	10	10						
OM	3	2	2			1			
P	40	37	30		7	3			
PM	5	4	3		1				1
PTH	27	23	20		3	1	1	1	1
R	10	9	9						1
RO	7	7	6		1				
OTH	2	1	1			1			
UNSP	5	5	4	1					
Not Class	9								
Inactive	182								

Note: Excludes Address Unknown.

Subspecialties in this table are condensed into major specialties. See Appendix A.

Table 3.7

Physicians by State, Self-Designated Specialty, and Activity, 2006, continued
Pacific Islands

Specialty	Total Physicians	Patient Care		Hospital Based		Other Professional Activity			
		Total Patient Care	Office Based	Resid./ Fellows	Phys. Staff	Admin.	Med. Teach.	Research	Other
Total Physicians	238	193	143	3	47	7			4
GP/FM Prac.	48	48	42	1	5				
FM	39	39	34	1	4				
GP	9	9	8		1				
Med. Prac.	69	69	50	2	17				
CD	2	2	2						
D	45	45	34	2	9				
IM	20	20	12		8				
PD	2	2	2						
PUD									
	39	39	31		8				
Sur. Spec.	10	10	9		1				
GS	18	18	14		4				
OBG	2	2	1		1				
OPH	4	4	3		1				
ORS	2	2	1		1				
OTO	1	1	1						
PS	2	2	2						
U									
	48	37	20		17	7			4
Oth. Spec.	2	1			1	1			
AN	8	7	3		4	1			
DR	5	5	3		2				
EM	9	9	3		6				
N	2	2	2						
OM	1								1
P	10	8	6		2	1			1
PHP	3					2			1
PTH	4	2	1		1	1			1
R	1	1	1						
OTH	1					1			
UNSP	2	2	1		1				
Not Class	16								
Inactive	18								

Note: Excludes Address Unknown.

Subspecialties in this table are condensed into major specialties. See Appendix A.

Table 3.8

Female Physicians by State, Self-Designated Specialty, and Activity, 2006
Alabama

| | | Patient Care | | | | Other Professional Activity | | | |
| | | | | Hospital Based | | | | | |
Specialty	Total Physicians	Total Patient Care	Office Based	Resid./ Fellows	Phys. Staff	Admin.	Med. Teach.	Research	Other
Total Physicians	2,431	2,104	1,496	437	171	19	15	22	9
GP/FM Prac.	350	345	264	56	25	3	2		
FM	335	330	251	56	23	3	2		
GP	15	15	13		2				
Med. Spec.	979	948	683	204	61	5	8	15	3
AI	14	14	12	2					
CD	21	20	19		1			1	
D	50	50	42	8					
GE	14	13	10	3				1	
IM	467	448	297	118	33	3	7	7	2
PD	397	389	290	72	27	1	1	5	1
PDC	4	4	4						
PUD	12	10	9	1		1		1	
Sur. Spec.	288	284	193	70	21		3		1
GS	58	56	27	20	9		1		1
NS	3	3	1	1	1				
OBG	167	165	123	34	8		2		
OPH	27	27	19	6	2				
ORS	11	11	6	5					
OTO	13	13	9	4					
PS	2	2	2						
TS	2	2	1		1				
U	5	5	5						
Oth. Spec.	552	527	356	107	64	11	2	7	5
AN	83	82	58	17	7	1			
CHP	36	35	29	3	3			1	
DR	57	55	41	12	2			1	1
EM	52	51	28	10	13			1	
FOP	1								1
GPM	5	5	5						
MG	2	2		2					
N	33	32	22	7	3			1	
NM	3	3	2	1					
OM	3	3	2		1				
P	104	100	66	15	19	2	1	1	
PHP	5	1	1			4			
PM	26	24	18	4	2	2			
PTH	87	85	51	26	8		1		1
R	15	13	12		1	1			1
RO	10	8	8					2	
OTH	14	12	9		3	1			1
UNSP	16	16	4	10	2				
Not Class	150								
Inactive	112								

Note: Excludes Address Unknown.

Subspecialties in this table are condensed into major specialties. See Appendix A.

Table 3.8

Female Physicians by State, Self-Designated Specialty, and Activity, 2006, continued
Alaska

Specialty	Total Physicians	Patient Care				Other Professional Activity			
		Total Patient Care	Office Based	Hospital Based		Admin.	Med. Teach.	Research	Other
				Resid./ Fellows	Phys. Staff				
Total Physicians	510	449	373	21	55	9	3	7	3
GP/FM Prac.	169	164	129	16	19	2	1	2	
FM	164	159	124	16	19	2	1	2	
GP	5	5	5						
Med. Spec.	126	122	104		18	2		2	
AI	2	2			2				
CD	2	2	2						
D	3	3	3						
IM	60	60	52		8				
PD	57	53	46		7	2		2	
PUD	2	2	1		1				
Sur. Spec.	68	67	60	2	5				1
CRS	1	1	1						
GS	13	12	10		2				1
OBG	42	42	39	2	1				
OPH	4	4	3		1				
ORS	1	1	1						
OTO	4	4	3		1				
PS	2	2	2						
U	1	1	1						
Oth. Spec.	108	96	80	3	13	5	2	3	2
AM	1	1			1				
AN	18	17	14	1	2		1		
CHP	5	5	5						
DR	6	6	5		1				
EM	28	26	22	1	3	2			
N	5	5	5						
OM	1							1	
P	23	22	19		3			1	
PHP	3					2			1
PM	6	6	6						
PTH	8	5	2		3		1	1	1
RO	1	1	1						
OTH	1					1			
UNSP	2	2	1	1					
Not Class	15								
Inactive	24								

Note: Excludes Address Unknown.

Subspecialties in this table are condensed into major specialties. See Appendix A.

Table 3.8

Female Physicians by State, Self-Designated Specialty, and Activity, 2006, continued
Arizona

Specialty	Total Physicians	Patient Care				Other Professional Activity			
		Total Patient Care	Office Based	Hospital Based		Admin.	Med. Teach.	Research	Other
				Resid./ Fellows	Phys. Staff				
Total Physicians	3,796	3,177	2,494	426	257	37	46	29	12
GP/FM Prac.	501	487	399	52	36	8	4	1	1
FM	477	464	380	52	32	7	4	1	1
GP	24	23	19		4	1			
Med. Spec.	1,412	1,349	1,037	197	115	16	30	12	5
AI	12	12	10	1	1				
CD	34	33	28	4	1			1	
D	64	62	54	5	3		1	1	
GE	32	32	23	7	2				
IM	678	649	494	92	63	6	13	7	3
PD	560	532	405	84	43	10	14	2	2
PDC	5	3	3				2		
PUD	27	26	20	4	2			1	
Sur. Spec.	505	497	377	89	31	2	1	4	1
CRS	6	6	5		1				
GS	106	105	62	34	9	1			
NS	5	5	2	3					
OBG	290	285	227	45	13	1	1	3	
OPH	40	39	34	1	4			1	
ORS	15	14	11	2	1				1
OTO	8	8	7		1				
PS	16	16	14	1	1				
TS	4	4	3		1				
U	15	15	12	3					
Oth. Spec.	883	844	681	88	75	11	11	12	5
AM	1							1	
AN	155	148	130	8	10	2	4		1
CHP	51	48	41	3	4		1	1	1
DR	84	84	68	12	4				
EM	129	128	93	15	20		1		
FOP	1	1	1						
GPM	16	14	14					2	
N	55	53	46	7			1	1	
NM	3	3	3						
OM	8	6	6			2			
P	196	189	140	23	26	5	1	1	
PHP	4	1	1			2		1	
PM	26	25	24		1			1	
PTH	85	80	62	11	7		2	2	1
R	20	20	19		1				
RO	15	15	14	1					
OTH	20	15	14		1		1	2	2
UNSP	14	14	5	8	1				
Not Class	244								
Inactive	251								

Note: Excludes Address Unknown.

Subspecialties in this table are condensed into major specialties. See Appendix A.

Table 3.8

Female Physicians by State, Self-Designated Specialty, and Activity, 2006, continued
Arkansas

Specialty	Total Physicians	Patient Care		Hospital Based		Other Professional Activity			
		Total Patient Care	Office Based	Resid./Fellows	Phys. Staff	Admin.	Med. Teach.	Research	Other
Total Physicians	1,391	1,216	846	260	110	13	25	5	5
GP/FM Prac.	268	257	188	57	12	1	9	1	
FM	259	248	179	57	12	1	9	1	
GP	9	9	9						
Med. Spec.	476	456	323	92	41	4	10	4	2
AI	10	10	10						
CD	9	8	8					1	
D	14	14	8	6					
GE	7	6	5		1		1		
IM	178	170	113	36	21	1	5	1	1
PD	243	235	169	48	18	3	3	2	
PDC	4	4	4						
PUD	11	9	6	2	1		1		1
Sur. Spec.	161	158	116	35	7	1	2		
CRS	2	2	2						
GS	31	30	18	12		1			
OBG	80	78	65	12	1		2		
OPH	21	21	16	3	2				
ORS	8	8	4	4					
OTO	11	11	6	3	2				
PS	3	3	3						
TS	1	1			1				
U	4	4	2	1	1				
Oth. Spec.	359	345	219	76	50	7	4		3
AM	1					1			
AN	69	69	41	19	9				
CHP	15	14	9	2	3		1		
DR	34	33	18	12	3		1		
EM	41	39	25	6	8	1	1		
GPM	3	3	2		1				
MG	1	1	1						
N	28	28	19	6	3				
NM	3	3	1	1	1				
OM	1	1	1						
P	69	67	40	12	15	1	1		
PHP	2					2			
PM	23	23	13	7	3				
PTH	44	43	28	11	4				1
R	9	8	8						1
RO	5	5	5						
OTH	5	2	2			2			1
UNSP	6	6	6						
Not Class	58								
Inactive	69								

Note: Excludes Address Unknown.

Subspecialties in this table are condensed into major specialties. See Appendix A.

Table 3.8

Female Physicians by State, Self-Designated Specialty, and Activity, 2006, continued
California

Specialty	Total Physicians	Patient Care				Other Professional Activity			
		Total Patient Care	Office Based	Hospital Based		Admin.	Med. Teach.	Research	Other
				Resid./ Fellows	Phys. Staff				
Total Physicians	31,083	25,728	19,963	3,908	1,857	325	250	387	155
GP/FM Prac.	3,678	3,593	2,943	459	191	25	34	13	13
FM	3,337	3,261	2,655	459	147	21	32	12	11
GP	341	332	288		44	4	2	1	2
Med. Spec.	12,049	11,544	9,042	1,737	765	121	106	234	44
AI	127	116	96	6	14		1	9	1
CD	245	224	183	21	20	5	6	10	
D	602	591	505	56	30	1	2	7	1
GE	176	169	119	37	13		1	6	
IM	5,876	5,613	4,380	867	366	56	48	136	23
PD	4,802	4,621	3,599	717	305	59	47	56	19
PDC	67	64	48	12	4			3	
PUD	154	146	112	21	13		1	7	
Sur. Spec.	3,977	3,911	3,007	674	230	23	22	16	5
CRS	22	21	17	2	2	1			
GS	677	667	409	216	42	4		4	2
NS	41	41	30	9	2				
OBG	2,249	2,208	1,786	305	117	15	17	7	2
OPH	428	420	360	31	29	3	2	3	
ORS	149	147	107	32	8		1		1
OTO	176	176	125	40	11				
PS	129	128	101	18	9		1		
TS	33	33	27	3	3				
U	73	70	45	18	7		1	2	
Oth. Spec.	7,141	6,680	4,971	1,038	671	156	88	124	93
AM	2	2	1		1				
AN	1,133	1,096	862	136	98	9	14	10	4
CHP	359	347	300	27	20	4	3	5	
DR	608	588	430	100	58		11	3	6
EM	837	817	582	158	77	8	8	2	2
FOP	18	14	14			1			3
GPM	131	102	81	13	8	10	4	7	8
MG	35	25	16	4	5	3	1	6	
N	395	371	303	42	26	3	3	15	3
NM	50	45	32	4	9			2	3
OM	81	62	55	2	5	8	3	5	3
P	1,713	1,645	1,197	246	202	27	15	21	5
PHP	57	12	10		2	29	5	6	5
PM	268	260	200	24	36	6	1		1
PTH	686	605	449	95	61	24	9	14	34
R	162	155	131	8	16		5	1	1
RO	130	128	97	21	10			2	
TTS	2	2	2						
OTH	135	77	68		9	21	3	21	13
UNSP	339	327	141	158	28	3	3	4	2
Not Class	2,315								
Inactive	1,923								

Note: Excludes Address Unknown.

Subspecialties in this table are condensed into major specialties. See Appendix A.

Table 3.8

Female Physicians by State, Self-Designated Specialty, and Activity, 2006, continued
Colorado

Specialty	Total Physicians	Patient Care		Hospital Based		Other Professional Activity			
		Total Patient Care	Office Based	Resid./ Fellows	Phys. Staff	Admin.	Med. Teach.	Research	Other
Total Physicians	4,096	3,523	2,776	505	242	41	38	40	20
GP/FM Prac.	679	657	531	79	47	9	10		3
FM	666	645	520	79	46	8	10		3
GP	13	12	11		1	1			
Med. Spec.	1,477	1,423	1,093	243	87	13	11	24	6
AI	37	34	22	10	2	1	1		1
CD	29	29	22	6	1				
D	70	68	59	7	2			2	
GE	21	21	14	6	1				
IM	701	679	524	108	47	3	3	13	3
PD	575	552	429	90	33	9	7	5	2
PDC	9	9	2	7					
PUD	35	31	21	9	1			4	
Sur. Spec.	569	563	455	77	31	1	3	2	
CRS	3	3	3						
GS	95	94	63	25	6		1		
NS	3	3	3						
OBG	348	344	286	41	17	1	2	1	
OPH	46	46	39	4	3				
ORS	26	25	20	3	2			1	
OTO	23	23	19	2	2				
PS	13	13	11	1	1				
U	12	12	11	1					
Oth. Spec.	937	880	697	106	77	18	14	14	11
AN	158	151	132	12	7		5	1	1
CHP	63	59	50	5	4	2	2		
DR	64	62	45	7	10	1	1		
EM	151	148	110	21	17	2	1		
FOP	3	2	2						1
GPM	25	18	17		1	4		2	1
MG	5	5	4	1					
N	55	52	45	6	1			3	
OM	9	7	7				1		1
P	199	189	150	18	21	2	1	4	3
PHP	10	2	2			5		2	1
PM	48	45	34	6	5		1		2
PTH	73	71	50	14	7	1	1		
R	20	18	16	1	1		1	1	
RO	14	14	11	2	1				
OTH	13	10	9		1	1		1	1
UNSP	27	27	13	13	1				
Not Class	196								
Inactive	238								

Note: Excludes Address Unknown.

Subspecialties in this table are condensed into major specialties. See Appendix A.

Table 3.8

Female Physicians by State, Self-Designated Specialty, and Activity, 2006, continued
Connecticut

Specialty	Total Physicians	Patient Care				Other Professional Activity			
		Total Patient Care	Office Based	Hospital Based		Admin.	Med. Teach.	Research	Other
				Resid./ Fellows	Phys. Staff				
Total Physicians	4,236	3,517	2,357	831	329	48	38	67	20
GP/FM Prac.	196	194	160	24	10	1	1		
FM	182	180	148	24	8	1	1		
GP	14	14	12		2				
Med. Spec.	1,879	1,774	1,169	445	160	28	26	42	9
AI	12	10	9	1				1	1
CD	40	38	28	8	2	2			
D	83	82	68	9	5			1	
GE	39	36	24	11	1		3		
IM	1,055	992	615	281	96	19	13	26	5
PD	595	568	395	121	52	5	8	11	3
PDC	7	6	4	2			1		
PUD	48	42	26	12	4	2	1	3	
Sur. Spec.	558	557	401	136	20			1	
CRS	6	6	6						
GS	102	101	51	48	2			1	
NS	6	6	4	2					
OBG	330	330	252	64	14				
OPH	63	63	57	5	1				
ORS	10	10	6	4					
OTO	12	12	7	3	2				
PS	13	13	10	2	1				
TS	2	2	1	1					
U	14	14	7	7					
Oth. Spec.	1,057	992	627	226	139	19	11	24	11
AM	1	1	1						
AN	150	149	106	28	15		1		
CHP	64	61	49	9	3		1	2	
DR	110	108	75	25	8		1		1
EM	98	94	34	34	26	2	2		
FOP	2	1	1						1
GPM	12	8	6	2		1	1	2	
MG	4	2	2			1		1	
N	56	52	37	9	6			3	1
NM	7	7	6	1					
OM	10	6	4		2	1	1	1	1
P	307	293	184	60	49	5	2	6	1
PHP	4	2	2			1			1
PM	24	23	20	1	2				1
PTH	132	121	65	36	20	4	1	3	3
R	14	14	11	1	2				
RO	17	16	11	3	2			1	
TTS	1	1	1						
OTH	22	11	8		3	4	1	5	1
UNSP	22	22	4	17	1				
Not Class	345								
Inactive	201								

Note: Excludes Address Unknown.

Subspecialties in this table are condensed into major specialties. See Appendix A.

Table 3.8

Female Physicians by State, Self-Designated Specialty, and Activity, 2006, continued
Delaware

| Specialty | Total Physicians | Patient Care | | | | Other Professional Activity | | | |
| | | Total Patient Care | Office Based | Hospital Based | | Admin. | Med. Teach. | Research | Other |
				Resid./ Fellows	Phys. Staff				
Total Physicians	724	616	439	109	68	8	6	7	1
GP/FM Prac.	109	103	77	14	12	3	2	1	
FM	107	101	76	14	11	3	2	1	
GP	2	2	1		1				
Med. Spec.	271	262	188	49	25	3	2	3	1
CD	3	3	3						
D	6	6	6						
GE	3	3	3						
IM	114	110	82	18	10	2	1	1	
PD	136	131	88	28	15	1	1	2	1
PDC	3	3		3					
PUD	6	6	6						
Sur. Spec.	98	98	69	22	7				
CRS	1	1	1						
GS	25	25	14	10	1				
OBG	54	54	41	9	4				
OPH	9	9	7	1	1				
ORS	1	1			1				
OTO	3	3	1	2					
PS	3	3	3						
U	2	2	2						
Oth. Spec.	160	153	105	24	24	2	2	3	
AN	26	26	21	2	3				
CHP	6	6	4		2				
DR	16	15	11	3	1	1			
EM	29	29	15	10	4				
FOP	1	1			1				
GPM	1	1			1				
MG	2	1	1				1		
N	3	3	3						
NM	1	1	1						
P	38	36	25	5	6		1	1	
PHP	2	1	1			1			
PM	7	7	6		1				
PTH	12	12	9		3				
R	4	4	3		1				
RO	2	2	2						
OTH	2	1	1					1	
UNSP	8	7	2	4	1			1	
Not Class	42								
Inactive	44								

Note: Excludes Address Unknown.

Subspecialties in this table are condensed into major specialties. See Appendix A.

Table 3.8

Female Physicians by State, Self-Designated Specialty, and Activity, 2006, continued
District of Columbia

Specialty	Total Physicians	Patient Care				Other Professional Activity			
		Total Patient Care	Office Based	Hospital Based		Admin.	Med. Teach.	Research	Other
				Resid./ Fellows	Phys. Staff				
Total Physicians	1,846	1,450	783	487	180	44	28	43	13
GP/FM Prac.	84	79	56	15	8	3	2		
FM	79	75	53	15	7	2	2		
GP	5	4	3		1	1			
Med. Spec.	783	712	382	243	87	23	14	28	6
AI	11	8	7	1		1		2	
CD	31	28	13	8	7	1		2	
D	35	34	22	9	3				1
GE	8	8	4	2	2				
IM	380	344	184	125	35	12	8	13	3
PD	299	274	143	95	36	8	6	9	2
PDC	7	6	4	2		1			
PUD	12	10	5	1	4			2	
Sur. Spec.	261	256	116	118	22	1		3	1
CRS	4	4	2	1	1				
GS	61	58	21	36	1			2	1
NS	3	3	1	1	1				
OBG	124	123	59	50	14	1			
OPH	38	37	19	15	3			1	
ORS	15	15	3	10	2				
OTO	7	7	5	2					
PS	6	6	4	2					
TS	3	3	2	1					
Oth. Spec.	450	403	229	111	63	17	12	12	6
AM	1					1			
AN	53	49	29	10	10		4		
CHP	27	22	19		3	1	2	2	
DR	56	56	26	22	8				
EM	43	42	24	13	5		1		
FOP	2	1	1						1
GPM	6	3	2	1				1	2
MG	2	2	1	1					
N	31	29	13	12	4			2	
NM	3	3	1		2				
OM	1	1			1				
P	106	100	66	23	11	4	2		
PHP	6					5		1	
PM	14	13	8	2	3		1		
PTH	55	41	20	12	9	5	2	4	3
R	11	11	8		3				
RO	3	3	1	1	1				
OTH	12	9	7		2	1		2	
UNSP	18	18	3	14	1				
Not Class	186								
Inactive	82								

Note: Excludes Address Unknown.

Subspecialties in this table are condensed into major specialties. See Appendix A.

Table 3.8

Female Physicians by State, Self-Designated Specialty, and Activity, 2006, continued
Florida

Specialty	Total Physicians	Patient Care				Other Professional Activity			
		Total Patient Care	Office Based	Hospital Based		Admin.	Med. Teach.	Research	Other
				Resid./ Fellows	Phys. Staff				
Total Physicians	11,601	9,595	7,492	1,262	841	108	107	78	53
GP/FM Prac.	1,387	1,342	1,104	151	87	13	23	1	8
FM	1,203	1,167	946	151	70	10	22		4
GP	184	175	158		17	3	1	1	4
Med. Spec.	4,516	4,369	3,427	570	372	38	50	49	10
AI	51	50	45	2	3			1	
CD	98	93	78	10	5	2		2	1
D	241	240	204	33	3			1	
GE	61	58	45	11	2	2	1		
IM	2,069	2,003	1,556	242	205	17	23	23	3
PD	1,910	1,844	1,438	263	143	16	25	19	6
PDC	26	25	18	3	4			1	
PUD	60	56	43	6	7	1	1	2	
Sur. Spec.	1,316	1,303	1,031	193	79	3	8		2
CRS	16	15	11	3	1	1			
GS	178	177	112	43	22	1			
NS	22	22	12	6	4				
OBG	754	746	611	104	31		7		1
OPH	173	172	147	17	8		1		
ORS	45	45	31	8	6				
OTO	56	56	49	5	2				
PS	52	51	44	6	1				1
TS	7	6	5		1	1			
U	13	13	9	1	3				
Oth. Spec.	2,722	2,581	1,930	348	303	54	26	28	33
AM	2	1			1	1			
AN	508	498	373	80	45	1	6	3	
CHP	129	126	105	11	10	1	2		
DR	295	289	229	37	23	1	2		3
EM	314	310	226	39	45	3			1
FOP	19	16	16			1			2
GPM	29	23	15	4	4	4		1	1
MG	7	5	2	2	1		1	1	
N	162	154	124	17	13	1	2	5	
NM	7	6	4	1	1				1
OM	20	13	7		6	5		1	1
P	515	492	346	60	86	12	6	4	1
PHP	13	4	4			7	1	1	
PM	89	85	71	4	10	3		1	
PTH	331	291	209	48	34	9	4	7	20
R	69	66	56	3	7	1	1	1	
RO	58	57	46	7	4		1		
TTS	1	1			1				
OTH	26	21	18		3	3			2
UNSP	128	123	79	35	9	1		3	1
Not Class	662								
Inactive	998								

Note: Excludes Address Unknown.

Subspecialties in this table are condensed into major specialties. See Appendix A.

Table 3.8

Female Physicians by State, Self-Designated Specialty, and Activity, 2006, continued
Georgia

| Specialty | Total Physicians | Patient Care | | Hospital Based | | Other Professional Activity | | | |
		Total Patient Care	Office Based	Resid./ Fellows	Phys. Staff	Admin.	Med. Teach.	Research	Other
Total Physicians	6,106	5,227	4,007	809	411	75	59	86	38
GP/FM Prac.	745	723	573	106	44	8	11	2	1
FM	706	689	547	106	36	5	10	2	
GP	39	34	26		8	3	1		1
Med. Spec.	2,497	2,395	1,839	354	202	28	28	33	13
AI	22	20	18	1	1		1	1	
CD	44	43	34	6	3		1		
D	101	100	79	16	5		1		
GE	33	33	27	6					
IM	1,211	1,162	840	211	111	17	13	16	3
PD	1,038	992	806	105	81	11	12	13	10
PDC	9	9	7	2					
PUD	39	36	28	7	1			3	
Sur. Spec.	832	823	638	151	34	6	1		2
CRS	5	5	5						
GS	117	116	54	54	8		1		
NS	11	11	8	1	2				
OBG	565	558	467	74	17	5			2
OPH	58	58	43	12	3				
ORS	16	15	13	2		1			
OTO	28	28	22	3	3				
PS	19	19	18	1					
TS	3	3	1	2					
U	10	10	7	2	1				
Oth. Spec.	1,411	1,286	957	198	131	33	19	51	22
AM	2					2			
AN	204	202	159	27	16	1	1		
CHP	77	72	59	8	5		5		
DR	117	114	86	17	11		1		2
EM	200	192	139	31	22	3	3	1	1
FOP	7	5	2	1	2				2
GPM	62	50	32	3	15	2	1	7	2
MG	3	2	2					1	
N	72	67	56	9	2	1		4	
NM	3	3	2		1				
OM	17	9	9			4	1	2	1
P	282	271	197	38	36	1	4	5	1
PHP	39	7	2		5	11	1	19	1
PM	43	41	33	4	4	1		1	
PTH	143	126	99	24	3	4	1	4	8
R	39	38	29	5	4			1	
RO	27	27	22	5					
OTH	21	11	9		2	1	1	4	4
UNSP	53	49	20	26	3	2		2	
Not Class	359								
Inactive	262								

Note: Excludes Address Unknown.

Subspecialties in this table are condensed into major specialties. See Appendix A.

Table 3.8

Female Physicians by State, Self-Designated Specialty, and Activity, 2006, continued
Hawaii

| Specialty | Total Physicians | Patient Care | | | | Other Professional Activity | | | |
		Total Patient Care	Office Based	Resid./ Fellows	Phys. Staff	Admin.	Med. Teach.	Research	Other
Total Physicians	1,261	1,032	782	146	104	16	22	8	7
GP/FM Prac.	155	147	119	13	15	2	5		1
FM	142	134	107	13	14	2	5		1
GP	13	13	12		1				
Med. Spec.	475	455	354	57	44	5	9	4	2
AI	2	2	2						
CD	4	3	3					1	
D	19	17	14		3	1		1	
GE	2	2	2						
IM	237	230	178	33	19	1	6		
PD	203	194	149	23	22	2	3	2	2
PUD	8	7	6	1		1			
Sur. Spec.	183	174	129	36	9	2	5	2	
GS	34	32	21	9	2	1	1		
NS	2	2	1		1				
OBG	119	112	83	25	4	1	4	2	
OPH	15	15	14		1				
ORS	5	5	4	1					
OTO	3	3	1	1	1				
U	5	5	5						
Oth. Spec.	272	256	180	40	36	7	3	2	4
AM	2	2	1		1				
AN	31	31	26		5				
CHP	22	21	16	4	1	1			
DR	18	18	9	3	6				
EM	31	29	25	1	3	2			
FOP	3	2	1	1					1
GPM	9	8	6		2			1	
N	15	14	10		4			1	
OM	5	4	4			1			
P	80	76	45	22	9	3	1		
PHP	4	3	2		1		1		
PM	10	9	9						1
PTH	22	20	10	7	3				2
R	7	6	6				1		
RO	1	1	1						
OTH	5	5	5						
UNSP	7	7	4	2	1				
Not Class	70								
Inactive	106								

Note: Excludes Address Unknown.

Subspecialties in this table are condensed into major specialties. See Appendix A.

Table 3.8

Female Physicians by State, Self-Designated Specialty, and Activity, 2006, continued
Idaho

Specialty	Total Physicians	Patient Care				Other Professional Activity			
		Total Patient Care	Office Based	Hospital Based		Admin.	Med. Teach.	Research	Other
				Resid./ Fellows	Phys. Staff				
Total Physicians	547	491	409	36	46	2	4	1	1
GP/FM Prac.	150	147	117	22	8	1	2		
FM	146	143	114	22	7	1	2		
GP	4	4	3		1				
Med. Spec.	170	165	134	10	21	1	2	1	1
CD	3	3	3						
D	6	6	5		1				
GE	5	5	5						
IM	97	95	75	8	12	1	1		
PD	51	49	40	2	7		1		1
PDC	1	1	1						
PUD	7	6	5		1			1	
Sur. Spec.	79	79	76	1	2				
CRS	1	1	1						
GS	15	15	13	1	1				
OBG	48	48	47		1				
OPH	5	5	5						
ORS	3	3	3						
OTO	3	3	3						
PS	2	2	2						
U	2	2	2						
Oth. Spec.	100	100	82	3	15				
AN	16	16	14	1	1				
CHP	4	4	4						
DR	19	19	17		2				
EM	17	17	13	1	3				
N	7	7	7						
OM	1	1			1				
P	20	20	15		5				
PHP	1	1	1						
PM	5	5	4		1				
PTH	4	4	3		1				
R	2	2	2						
RO	2	2	2						
UNSP	2	2		1	1				
Not Class	15								
Inactive	33								

Note: Excludes Address Unknown.

Subspecialties in this table are condensed into major specialties. See Appendix A.

Table 3.8

Female Physicians by State, Self-Designated Specialty, and Activity, 2006, continued
Illinois

Specialty	Total Physicians	Patient Care				Other Professional Activity			
		Total Patient Care	Office Based	Hospital Based		Admin.	Med. Teach.	Research	Other
				Resid./ Fellows	Phys. Staff				
Total Physicians	12,505	10,517	7,140	2,533	844	128	132	106	63
GP/FM Prac.	1,451	1,406	1,043	274	89	15	24	3	3
FM	1,348	1,309	965	274	70	12	24	2	1
GP	103	97	78		19	3		1	2
Med. Spec.	5,034	4,836	3,248	1,253	335	64	52	67	15
AI	85	78	67	8	3	1	1	5	
CD	106	98	69	22	7	2	2	4	
D	190	186	139	40	7	1	1	2	
GE	68	65	44	17	4		2	1	
IM	2,714	2,610	1,686	739	185	39	26	35	4
PD	1,776	1,715	1,187	409	119	16	20	17	8
PDC	24	21	16	3	2	1		1	1
PUD	71	63	40	15	8	4		2	2
Sur. Spec.	1,580	1,552	1,072	392	88	6	12	8	2
CRS	6	6	4	1	1				
GS	267	264	128	121	15			2	1
NS	16	16	9	5	2				
OBG	917	901	685	162	54	6	5	5	
OPH	184	178	142	30	6		4	1	1
ORS	50	50	24	24	2				
OTO	61	60	36	18	6		1		
PS	41	40	24	16			1		
TS	11	11	9	1	1				
U	27	26	11	14	1		1		
Oth. Spec.	2,881	2,723	1,777	614	332	43	44	28	43
AM	1	1	1						
AN	511	498	338	107	53	2	8	2	1
CHP	116	110	90	15	5	2	2		2
DR	246	239	153	69	17	1	3		3
EM	390	385	219	109	57		3	1	1
FOP	11	9	9				1		1
GPM	18	14	13	1		2	1	1	
MG	8	7	6		1			1	
N	184	175	114	43	18	1	1	6	1
NM	12	11	8	1	2				1
OM	33	25	22	1	2	4		1	3
P	567	540	382	88	70	12	9	1	5
PHP	9	3	2		1	3	1	2	
PM	161	155	93	31	31	3	2		1
PTH	360	316	193	73	50	6	11	8	19
R	51	49	31	6	12	1	1		
RO	39	39	29	6	4				
TTS	1							1	
OTH	45	30	27		3	6	1	4	4
UNSP	117	116	46	64	6				1
VM	1	1	1						
Not Class	955								
Inactive	604								

Note: Excludes Address Unknown.

Subspecialties in this table are condensed into major specialties. See Appendix A.

Table 3.8

Female Physicians by State, Self-Designated Specialty, and Activity, 2006, continued
Indiana

| Specialty | Total Physicians | Patient Care | | Hospital Based | | Other Professional Activity | | | |
		Total Patient Care	Office Based	Resid./ Fellows	Phys. Staff	Admin.	Med. Teach.	Research	Other
Total Physicians	3,812	3,330	2,476	566	288	26	31	41	16
GP/FM Prac.	705	692	524	119	49	3	8		2
FM	686	674	508	119	47	3	8		1
GP	19	18	16		2				1
Med. Spec.	1,382	1,333	957	240	136	11	10	24	4
AI	12	11	11					1	
CD	28	26	22	3	1		1	1	
D	56	56	46	9	1				
GE	11	10	7	2	1			1	
IM	620	593	423	98	72	8	5	11	3
PD	631	614	435	125	54	3	4	9	1
PDC	8	8	6	1	1				
PUD	16	15	7	2	6			1	
Sur. Spec.	475	466	356	85	25	1	8		
CRS	3	3	3						
GS	61	59	32	23	4		2		
NS	4	4	4						
OBG	303	296	237	43	16	1	6		
OPH	44	44	37	7					
ORS	13	13	9	2	2				
OTO	21	21	16	3	2				
PS	14	14	11	2	1				
TS	3	3	2	1					
U	9	9	5	4					
Oth. Spec.	882	839	639	122	78	11	5	17	10
AN	181	179	150	18	11		1		1
CHP	44	44	39	2	3				
DR	71	70	55	12	3	1			
EM	122	122	86	22	14				
GPM	1								1
MG	5	4	3		1			1	
N	5	4	3	1				1	
NM	59	53	40	11	2		1	4	1
OM	3	3	2		1				
P	12	10	9		1	1			1
PHP	149	140	105	12	23	1	1	6	1
PM	3					2		1	
PTH	35	33	28	2	3	2			
R	95	83	59	14	10	3	2	3	4
RO	34	34	30	2	2				
OTH	20	20	15	2	3				
UNSP	16	13	12	1		1		1	1
	27	27	3	23	1				
Not Class									
Inactive	167								

Note: Excludes Address Unknown.

Subspecialties in this table are condensed into major specialties. See Appendix A.

Table 3.8

Female Physicians by State, Self-Designated Specialty, and Activity, 2006, continued
Iowa

Specialty	Total Physicians	Patient Care Total Patient Care	Office Based	Hospital Based Resid./ Fellows	Phys. Staff	Other Professional Activity Admin.	Med. Teach.	Research	Other
Total Physicians	1,471	1,232	890	254	88	14	19	18	6
GP/FM Prac.	341	326	252	55	19	4	7	1	3
FM	331	318	246	55	17	2	7	1	3
GP	10	8	6		2	2			
Med. Spec.	451	430	315	86	29	5	7	8	1
AI	7	5	4	1		1		1	
CD	15	15	12	2	1				
D	27	27	18	9					
GE	5	4	4					1	
IM	189	183	132	34	17	2	2	2	
PD	189	180	138	34	8	2	4	2	1
PDC	7	6	3	2	1		1		
PUD	12	10	4	4	2			2	
Sur. Spec.	193	188	134	40	14	1	2	2	
CRS	1	1	1						
GS	37	36	17	15	4	1			
NS	1	1	1						
OBG	99	95	75	15	5		2	2	
OPH	33	33	27	5	1				
ORS	9	9	6	3					
OTO	8	8	4	1	3				
PS	3	3	2		1				
TS	1	1		1					
U	1	1	1						
Oth. Spec.	304	288	189	73	26	4	3	7	2
AN	47	46	34	11	1		1		
CHP	19	19	13	4	2				
DR	25	25	16	6	3				
EM	17	16	7	6	3		1		
FOP	2	2	2						
GPM	3	3	2	1					
MG	2	2	2						
N	23	22	15	6	1			1	
NM	2	2	2						
OM	5	4	4					1	
P	60	58	31	15	12			2	
PHP	3							2	1
PM	13	11	9	1	1	2			
PTH	44	42	31	11		1	1		
R	3	3	2		1				
RO	13	13	11	1	1				
OTH	7	5	4		1	1			1
UNSP	16	15	4	11				1	
Not Class	111								
Inactive	71								

Note: Excludes Address Unknown.

Subspecialties in this table are condensed into major specialties. See Appendix A.

Table 3.8

Female Physicians by State, Self-Designated Specialty, and Activity, 2006, continued
Kansas

| Specialty | Total Physicians | Patient Care | | Hospital Based | | Other Professional Activity | | | |
		Total Patient Care	Office Based	Resid./ Fellows	Phys. Staff	Admin.	Med. Teach.	Research	Other
Total Physicians	1,761	1,526	1,107	270	149	11	23	6	9
GP/FM Prac.	331	322	257	44	21	1	8		
FM	318	310	250	44	16		8		
GP	13	12	7		5	1			
Med. Spec.	584	567	403	107	57	2	9	2	4
AI	8	8	6	2					
CD	13	13	12	1					
D	25	25	21	4					
GE	5	5	3	2					
IM	270	260	180	52	28	1	5	2	2
PD	253	246	175	44	27	1	4		2
PDC	1	1	1						
PUD	9	9	5	2	2				
Sur. Spec.	238	233	178	45	10	1	4		
CRS	1	1	1						
GS	48	47	30	12	5	1			
NS	1						1		
OBG	140	137	106	28	3		3		
OPH	24	24	22	1	1				
ORS	7	7	6	1					
OTO	7	7	5	2					
PS	7	7	6	1					
U	3	3	2		1				
Oth. Spec.	422	404	269	74	61	7	2	4	5
AN	73	73	48	17	8				
CHP	31	30	18	4	8	1			
DR	33	33	26	4	3				
EM	44	44	31	4	9				
FOP	2	2	2						
GPM	1	1	1						
MG	1	1			1				
N	25	25	23	1	1				
NM	1	1			1				
OM	3	2	1		1				1
P	101	96	57	25	14	2	1	2	
PHP	3	1	1			2			
PM	21	21	13	2	6				
PTH	54	49	29	11	9	1		1	3
R	5	4	4						1
RO	11	11	10	1					
OTH	5	3	3				1	1	
UNSP	8	7	2	5		1			
Not Class	96								
Inactive	90								

Note: Excludes Address Unknown.

Subspecialties in this table are condensed into major specialties. See Appendix A.

Table 3.8

Female Physicians by State, Self-Designated Specialty, and Activity, 2006, continued
Kentucky

Specialty	Total Physicians	Patient Care		Hospital Based		Other Professional Activity			
		Total Patient Care	Office Based	Resid./ Fellows	Phys. Staff	Admin.	Med. Teach.	Research	Other
Total Physicians	2,683	2,282	1,684	416	182	20	31	16	7
GP/FM Prac.	363	355	290	42	23	5	3		
FM	339	331	268	42	21	5	3		
GP	24	24	22		2				
Med. Spec.	963	936	692	171	73	4	14	9	
AI	11	11	10		1				
CD	23	23	15	4	4				
D	44	44	39	5					
GE	10	9	7	2				1	
IM	431	418	296	78	44	2	5	6	
PD	426	413	310	81	22	2	9	2	
PDC	3	3	3						
PUD	15	15	12	1	2				
Sur. Spec.	360	356	267	71	18	1	2	1	
CRS	1	1	1						
GS	62	60	36	21	3		1	1	
NS	6	6	3	2	1				
OBG	214	212	166	36	10	1	1		
OPH	29	29	27	1	1				
ORS	16	16	9	4	3				
OTO	6	6	4	2					
PS	16	16	14	2					
U	10	10	7	3					
Oth. Spec.	670	635	435	132	68	10	12	6	7
AN	123	118	86	20	12	1	4		
CHP	41	38	31	4	3		1	1	1
DR	57	57	46	10	1				
EM	81	79	53	13	13		2		
FOP	6	3	3						3
GPM	1	1		1					
MG	3	3	1	1	1				
N	26	24	20	3	1	1		1	
NM	1	1	1						
OM	6	4	4					2	
P	141	133	79	33	21	3	2	1	2
PHP	3	1	1			2			
PM	27	27	20	4	3				
PTH	88	86	51	26	9	1			1
R	11	10	10				1		
RO	18	17	12	3	2		1		
OTH	13	10	10			2		1	
UNSP	24	23	7	14	2		1		
Not Class	182								
Inactive	145								

Note: Excludes Address Unknown.

Subspecialties in this table are condensed into major specialties. See Appendix A.

Table 3.8

Female Physicians by State, Self-Designated Specialty, and Activity, 2006, continued
Louisiana

Specialty	Total Physicians	Patient Care		Hospital Based		Other Professional Activity			
		Total Patient Care	Office Based	Resid./ Fellows	Phys. Staff	Admin.	Med. Teach.	Research	Other
Total Physicians	3,057	2,605	1,839	588	178	22	48	13	5
GP/FM Prac.	326	321	226	63	32	2	3		
FM	304	299	208	63	28	2	3		
GP	22	22	18		4				
Med. Spec.	1,222	1,173	849	250	74	9	29	10	1
AI	15	14	12	2			1		
CD	26	25	20	5			1		
D	74	74	54	19	1				
GE	15	14	10	4				1	
IM	507	484	332	117	35	4	15	3	1
PD	563	542	401	103	38	5	10	6	
PDC	1	1	1						
PUD	21	19	19				2		
Sur. Spec.	455	449	312	123	14		5		1
CRS	2	2	1	1					
GS	78	76	37	37	2		1		1
NS	7	7	5	2					
OBG	243	240	175	56	9		3		
OPH	47	47	37	9	1				
ORS	16	15	8	6	1		1		
OTO	36	36	29	6	1				
PS	11	11	9	2					
TS	4	4	4						
U	11	11	7	4					
Oth. Spec.	690	662	452	152	58	11	11	3	3
AN	109	107	78	22	7		2		
CHP	32	31	23	6	2		1		
DR	66	65	43	18	4		1		
EM	97	96	56	31	9		1		
FOP	2	2	2						
GPM	6	5	4	1		1			
MG	2	1	1				1		
N	61	59	39	13	7		2		
NM	2	2	1		1				
OM	2	2			2				
P	153	145	101	30	14	8			
PHP	4	1	1			2		1	
PM	28	28	22	4	2				
PTH	87	81	54	19	8		2	1	3
R	11	10	9		1		1		
RO	7	7	7						
OTH	5	4	4					1	
UNSP	16	16	7	8	1				
Not Class	220								
Inactive	144								

Note: Excludes Address Unknown.

Subspecialties in this table are condensed into major specialties. See Appendix A.

Table 3.8

Female Physicians by State, Self-Designated Specialty, and Activity, 2006, continued
Maine

| Specialty | Total Physicians | Patient Care | | | | Other Professional Activity | | | |
		Total Patient Care	Office Based	Resid./ Fellows	Phys. Staff	Admin.	Med. Teach.	Research	Other
Total Physicians	1,128	971	750	112	109	14	8	4	4
GP/FM Prac.	223	218	166	28	24	2	3		
FM	221	217	165	28	24	1	3		
GP	2	1	1			1			
Med. Spec.	349	340	275	32	33	4	3	2	
AI	2	2	1		1				
CD	7	7	7						
D	8	8	6		2				
GE	1							1	
IM	192	185	147	17	21	3	3	1	
PD	126	125	103	14	8	1			
PDC	3	3	2		1				
PUD	10	10	9	1					
Sur. Spec.	153	148	119	22	7	1	2	1	1
CRS	1	1	1						
GS	35	35	21	11	3				
NS	1	1	1						
OBG	86	84	70	11	3	1			1
OPH	12	10	9		1		2		
ORS	11	11	11						
OTO	2	2	2						
PS	3	3	3						
TS	1							1	
U	1	1	1						
Oth. Spec.	276	265	190	30	45	7		1	3
AN	40	39	30	5	4			1	
CHP	28	27	23		4	1			
DR	21	21	12	4	5				
EM	51	51	29	10	12				
FOP	2	1	1						1
MG	1	1			1				
N	9	9	8		1				
OM	4	4	3		1				
P	80	77	56	9	12	2			1
PHP	3					2			1
PM	7	7	4		3				
PTH	15	15	13		2				
R	1	1	1						
RO	3	3	3						
OTH	3	1	1			2			
UNSP	8	8	6	2					
Not Class	48								
Inactive	79								

Note: Excludes Address Unknown.

Subspecialties in this table are condensed into major specialties. See Appendix A.

Table 3.8

Female Physicians by State, Self-Designated Specialty, and Activity, 2006, continued
Maryland

Specialty	Total Physicians	Patient Care				Other Professional Activity			
		Total Patient Care	Office Based	Hospital Based		Admin.	Med. Teach.	Research	Other
				Resid./ Fellows	Phys. Staff				
Total Physicians	8,380	6,611	4,586	1,243	782	179	86	271	65
GP/FM Prac.	561	540	436	54	50	7	5	4	5
FM	523	504	409	54	41	7	5	4	3
GP	38	36	27		9				2
Med. Spec.	3,517	3,212	2,179	677	356	74	49	160	22
AI	55	45	37	5	3		2	8	
CD	77	71	56	9	6	1		5	
D	121	117	93	17	7		1	2	1
GE	48	45	30	11	4		1	2	
IM	1,834	1,673	1,076	419	178	37	25	90	9
PD	1,311	1,196	851	198	147	36	19	48	12
PDC	13	12	7	2	3		1		
PUD	58	53	29	16	8			5	
Sur. Spec.	953	926	646	192	88	7	3	13	4
CRS	8	7	6	1		1			
GS	148	145	65	66	14	1	1	1	
NS	10	8	5	2	1	1		1	
OBG	528	514	394	72	48	3	2	6	3
OPH	127	123	96	16	11			3	1
ORS	34	34	21	8	5				
OTO	43	43	25	15	3				
PS	27	25	20	4	1	1		1	
TS	8	8	7	1					
U	20	19	7	7	5			1	
Oth. Spec.	2,181	1,933	1,325	320	288	91	29	94	34
AM	1					1			
AN	297	287	207	38	42	2	5	2	1
CHP	138	132	104	8	20	2	1	2	1
DR	170	166	118	22	26	1	1	2	
EM	213	206	144	35	27	4	1		2
FOP	11	9	6	1	2			1	1
GPM	93	66	42	17	7	9	3	12	3
MG	19	15	7	5	3	2		2	
N	147	126	73	33	20	6	2	13	
NM	12	10	6	3	1	2			
OM	25	15	11		4	8		1	1
P	508	473	338	69	66	12	6	13	4
PHP	39	4	4			23	1	9	2
PM	74	66	43	15	8	3	2	3	
PTH	235	190	119	32	39	7	5	19	14
R	43	39	28	4	7	1	2		1
RO	38	37	30	4	3			1	
OTH	45	22	17		5	7		13	3
UNSP	73	70	28	34	8	1		1	1
Not Class	736								
Inactive	432								

Note: Excludes Address Unknown.

Subspecialties in this table are condensed into major specialties. See Appendix A.

Table 3.8

Female Physicians by State, Self-Designated Specialty, and Activity, 2006, continued
Massachusetts

Specialty	Total Physicians	Patient Care				Other Professional Activity			
		Total Patient Care	Office Based	Hospital Based		Admin.	Med. Teach.	Research	Other
				Resid./ Fellows	Phys. Staff				
Total Physicians	**11,055**	**8,966**	**5,954**	**2,085**	**927**	**94**	**92**	**288**	**49**
GP/FM Prac.	596	578	457	78	43	8	6	1	3
FM	562	549	436	78	35	6	6		1
GP	34	29	21		8	2		1	2
Med. Spec.	4,786	4,496	3,004	1,061	431	40	43	190	17
AI	35	24	13	8	3	1		10	
CD	132	118	69	34	15		1	11	2
D	165	160	121	26	13	1		3	1
GE	82	77	46	22	9			5	
IM	2,699	2,532	1,657	650	225	22	26	112	7
PD	1,551	1,471	1,030	286	155	15	14	44	7
PDC	41	41	24	12	5				
PUD	81	73	44	23	6	1	2	5	
Sur. Spec.	1,224	1,201	801	308	92	7	4	11	1
CRS	2	2	2						
GS	276	270	115	132	23	2		3	1
NS	7	7	3	1	3				
OBG	640	627	476	101	50	5	3	5	
OPH	124	122	98	15	9			2	
ORS	64	64	34	28	2				
OTO	41	40	28	11	1			1	
PS	39	38	28	8	2		1		
TS	8	8	3	3	2				
U	23	23	14	9					
Oth. Spec.	2,883	2,691	1,692	638	361	39	39	86	28
AN	412	393	237	111	45	2	11	4	2
CHP	168	161	120	22	19	1	2	3	1
DR	251	244	147	64	33	1	4	2	
EM	283	276	153	88	35	3	3	1	
FOP	7	6	6						1
GPM	29	22	13	6	3	1	1	5	
MG	18	15	7	5	3			3	
N	201	185	119	36	30	1	2	12	1
NM	10	8	6	2			1	1	
OM	12	6	5	1		1		2	3
P	812	764	515	135	114	15	9	20	4
PHP	13	3	1		2	3	1	4	2
PM	74	73	42	12	19	1			
PTH	313	288	176	79	33	6	2	9	8
R	84	76	53	14	9	1	1	4	2
RO	55	54	34	12	8				1
TTS	1	1	1						
OTH	38	18	13	2	3	3	1	13	3
UNSP	101	97	43	49	5		1	3	
VM	1	1	1						
Not Class	1,116								
Inactive	450								

Note: Excludes Address Unknown.

Subspecialties in this table are condensed into major specialties. See Appendix A.

Table 3.8

Female Physicians by State, Self-Designated Specialty, and Activity, 2006, continued
Michigan

Specialty	Total Physicians	Patient Care				Other Professional Activity			
		Total Patient Care	Office Based	Hospital Based		Admin.	Med. Teach.	Research	Other
				Resid./ Fellows	Phys. Staff				
Total Physicians	8,097	6,787	4,571	1,679	537	83	95	84	24
GP/FM Prac.	1,083	1,052	780	194	78	10	16	4	1
FM	1,036	1,008	742	194	72	7	16	4	1
GP	47	44	38		6	3			
Med. Spec.	3,083	2,946	2,018	724	204	33	47	53	4
AI	40	39	34	4	1	1			
CD	48	48	32	14	2				
D	118	118	79	33	6				
GE	38	36	26	9	1		1	1	
IM	1,610	1,528	1,045	392	91	25	22	33	2
PD	1,182	1,134	780	255	99	7	23	16	2
PDC	17	17	9	7	1				
PUD	30	26	13	10	3		1	3	
Sur. Spec.	1,059	1,049	664	325	60		4	6	
CRS	9	9	8	1					
GS	208	207	89	106	12		1		
NS	9	9	5	2	2				
OBG	626	619	422	162	35		3	4	
OPH	106	105	75	24	6			1	
ORS	36	36	21	13	2				
OTO	25	25	16	7	2				
PS	26	25	19	5	1			1	
TS	1	1	1						
U	13	13	8	5					
Oth. Spec.	1,848	1,740	1,109	436	195	40	28	21	19
AM	2							2	
AN	211	203	143	39	21		5	3	
CHP	105	97	65	14	18	3	4	1	
DR	164	158	100	41	17		4		2
EM	301	297	169	112	16	2	2		
FOP	3	3	2		1				
GPM	10	8	7	1		2			
MG	8	8	4	2	2				
N	113	106	71	29	6		3	3	1
NM	13	13	5	2	6				
OM	23	20	16		4	3			
P	385	362	260	56	46	13	5	3	2
PHP	8	2	2			4		1	1
PM	91	88	68	13	7		1		2
PTH	197	170	97	45	28	9	3	6	9
R	39	37	27	4	6		1		1
RO	47	46	28	8	10	1			
TTS	2	1	1						1
OTH	26	21	16	2	3	3		2	
UNSP	100	100	28	68	4				
Not Class	626								
Inactive	398								

Note: Excludes Address Unknown.

Subspecialties in this table are condensed into major specialties. See Appendix A.

Table 3.8

Female Physicians by State, Self-Designated Specialty, and Activity, 2006, continued
Minnesota

| Specialty | Total Physicians | Patient Care | | | | Other Professional Activity | | | |
		Total Patient Care	Office Based	Resid./ Fellows	Phys. Staff	Admin.	Med. Teach.	Research	Other
Total Physicians	4,753	4,106	3,040	801	265	42	36	50	16
GP/FM Prac.	1,008	987	818	116	53	7	8	4	2
FM	993	973	806	116	51	6	8	4	2
GP	15	14	12		2	1			
Med. Spec.	1,669	1,601	1,146	348	107	16	17	30	5
AI	18	17	16	1				1	
CD	67	65	47	15	3			2	
D	103	102	73	27	2		1		
GE	35	32	21	9	2		1	2	
IM	782	747	511	176	60	10	7	15	3
PD	623	600	449	112	39	5	8	8	2
PDC	8	8	7	1					
PUD	33	30	22	7	1	1		2	
Sur. Spec.	590	585	424	140	21		3	2	
CRS	8	8	7	1					
GS	110	107	54	49	4		1	2	
NS	11	11	6	4	1				
OBG	308	306	258	42	6		2		
OPH	59	59	44	11	4				
ORS	42	42	21	19	2				
OTO	26	26	16	7	3				
PS	11	11	7	3	1				
TS	4	4	4						
U	11	11	7	4					
Oth. Spec.	983	933	652	197	84	19	8	14	9
AN	100	98	66	24	8		1	1	
CHP	51	50	41	5	4			1	
DR	104	104	77	18	9				
EM	118	116	71	31	14		2		
FOP	7	4	3		1		1		2
GPM	14	13	12		1	1			
MG	9	8	6	1	1			1	
N	80	75	53	19	3	1	1	3	
NM	3	3	3						
OM	21	13	9	3	1	5	1		2
P	186	182	131	34	17	2	1	1	
PHP	7	2	1		1	2		2	1
PM	74	73	52	13	8				1
PTH	123	114	79	27	8	4		3	2
R	16	15	11	2	2				1
RO	19	18	14	3	1		1		
OTH	10	4	2	1	1	4		2	
UNSP	41	41	21	16	4				
Not Class	293								
Inactive	210								

Note: Excludes Address Unknown.

Subspecialties in this table are condensed into major specialties. See Appendix A.

Table 3.8

Female Physicians by State, Self-Designated Specialty, and Activity, 2006, continued
Mississippi

| Specialty | Total Physicians | Patient Care | | | | Other Professional Activity | | | |
| | | Total Patient Care | Office Based | Hospital Based | | Admin. | Med. Teach. | Research | Other |
				Resid./ Fellows	Phys. Staff				
Total Physicians	1,158	968	697	137	134	17	15	8	8
GP/FM Prac.	169	155	118	14	23	6	6	1	1
FM	155	143	107	14	22	5	6	1	
GP	14	12	11		1	1			1
Med. Spec.	411	396	303	48	45	6	4	4	1
AI	5	4	3	1					1
CD	8	7	6		1	1			
D	9	9	8	1					
GE	9	9	6	1	2				
IM	185	180	130	22	28	1	1	3	
PD	185	177	142	22	13	4	3	1	
PDC	1	1	1						
PUD	9	9	7	1	1				
Sur. Spec.	155	152	107	29	16		3		
CRS	1	1	1						
GS	26	24	9	8	7		2		
OBG	93	92	71	15	6		1		
OPH	16	16	14	2					
ORS	6	6	4	1	1				
OTO	7	7	4	2	1				
PS	3	3	2	1					
TS	1	1			1				
U	2	2	2						
Oth. Spec.	281	265	169	46	50	5	2	3	6
AM	1	1	1						
AN	41	41	25	6	10				
CHP	16	15	11	1	3			1	
DR	21	21	16	4	1				
EM	31	28	20	4	4	1	1		1
GPM	1	1	1						
N	25	23	17	5	1		1	1	
NM	3	3	1		2				
P	73	70	36	15	19	2		1	
PHP	3	2	1		1	1			
PM	6	6	6						
PTH	45	40	23	9	8	1			4
R	7	7	6		1				
RO	1	1	1						
OTH	2	2	2						
UNSP	5	4	2	2					1
Not Class	72								
Inactive	70								

Note: Excludes Address Unknown.

Subspecialties in this table are condensed into major specialties. See Appendix A.

Table 3.8

Female Physicians by State, Self-Designated Specialty, and Activity, 2006, continued
Missouri

Specialty	Total Physicians	Patient Care				Other Professional Activity			
		Total Patient Care	Office Based	Hospital Based		Admin.	Med. Teach.	Research	Other
				Resid./ Fellows	Phys. Staff				
Total Physicians	4,159	3,547	2,379	856	312	34	44	45	19
GP/FM Prac.	455	446	346	70	30	4	4		1
FM	439	430	332	70	28	4	4		1
GP	16	16	14		2				
Med. Spec.	1,705	1,637	1,064	415	158	17	18	27	6
AI	32	31	21	9	1				1
CD	36	32	20	10	2	1		2	1
D	85	85	57	23	5				
GE	23	22	14	7	1			1	
IM	795	763	502	191	70	8	8	13	3
PD	691	664	419	169	76	7	9	10	1
PDC	12	12	6	4	2				
PUD	31	28	25	2	1	1	1	1	
Sur. Spec.	537	529	346	154	29	2	6		
CRS	4	4	4						
GS	84	82	47	33	2		2		
NS	4	4	1	1	2				
OBG	306	300	212	70	18	2	4		
OPH	50	50	37	11	2				
ORS	24	24	12	10	2				
OTO	22	22	12	7	3				
PS	23	23	12	11					
TS	6	6	5	1					
U	14	14	4	10					
Oth. Spec.	992	935	623	217	95	11	16	18	12
AN	166	164	120	31	13		1	1	
CHP	61	55	40	9	6		1	5	
DR	110	106	59	36	11		3	1	
EM	99	97	55	23	19		2		
FOP	3	1	1						2
GPM	6	6	5		1				
MG	5	3	1	1	1		2		
N	69	61	39	17	5	3	1	4	
NM	5	3	2	1			1	1	
OM	7	6	6			1			
P	199	192	133	39	20	2	2	1	2
PHP	3	2	1		1	1			
PM	48	47	34	9	4	1			
PTH	135	122	79	33	10	3	2	2	6
R	24	22	19		3		1	1	
RO	19	19	14	4	1				
OTH	8	5	5					1	2
UNSP	25	24	10	14				1	
Not Class	301								
Inactive	169								

Note: Excludes Address Unknown.

Subspecialties in this table are condensed into major specialties. See Appendix A.

Table 3.8

Female Physicians by State, Self-Designated Specialty, and Activity, 2006, continued
Montana

| Specialty | Total Physicians | Patient Care | | | | Other Professional Activity | | | |
		Total Patient Care	Office Based	Resid./ Fellows	Phys. Staff	Admin.	Med. Teach.	Research	Other
Total Physicians	531	471	384	14	73	2	7	1	1
GP/FM Prac.	137	133	102	8	23	1	3		
FM	134	131	101	8	22		3		
GP	3	2	1		1	1			
Med. Spec.	169	167	138	4	25		2		
AI	2	2	2						
CD	6	6	6						
D	10	10	10						
GE	1	1	1						
IM	84	83	65	3	15		1		
PD	63	62	51	1	10		1		
PUD	3	3	3						
Sur. Spec.	71	70	67	1	2				1
GS	13	13	12	1					
OBG	41	40	38		2				1
OPH	4	4	4						
ORS	6	6	6						
OTO	2	2	2						
PS	1	1	1						
U	4	4	4						
Oth. Spec.	105	101	77	1	23	1	2	1	
AN	16	15	12		3		1		
CHP	3	3	3						
DR	5	5	4		1				
EM	21	21	10	1	10				
MG	1	1			1				
N	6	6	6						
OM	1	1			1				
P	28	26	24		2	1	1		
PM	6	6	5		1				
PTH	7	7	6		1				
RO	4	4	4						
OTH	5	4	2		2			1	
UNSP	2	2	1		1				
Not Class	9								
Inactive	40								

Note: Excludes Address Unknown.

Subspecialties in this table are condensed into major specialties. See Appendix A.

Table 3.8

Female Physicians by State, Self-Designated Specialty, and Activity, 2006, continued
Nebraska

| Specialty | Total Physicians | Patient Care | | | | Other Professional Activity | | | |
		Total Patient Care	Office Based	Resid./ Fellows	Phys. Staff	Admin.	Med. Teach.	Research	Other
Total Physicians	1,193	1,034	740	223	71	9	16	7	3
GP/FM Prac.	218	213	159	38	16	3	2		
FM	215	210	157	38	15	3	2		
GP	3	3	2		1				
Med. Spec.	405	393	272	94	27	3	5	3	1
AI	3	3	3						
CD	15	15	7	7	1				
D	9	9	9						
GE	5	5	4	1					
IM	201	195	123	58	14	1	2	3	
PD	166	162	123	27	12	2	1		1
PDC	1	1	1						
PUD	5	3	2	1			2		
Sur. Spec.	158	153	118	33	2	2	2	1	
CRS	2	2	2						
GS	33	31	19	12		1		1	
NS	1	1	1						
OBG	79	77	60	15	2		2		
OPH	18	17	15	2		1			
ORS	5	5	3	2					
OTO	13	13	11	2					
PS	6	6	6						
U	1	1	1						
Oth. Spec.	288	275	191	58	26	1	7	3	2
AN	62	60	40	17	3		2		
CHP	18	18	16	1	1				
DR	37	35	24	9	2		1		1
EM	23	23	14	7	2				
GPM	3	2	2					1	
N	13	12	11		1		1		
NM	3	3	3						
OM	2	1	1			1			
P	61	61	39	15	7				
PM	9	9	7		2				
PTH	33	29	19	6	4		2	2	
R	7	7	5	1	1				
RO	6	6	5		1				
OTH	5	4	3		1				1
UNSP	6	5	2	2	1		1		
Not Class	84								
Inactive	40								

Note: Excludes Address Unknown.

Subspecialties in this table are condensed into major specialties. See Appendix A.

Table 3.8

Female Physicians by State, Self-Designated Specialty, and Activity, 2006, continued
Nevada

| Specialty | Total Physicians | Patient Care | | | | Other Professional Activity | | | |
| | | Total Patient Care | Office Based | Hospital Based | | Admin. | Med. Teach. | Research | Other |
				Resid./ Fellows	Phys. Staff				
Total Physicians	1,205	1,018	821	101	96	11	9	4	2
GP/FM Prac.	163	158	130	14	14	1	3		1
FM	154	149	124	14	11	1	3		1
GP	9	9	6		3				
Med. Spec.	482	469	380	55	34	6	5	2	
AI	2	1	1					1	
CD	14	14	13		1				
D	9	9	9						
GE	4	4	4						
IM	269	260	203	38	19	5	4		
PD	176	173	144	17	12	1	1	1	
PDC	3	3	3						
PUD	5	5	3		2				
Sur. Spec.	152	149	121	16	12	1	1		1
CRS	2	2	1	1					
GS	32	32	21	6	5				
NS	2	2	2						
OBG	85	82	69	9	4	1	1		1
OPH	12	12	11		1				
ORS	3	3	3						
OTO	3	3	2		1				
PS	6	6	6						
TS	2	2	2						
U	5	5	4		1				
Oth. Spec.	247	242	190	16	36	3		2	
AN	40	40	36	1	3				
CHP	16	15	12	2	1			1	
DR	24	24	22	1	1				
EM	36	36	27	3	6				
FOP	6	6	6						
GPM	5	5	4		1				
MG	1							1	
N	14	14	11		3				
OM	3	3	3						
P	48	48	26	8	14				
PM	14	13	11		2	1			
PTH	20	18	16		2	2			
R	2	2	2						
RO	7	7	7						
OTH	4	4	1		3				
UNSP	7	7	6	1					
Not Class	68								
Inactive	93								

Note: *Excludes Address Unknown.*

Subspecialties in this table are condensed into major specialties. See Appendix A.

Table 3.8

Female Physicians by State, Self-Designated Specialty, and Activity, 2006, continued
New Hampshire

Specialty	Total Physicians	Patient Care				Other Professional Activity			
		Total Patient Care	Office Based	Hospital Based		Admin.	Med. Teach.	Research	Other
				Resid./ Fellows	Phys. Staff				
Total Physicians	1,069	913	699	108	106	6	6	8	5
GP/FM Prac.	158	156	121	10	25			1	1
FM	155	153	119	10	24			1	1
GP	3	3	2		1				
Med. Spec.	392	378	290	48	40	2	5	4	3
AI	1	1	1						
CD	8	8	8						
D	11	11	6	4	1				
GE	4	4	4						
IM	200	192	139	29	24	1	2	4	1
PD	160	154	124	15	15	1	3		2
PDC	1	1	1						
PUD	7	7	7						
Sur. Spec.	173	172	141	14	17		1		
GS	28	28	19	4	5				
NS	4	4	3		1				
OBG	108	107	93	8	6		1		
OPH	13	13	13						
ORS	7	7	3	1	3				
OTO	5	5	5						
PS	4	4	3		1				
U	4	4	2	1	1				
Oth. Spec.	215	207	147	36	24	4		3	1
AN	33	33	21	8	4				
CHP	13	13	11	1	1				
DR	17	17	12	3	2				
EM	28	28	21	1	6				
GPM	6	5		5		1			
N	10	10	10						
NM	1	1	1						
OM	4	1	1			3			
P	53	51	40	7	4			2	
PHP	1	1	1						
PM	4	4	4						
PTH	24	23	17	5	1				1
R	5	5	3	1	1				
RO	2	2	1		1				
OTH	3	2	1		1			1	
UNSP	11	11	3	5	3				
Not Class	62								
Inactive	69								

Note: Excludes Address Unknown.

Subspecialties in this table are condensed into major specialties. See Appendix A.

Table 3.8

Female Physicians by State, Self-Designated Specialty, and Activity, 2006, continued
New Jersey

Specialty	Total Physicians	Patient Care				Other Professional Activity			
		Total Patient Care	Office Based	Hospital Based		Admin.	Med. Teach.	Research	Other
				Resid./ Fellows	Phys. Staff				
Total Physicians	9,441	7,823	5,686	1,257	880	117	102	124	66
GP/FM Prac.	635	606	443	116	47	5	18	4	2
FM	571	546	401	116	29	3	18	3	1
GP	64	60	42		18	2		1	1
Med. Spec.	4,257	4,045	2,912	685	448	58	57	70	27
AI	53	51	43	4	4	1			1
CD	84	80	62	9	9	1	1	1	1
D	138	135	117	11	7		1	2	
GE	52	49	39	4	6	1		1	1
IM	2,113	1,985	1,366	418	201	36	29	45	18
PD	1,727	1,661	1,223	233	205	18	23	19	6
PDC	20	19	14		5		1		
PUD	70	65	48	6	11	1	2	2	
Sur. Spec.	1,066	1,045	823	168	54	7	7	3	4
CRS	5	5	3	2					
GS	158	154	93	51	10	2	1	1	
NS	5	5	3	1	1				
OBG	674	661	531	92	38	4	6	1	2
OPH	126	124	116	7	1			1	1
ORS	26	26	18	8					
OTO	26	26	23	2	1				
PS	28	28	24	2	2				
TS	7	5	4	1		1			1
U	11	11	8	2	1				
Oth. Spec.	2,274	2,127	1,508	288	331	47	20	47	33
AN	408	398	312	39	47		2	4	4
CHP	126	119	95	8	16	2	1	3	1
DR	213	208	157	34	17		1	1	3
EM	176	173	109	39	25	1	2		
FOP	7	4	4			2		1	
GPM	25	22	18	2	2	1	1	1	
MG	8	6	2	1	3		1	1	
N	145	135	103	19	13	1	2	6	1
NM	9	8	5		3				1
OM	23	16	13	1	2	5			2
P	564	535	342	70	123	12	4	8	5
PHP	8	2	2			3	1		2
PM	144	142	96	17	29	2			
PTH	238	211	145	31	35	7	3	7	10
R	49	45	42		3		1	1	2
RO	39	38	31	1	6			1	
TTS	1							1	
OTH	50	24	19	1	4	11	1	12	2
UNSP	41	41	13	25	3				
Not Class	648								
Inactive	561								

Note: Excludes Address Unknown.

Subspecialties in this table are condensed into major specialties. See Appendix A.

Table 3.8

Female Physicians by State, Self-Designated Specialty, and Activity, 2006, continued
New Mexico

Specialty	Total Physicians	Patient Care		Hospital Based		Other Professional Activity			
		Total Patient Care	Office Based	Resid./ Fellows	Phys. Staff	Admin.	Med. Teach.	Research	Other
Total Physicians	1,682	1,383	1,034	207	142	22	24	21	15
GP/FM Prac.	316	309	250	29	30		3	2	2
FM	301	295	239	29	27		3	2	1
GP	15	14	11		3				1
Med. Spec.	555	523	386	74	63	11	11	7	3
AI	3	3	3						
CD	20	20	16	1	3				
D	17	17	12	4	1				
GE	7	7	5	1	1				
IM	287	270	198	40	32	7	6	4	
PD	208	195	143	26	26	3	4	3	3
PDC	2	2	2						
PUD	11	9	7	2		1	1		
Sur. Spec.	184	180	132	40	8	1	2		1
GS	1	1	1						
NS	39	39	24	11	4				
OBG	1	1		1					
OPH	107	104	83	20	1		2		1
ORS	8	8	8						
OTO	15	15	6	6	3				
PS	7	7	5	2					
TS	2	2	2						
U	4	3	3			1			
Oth. Spec.	410	371	266	64	41	10	8	12	9
AM	2	1	1			1			
AN	51	51	36	11	4				
CHP	26	23	21	2		1	1	1	
DR	23	20	12	6	2		1		2
EM	70	69	46	11	12		1		
FOP	2	2	2						
GPM	7	6	3	1	2			1	
MG	2	2	2						
N	18	15	12	2	1		2	1	
OM	7	6	5		1	1			
P	102	94	63	16	15	3	2	2	1
PHP	4	1	1			3			
PM	10	10	10						
PTH	53	45	32	12	1		1	4	3
R	3	3	3						
RO	4	4	3		1				
OTH	13	7	7			1		3	2
UNSP	13	12	7	3	2				1
Not Class	111								
Inactive	106								

Note: Excludes Address Unknown.

Subspecialties in this table are condensed into major specialties. See Appendix A.

Table 3.8

Female Physicians by State, Self-Designated Specialty, and Activity, 2006, continued
New York

| Specialty | Total Physicians | Patient Care | | | | Other Professional Activity | | | |
| | | Total Patient Care | Office Based | Hospital Based | | Admin. | Med. Teach. | Research | Other |
				Resid./ Fellows	Phys. Staff				
Total Physicians	26,763	21,662	13,039	6,033	2,590	347	301	369	118
GP/FM Prac.	1,365	1,329	946	277	106	16	17	1	2
FM	1,281	1,250	881	277	92	12	17	1	1
GP	84	79	65		14	4			1
Med. Spec.	11,445	10,838	6,352	3,345	1,141	162	167	225	53
AI	126	118	90	18	10		2	6	
CD	258	250	176	50	24	2	1	5	
D	397	388	301	69	18	2	5	1	1
GE	150	141	88	38	15		3	6	
IM	6,108	5,768	3,157	2,053	558	95	85	128	32
PD	4,164	3,947	2,405	1,064	478	61	65	72	19
PDC	62	57	31	10	16		1	4	
PUD	180	169	104	43	22	2	5	3	1
Sur. Spec.	3,182	3,128	1,945	935	248	11	24	17	2
CRS	21	21	16	3	2				
GS	587	579	231	300	48	2	5	1	
NS	23	23	14	8	1				
OBG	1,760	1,726	1,169	414	143	9	14	10	1
OPH	379	369	273	69	27		5	5	
ORS	117	116	51	58	7			1	
OTO	128	128	77	40	11				
PS	83	82	69	10	3				1
TS	22	22	11	7	4				
U	62	62	34	26	2				
Oth. Spec.	6,805	6,367	3,796	1,476	1,095	158	93	126	61
AN	926	891	596	182	113	7	14	11	3
CHP	431	396	268	51	77	16	6	11	2
DR	624	608	382	143	83	3	5	1	7
EM	602	592	291	203	98	6	3	1	
FOP	21	15	14	1		1			5
GPM	77	65	44	17	4	6	2	3	1
MG	17	12	4	5	3		1	3	1
N	440	410	238	114	58	8	7	15	
NM	48	44	27	9	8	1	1		2
OM	26	18	14	1	3	7		1	
P	2,015	1,908	1,087	432	389	38	29	31	9
PHP	48	20	15		5	19		9	
PM	360	343	227	57	59	6	6	1	4
PTH	655	592	317	149	126	18	11	16	18
R	170	159	112	11	36	3	4	2	2
RO	100	97	63	23	11		1	1	1
TTS	1	1	1						
OTH	91	48	36	1	11	16	2	19	6
UNSP	153	148	60	77	11	3	1	1	
Not Class	2,521								
Inactive	1,445								

Note: Excludes Address Unknown.

Subspecialties in this table are condensed into major specialties. See Appendix A.

Table 3.8

Female Physicians by State, Self-Designated Specialty, and Activity, 2006, continued
North Carolina

| Specialty | Total Physicians | Patient Care | | | | Other Professional Activity | | | |
| | | Total Patient Care | Office Based | Hospital Based | | Admin. | Med. Teach. | Research | Other |
				Resid./ Fellows	Phys. Staff				
Total Physicians	6,773	5,673	4,169	1,063	441	72	90	99	31
GP/FM Prac.	973	946	751	127	68	9	13	4	1
FM	950	923	730	127	66	9	13	4	1
GP	23	23	21		2				
Med. Spec.	2,567	2,424	1,774	471	179	24	43	67	9
AI	30	25	21	3	1		2	3	
CD	48	45	36	8	1	1	1	1	
D	128	128	103	21	4				
GE	42	37	28	5	4		3	1	1
IM	1,210	1,143	826	221	96	13	13	37	4
PD	1,067	1,006	733	202	71	10	24	23	4
PDC	6	6	5	1					
PUD	36	34	22	10	2			2	
Sur. Spec.	852	837	627	174	36	2	11	2	
GS	127	124	68	53	3	1	1	1	
NS	12	12	6	4	2				
OBG	546	535	421	90	24	1	10		
OPH	82	82	74	7	1				
ORS	27	27	12	12	3				
OTO	32	31	26	3	2			1	
PS	16	16	14	2					
TS	2	2		2					
U	8	8	6	1	1				
Oth. Spec.	1,573	1,466	1,017	291	158	37	23	26	21
AN	215	203	119	63	21	3	6	3	
CHP	89	84	64	8	12	2	1	2	
DR	138	133	102	23	8		3	1	1
EM	225	218	148	44	26	2	4		1
FOP	4	3	2	1					1
GPM	36	30	21	6	3	2		3	1
MG	8	6	4	1	1	1	1		
N	97	97	74	17	6				
NM	7	5	3	1	1	1		1	
OM	11	5	4		1	6			
P	379	362	264	58	40	4	5	5	3
PHP	14	6	6			7			1
PM	62	58	36	14	8	2	1	1	
PTH	159	142	92	34	16	3	1	7	6
R	33	30	23	4	3		1		2
RO	40	39	32	5	2				1
OTH	23	14	10		4	4		3	2
UNSP	33	31	13	12	6				2
Not Class	479								
Inactive	329								

Note: Excludes Address Unknown.

Subspecialties in this table are condensed into major specialties. See Appendix A.

Table 3.8

Female Physicians by State, Self-Designated Specialty, and Activity, 2006, continued
North Dakota

Specialty	Total Physicians	Patient Care				Other Professional Activity			
		Total Patient Care	Office Based	Hospital Based		Admin.	Med. Teach.	Research	Other
				Resid./ Fellows	Phys. Staff				
Total Physicians	366	335	250	46	39	6	3		2
GP/FM Prac.	110	106	72	20	14	2	1		1
FM	106	103	69	20	14	2	1		
GP	4	3	3						1
Med. Spec.	106	102	82	10	10	3	1		
AI	1	1	1						
CD	1	1	1						
D	5	5	4		1				
GE	1	1	1						
IM	60	56	38	10	8	3	1		
PD	36	36	35		1				
PUD	2	2	2						
Sur. Spec.	41	41	35	3	3				
GS	10	10	7	3					
OBG	22	22	20		2				
OPH	3	3	3						
ORS	2	2	2						
OTO	3	3	2		1				
PS	1	1	1						
Oth. Spec.	89	86	61	13	12	1	1		1
AN	14	14	10	2	2				
CHP	8	7	6		1				1
DR	6	6	6						
EM	4	4	3		1				
N	9	9	6	1	2				
OM	1	1			1				
P	23	23	16	5	2				
PM	3	3	2		1				
PTH	13	12	9	1	2		1		
R	1	1	1						
RO	1	1	1						
OTH	1					1			
UNSP	5	5	1	4					
Not Class	12								
Inactive	8								

Note: Excludes Address Unknown.

Subspecialties in this table are condensed into major specialties. See Appendix A.

Table 3.8

Female Physicians by State, Self-Designated Specialty, and Activity, 2006, continued
Ohio

Specialty	Total Physicians	Patient Care		Hospital Based		Other Professional Activity			
		Total Patient Care	Office Based	Resid./ Fellows	Phys. Staff	Admin.	Med. Teach.	Research	Other
Total Physicians	9,416	7,924	5,394	1,832	698	72	104	83	31
GP/FM Prac.	1,193	1,158	868	206	84	12	20	2	1
FM	1,127	1,095	826	206	63	10	20	2	
GP	66	63	42		21	2			1
Med. Spec.	3,690	3,557	2,350	876	331	24	51	48	10
AI	36	34	26	6	2		1	1	
CD	82	76	53	16	7	1	3	2	
D	151	149	106	37	6		2		
GE	52	50	35	11	4		2		
IM	1,661	1,598	1,061	397	140	17	24	18	4
PD	1,631	1,578	1,024	391	163	6	19	22	6
PDC	29	27	15	9	3			2	
PUD	48	45	30	9	6			3	
Sur. Spec.	1,146	1,131	758	321	52	3	8	3	1
CRS	3	3	3						
GS	233	225	117	96	12	3	4	1	
NS	16	16	8	7	1				
OBG	641	639	469	141	29		1	1	
OPH	120	116	86	25	5		2	1	1
ORS	36	36	21	13	2				
OTO	38	38	20	17	1				
PS	29	28	18	10			1		
TS	8	8	6		2				
U	22	22	10	12					
Oth. Spec.	2,185	2,078	1,418	429	231	33	25	30	19
AM	1					1			
AN	345	341	232	73	36	2		1	1
CHP	113	111	81	18	12	1			1
DR	184	182	127	35	20	1		1	
EM	279	273	175	66	32	2	3	1	
FOP	9	8	7	1					1
GPM	13	12	11	1			1		
MG	11	6	3	2	1		1	3	1
N	126	120	73	33	14		1	4	1
NM	5	5	4		1				
OM	24	19	15	1	3	1		2	2
P	458	438	299	86	53	9	5	4	2
PHP	8	3	2		1	3	2		
PM	84	81	53	17	11	1		1	1
PTH	291	261	186	45	30	10	8	5	7
R	71	68	58	2	8		1	1	1
RO	39	38	29	5	4		1		
TTS	2	2	2						
OTH	34	24	20		4	1	1	7	1
UNSP	86	84	39	44	1	1	1		
VM	2	2	2						
Not Class	737								
Inactive	465								

Note: Excludes Address Unknown.

Subspecialties in this table are condensed into major specialties. See Appendix A.

Table 3.8

Female Physicians by State, Self-Designated Specialty, and Activity, 2006, continued
Oklahoma

Specialty	Total Physicians	Patient Care				Other Professional Activity			
		Total Patient Care	Office Based	Hospital Based		Admin.	Med. Teach.	Research	Other
				Resid./ Fellows	Phys. Staff				
Total Physicians	1,584	1,336	965	255	116	17	30	9	9
GP/FM Prac.	254	248	162	60	26	2	2		2
FM	235	230	146	60	24	2	2		1
GP	19	18	16		2				1
Med. Spec.	563	533	390	104	39	5	17	6	2
AI	6	6	5		1				
CD	15	15	9	3	3				
D	24	24	16	7	1				
GE	7	7	7						
IM	258	243	181	40	22	3	8	3	1
PD	241	226	162	53	11	2	9	3	1
PDC	3	3	3						
PUD	9	9	7	1	1				
Sur. Spec.	211	206	151	44	11		4	1	
CRS	3	3	2		1				
GS	43	43	25	15	3				
NS	2	2	2						
OBG	123	118	90	21	7		4	1	
OPH	21	21	21						
ORS	8	8	3	5					
OTO	3	3	1	2					
PS	2	2	2						
TS	3	3	3						
U	3	3	2	1					
Oth. Spec.	373	349	262	47	40	10	7	2	5
AN	53	51	42	5	4		1		1
CHP	18	16	11		5	1	1		
DR	48	46	35	8	3				2
EM	26	25	20		5	1			
FOP	2	1	1						1
GPM	3	3	2		1				
MG	1						1		
N	23	23	16	5	2				
NM	1	1	1						
OM	9	7	5		2	2			
P	100	95	63	18	14	2	2	1	
PHP	2	1	1			1			
PM	11	11	11						
PTH	42	38	29	7	2	1	2		1
R	11	11	9		2				
RO	10	9	9			1			
OTH	2						1	1	
UNSP	11	11	7	4					
Not Class	84								
Inactive	99								

Note: Excludes Address Unknown.

Subspecialties in this table are condensed into major specialties. See Appendix A.

Table 3.8

Female Physicians by State, Self-Designated Specialty, and Activity, 2006, continued
Oregon

| Specialty | Total Physicians | Patient Care | | Hospital Based | | Other Professional Activity | | | |
		Total Patient Care	Office Based	Resid./ Fellows	Phys. Staff	Admin.	Med. Teach.	Research	Other
Total Physicians	3,270	2,831	2,230	372	229	32	24	27	14
GP/FM Prac.	495	482	407	46	29	7	1	3	2
FM	480	470	396	46	28	5	1	2	2
GP	15	12	11		1	2		1	
Med. Spec.	1,226	1,192	924	176	92	8	11	14	1
AI	7	7	7						
CD	32	31	24	3	4	1			
D	54	54	46	6	2				
GE	22	21	18	3			1		
IM	704	683	503	118	62	4	6	10	1
PD	386	377	315	43	19	3	4	2	
PDC	6	6	3	1	2				
PUD	15	13	8	2	3			2	
Sur. Spec.	482	475	372	80	23	2	2	2	1
CRS	1	1	1						
GS	100	99	45	44	10				1
NS	10	10	9	1					
OBG	281	276	244	23	9	2	1	2	
OPH	35	35	30	3	2				
ORS	19	19	15	3	1				
OTO	19	18	14	3	1		1		
PS	8	8	6	2					
TS	1	1	1						
U	8	8	7	1					
Oth. Spec.	725	682	527	70	85	15	10	8	10
AN	126	122	97	8	17		4		
CHP	39	39	34	1	4				
DR	52	50	42	5	3	1			1
EM	112	110	86	9	15	1	1		
FOP	4	3	3				1		
GPM	13	10	9		1	1		2	
MG	4	3	2	1				1	
N	44	43	36	4	3	1			
NM	3	3	2	1					
OM	3	1	1			2			
P	163	156	115	16	25	2	3	1	1
PHP	8	4	3		1	2		1	1
PM	25	23	20		3	2			
PTH	60	54	37	10	7			2	4
R	15	14	11	3			1		
RO	18	18	16	2					
OTH	16	9	7		2	3		1	3
UNSP	20	20	6	10	4				
Not Class	174								
Inactive	168								

Note: Excludes Address Unknown.

Subspecialties in this table are condensed into major specialties. See Appendix A.

Table 3.8

Female Physicians by State, Self-Designated Specialty, and Activity, 2006, continued
Pennsylvania

| Specialty | Total Physicians | Patient Care | | | | Other Professional Activity | | | |
		Total Patient Care	Office Based	Resid./ Fellows	Phys. Staff	Admin.	Med. Teach.	Research	Other
Total Physicians	11,840	9,621	6,265	2,461	895	148	145	177	58
GP/FM Prac.	1,276	1,226	865	279	82	15	29	4	2
FM	1,212	1,166	821	279	66	14	29	2	1
GP	64	60	44		16	1		2	1
Med. Spec.	4,548	4,291	2,765	1,158	368	60	62	120	15
AI	51	45	40	5				5	1
CD	126	120	80	30	10		1	5	
D	195	191	143	41	7		2	2	
GE	91	86	58	26	2		2	2	1
IM	2,340	2,199	1,352	659	188	41	26	67	7
PD	1,631	1,544	1,034	364	146	19	30	32	6
PDC	26	24	11	8	5			2	
PUD	88	82	47	25	10		1	5	
Sur. Spec.	1,425	1,392	902	404	86	10	9	7	7
CRS	11	11	10	1					
GS	278	272	125	125	22	1	2	2	1
NS	13	13	5	7	1				
OBG	770	752	509	192	51	6	6	3	3
OPH	183	176	147	25	4	2	1	2	2
ORS	50	49	27	20	2	1			
OTO	53	52	36	14	2				1
PS	32	32	17	13	2				
TS	10	10	9	1					
U	25	25	17	6	2				
Oth. Spec.	2,900	2,712	1,733	620	359	63	45	46	34
AN	400	385	274	68	43	4	8	3	
CHP	138	127	105	10	12	3	4	2	2
DR	331	324	213	75	36		3	1	3
EM	338	326	173	105	48	5	4	3	
FOP	6	2	2						4
GPM	28	20	16	3	1	1	2	2	3
MG	11	11	5	4	2				
N	177	167	107	47	13	2	1	7	
NM	18	15	12	1	2	2		1	
OM	18	12	10		2	5			1
P	678	638	411	133	94	17	12	9	2
PHP	11	2	1		1	6		2	1
PM	153	148	106	15	27	2		2	1
PTH	324	291	162	81	48	10	8	2	13
R	75	74	55	5	14		1		
RO	51	51	33	13	5				
TTS	1	1	1						
OTH	49	30	22	1	7	4	2	9	4
UNSP	92	87	24	59	4	2		3	
VM	1	1	1						
Not Class	922								
Inactive	769								

Note: Excludes Address Unknown.

Subspecialties in this table are condensed into major specialties. See Appendix A.

Table 3.8

Female Physicians by State, Self-Designated Specialty, and Activity, 2006, continued
Puerto Rico

Specialty	Total Physicians	Patient Care		Hospital Based		Other Professional Activity			
		Total Patient Care	Office Based	Resid./Fellows	Phys. Staff	Admin.	Med. Teach.	Research	Other
Total Physicians	3,848	2,899	2,189	376	334	73	43	15	13
GP/FM Prac.	666	640	536	19	85	18	6		2
FM	301	288	243	19	26	9	3		1
GP	365	352	293		59	9	3		1
Med. Spec.	1,151	1,088	760	199	129	31	20	6	6
AI	1	1	1						
CD	20	20	17	2	1				
D	41	41	31	7	3				
GE	18	16	12	2	2		1	1	
IM	475	460	289	127	44	4	8	1	2
PD	579	534	396	60	78	27	10	4	4
PDC	3	3	3						
PUD	14	13	11	1	1		1		
Sur. Spec.	211	205	151	37	17	3	1	1	1
GS	37	36	21	13	2	1			
NS	1	1	1						
OBG	113	109	82	16	11	1	1	1	1
OPH	35	35	30	1	4				
ORS	6	5	2	3		1			
OTO	7	7	4	3					
PS	5	5	4	1					
TS	1	1	1						
U	6	6	6						
Oth. Spec.	1,015	966	742	121	103	21	16	8	4
AN	49	47	30	9	8		1		1
CHP	35	32	26	4	2	1	2		
DR	60	56	46	3	7	2	2		
EM	41	40	23	14	3		1		
FOP	3	3	3						
GPM	8	5	4		1	2		1	
MG	1	1	1						
N	47	44	27	10	7		2	1	
NM	11	9	9			1			1
OM	14	11	9		2	3			
P	171	159	107	27	25	4	3	4	1
PHP	1					1			
PM	87	86	68	9	9		1		
PTH	43	39	30	7	2	1	2	1	
R	19	18	15	1	2			1	
RO	6	5	5			1			
OTH	24	17	13		4	5	2		
UNSP	395	394	326	37	31				1
Not Class	663								
Inactive	142								

Note: Excludes Address Unknown.

Subspecialties in this table are condensed into major specialties. See Appendix A.

Table 3.8

Female Physicians by State, Self-Designated Specialty, and Activity, 2006, continued
Rhode Island

Specialty	Total Physicians	Patient Care				Other Professional Activity			
		Total Patient Care	Office Based	Hospital Based		Admin.	Med. Teach.	Research	Other
				Resid./ Fellows	Phys. Staff				
Total Physicians	1,400	1,164	717	333	114	14	10	22	8
GP/FM Prac.	112	109	86	17	6	2	1		
FM	109	106	83	17	6	2	1		
GP	3	3	3						
Med. Spec.	611	587	361	176	50	3	7	9	5
AI	1	1	1						
CD	10	10	9		1				
D	32	31	20	10	1		1		
GE	11	11	7	2	2				
IM	305	296	169	99	28		1	6	2
PD	238	225	144	65	16	3	5	2	3
PDC	4	4	3		1				
PUD	10	9	8		1			1	
Sur. Spec.	178	172	109	53	10	2		3	1
GS	1	1		1					
NS	37	33	15	18		1		3	
OBG	4	4	2	1	1				
OPH	107	105	74	25	6	1			1
ORS	10	10	6	1	3				
OTO	5	5	3	2					
PS	5	5	5						
U	5	5	4	1					
	4	4		4					
Oth. Spec.									
AN	317	296	161	87	48	7	2	10	2
CHP	30	29	24		5	1			
DR	20	17	10	5	2			2	1
EM	37	35	21	11	3			1	1
FOP	44	44	20	19	5				
GPM	2	1			1	1			
MG	1	1	1						
N	2	2		1	1				
NM	24	23	12	10	1		1		
OM	3	3	2		1				
P	92	87	39	31	17	3		2	
PHP	1					1			
PM	3	3			3				
PTH	34	29	17	4	8	1	1	3	
R	2	2	2						
RO	5	5	4	1					
OTH	7	5	5					2	
UNSP	10	10	4	5	1				
Not Class	120								
Inactive	62								

Note: Excludes Address Unknown.

Subspecialties in this table are condensed into major specialties. See Appendix A.

Table 3.8

Female Physicians by State, Self-Designated Specialty, and Activity, 2006, continued
South Carolina

Specialty	Total Physicians	Patient Care				Other Professional Activity			
		Total Patient Care	Office Based	Hospital Based		Admin.	Med. Teach.	Research	Other
				Resid./ Fellows	Phys. Staff				
Total Physicians	2,572	2,273	1,605	455	213	24	37	20	10
GP/FM Prac.	430	415	305	80	30	4	7	2	2
FM	410	398	289	80	29	3	7	2	
GP	20	17	16		1	1			2
Med. Spec.	952	916	634	182	100	5	18	10	3
AI	13	12	11	1			1		
CD	15	15	15						
D	47	47	38	7	2				
GE	10	10	9	1					
IM	436	418	282	83	53	4	5	8	1
PD	416	399	270	84	45	1	12	2	2
PDC	7	7	4	3					
PUD	8	8	5	3					
Sur. Spec.	365	357	257	86	14		6		2
GS	48	46	22	22	2		1		1
NS	4	4	3	1					
OBG	234	229	174	43	12		4		1
OPH	39	39	32	7					
ORS	12	12	6	6					
OTO	13	12	8	4			1		
PS	12	12	9	3					
TS	2	2	2						
U	1	1	1						
Oth. Spec.	617	585	409	107	69	15	6	8	3
AN	84	80	67	10	3	1	2	1	
CHP	59	57	36	12	9			2	
DR	44	44	33	8	3				
EM	79	76	59	8	9	3			
FOP	2	2	1		1				
GPM	4	4	3		1				
MG	1	1	1						
N	25	23	16	5	2	1	1		
NM	4	3	2		1			1	
OM	1	1	1						
P	180	175	111	35	29	2		2	1
PHP	8	2	1		1	5		1	
PM	14	14	13		1				
PTH	68	61	40	17	4	2	2	1	2
R	11	11	8		3				
RO	10	10	10						
OTH	3	1			1	1	1		
UNSP	20	20	7	12	1				
Not Class	113								
Inactive	95								

Note: Excludes Address Unknown.

Subspecialties in this table are condensed into major specialties. See Appendix A.

Table 3.8

Female Physicians by State, Self-Designated Specialty, and Activity, 2006, continued
South Dakota

| Specialty | Total Physicians | Patient Care | | | | Other Professional Activity | | | |
| | | Total Patient Care | Office Based | Hospital Based | | Admin. | Med. Teach. | Research | Other |
				Resid./ Fellows	Phys. Staff				
Total Physicians	429	383	303	43	37	3	1		1
GP/FM Prac.	116	115	88	14	13		1		
FM	114	113	87	14	12		1		
GP	2	2	1		1				
Med. Spec.	126	123	101	13	9	2			1
AI	1	1	1						
CD	2	2	2						
D	9	9	9						
GE	2	2	2						
IM	66	64	43	13	8	2			
PD	43	42	41		1				1
PDC	1	1	1						
PUD	2	2	2						
Sur. Spec.	63	63	52	2	9				
GS	10	10	7		3				
OBG	41	41	34	2	5				
OPH	5	5	5						
ORS	1	1	1						
OTO	2	2	1		1				
PS	2	2	2						
U	2	2	2						
Oth. Spec.	83	82	62	14	6	1			
AN	6	6	5		1				
CHP	7	6	2	3	1	1			
DR	12	12	12						
EM	12	12	12						
MG	1	1	1						
N	8	8	7		1				
OM	1	1	1						
P	18	18	8	8	2				
PM	3	3	3						
PTH	10	10	9		1				
RO	1	1	1						
UNSP	4	4	1	3					
Not Class	20								
Inactive	21								

Note: Excludes Address Unknown.

Subspecialties in this table are condensed into major specialties. See Appendix A.

Table 3.8

Female Physicians by State, Self-Designated Specialty, and Activity, 2006, continued
Tennessee

Specialty	Total Physicians	Patient Care				Other Professional Activity			
		Total Patient Care	Office Based	Hospital Based		Admin.	Med. Teach.	Research	Other
				Resid./ Fellows	Phys. Staff				
Total Physicians	4,125	3,567	2,583	750	234	39	37	42	12
GP/FM Prac.	479	465	373	68	24	6	7	1	
FM	457	443	352	68	23	6	7	1	
GP	22	22	21		1				
Med. Spec.	1,718	1,651	1,183	360	108	14	19	33	1
AI	15	15	13	2					
CD	31	30	22	6	2			1	
D	59	59	49	7	3				
GE	13	13	10	2	1				
IM	813	783	551	182	50	5	12	12	1
PD	745	711	505	156	50	9	7	18	
PDC	10	9	7	1	1			1	
PUD	32	31	26	4	1			1	
Sur. Spec.	611	605	424	157	24	2	3	1	
CRS	3	3	3						
GS	121	121	58	59	4				
NS	6	6	4	2					
OBG	365	360	274	73	13	1	3	1	
OPH	52	52	43	7	2				
ORS	14	14	12	1	1				
OTO	23	23	13	8	2				
PS	13	13	11	1	1				
TS	5	4	2	1	1	1			
U	9	9	4	5					
Oth. Spec.	889	846	603	165	78	17	8	7	11
AN	143	140	106	23	11	2		1	
CHP	34	30	26	1	3	2	2		
DR	97	95	63	26	6	1			1
EM	93	92	60	21	11		1		
FOP	6	5	4		1				1
GPM	8	6	5	1		1	1		
MG	5	5	3		2				
N	55	53	47	5	1		1	1	
NM	5	5	4	1					
OM	11	9	8	1		2			
P	193	191	127	42	22	1	1		
PHP	11	3	3			6		1	1
PM	20	20	16		4				
PTH	125	113	79	26	8	1	2	2	7
R	28	28	25		3				
RO	11	11	8		3				
OTH	13	9	7		2	1		2	1
UNSP	31	31	12	18	1				
Not Class	237								
Inactive	191								

Note: Excludes Address Unknown.

Subspecialties in this table are condensed into major specialties. See Appendix A.

Table 3.8

Female Physicians by State, Self-Designated Specialty, and Activity, 2006, continued

Texas

| Specialty | Total Physicians | Patient Care | | | | Other Professional Activity | | | |
		Total Patient Care	Office Based	Resid./ Fellows	Phys. Staff	Admin.	Med. Teach.	Research	Other
Total Physicians	14,675	12,526	9,157	2,525	844	136	159	115	55
GP/FM Prac.	1,868	1,813	1,443	280	90	21	24	5	5
FM	1,773	1,723	1,367	280	76	18	24	5	3
GP	95	90	76		14	3			2
Med. Spec.	5,654	5,458	3,992	1,079	387	45	69	71	11
AI	85	80	71	6	3			5	
CD	119	117	92	18	7		1	1	
D	276	274	201	56	17	1	1		
GE	84	82	65	12	5			2	
IM	2,459	2,354	1,682	486	186	21	39	40	5
PD	2,511	2,435	1,791	485	159	22	27	21	6
PDC	41	41	34	5	2				
PUD	79	75	56	11	8	1	1	2	
Sur. Spec.	2,049	2,005	1,451	482	72	12	24	6	2
CRS	9	9	7	2					
GS	340	334	182	142	10		5	1	
NS	16	16	10	6					
OBG	1,214	1,188	919	236	33	6	15	4	1
OPH	207	198	160	25	13	4	3	1	1
ORS	62	62	34	22	6				
OTO	87	86	64	19	3	1			
PS	60	59	40	14	5	1			
TS	6	6	6						
U	48	47	29	16	2		1		
Oth. Spec.	3,420	3,250	2,271	684	295	58	42	33	37
AM	10	6	2	1	3	3			1
AN	663	643	475	125	43	6	9	3	2
CHP	207	195	149	33	13	6	4	1	1
DR	324	322	239	59	24		1	1	
EM	280	272	197	53	22	3	2		3
FOP	15	11	9	2		1			3
GPM	23	20	15	4	1	2		1	
MG	17	14	12	1	1	1		2	
N	199	191	137	42	12	2	3	3	
NM	19	17	12	3	2			2	
OM	23	17	14		3	4	1		1
P	655	629	419	132	78	11	4	4	7
PHP	17	5	4		1	9	1	2	
PM	187	183	135	33	15	3			1
PTH	472	437	282	107	48	4	10	7	14
R	87	81	58	7	16		3	3	
RO	67	66	47	13	6		1		
TTS	1	1	1						
OTH	36	24	22		2	3	3	3	3
UNSP	118	116	42	69	5			1	1
Not Class	1,066								
Inactive	618								

Note: Excludes Address Unknown.

Subspecialties in this table are condensed into major specialties. See Appendix A.

Table 3.8

Female Physicians by State, Self-Designated Specialty, and Activity, 2006, continued
Utah

Specialty	Total Physicians	Patient Care				Other Professional Activity			
		Total Patient Care	Office Based	Hospital Based		Admin.	Med. Teach.	Research	Other
				Resid./ Fellows	Phys. Staff				
Total Physicians	1,223	1,048	766	219	63	12	10	17	9
GP/FM Prac.	148	146	121	15	10	1	1		
FM	145	143	119	15	9	1	1		
GP	3	3	2		1				
Med. Spec.	460	435	320	89	26	4	3	14	4
AI	4	4	3		1				
CD	8	5	3	2			1	2	
D	15	11	7	4			1	3	
GE	9	9	7	2					
IM	184	178	133	35	10	1		3	2
PD	223	213	155	44	14	3	1	4	2
PDC	3	3	2		1				
PUD	14	12	10	2				2	
Sur. Spec.	171	168	115	48	5	1	1		1
CRS	1	1	1						
GS	36	35	17	16	2	1			
NS	5	5	1	4					
OBG	92	90	72	16	2		1		1
OPH	11	11	8	3					
ORS	9	9	5	3	1				
OTO	4	4	1	3					
PS	8	8	7	1					
TS	1	1	1						
U	4	4	2	2					
Oth. Spec.	317	299	210	67	22	6	5	3	4
AM	1	1			1				
AN	46	43	30	13			3		
CHP	19	18	16	1	1	1			
DR	23	22	18	3	1				1
EM	54	54	42	8	4				
FOP	1	1	1						
GPM	5	5	4		1				
MG	2	2		1	1				
N	37	35	29	5	1			2	
NM	1	1		1					
OM	4	4	3	1					
P	51	50	28	12	10	1			
PHP	2					2			
PM	16	16	11	4	1				
PTH	32	27	15	11	1	1	1	1	2
R	5	3	2	1		1	1		
RO	6	6	6						
OTH	3	3	3						
UNSP	9	8	2	6					1
Not Class	84								
Inactive	43								

Note: Excludes Address Unknown.

Subspecialties in this table are condensed into major specialties. See Appendix A.

Table 3.8

Female Physicians by State, Self-Designated Specialty, and Activity, 2006, continued
Vermont

| Specialty | Total Physicians | Patient Care | | Hospital Based | | Other Professional Activity | | | |
		Total Patient Care	Office Based	Resid./ Fellows	Phys. Staff	Admin.	Med. Teach.	Research	Other
Total Physicians	803	667	459	131	77	8	11	10	6
GP/FM Prac.	133	131	103	11	17	2			
FM	131	129	101	11	17	2			
GP	2	2	2						
Med. Spec.	270	255	177	54	24	2	5	6	2
AI	3	3	3						
CD	5	5	2	3					
D	7	7	6	1					
GE	3	3	1	2					
IM	151	142	91	34	17		4	5	
PD	95	90	71	14	5	2	1		2
PDC	2	2	1		1				
PUD	4	3	2		1			1	
Sur. Spec.	101	99	65	26	8		2		
GS	20	19	8	11			1		
NS	2	2	1	1					
OBG	63	62	45	12	5		1		
OPH	3	3	3						
ORS	4	4	2		2				
OTO	3	3	1	2					
PS	4	4	4						
U	2	2	1		1				
Oth. Spec.	198	182	114	40	28	4	4	4	4
AN	27	26	15	8	3		1		
CHP	13	13	11	1	1				
DR	17	16	8	4	4		1		
EM	16	16	8	1	7				
GPM	5	4	2	2		1			
N	9	7	3	3	1			1	1
P	57	55	43	6	6			1	1
PHP	1								1
PM	3	2	2			1			
PTH	33	29	14	10	5	2		1	1
R	2	2	2						
RO	3	3	2	1					
OTH	4	2	2					1	1
UNSP	8	7	2	4	1		1		
Not Class	54								
Inactive	47								

Note: *Excludes Address Unknown.*

Subspecialties in this table are condensed into major specialties. See Appendix A.

Table 3.8

Female Physicians by State, Self-Designated Specialty, and Activity, 2006, continued
Virginia

| Specialty | Total Physicians | Patient Care | | | | Other Professional Activity | | | |
| | | Total Patient Care | Office Based | Resid./ Fellows | Phys. Staff | Admin. | Med. Teach. | Research | Other |
				Hospital Based					
Total Physicians	6,789	5,739	4,206	1,002	531	60	68	51	53
GP/FM Prac.	891	859	663	129	67	8	20		4
FM	828	802	626	129	47	6	17		3
GP	63	57	37		20	2	3		1
Med. Spec.	2,591	2,492	1,862	403	227	21	23	31	24
AI	32	30	23	5	2			2	
CD	51	49	38	9	2			1	1
D	123	121	99	16	6		1		1
GE	36	36	30	3	3				
IM	1,206	1,147	817	211	119	14	12	19	14
PD	1,091	1,059	818	153	88	7	10	8	7
PDC	12	11	7	2	2			1	
PUD	40	39	30	4	5				1
Sur. Spec.	929	909	687	171	51	4	10	2	4
CRS	3	3	3						
GS	144	140	69	60	11	1	2	1	
NS	11	11	7	2	2				
OBG	580	567	461	82	24	3	5	1	4
OPH	94	92	78	9	5		2		
ORS	31	31	19	9	3				
OTO	29	29	24	3	2				
PS	23	22	17	3	2		1		
TS	2	2	2						
U	12	12	7	3	2				
Oth. Spec.	1,560	1,479	994	299	186	27	15	18	21
AM	2	2	2						
AN	248	244	163	38	43	1	3		
CHP	77	77	62	7	8				
DR	150	146	114	19	13		1	1	2
EM	206	205	126	56	23				1
FOP	7	5	5			1			1
GPM	19	16	14	2		1	1	1	
MG	4	4	3		1				
N	75	71	48	18	5	1		3	
NM	6	5	4		1			1	
OM	10	4	1		3	4	1		1
P	382	370	237	74	59	4	4	2	2
PHP	15	5	3		2	8		1	1
PM	70	67	46	13	8	2		1	
PTH	146	126	83	31	12	4	4	4	8
R	28	26	23	2	1		1		1
RO	22	22	17	4	1				
OTH	25	18	16		2	1		4	2
UNSP	68	66	27	35	4				2
Not Class	417								
Inactive	401								

Note: Excludes Address Unknown.

Subspecialties in this table are condensed into major specialties. See Appendix A.

Table 3.8

Female Physicians by Self-Designated State, Specialty, and Activity, 2006, continued
Virgin Islands

Specialty	Total Physicians	Patient Care				Other Professional Activity			
		Total Patient Care	Office Based	Hospital Based		Admin.	Med. Teach.	Research	Other
				Resid./ Fellows	Phys. Staff				
Total Physicians	62	50	35	3	12				
GP/FM Prac.	7	7	4	2	1				
FM	6	6	4	2					
GP	1	1			1				
Med. Spec.	20	20	13	1	6				
AI	1	1	1						
D	1	1	1						
IM	9	9	6	1	2				
PD	9	9	5		4				
Sur. Spec.	13	13	12		1				
GS	2	2	2						
OBG	9	9	8		1				
OPH	1	1	1						
ORS	1	1	1						
Oth. Spec.	10	10	6		4				
AN	2	2	2						
DR	1	1	1						
EM	3	3			3				
GPM	1	1	1						
P	2	2	1		1				
UNSP	1	1	1						
Not Class	7								
Inactive	5								

Note: Excludes Address Unknown.

Subspecialties in this table are condensed into major specialties. See Appendix A.

Table 3.8

Female Physicians by State, Self-Designated Specialty, and Activity, 2006, continued
Washington

Specialty	Total Physicians	Patient Care				Other Professional Activity			
		Total Patient Care	Office Based	Hospital Based		Admin.	Med. Teach.	Research	Other
				Resid./ Fellows	Phys. Staff				
Total Physicians	5,579	4,685	3,710	625	350	54	46	81	27
GP/FM Prac.	1,100	1,073	899	114	60	7	12	5	3
FM	1,059	1,033	867	114	52	6	12	5	3
GP	41	40	32		8	1			
Med. Spec.	1,916	1,825	1,418	263	144	18	16	53	4
AI	16	14	13	1		1		1	
CD	29	26	22	2	2			3	
D	90	89	76	6	7	1			
GE	37	35	25	6	4			2	
IM	1,035	986	767	142	77	11	9	27	2
PD	672	641	489	99	53	5	6	18	2
PDC	6	5	5				1		
PUD	31	29	21	7	1			2	
Sur. Spec.	674	666	543	86	37	1	4	3	
CRS	3	3	3						
GS	129	127	82	40	5		2		
NS	9	9	6	2	1				
OBG	367	362	314	28	20	1	2	2	
OPH	60	60	51	5	4				
ORS	33	33	24	6	3				
OTO	27	27	24		3				
PS	25	25	23	2					
TS	4	3	3					1	
U	17	17	13	3	1				
Oth. Spec.	1,203	1,121	850	162	109	28	14	20	20
AM	1	1	1						
AN	231	221	171	33	17	2	6	1	1
CHP	41	39	31	4	4	1	1		
DR	131	127	101	19	7		2		2
EM	113	111	92	5	14	2			
FOP	3	1	1						2
GPM	27	25	18	5	2	1		1	
MG	8	3	3			1	3		1
N	72	66	49	12	5	1		2	3
NM	5	4	3	1				1	
OM	15	13	10		3	1			1
P	257	245	181	36	28	3	1	5	3
PHP	14	5	5			4	1	3	1
PM	67	63	49	5	9	3	1		
PTH	100	91	66	16	9	2	2	2	3
R	32	32	21	7	4				
RO	18	18	14	3	1				
TTS	1	1			1				
OTH	20	10	10			6		2	2
UNSP	47	45	24	16	5	1			1
Not Class	321								
Inactive	365								

Note: Excludes Address Unknown.

Subspecialties in this table are condensed into major specialties. See Appendix A.

Table 3.8

Female Physicians by State, Self-Designated Specialty, and Activity, 2006, continued
West Virginia

| Specialty | Total Physicians | Patient Care | | Hospital Based | | Other Professional Activity | | | |
		Total Patient Care	Office Based	Resid./ Fellows	Phys. Staff	Admin.	Med. Teach.	Research	Other
Total Physicians	1,051	872	607	186	79	12	14	5	7
GP/FM Prac.	189	184	134	40	10	1	3		1
FM	178	173	125	40	8	1	3		1
GP	11	11	9		2				
Med. Spec.	379	361	253	78	30	4	10	3	1
AI	4	4	4						
CD	8	8	6	2					
D	14	13	11	1	1		1		
GE	1	1	1						
IM	175	169	116	34	19	2	3		1
PD	167	157	108	39	10	2	5	3	
PDC	1	1	1						
PUD	9	8	6	2			1		
Sur. Spec.	121	120	74	40	6				1
GS	29	29	18	11					
NS	66	66	43	20	3				
OBG	13	12	8	3	1				1
OPH	3	3	1	1	1				
ORS	4	4	1	3					
OTO	3	3	2	1					
PS	2	2	1		1				
TS	1	1		1					
Oth. Spec.	221	207	146	28	33	7	1	2	4
AN	22	22	17		5				
CHP	13	12	11		1	1			
DR	23	23	16	5	2				
EM	25	23	16	1	6		1	1	
GPM	2	2	2						
MG	1	1	1						
N	17	17	14	3					
OM	3	2	2					1	
P	43	43	25	11	7				
PHP	2					1			1
PM	8	8	8						
PTH	43	37	24	5	8	3			3
R	4	4	2		2				
RO	1	1	1						
OTH	5	3	3			2			
UNSP	9	9	4	3	2				
Not Class	80								
Inactive	61								

Note: Excludes Address Unknown.

Subspecialties in this table are condensed into major specialties. See Appendix A.

Table 3.8

Female Physicians by State, Self-Designated Specialty, and Activity, 2006, continued
Wisconsin

| Specialty | Total Physicians | Patient Care | | Hospital Based | | Other Professional Activity | | | |
		Total Patient Care	Office Based	Resid./ Fellows	Phys. Staff	Admin.	Med. Teach.	Research	Other
Total Physicians	4,240	3,700	2,833	605	262	26	54	41	20
GP/FM Prac.	813	791	655	95	41	5	12	2	3
FM	794	774	640	95	39	5	12	2	1
GP	19	17	15		2				2
Med. Spec.	1,489	1,429	1,088	250	91	13	20	22	5
AI	29	28	20	7	1				1
CD	35	33	29	3	1			2	
D	77	77	56	15	6				
GE	22	22	14	8					
IM	719	687	514	122	51	7	9	13	3
PD	579	556	433	93	30	6	11	5	1
PDC	10	10	10						
PUD	18	16	12	2	2			2	
Sur. Spec.	561	553	407	111	35		4	4	
CRS	2	2	2						
GS	97	96	53	38	5			1	
NS	10	10	4	4	2				
OBG	314	311	245	43	23		2	1	
OPH	60	58	49	6	3			2	
ORS	22	22	15	6	1				
OTO	25	24	19	4	1		1		
PS	10	10	7	3					
TS	6	6	4	2					
U	15	14	9	5			1		
Oth. Spec.	978	927	683	149	95	8	18	13	12
AN	201	191	132	36	23	1	7	2	
CHP	45	45	36	6	3				
DR	79	79	64	11	4				
EM	91	90	68	11	11	1			
FOP	4	3	3			1			
GPM	8	5	5				1	1	1
MG	5	4	3		1			1	
N	66	64	52	11	1		1	1	
NM	5	5	5						
OM	11	10	9		1		1		
P	201	193	143	24	26	2	3	3	
PHP	2	1			1				1
PM	63	63	51	6	6				
PTH	110	94	68	14	12	3	3	1	9
R	23	21	18	2	1		2		
RO	19	19	15	4					
OTH	13	9	6		3			4	
UNSP	32	31	5	24	2				1
Not Class	193								
Inactive	206								

Note: Excludes Address Unknown.

Subspecialties in this table are condensed into major specialties. See Appendix A.

Table 3.8

Female Physicians by State, Self-Designated Specialty, and Activity, 2006, continued
Wyoming

| Specialty | Total Physicians | Patient Care | | Hospital Based | | Other Professional Activity | | | |
		Total Patient Care	Office Based	Resid./ Fellows	Phys. Staff	Admin.	Med. Teach.	Research	Other
Total Physicians	217	192	158	13	21		2	3	
GP/FM Prac.	69	67	48	10	9		2		
FM	65	64	46	10	8		1		
GP	4	3	2		1		1		
Med. Spec.	57	55	51	1	3			2	
D	2	2	2						
IM	31	30	28		2			1	
PD	21	20	19		1			1	
PUD	3	3	2	1					
Sur. Spec.	32	32	30	1	1				
GS	6	6	5	1					
NS	1	1	1						
OBG	17	17	16		1				
OPH	3	3	3						
ORS	3	3	3						
OTO	1	1	1						
U	1	1	1						
Oth. Spec.	39	38	29	1	8			1	
AN	5	5	4		1				
CHP	3	3	2		1				
EM	7	7	6		1				
N	1	1	1						
P	13	13	9		4				
PM	1	1	1						
PTH	5	4	4					1	
R	1	1	1						
RO	2	2	1		1				
UNSP	1	1		1					
Not Class	6								
Inactive	14								

Note: Excludes Address Unknown.

Subspecialties in this table are condensed into major specialties. See Appendix A.

Table 3.8

Female Physicians by State, Self-Designated Specialty, and Activity, 2006, continued
Pacific Islands

| Specialty | Total Physicians | Patient Care | | Hospital Based | | Other Professional Activity | | | |
		Total Patient Care	Office Based	Resid./ Fellows	Phys. Staff	Admin.	Med. Teach.	Research	Other
Total Physicians	54	47	31	1	15	1			1
GP/FM Prac.	13	13	10		3				
FM	11	11	8		3				
GP	2	2	2						
Med. Spec.	19	19	13	1	5				
IM	1	1	1						
PD	7	7	5	1	1				
PUD	10	10	6		4				
	1	1	1						
Sur. Spec.									
GS	6	6	5		1				
OBG	6	6	5		1				
Oth. Spec.	11	9	3		6	1			1
AN	5	4	1		3	1			
EM	1	1			1				
OM	1								1
P	4	4	2		2				
Not Class	3								
Inactive	2								

Note: Excludes Address Unknown.

Subspecialties in this table are condensed into major specialties. See Appendix A.

Table 3.9

Physicians by Census Division and County Group, 2006

Division County Group	Total Physicians	Total Patient Care	FM/GP Practice	Medical Specialties	Surgical Specialties	Other Specialties	Hospital Based Practice	Other Professional Activity	Inactive	Not Classified
				Major Professional Activity						
				Patient Care						
				Office-Based Practice						
Total Divisions	921,432	722,764	74,900	207,310	127,118	150,729	162,707	43,718	108,344	46,252
New England	62,366	47,724	2,842	14,559	7,391	9,821	13,111	3,941	6,503	4,177
0	7,377	5,763	316	1,759	979	1,050	1,659	433	714	462
1	44	29	7	6	2	12	2	3	11	1
2	120	79	23	13	10	15	18	6	34	1
3	1,716	1,245	207	350	220	258	210	66	378	27
4	2,489	1,870	225	432	337	348	528	136	382	101
6	12,090	9,465	968	3,072	1,741	2,040	1,644	498	1,798	327
7	31,173	23,656	894	7,091	3,382	4,664	7,625	2,227	2,496	2,783
8	7,357	5,617	202	1,836	720	1,434	1,425	572	690	475
Mid-Atlantic	156,213	121,614	6,905	36,075	19,592	23,572	35,470	8,370	16,423	9,744
0	19,160	14,937	857	4,613	2,426	2,928	4,113	1,100	1,988	1,130
1	13	5	1	4					7	1
2	344	273	24	68	42	43	96	11	42	18
3	1,336	1,020	229	273	187	180	151	25	264	27
4	3,646	2,877	455	833	579	596	414	99	592	77
6	34,942	27,626	2,599	8,456	5,228	5,669	5,674	1,542	4,454	1,309
7	36,066	28,072	1,316	9,305	4,715	5,767	6,969	2,122	4,009	1,847
8	60,706	46,804	1,424	12,523	6,415	8,389	18,053	3,471	5,067	5,335
E N Central	132,591	105,863	11,839	29,278	17,657	21,378	25,711	5,583	14,393	6,715
0	17,543	13,821	1,205	3,810	2,407	2,801	3,598	733	1,811	1,172
1	164	121	55	28	15	5	18	4	38	1
2	1,489	1,106	472	193	141	146	154	29	331	22
3	5,551	4,491	1,286	1,049	817	744	595	122	852	86
4	5,453	4,411	835	1,199	922	849	606	125	810	106
6	41,885	33,822	4,422	9,412	6,093	7,542	6,353	1,596	5,024	1,435
7	22,063	17,803	1,570	5,128	2,916	3,767	4,422	1,083	2,192	978
8	17,916	14,104	958	3,959	2,146	2,619	4,422	839	1,701	1,264
9	20,527	16,184	1,036	4,500	2,200	2,905	5,543	1,052	1,634	1,651
W N Central	54,421	43,386	6,495	10,954	7,513	8,504	9,920	2,387	6,283	2,346
0	9,744	7,789	867	2,147	1,230	1,656	1,889	513	936	498
1	985	748	428	93	52	49	126	8	203	26
2	2,751	2,134	954	295	333	265	287	52	523	42
3	4,140	3,341	991	713	723	540	374	78	654	67
4	1,616	1,324	238	336	331	271	148	34	232	26
6	24,902	19,796	2,372	4,880	3,324	3,994	5,226	1,179	2,635	1,284
7	5,630	4,597	230	1,474	853	976	1,064	225	580	227
8	4,653	3,657	415	1,016	667	753	806	298	520	176
S Atlantic	174,658	134,873	13,440	40,280	24,993	28,129	28,031	8,794	23,224	7,699
0	28,070	20,639	1,949	6,288	3,810	4,453	4,139	1,849	4,076	1,492
1	594	445	147	116	67	55	60	8	128	13
2	4,068	3,100	771	866	518	501	444	102	777	87
3	6,777	5,302	1,003	1,383	1,005	951	960	165	1,121	187
4	8,479	6,751	930	2,050	1,577	1,432	762	193	1,386	148
6	65,262	51,318	5,386	14,679	9,612	10,539	11,102	2,712	8,617	2,597
7	49,357	38,489	2,543	11,946	6,683	8,320	8,997	3,328	4,958	2,556
8	12,051	8,829	711	2,952	1,721	1,878	1,567	437	2,161	619
E S Central	45,503	37,236	4,502	10,620	7,494	7,308	7,312	1,691	4,865	1,692
0	6,031	4,830	467	1,346	847	960	1,210	330	549	319
1	169	142	68	32	15	13	14		27	
2	1,536	1,246	538	272	166	133	137	20	235	35
3	4,075	3,332	788	956	696	520	372	62	572	108
4	2,884	2,457	369	768	614	497	209	43	342	40
6	18,254	15,091	1,675	4,294	3,205	3,113	2,804	633	1,956	568
7	12,554	10,138	597	2,952	1,951	2,072	2,566	603	1,184	622

Table 3.9

Physicians by Census Division and County Group, 2006, continued

		Major Professional Activity								
		Patient Care								
		Total Patient Care	Office-Based Practice				Hospital Based Practice	Other Professional Activity	Inactive	Not Classified
Division County Group	Total Physicians		FM/GP Practice	Medical Specialties	Surgical Specialties	Other Specialties				
W S Central	81,189	66,156	8,054	18,072	12,684	13,695	13,651	3,184	8,153	3,663
0	7,330	5,851	646	1,450	1,042	1,200	1,513	423	685	367
1	321	243	149	34	16	16	28	11	64	3
2	1,753	1,379	662	234	200	117	166	17	329	28
3	3,478	2,841	713	707	627	439	355	69	512	56
4	1,672	1,351	254	419	327	224	127	30	268	23
6	31,763	26,247	3,029	7,285	5,127	5,411	5,395	1,062	3,156	1,291
7	9,166	7,476	838	2,180	1,447	1,715	1,296	382	955	347
8	25,706	20,768	1,763	5,763	3,898	4,573	4,771	1,190	2,184	1,548
Mountain	52,817	41,384	5,495	11,150	7,884	9,795	7,060	2,129	7,516	1,772
0	9,823	7,585	841	1,914	1,387	1,781	1,662	556	1,236	442
1	568	421	207	42	53	57	62	17	119	11
2	1,465	1,115	369	187	235	188	136	28	298	23
3	2,460	1,914	425	415	429	429	216	56	446	43
4	3,124	2,436	457	584	524	527	344	66	548	74
6	15,772	12,613	1,654	3,333	2,509	3,007	2,110	675	2,062	417
7	7,045	5,422	554	1,534	884	1,387	1,063	343	1,010	267
8	12,560	9,878	988	3,141	1,863	2,419	1,467	388	1,797	495
Pacific	148,307	114,102	13,411	33,852	20,546	26,252	20,041	7,146	20,119	6,866
0	15,228	11,423	1,175	3,269	1,881	2,667	2,431	1,066	1,819	915
1	172	139	69	9	9	17	35	4	25	4
2	732	541	197	81	90	106	67	24	148	18
3	1,192	894	281	176	167	169	101	33	252	13
4	5,485	4,254	890	1,101	873	1,000	390	156	974	97
6	24,028	18,620	2,982	5,242	3,570	4,531	2,295	838	4,022	537
7	26,102	20,233	1,952	6,258	3,528	4,634	3,861	1,238	3,317	1,299
8	49,896	38,212	4,022	11,435	6,736	8,746	7,273	2,605	6,465	2,591
9	25,472	19,786	1,843	6,281	3,692	4,382	3,588	1,182	3,097	1,392
Possessions	13,367	10,426	1,917	2,470	1,364	2,275	2,400	493	865	1,578
0	7,726	5,987	1,102	1,353	729	1,313	1,490	262	411	1,062
1	45	30	11	4	4	2	9	3	7	5
2	135	106	39	24	7	14	22	2	5	22
3	734	566	159	126	68	101	112	20	56	92
4	139	118	31	25	16	13	33	5	12	4
6	4,586	3,617	574	938	540	832	733	201	374	393
8	1	1					1			
9	1	1	1							

Table 3.10

Physicians by Census Division, State, and County Group, 2006

				Major Professional Activity						
				Patient Care						
				Office-Based Practice						
Division County Group	Total Physicians	Total Patient Care	FM/GP Practice	Medical Specialties	Surgical Specialties	Other Specialties	Hospital Based Practice	Other Professional Activity	Inactive	Not Classified
Total Divisions	921,432	722,764	74,900	207,310	127,118	150,729	162,707	43,718	108,344	46,252
New England	62,366	47,724	2,842	14,559	7,391	9,821	13,111	3,941	6,503	4,177
Connecticut	14,488	11,219	492	3,621	1,978	2,243	2,885	894	1,587	783
0	1,983	1,545	49	488	324	259	425	123	209	105
6	1,980	1,502	169	515	268	294	256	102	329	47
7	10,524	8,172	274	2,618	1,386	1,690	2,204	669	1,049	630
8	1									1
Maine	4,197	3,249	461	855	592	697	644	203	628	116
0	635	492	80	137	81	104	90	31	97	15
2	1	1				1				
3	600	399	83	102	73	84	57	25	166	10
4	655	524	99	104	112	92	117	25	88	18
6	2,306	1,833	199	512	326	416	380	122	277	73
Massachusetts	32,575	24,646	1,065	7,636	3,363	5,216	7,366	2,319	2,819	2,780
0	2,894	2,264	87	724	366	446	641	180	235	212
1	21	10	4	1	1	2	2	2	9	
2	46	27	4	7	4	4	8	5	14	
6	3,953	3,098	230	1,124	549	654	541	128	615	112
7	18,305	13,630	538	3,944	1,723	2,676	4,749	1,432	1,256	1,982
8	7,356	5,617	202	1,836	720	1,434	1,425	572	690	474
New Hampshire	4,079	3,175	392	887	605	676	615	161	616	126
0	71	50	8	9	12	12	9	2	19	
3	281	204	37	42	31	41	53	7	66	4
4	1,332	975	79	228	163	187	318	88	198	71
6	2,395	1,946	268	608	399	436	235	64	333	51
Rhode Island	4,368	3,456	173	1,088	544	612	1,039	209	457	244
0	909	750	38	256	111	129	216	44	68	47
3	295	233	9	96	32	61	35	12	42	8
6	821	620	44	207	128	124	117	27	156	18
7	2,343	1,853	82	529	273	298	671	126	191	171
Vermont	2,659	1,979	259	472	309	377	562	155	396	128
0	885	662	54	145	85	100	278	53	86	83
1	23	19	3	5	1	10		1	2	1
2	73	51	19	6	6	10	10	1	20	1
3	540	409	78	110	84	72	65	22	104	5
4	502	371	47	100	62	69	93	23	96	12
6	635	466	58	106	71	116	115	55	88	26
7	1	1					1			
Mid-Atlantic	156,213	121,614	6,905	36,075	19,592	23,572	35,470	8,370	16,423	9,744
New Jersey	30,183	24,120	1,222	8,441	4,358	4,845	5,254	1,520	3,092	1,443
0	4,358	3,551	212	1,286	634	730	689	179	459	169
6	9,588	7,618	500	2,662	1,440	1,597	1,419	511	1,061	395
7	16,236	12,950	510	4,492	2,284	2,518	3,146	830	1,572	879
8	1	1		1						
New York	83,826	65,183	2,875	18,880	9,951	12,242	21,235	4,507	8,083	6,012
0	7,908	6,182	269	1,884	972	1,204	1,853	468	690	565
1	3	2	1	1					1	
2	50	35	11	9	4	8	3		14	1
3	468	358	82	103	62	64	47	11	89	10
4	2,009	1,576	245	454	310	343	224	64	323	46
6	12,977	10,321	825	3,179	1,973	2,074	2,270	557	1,578	515
7	12,210	9,427	445	2,958	1,490	1,880	2,654	726	1,391	657
8	48,201	37,282	997	10,292	5,140	6,669	14,184	2,681	3,997	4,218

Table 3.10

Physicians by Census Division, State, and County Group, 2006, continued

Division County Group	Total Physicians	Total Patient Care	FM/GP Practice	Medical Specialties	Surgical Specialties	Other Specialties	Hospital Based Practice	Other Professional Activity	Inactive	Not Classified
Pennsylvania	42,204	32,311	2,808	8,754	5,283	6,485	8,981	2,343	5,248	2,289
0	6,894	5,204	376	1,443	820	994	1,571	453	839	396
1	10	3		3					6	1
2	294	238	13	59	38	35	93	11	28	17
3	868	662	147	170	125	116	104	14	175	17
4	1,637	1,301	210	379	269	253	190	35	269	31
6	12,377	9,687	1,274	2,615	1,815	1,998	1,985	474	1,815	399
7	7,620	5,695	361	1,855	941	1,369	1,169	566	1,046	311
8	12,504	9,521	427	2,230	1,275	1,720	3,869	790	1,070	1,117
E N Central	132,591	105,863	11,839	29,278	17,657	21,378	25,711	5,583	14,393	6,715
Illinois	39,240	31,358	3,004	9,172	5,014	6,196	7,972	1,699	3,929	2,245
0	3,332	2,691	282	867	503	635	404	124	409	108
1	73	58	27	13	7	4	7	1	14	
2	420	329	134	70	43	36	46	8	79	4
3	975	819	202	206	178	133	100	13	128	15
4	1,091	860	166	215	178	151	150	25	175	31
6	6,903	5,580	718	1,690	1,118	1,150	904	227	873	220
7	5,919	4,837	439	1,611	787	1,182	818	249	617	216
9	20,527	16,184	1,036	4,500	2,200	2,905	5,543	1,052	1,634	1,651
Indiana	15,229	12,555	1,943	3,213	2,301	2,744	2,354	580	1,662	427
0	616	507	83	134	86	125	79	37	57	15
1	15	10	6	2			2		4	1
2	220	178	104	23	13	15	23	6	30	6
3	1,620	1,324	377	282	214	238	213	41	227	28
4	658	539	97	132	125	116	69	12	98	9
6	8,039	6,748	1,015	1,837	1,350	1,637	909	205	915	170
7	4,061	3,249	261	803	513	613	1,059	279	331	198
Michigan	27,877	21,994	2,156	6,129	3,593	4,224	5,892	1,235	3,135	1,504
0	3,452	2,815	272	802	532	520	689	102	377	156
1	53	35	15	6	5	1	8	3	15	
2	436	289	85	64	43	50	47	9	131	6
3	893	715	163	185	157	134	76	18	146	14
4	817	659	121	176	137	137	88	23	121	14
6	10,027	7,760	804	2,086	1,237	1,550	2,083	588	1,173	502
7	1,638	1,381	192	459	231	263	236	28	171	58
8	10,561	8,340	504	2,351	1,251	1,569	2,665	464	1,001	754
Ohio	34,091	26,832	2,742	7,321	4,496	5,295	6,978	1,392	3,770	2,085
0	8,760	6,663	431	1,743	1,092	1,331	2,066	383	864	846
2	41	31	16	4	2		9		10	
3	1,082	866	269	212	148	126	111	28	165	23
4	1,420	1,140	203	332	260	220	125	26	225	28
6	8,179	6,588	900	1,847	1,148	1,414	1,279	231	1,038	322
7	7,254	5,780	469	1,575	951	1,154	1,631	349	768	356
8	7,355	5,764	454	1,608	895	1,050	1,757	375	700	510
Wisconsin	16,154	13,124	1,994	3,443	2,253	2,919	2,515	677	1,897	454
0	1,383	1,145	137	264	194	190	360	87	104	47
1	23	18	7	7	3		1		5	
2	372	279	133	32	40	45	29	6	81	6
3	981	767	275	164	120	113	95	22	186	6
4	1,467	1,213	248	344	222	225	174	39	191	24
6	8,737	7,146	985	1,952	1,240	1,791	1,178	345	1,025	221
7	3,191	2,556	209	680	434	555	678	178	305	150

Table 3.10

Physicians by Census Division, State, and County Group, 2006, continued

Division County Group	Total Physicians	Total Patient Care	FM/GP Practice	Medical Specialties	Surgical Specialties	Other Specialties	Hospital Based Practice	Other Professional Activity	Inactive	Not Classified
				Office-Based Practice						
W N Central	54,421	43,386	6,495	10,954	7,513	8,504	9,920	2,387	6,283	2,346
Iowa	6,428	4,953	896	1,086	913	987	1,071	309	861	301
0	360	282	67	75	49	55	36	11	59	7
1	59	48	34	2	3	4	5		11	
2	652	481	256	35	74	55	61	11	150	10
3	801	635	151	141	138	125	80	14	138	14
4	173	147	22	40	35	37	13	1	24	1
6	4,383	3,360	366	793	614	711	876	272	479	269
Kansas	7,079	5,601	888	1,371	1,037	1,177	1,128	259	975	243
0	1,887	1,546	168	393	287	340	358	107	149	85
1	244	188	94	26	18	16	34	2	46	8
2	254	191	87	22	31	26	25	3	53	7
3	590	454	116	104	109	67	58	9	115	12
4	441	356	56	96	96	76	32	7	67	11
6	3,663	2,866	367	730	496	652	621	131	545	120
Minnesota	16,756	13,310	2,342	3,377	2,049	2,571	2,971	750	1,943	745
0	3,878	3,047	383	837	407	692	728	202	427	198
1	85	58	39	8	3	2	6		24	3
2	552	438	265	51	48	27	47	10	97	7
3	1,128	890	370	173	153	103	91	30	197	11
4	437	349	92	80	80	70	27	8	75	5
6	6,022	4,870	778	1,212	691	924	1,265	202	603	345
7	1	1					1			
8	4,653	3,657	415	1,016	667	753	806	298	520	176
Missouri	15,586	12,588	1,100	3,523	2,206	2,470	3,289	745	1,468	783
0	2,866	2,325	184	697	385	464	595	121	255	165
1	58	42	22	7	2	5	6		14	2
2	529	420	118	89	73	75	65	12	87	10
3	866	735	205	171	137	122	100	16	99	16
4	292	243	34	72	68	46	23	12	32	5
6	5,347	4,228	307	1,013	688	783	1,437	359	401	358
7	5,628	4,595	230	1,474	853	975	1,063	225	580	227
Nebraska	4,852	3,872	689	873	714	714	882	209	579	190
0	388	283	16	66	38	51	112	63	13	27
1	247	189	125	16	10	11	27		50	8
2	204	157	104	9	9	15	20	7	36	4
3	573	478	112	94	142	100	30	5	78	12
4	118	100	19	21	28	21	11	2	16	
6	3,321	2,664	313	667	487	515	682	132	386	139
7	1	1					1			
North Dakota	1,745	1,436	278	342	243	279	294	62	201	45
0	258	209	23	68	30	38	50	9	26	13
1	127	102	56	16	7	3	20	4	19	2
2	221	173	63	28	33	22	27	4	43	1
4	155	129	15	27	24	21	42	4	18	4
6	984	823	121	203	149	195	155	41	95	25
South Dakota	1,975	1,626	302	382	351	306	285	53	256	39
0	107	97	26	11	34	16	10		7	3
1	165	121	58	18	9	8	28	2	39	3
2	339	274	61	61	65	45	42	5	57	3
3	182	149	37	30	44	23	15	4	27	2
6	1,182	985	120	262	199	214	190	42	126	28

Table 3.10

Physicians by Census Division, State, and County Group, 2006, continued

		Major Professional Activity								
		Patient Care								
		Total Patient Care	Office-Based Practice				Hospital Based Practice	Other Professional Activity	Inactive	Not Classified
Division County Group	Total Physicians		FM/GP Practice	Medical Specialties	Surgical Specialties	Other Specialties				
S Atlantic	174,658	134,873	13,440	40,280	24,993	28,129	28,031	8,794	23,224	7,699
Delaware	2,414	1,926	187	581	363	389	406	95	281	111
0	219	176	12	48	24	53	39	11	17	14
4	287	237	33	82	50	52	20	12	32	6
6	1,908	1,513	142	451	289	284	347	72	232	91
DC	5,023	3,707	132	923	473	665	1,514	513	377	423
0	732	487	25	96	39	59	268	124	46	75
7	4,290	3,219	106	827	434	606	1,246	389	331	348
8	1	1	1							
Florida	53,566	40,192	4,043	13,121	7,850	8,830	6,348	1,808	9,682	1,865
0	12,143	9,003	932	3,076	1,817	2,012	1,166	350	2,391	395
1	7	3	1			2			4	
2	167	134	46	36	15	16	21	3	27	3
3	378	250	58	59	30	51	52	13	108	7
4	1,234	873	98	303	195	201	76	28	315	18
6	16,402	12,120	1,366	3,827	2,443	2,667	1,817	550	3,314	412
7	11,186	8,982	832	2,869	1,629	2,003	1,649	427	1,362	411
8	12,049	8,827	710	2,951	1,721	1,878	1,567	437	2,161	619
Georgia	22,805	18,410	1,858	5,607	3,711	3,840	3,394	1,055	2,455	877
0	2,493	2,008	213	605	334	456	400	109	233	142
1	153	106	45	26	8	8	19	4	38	5
2	1,000	784	265	206	105	109	99	12	189	15
3	1,216	999	157	308	236	178	120	24	167	26
4	1,570	1,299	150	411	357	274	107	23	228	20
6	6,515	5,349	534	1,569	1,133	1,022	1,091	235	717	214
7	9,858	7,865	494	2,482	1,538	1,793	1,558	648	883	455
Maryland	25,969	19,195	1,060	5,893	3,066	4,026	5,150	2,458	2,638	1,668
0	4,961	3,449	151	1,031	610	717	940	700	444	368
2	112	69	14	27	10	10	8	4	38	1
3	406	287	43	91	56	61	36	18	94	7
4	425	347	25	132	81	80	29	10	60	8
6	4,904	3,878	365	1,271	626	882	734	260	508	256
7	15,161	11,165	462	3,341	1,683	2,276	3,403	1,466	1,494	1,028
North Carolina	25,385	20,004	2,334	5,679	3,784	4,068	4,139	1,256	2,979	1,135
0	3,155	2,264	200	618	454	488	504	330	314	241
1	58	44	14	13	2	9	6		12	2
2	416	296	104	70	46	36	40	8	103	9
3	1,216	923	236	248	188	151	100	33	242	18
4	2,439	1,984	295	629	482	401	177	36	391	28
6	13,104	10,362	1,084	2,743	1,762	2,061	2,712	647	1,405	687
7	4,996	4,130	401	1,357	850	922	600	202	512	150
8	1	1	1		1					
South Carolina	11,241	9,148	1,224	2,338	1,798	1,900	1,888	401	1,354	331
0	813	513	95	123	97	112	86	25	253	21
1	6	4	3			1			2	
2	102	81	42	10	12	8	9	1	18	2
3	451	387	106	97	85	49	50	2	54	8
4	982	784	181	197	161	164	81	22	161	14
6	8,887	7,379	797	1,911	1,443	1,566	1,662	351	866	286

Table 3.10

Physicians by Census Division, State, and County Group, 2006, continued

Division County Group	Total Physicians	Total Patient Care	FM/GP Practice	Medical Specialties	Surgical Specialties	Other Specialties	Hospital Based Practice	Other Professional Activity	Inactive	Not Classified
Major Professional Activity										
Patient Care										
Office-Based Practice										
Virginia	23,545	18,529	2,097	5,216	3,281	3,703	4,232	1,019	2,914	1,074
0	2,562	1,941	215	501	341	412	472	169	291	160
1	339	267	75	73	57	33	29	3	65	4
2	2,123	1,630	266	492	313	310	249	68	370	53
3	2,360	1,857	280	447	305	351	474	60	340	101
4	432	341	67	69	74	93	38	4	77	10
6	11,863	9,365	946	2,564	1,642	1,784	2,429	519	1,395	582
7	3,866	3,128	248	1,070	549	720	541	196	376	164
West Virginia	4,710	3,762	505	922	667	708	960	189	544	215
0	992	798	106	190	94	144	264	31	87	76
1	31	21	9	4		2	6	1	7	2
2	148	106	34	25	17	12	18	6	32	4
3	750	599	123	133	105	110	128	15	116	20
4	1,110	886	81	227	177	167	234	58	122	44
6	1,679	1,352	152	343	274	273	310	78	180	69
E S Central	45,503	37,236	4,502	10,620	7,494	7,308	7,312	1,691	4,865	1,692
Alabama	10,994	9,090	1,073	2,569	1,901	1,706	1,841	397	1,101	405
0	2,022	1,597	96	410	237	351	503	110	192	123
1	6	5	1	3			1		1	
2	240	196	95	36	22	17	26	8	34	2
3	440	366	107	102	70	48	39	7	56	11
4	469	414	100	111	108	63	32	6	43	6
6	5,300	4,470	566	1,325	1,041	888	650	129	578	123
7	2,517	2,042	108	582	423	339	590	137	197	140
Kentucky	10,828	8,820	1,141	2,494	1,702	1,857	1,626	373	1,157	473
0	1,546	1,282	159	371	256	238	258	62	104	97
1	86	75	40	13	10	7	5		11	
2	570	481	195	101	60	76	49	5	72	12
3	1,710	1,411	259	432	283	261	176	32	208	59
4	759	647	81	214	154	151	47	8	94	10
6	2,696	2,168	216	577	414	476	485	98	290	139
7	3,461	2,756	191	786	525	648	606	168	378	156
Mississippi	5,890	4,779	659	1,252	1,024	883	961	191	741	176
0	301	239	33	75	61	33	37	5	49	8
1	43	37	14	11	3	3	6		6	
2	375	293	121	64	50	18	40	2	69	11
3	802	640	155	156	149	96	84	10	135	17
4	866	723	83	223	192	147	78	16	112	14
6	3,503	2,847	253	723	569	586	716	158	370	126
Tennessee	17,791	14,547	1,629	4,305	2,867	2,862	2,884	730	1,866	638
0	2,162	1,712	179	490	293	338	412	153	204	91
1	34	25	13	5	2	3	2		9	
2	351	276	127	71	34	22	22	5	60	10
3	1,123	915	267	266	194	115	73	13	173	21
4	790	673	105	220	160	136	52	13	93	10
6	6,755	5,606	640	1,669	1,181	1,163	953	248	718	180
7	6,576	5,340	298	1,584	1,003	1,085	1,370	298	609	326

Table 3.10

Physicians by Census Division, State, and County Group, 2006, continued

			Major Professional Activity							
			Patient Care							
			Office-Based Practice							
Division County Group	Total Physicians	Total Patient Care	FM/GP Practice	Medical Specialties	Surgical Specialties	Other Specialties	Hospital Based Practice	Other Professional Activity	Inactive	Not Classified
W S Central	81,189	66,156	8,054	18,072	12,684	13,695	13,651	3,184	8,153	3,663
Arkansas	6,464	5,315	983	1,251	983	998	1,100	224	761	163
0	321	260	57	40	40	49	74	6	45	10
1	31	23	16	4		1	2	2	6	
2	498	391	220	48	57	24	42	5	97	5
3	598	509	130	124	102	81	72	7	72	10
4	556	440	90	123	101	89	37	11	101	4
6	4,460	3,692	470	912	683	754	873	193	440	134
Louisiana	12,643	10,388	1,038	2,910	2,122	2,012	2,306	459	1,214	577
0	108	87	25	17	11	13	21		17	4
1	17	11	4	2	1	1	3	1	5	
2	283	232	102	52	32	17	29	1	40	10
3	525	453	114	127	99	61	52	10	54	8
4	420	349	68	109	90	36	46	8	54	9
6	11,290	9,256	725	2,603	1,889	1,884	2,155	439	1,044	546
Oklahoma	7,111	5,662	800	1,455	1,101	1,181	1,125	272	947	225
0	474	369	32	100	108	69	60	22	73	9
1	51	36	27	2	2	1	4		13	2
2	216	172	75	29	29	11	28	3	35	6
3	756	611	156	144	134	85	92	17	119	9
4	241	179	21	67	46	27	18	7	52	3
6	1,062	871	148	188	151	179	205	20	144	27
7	4,311	3,424	341	925	631	809	718	203	511	169
Texas	54,971	44,791	5,233	12,456	8,478	9,504	9,120	2,229	5,231	2,698
0	6,427	5,135	532	1,293	883	1,069	1,358	395	550	344
1	222	173	102	26	13	13	19	8	40	1
2	756	584	265	105	82	65	67	8	157	7
3	1,599	1,268	313	312	292	212	139	35	267	29
4	455	383	75	120	90	72	26	4	61	7
6	14,951	12,428	1,686	3,582	2,404	2,594	2,162	410	1,528	584
7	4,855	4,052	497	1,255	816	906	578	179	444	178
8	25,706	20,768	1,763	5,763	3,898	4,573	4,771	1,190	2,184	1,548
Mountain	52,817	41,384	5,495	11,150	7,884	9,795	7,060	2,129	7,516	1,772
Arizona	15,127	11,617	1,269	3,428	2,146	2,819	1,955	580	2,330	595
0	1,519	1,069	100	271	195	276	227	104	275	70
1	8	5	3			1	1		2	1
2	14	12	4	3	2	1	2		2	2
3	161	110	42	29	18	11	10	6	42	3
4	677	507	108	142	88	96	73	18	128	24
6	669	527	81	162	111	119	54	14	110	18
7	3,026	2,313	214	641	397	615	446	124	478	109
8	9,053	7,074	717	2,180	1,335	1,700	1,142	314	1,293	370
Colorado	14,175	11,176	1,470	2,956	2,107	2,688	1,955	680	1,879	436
0	3,597	2,846	324	754	614	706	448	158	485	108
1	153	106	54	12	8	15	17	8	35	4
2	501	362	103	55	81	82	41	11	117	10
3	550	418	96	73	108	109	32	15	108	9
6	8,675	6,908	809	1,885	1,229	1,635	1,350	463	1,014	287
7	699	536	84	177	67	141	67	25	120	18

Table 3.10

Physicians by Census Division, State, and County Group, 2006, continued

Division County Group	Total Physicians	Total Patient Care	FM/GP Practice	Medical Specialties	Surgical Specialties	Other Specialties	Hospital Based Practice	Other Professional Activity	Inactive	Not Classified
Idaho	2,934	2,372	483	518	550	535	286	68	455	38
0	252	202	41	40	32	53	36	10	36	3
1	114	84	42	8	11	12	11	1	25	4
2	226	160	70	22	35	21	12	3	62	1
3	246	182	43	39	45	33	22	9	50	5
4	683	562	98	125	138	155	46	9	101	11
6	1,413	1,182	189	284	289	261	159	36	181	14
Montana	2,548	1,991	365	460	443	460	263	66	462	29
0	195	159	33	39	39	32	16	4	30	2
1	165	127	57	13	19	16	22	5	32	1
2	223	176	62	29	34	19	32	4	40	3
3	175	125	37	28	31	17	12	3	46	1
4	597	437	79	87	91	117	63	20	132	8
6	1,193	967	97	264	229	259	118	30	182	14
Nevada	5,384	4,305	485	1,359	822	1,092	547	131	773	173
0	425	334	64	98	35	70	67	15	54	21
1	12	10	5	1	1	2	1		2	
2	55	51	15	14	10	2	10		3	1
3	343	267	44	73	55	67	28	6	62	7
4	9	7	3	4				1	1	
6	1,033	832	83	208	193	232	116	35	147	19
8	3,507	2,804	271	961	528	719	325	74	504	125
New Mexico	5,424	4,160	617	1,052	646	893	952	280	743	239
0	882	650	81	126	78	144	221	70	92	70
1	9	7	3	2	1	1			2	
2	160	126	38	32	21	18	17	2	30	2
3	347	286	66	70	57	51	42	4	50	7
4	730	588	119	146	114	84	125	12	105	25
6	1,025	756	151	197	123	194	91	53	185	30
7	2,271	1,747	159	479	252	401	456	139	279	105
Utah	6,093	4,860	621	1,202	955	1,103	979	286	692	253
0	2,749	2,167	166	556	360	467	618	185	229	167
1	51	39	21	3	6	5	4	1	10	1
2	123	106	47	17	21	14	7	2	10	5
3	285	225	43	49	41	64	28	7	43	10
4	428	335	50	80	93	75	37	6	81	6
6	1,408	1,162	197	260	266	248	191	30	186	29
7	1,049	826	97	237	168	230	94	55	133	35
Wyoming	1,132	903	185	175	215	205	123	38	182	9
0	204	158	32	30	34	33	29	10	35	1
1	56	43	22	3	7	5	6	2	11	
2	163	122	30	15	31	31	15	6	34	1
3	353	301	54	54	74	77	42	6	45	1
6	356	279	47	73	69	59	31	14	57	6
Pacific	148,307	114,102	13,411	33,852	20,546	26,252	20,041	7,146	20,119	6,866
Alaska	1,697	1,436	295	282	276	311	272	73	150	37
0	21	16	4	1	3	2	6	1	4	
1	101	84	41	5	3	10	25	2	11	4
2	76	64	26	12	6	4	16	5	4	3
3	181	156	48	24	27	38	19	5	19	1
4	302	265	54	47	60	58	46	6	24	7
6	1,016	851	122	193	177	199	160	54	88	22

Table 3.10

Physicians by Census Division, State, and County Group, 2006, continued

Division County Group	Total Physicians	Total Patient Care	FM/GP Practice	Medical Specialties	Surgical Specialties	Other Specialties	Hospital Based Practice	Other Professional Activity	Inactive	Not Classified
California	110,406	84,858	9,139	25,991	15,367	19,537	14,824	5,281	14,730	5,488
0	12,460	9,431	920	2,781	1,552	2,242	1,936	811	1,495	719
1	10	6	3			2	1	1	3	
2	138	107	42	15	15	19	16	2	26	3
3	357	271	83	56	53	52	27	12	71	3
4	1,406	1,110	237	282	221	267	103	43	229	22
6	13,085	10,045	1,623	2,905	1,896	2,500	1,121	432	2,305	300
7	16,610	12,701	1,213	4,052	2,235	2,906	2,295	809	2,128	964
8	40,869	31,402	3,175	9,620	5,703	7,167	5,737	1,989	5,376	2,085
9	25,471	19,785	1,843	6,280	3,692	4,382	3,588	1,182	3,097	1,392
Hawaii	4,599	3,625	337	1,104	617	828	739	216	603	152
0	119	100	8	19	16	15	42	4	4	11
4	927	709	134	213	126	189	47	31	167	20
7	3,552	2,815	195	871	475	624	650	181	432	121
9	1	1		1						
Oregon	11,741	9,029	1,192	2,534	1,728	2,077	1,498	510	1,737	458
0	1,514	1,084	111	284	193	206	290	127	160	142
1	38	34	18	2	5	2	7		4	
2	339	254	82	36	53	61	22	13	61	10
3	219	162	35	35	38	32	22	2	52	3
4	1,384	1,060	199	271	247	232	111	35	255	34
6	5,176	4,004	581	1,169	795	964	495	174	878	118
7	3,071	2,431	166	737	397	580	551	159	327	151
Washington	19,864	15,154	2,448	3,941	2,558	3,499	2,708	1,066	2,899	731
0	1,114	792	132	184	117	202	157	123	156	43
1	23	15	7	2	1	3	2	1	7	
2	179	116	47	18	16	22	13	4	57	2
3	435	305	115	61	49	47	33	14	110	6
4	1,466	1,110	266	288	219	254	83	41	299	14
6	4,751	3,720	656	975	702	868	519	178	751	97
7	2,869	2,286	378	598	421	524	365	89	430	63
8	9,027	6,810	847	1,815	1,033	1,579	1,536	616	1,089	506
Possessions	13,367	10,426	1,917	2,470	1,364	2,275	2,400	493	865	1,578
Puerto Rico	11,900	9,169	1,742	2,281	1,180	2,111	1,855	428	805	1,494
0	6,554	4,973	975	1,212	595	1,175	1,016	206	384	988
1	18	12	5		1	2	4	1	3	2
2	135	106	39	24	7	14	22	2	5	22
3	607	461	148	107	38	88	80	18	39	89
6	4,585	3,616	574	938	539	832	733	201	374	393
9	1	1	1							
Virgin Islands	200	166	17	35	45	26	43	2	23	8
0	67	55	4	15	14	13	9		6	5
1	6	6	2	1	1		2			
3	127	105	11	19	30	13	32	2	17	3
Pacific Islands	1,267	1,091	158	154	139	138	502	63	37	76
0	1,105	959	123	126	120	125	465	56	21	69
1	21	12	4	3	2		3	2	4	3
4	139	118	31	25	16	13	33	5	12	4
6	1	1			1					
8	1	1					1			

Table 3.11

Physicians by State and County, 2006

State County	Total Physicians	Total Patient Care	FM/GP Practice	Medical Specialties	Surgical Specialties	Other Specialties	Hospital Based Practice	Other Professional Activity	Inactive	Not Classified
				Major Professional Activity						
				Patient Care						
				Office-Based Practice						
Total States-Possessions	921,423	723,111	74,899	207,306	127,118	151,082	162,706	43,718	108,342	46,252
Alabama	10,994	9,091	1,073	2,569	1,901	1,707	1,841	397	1,101	405
Autauga	38	34	13	10	1	6	4	2	2	
Baldwin	390	293	62	65	60	76	30	13	81	3
Barbour	18	13	5	5	2		1		4	1
Bibb	6	6	4	1			1			
Blount	21	16	6	5		2	3		5	
Bullock	11	9	2	5			2		1	1
Butler	18	16	2	6	6	1	1		2	
Calhoun	227	199	27	58	55	30	29	1	25	2
Chambers	37	34	6	15	9	3	1		1	2
Cherokee	11	8	5	1	1		1		3	
Chilton	20	14	5	6	2	1			5	1
Choctaw	9	7	6	1					2	
Clarke	16	15	10	4	1				1	
Clay	8	8	6				2			
Cleburne	1	1	1							
Coffee	62	53	6	14	16	9	8	2	6	1
Colbert	98	78	12	29	18	13	6	2	17	1
Conecuh	9	6	3			1	2		3	
Coosa	1	1	1							
Covington	41	36	13	10	9	3	1		5	
Crenshaw	8	5	1	1		1	2		3	
Cullman	112	102	18	31	29	17	7		10	
Dale	36	25	3	6	6	4	6	2	6	3
Dallas	76	57	12	19	12	6	8	2	14	3
De Kalb	48	40	10	9	12	6	3	1	7	
Elmore	46	32	9	10	3	5	5	4	9	1
Escambia	31	23	12	2	4	3	2		7	1
Etowah	210	182	29	61	49	35	8	3	21	4
Fayette	15	12	9	1	1	1		1	2	
Franklin	31	24	7	3	7	5	2		6	1
Geneva	14	12	7		3	1	1	2		
Greene	6	5	1	3			1		1	
Hale	9	8	3	2		3			1	
Henry	8	6	2	2		1	1		2	
Houston	350	307	25	98	84	84	16	3	37	3
Jackson	58	53	22	11	9	7	4		4	1
Jefferson	3,907	3,117	131	834	584	572	996	221	325	244
Lamar	3	2	2						1	
Lauderdale	186	157	14	57	46	33	7	2	27	
Lawrence	10	9	5	1	2		1		1	
Lee	203	181	23	64	44	29	21	3	17	2
Limestone	67	53	15	13	14	5	6	1	10	3
Lowndes	5	3		1		1	1	1	1	
Macon	23	19	2	4	4	2	7	2	2	
Madison	888	754	116	208	154	175	101	20	87	27
Marengo	18	17	9	1	3	2	2			1
Marion	27	26	6	7	4	3	6		1	
Marshall	103	91	27	23	17	13	11	3	7	2
Mobile	1,199	1,011	74	302	237	164	234	45	96	47
Monroe	21	16	8	4	3		1	1	4	
Montgomery	671	574	54	182	134	106	98	19	63	15
Morgan	222	192	33	58	50	41	10	2	26	2
Perry	5	4	3	1					1	
Pickens	10	10	8		1		1			

Table 3.11

Physicians by State and County, 2006, continued

State County	Total Physicians	Major Professional Activity						Other Professional Activity	Inactive	Not Classified
		Patient Care								
		Total Patient Care	Office-Based Practice				Hospital Based Practice			
			FM/GP Practice	Medical Specialties	Surgical Specialties	Other Specialties				
Pike	27	22	6	9	3	2	2	1	3	1
Randolph	8	6	4			1	1		2	
Russell	29	25	10	6	4	4	1		3	1
Shelby	471	404	46	128	64	102	64	11	40	16
St. Clair	40	34	10	8	4	4	8	2	4	
Sumter	5	5	2	2			1			
Talladega	73	62	11	19	18	11	3	1	7	3
Tallapoosa	61	51	11	12	14	10	4		9	1
Tuscaloosa	511	419	56	108	75	92	88	22	59	11
Walker	74	66	12	18	23	9	4	1	7	
Washington	8	5	2	2			1		3	
Wilcox	5	5	2	1		1	1			
Winston	14	11	6	2		1	2	1	2	
Alaska	1,697	1,437	295	282	276	312	272	73	150	37
Aleutians East	1								1	
Aleutians West	3	3	2	1						
Anchorage	1,016	852	122	193	177	200	160	54	88	22
Bethel	21	18	8	4	1		5	2		1
Bristol-Bay	1	1				1				
Dillingham	11	10	7				3			1
Fairbanks North Star	214	181	28	33	41	45	34	6	20	7
Haines	7	5	4				1		2	
Juneau	93	83	23	12	13	23	12	2	7	1
Kenai Peninsula	88	73	25	12	14	15	7	3	12	
Ketchikan Gateway	39	31	6	5	5	3	12	2	6	
Kodiak Island	24	19	8	3	3	3	2	1	2	2
Matanuska Susitna	91	86	26	14	19	13	14	1	4	
Nome	9	9	5			2	2			
North Slope	4	4	4							
Northwest Arctic	7	5	4				1			2
Prince Of Wales	5	5	3			1	1			
Sitka	39	34	7	4	3	6	14	2	2	1
Skagway Hoonah Angoon	1								1	
Southeast Fairbanks	4	3	2				1		1	
Valdez Cordova	8	8	7	1						
Wrangell Petersburg	11	7	4				3		4	
Arizona	15,127	11,622	1,269	3,428	2,146	2,824	1,955	580	2,330	595
Apache	75	58	8	21	6	8	15	2	6	9
Cochise	136	107	22	27	19	27	12	6	17	6
Coconino	350	296	51	64	67	70	44	10	37	7
Gila	89	66	22	17	12	8	7	3	20	
Graham	23	19	12	3	2	1	1		3	1
Greenlee	9	6	3			1	2		2	1
La Paz	14	12	4	3	2	1	2		2	
Maricopa	9,460	7,345	738	2,249	1,395	1,789	1,174	330	1,407	378
Mohave	242	207	27	70	44	54	12	3	26	6
Navajo	124	102	38	26	14	12	12	3	14	5
Pima	3,674	2,727	242	731	450	708	596	205	584	158
Pinal	150	108	21	32	18	19	18	1	37	4
Santa Cruz	50	26	8	9	4	2	3	3	19	2
Yavapai	496	341	54	93	66	86	42	13	135	7
Yuma	235	202	19	83	47	38	15	1	21	11
Arkansas	6,464	5,316	983	1,251	983	999	1,100	224	761	163
Arkansas	25	20	12	1	5	1	1	1	4	
Ashley	20	19	10	1	3	1	4		1	
Baxter	100	88	15	25	22	17	9		11	1
Benton	261	205	54	59	45	27	20	2	47	7
Boone	72	66	20	13	10	14	9	1	5	
Bradley	13	13	11		2					
Calhoun	1	1	1							

Table 3.11

Physicians by State and County, 2006, continued

State County	Total Physicians	Total Patient Care	FM/GP Practice	Medical Specialties	Surgical Specialties	Other Specialties	Hospital Based Practice	Other Professional Activity	Inactive	Not Classified
			Major Professional Activity							
			Patient Care							
			Office-Based Practice							
Carroll	32	22	13	1	5		3		9	1
Chicot	19	14	6	3	2	2	1		4	1
Clark	26	22	7	5	4	2	4		4	
Clay	7	6	4	1		1			1	
Cleburne	39	26	13	1	5	4	3		13	
Cleveland	1								1	
Columbia	25	16	7	3	1	1	4	1	7	1
Conway	19	17	10	3	2	1	1		2	
Craighead	306	261	39	70	65	55	32	11	33	1
Crawford	46	39	16	7	3	6	7	1	4	2
Crittenden	52	44	5	20	12	4	3		6	2
Cross	15	12	7	3			2		3	
Dallas	3	3	3							
Desha	10	7	6		1			1	2	
Drew	8	7	5	1		1			1	
Faulkner	149	133	29	35	35	24	10	1	12	3
Franklin	7	5	4		1				2	
Fulton	10	8	5	2		1			2	
Garland	309	229	36	67	49	51	26	8	70	2
Grant	8	5	4			1			3	
Greene	45	41	17	7	10	7			4	
Hempstead	20	15	6	5	4			1	4	
Hot Spring	15	11	6	3			2		4	
Howard	10	9	5	1	1		2			1
Independence	79	69	17	14	16	16	6		9	1
Izard	12	7	4	2			1		5	
Jackson	24	22	6	2	8	3	3		1	1
Jefferson	188	161	35	44	33	22	27	4	16	7
Johnson	26	23	15	2	4	1	1		3	
Lafayette	3	2	2					1		
Lawrence	11	11	6	2			3			
Lee	8	4	4						4	
Little River	10	8	4		1	2	1		2	
Logan	12	10	6	1	2	1			2	
Lonoke	31	26	13	1	1	5	6	1	3	1
Madison	7	3	2				1		4	
Marion	7	3	2				1		4	
Miller	50	43	9	6	4	3	21	1	4	2
Mississippi	41	35	12	13	6		4		5	1
Monroe	5	3	1	2					1	1
Montgomery	5	2	1	1					3	
Nevada	4	4	3				1			
Newton	3	2	1	1					1	
Ouachita	24	18	8	6	4				6	
Perry	2	2	1	1						
Phillips	26	19	8	3	4	3	1		5	2
Pike	8	6	4				2		2	
Poinsett	9	5	5						3	1
Polk	31	23	9	4	5	1	4	1	7	
Pope	98	84	20	20	25	18	1	2	12	
Prairie	3	3	3							
Pulaski	2,695	2,223	162	512	350	504	695	152	219	101
Randolph	18	15	9	1	2		3		3	
Saline	104	92	22	22	16	13	19		11	1
Scott	5	3	1	2					2	
Searcy	5	3	1			1	1	1	1	
Sebastian	422	329	62	99	72	54	42	13	67	13
Sevier	13	10	6	3		1			3	

Table 3.11

Physicians by State and County, 2006, continued

State County	Total Physicians	Total Patient Care	Office-Based Practice FM/GP Practice	Medical Specialties	Surgical Specialties	Other Specialties	Hospital Based Practice	Other Professional Activity	Inactive	Not Classified
Sharp	11	9	5	3			1		2	
St. Francis	20	18	6	6	3	2	1		1	1
Stone	9	9	6		2	1				
Union	110	92	20	21	17	15	19	4	14	
Van Buren	13	8	3	2		1	2	1	4	
Washington	506	432	69	93	100	89	81	14	54	6
White	109	93	22	23	21	20	7	1	14	1
Woodruff	5	5	3	1			1			
Yell	19	13	9	1		1	2		5	1
California	110,406	84,907	9,139	25,991	15,367	19,586	14,824	5,281	14,730	5,488
Alameda	4,976	3,927	315	1,396	639	898	679	237	559	253
Alpine	2	1				1		1		
Amador	69	48	12	10	7	15	4	3	18	
Butte	534	420	70	118	94	106	32	10	96	8
Calaveras	57	38	12	6	9	8	3	4	15	
Colusa	15	13	4	3	2	2	2		1	1
Contra Costa	3,181	2,448	250	863	449	581	305	114	510	109
Del Norte	47	41	9	11	9	8	4		6	
El Dorado	380	307	67	66	59	85	30	11	52	10
Fresno	1,942	1,541	194	473	286	320	268	75	239	87
Glenn	12	8	4	1	2		1		4	
Humboldt	336	270	65	51	50	79	25	9	56	1
Imperial	142	115	12	43	29	19	12	7	15	5
Inyo	52	36	12	8	5	6	5	1	13	2
Kern	1,209	1,021	143	326	181	205	166	35	124	29
Kings	146	118	33	22	19	19	25	1	16	11
Lake	96	79	22	25	14	13	5	4	13	
Lassen	41	31	14	5	5	3	4	1	7	2
Los Angeles	31,094	24,090	2,204	7,472	4,387	5,427	4,600	1,558	3,675	1,771
Madera	168	144	19	60	24	21	20	2	19	3
Marin	1,771	1,239	86	400	216	409	128	109	380	43
Mariposa	17	12	6	2		2	2		5	
Mendocino	242	185	44	47	42	37	15	9	47	1
Merced	259	220	60	55	45	24	36	6	26	7
Modoc	8	5	3			1	1		3	
Mono	35	29	4	4	5	10	6	1	3	2
Monterey	988	717	116	206	151	163	81	36	220	15
Napa	569	395	43	113	60	117	62	21	144	9
Nevada	298	225	42	53	44	67	19	9	59	5
Orange	10,088	7,895	956	2,481	1,515	1,872	1,071	374	1,430	389
Placer	1,051	815	127	267	156	199	66	22	187	27
Plumas	34	27	16	1	5	2	3		7	
Riverside	3,036	2,248	342	682	480	502	242	91	612	85
Sacramento	4,176	3,289	337	947	591	773	641	220	461	206
San Benito	48	42	12	8	10	8	4		6	
San Bernardino	3,748	2,963	371	776	507	589	720	126	415	244
San Diego	10,747	8,037	824	2,193	1,421	1,916	1,683	655	1,574	481
San Francisco	6,534	4,795	226	1,417	693	1,166	1,293	531	555	653
San Joaquin	1,114	927	136	300	186	178	127	19	125	43
San Luis Obispo	879	671	88	170	120	214	79	26	168	14
San Mateo	3,151	2,306	117	787	444	565	393	189	478	178
Santa Barbara	1,363	1,006	130	316	197	256	107	39	292	26
Santa Clara	7,121	5,376	361	1,852	932	1,171	1,060	431	782	532
Santa Cruz	797	623	126	168	107	166	56	22	137	15
Shasta	501	397	66	88	90	110	43	17	76	11
Siskiyou	93	70	21	15	13	13	8	5	17	1
Solano	914	764	96	233	133	147	155	25	79	46
Sonoma	1,527	1,145	244	285	233	278	105	51	309	22
Stanislaus	943	773	153	246	162	153	59	21	119	30

Table 3.11

Physicians by State and County, 2006, continued

State County	Total Physicians	Total Patient Care	FM/GP Practice	Medical Specialties	Surgical Specialties	Other Specialties	Hospital Based Practice	Other Professional Activity	Inactive	Not Classified
				Major Professional Activity						
				Patient Care						
				Office-Based Practice						
Sutter	204	166	39	55	28	31	13	2	34	2
Tehama	68	52	11	13	13	11	4	2	14	
Trinity	13	8	6		1		1		5	
Tulare	530	439	79	148	93	83	36	6	76	9
Tuolumne	148	117	18	38	15	33	13	5	25	1
Ventura	2,055	1,578	269	489	303	342	175	84	327	66
Yolo	776	603	91	160	77	151	124	54	88	31
Yuba	61	52	12	17	9	11	3		7	2
Colorado	14,175	11,180	1,470	2,956	2,107	2,692	1,955	680	1,879	436
Adams	412	344	68	113	54	68	41	22	31	15
Alamosa	35	27	6	6	6	5	4	1	6	1
Arapahoe	1,759	1,395	119	465	266	352	193	90	221	53
Archuleta	18	10	6	2		1	1	1	7	
Baca	4	3		2			1		1	
Bent	2								2	
Boulder	1,139	932	161	255	178	257	81	44	139	24
Broomfield	89	75	20	28	8	12	7	3	9	2
Chaffee	37	30	11	4	2	9	4		7	
Cheyenne	1	1	1							
Clear Creek	6	5	2	1		1	1		1	
Conejos	7	5	2			1	2		1	1
Costilla	3	1					1		2	
Crowley	2	1	1					1		
Custer	8	4	1	1	2			1	3	
Delta	52	37	14	7	5	7	4		13	2
Denver	4,072	3,178	178	824	510	705	961	294	375	225
Dolores	3	3	2				1			
Douglas	519	413	51	117	100	88	57	27	65	14
Eagle	168	126	19	26	35	27	19	6	34	2
El Paso	1,431	1,150	113	292	254	304	187	53	204	24
Elbert	2	1		1					1	
Fremont	48	40	14	7	9	7	3	1	7	
Garfield	110	80	18	12	20	28	2		28	2
Gilpin	1	1			1					
Grand	19	13	9		2	1	1		6	
Gunnison	26	19	6	1	7	4	1		7	
Hinsdale	5	2		1			1		3	
Huerfano	10	7	5			2			3	
Jackson	2	1	1						1	
Jefferson	1,345	1,052	168	329	181	278	96	54	215	24
Kiowa	2	2	1	1						
Kit Carson	4	3	3						1	
La Plata	222	167	26	34	41	57	9	7	45	3
Lake	4	3	2				1		1	
Larimer	739	597	135	142	122	131	67	21	109	12
Las Animas	20	17	5	3	4	2	3		2	1
Lincoln	4	4	4							
Logan	27	22	6	3	7	1	5		2	3
Mesa	402	313	53	60	63	80	57	16	67	6
Mineral	2	1	1					1		
Moffat	12	9	4	1	2	1	1		3	
Montezuma	48	38	10	4	9	10	5	1	8	1
Montrose	94	74	12	15	22	24	1	1	16	3
Morgan	33	27	13	3	8		3	1	5	
Otero	27	18	6	5	3	1	3	1	8	
Ouray	18	12	4	2	1	5		1	4	1
Park	12	4	2	2					8	
Phillips	6	4	4						1	1
Pitkin	79	53	5	12	15	16	5	2	22	2

Table 3.11

Physicians by State and County, 2006, continued

State County	Total Physicians	Total Patient Care	FM/GP Practice	Medical Specialties	Surgical Specialties	Other Specialties	Hospital Based Practice	Other Professional Activity	Inactive	Not Classified
				Major Professional Activity						
				Patient Care						
				Office-Based Practice						
Prowers	16	15	7	1	3		4		1	
Pueblo	433	350	51	84	64	96	55	8	72	3
Rio Blanco	12	9	5				4	1	2	
Rio Grande	9	6	4			1	1	1	2	
Routt	88	60	8	10	21	18	3	2	24	2
Saguache	5	4	2		1	1			1	
San Juan	1							1		
San Miguel	22	18	6	4	2	4	2	1	3	
Sedgwick	2	2	2							
Summit	93	70	19	11	17	18	5	3	20	
Teller	37	27	9	4	2	9	3	3	5	2
Weld	354	287	61	61	59	60	46	10	51	6
Yuma	13	8	4		1		3		4	1
Connecticut	14,488	11,224	492	3,621	1,978	2,248	2,885	894	1,587	783
Fairfield	3,755	2,943	103	1,029	589	627	595	175	466	171
Hartford	3,903	3,079	118	968	552	590	851	241	390	193
Litchfield	465	346	28	129	72	70	47	19	88	12
Middlesex	507	384	49	101	62	90	82	34	70	19
New Haven	4,707	3,586	83	1,083	547	716	1,157	370	381	370
New London	740	554	47	200	104	104	99	42	131	13
Tolland	245	196	34	68	25	29	40	8	37	4
Windham	166	136	30	43	27	22	14	5	24	1
Delaware	2,414	1,927	187	581	363	390	406	95	281	111
Kent	246	205	20	73	44	51	17	8	25	8
New Castle	1,784	1,407	126	398	251	267	365	72	212	93
Sussex	384	315	41	110	68	72	24	15	44	10
District Of Columbia	5,022	3,709	131	923	473	668	1,514	513	377	423
District Of Columbia	5,022	3,709	131	923	473	668	1,514	513	377	423
Florida	53,565	40,211	4,043	13,121	7,850	8,849	6,348	1,808	9,681	1,865
Alachua	2,107	1,624	109	373	206	297	639	168	179	136
Baker	12	10	5	2		1	2		2	
Bay	380	320	37	98	80	78	27	8	44	8
Bradford	18	14	6	4		1	3	1	3	
Brevard	1,344	1,082	136	366	233	253	94	28	200	34
Broward	4,917	3,844	285	1,461	785	886	427	139	779	155
Calhoun	7	6	1	2			3	1		
Charlotte	428	287	18	108	62	74	25	6	125	10
Citrus	306	210	26	77	39	52	16	3	89	4
Clay	396	320	60	82	50	63	65	10	55	11
Collier	1,253	694	50	244	171	174	55	37	501	21
Columbia	117	96	13	29	12	22	20	1	18	2
De Soto	31	25	6	7	5	4	3		6	
Dixie	3	1				1			2	
Duval	2,959	2,400	257	676	419	490	558	120	316	123
Escambia	1,004	814	92	208	152	181	181	40	131	19
Flagler	141	80	11	18	14	22	15	5	54	2
Franklin	11	5	2	2	1			1	4	1
Gadsden	43	30	11	1		7	11	6	7	
Gilchrist	4	3	1	1			1	1		
Glades	5	2				2			3	
Gulf	16	12	6	2	1	1	2		4	
Hamilton	6	4	3	1					1	1
Hardee	11	10	3	6	1				1	
Hendry	20	15	2	4	1	2	6		5	
Hernando	263	215	24	98	33	41	19	2	38	8
Highlands	204	152	18	61	37	30	6	6	40	6
Hillsborough	3,987	3,154	220	986	581	719	648	193	418	222
Holmes	13	11	6	3	1	1			2	

Table 3.11

Physicians by State and County, 2006, continued

State County	Total Physicians	Total Patient Care	FM/GP Practice	Medical Specialties	Surgical Specialties	Other Specialties	Hospital Based Practice	Other Professional Activity	Inactive	Not Classified
				Office-Based Practice						
Indian River	445	304	25	106	74	80	19	11	128	2
Jackson	52	39	11	11	8	3	6	1	9	3
Jefferson	7	5	2	1	1	1			2	
Lafayette	2	1	1						1	
Lake	586	441	59	154	89	106	33	12	120	13
Lee	1,523	1,008	82	341	251	234	100	42	449	24
Leon	810	616	108	148	113	130	117	48	123	23
Levy	24	20	10	3		3	4	1	3	
Madison	8	8	2	2		2	2			
Manatee	911	579	64	214	135	133	33	22	305	5
Marion	583	473	55	181	104	113	20	5	97	8
Martin	504	344	25	105	92	82	40	13	142	5
Miami Dade	9,495	6,985	696	2,188	1,207	1,430	1,464	371	1,506	633
Monroe	250	166	19	37	41	42	27	7	72	5
Nassau	115	56	13	16	8	15	4	6	48	5
Okaloosa	548	468	73	103	105	88	99	14	55	11
Okeechobee	48	44	3	21	8	5	7		3	1
Orange	2,932	2,420	254	772	456	554	384	87	341	84
Osceola	292	251	42	86	59	38	26	4	32	5
Palm Beach	4,525	3,140	191	1,204	733	715	297	122	1,167	96
Pasco	687	554	66	225	102	103	58	23	95	15
Pinellas	3,130	2,366	238	796	467	536	329	100	611	53
Polk	1,008	770	86	281	182	158	63	16	194	28
Putnam	88	66	8	23	18	10	7		19	3
Santa Rosa	300	257	51	58	36	70	42	6	32	5
Sarasota	1,549	1,007	101	353	242	241	70	34	497	11
Seminole	834	684	92	236	128	148	80	22	108	20
St. Johns	599	449	53	166	66	118	46	33	100	17
St. Lucie	378	279	31	92	66	70	20	5	86	8
Sumter	77	34	6	16	3	5	4		43	
Suwannee	21	12	4	3		2	3		8	1
Taylor	17	16	2	6	4	1	3		1	
Union	15	14	4	1	2	3	4		1	
Volusia	1,093	830	138	241	156	192	103	25	222	16
Wakulla	16	9	4	1		2	2		6	1
Walton	71	45	9	8	9	13	6	2	24	
Washington	16	11	7	2	1	1			4	1
Georgia	22,805	18,418	1,858	5,607	3,711	3,848	3,394	1,055	2,455	877
Appling	16	13	1	8	3		1		3	
Atkinson	2	1					1		1	
Bacon	15	13	6	3	3	1			1	1
Baldwin	133	108	9	28	21	22	28	4	18	3
Banks	3	3	1	1		1				
Barrow	34	27	10	8	4	5		2	5	
Bartow	107	93	20	21	25	19	8	1	10	3
Ben Hill	14	12	5	5		2			2	
Berrien	7	5	3	1	1				2	
Bibb	823	655	55	189	153	128	130	35	104	29
Bleckley	11	8	3	2	1		2		3	
Brantley	3	2	1				1			1
Brooks	8	6	1	3	1		1		2	
Bryan	52	45	5	16	7	6	11		4	3
Bulloch	103	92	13	30	29	12	8	1	9	1
Burke	19	16	9	2	1	1	3		3	
Butts	13	11	4	5	1	1			2	
Calhoun	4	3	1	2					1	
Camden	57	46	8	16	12	4	6	2	7	2
Candler	10	6	2	2	1		1		4	
Carroll	174	150	26	42	36	29	17	3	19	2

Table 3.11

Physicians by State and County, 2006, continued

State County	Total Physicians	Total Patient Care	Office-Based Practice FM/GP Practice	Office-Based Practice Medical Specialties	Office-Based Practice Surgical Specialties	Office-Based Practice Other Specialties	Hospital Based Practice	Other Professional Activity	Inactive	Not Classified
Catoosa	69	63	15	20	13	11	4		6	
Charlton	8	6	4	1		1			1	1
Chatham	1,015	808	60	227	184	176	161	33	147	27
Chattooga	9	7	5	1	1			1	1	
Cherokee	194	159	29	48	31	36	15	5	26	4
Clarke	376	320	22	88	90	79	41	9	43	4
Clay	3	2	1	1					1	
Clayton	265	224	14	88	65	41	16	11	24	6
Clinch	5	4	1	2			1			1
Cobb	1,390	1,169	94	417	264	283	111	37	143	41
Coffee	62	58	8	19	13	10	8	1	3	
Colquitt	54	47	9	11	11	11	5		7	
Columbia	707	579	46	133	46	116	238	25	58	45
Cook	14	12	10		1		1		2	
Coweta	124	103	17	33	28	17	8	1	18	2
Crawford	7	6	3	1			2		1	
Crisp	37	28	4	12	6	3	3		7	2
Dade	13	10	4	2		3	1		3	
Dawson	18	14	8	4		2			4	
De Kalb	3,548	2,666	139	791	336	582	818	374	267	241
Decatur	33	28	2	11	6	4	5		4	1
Dodge	27	24	3	9	6	5	1		2	1
Dooly	5	5	3		1		1			
Dougherty	304	260	22	90	64	52	32	8	30	6
Douglas	114	101	13	43	23	17	5	1	7	5
Early	7	6	4		2				1	
Effingham	19	17	7	4	4	1	1			2
Elbert	13	10	5	2	2		1	1	2	
Emanuel	16	13	3	3	3	3	1		2	1
Evans	9	8	3	2	2		1		1	
Fannin	24	20	7	5	3	2	3		3	1
Fayette	278	241	37	93	54	45	12	8	23	6
Floyd	379	317	54	80	69	63	51	8	44	10
Forsyth	118	100	21	27	26	19	7	4	11	3
Franklin	20	16	6	5	2	2	1		3	1
Fulton	5,213	4,189	210	1,262	898	1,043	776	285	493	246
Gilmer	27	19	7	5	4	3		1	7	
Glascock	1	1	1							
Glynn	263	193	15	58	55	50	15	6	61	3
Gordon	57	48	11	13	12	7	5	1	7	1
Grady	12	11	5	3	1	1	1		1	
Greene	29	20	6	4	6	4		1	8	
Gwinnett	951	822	99	315	154	150	104	28	67	34
Habersham	44	34	7	15	9	2	1	1	8	1
Hall	402	321	26	113	89	75	18	8	70	3
Hancock	6	2		1			1		3	1
Haralson	23	22	11	7	2	2			1	
Harris	31	22	6	3	2	4	7	1	7	1
Hart	22	18	7	5	2	1	3		4	
Henry	261	235	32	89	50	39	25	5	10	11
Houston	195	165	18	63	31	30	23	5	20	5
Irwin	5	4	1	1	1		1		1	
Jackson	49	41	10	17	2	7	5	2	5	1
Jasper	8	8	3	1	1	1	2			
Jeff Davis	8	8	3	3	2					
Jefferson	14	12	5	3	2		2		1	1
Jenkins	6	4	1	1			2		2	
Johnson	3	2	1	1				1		
Jones	13	10	4	1		2	3		3	
Lamar	14	12	5	1		3	3		2	

Table 3.11

Physicians by State and County, 2006, continued

State County	Total Physicians	Total Patient Care	Office-Based Practice				Hospital Based Practice	Other Professional Activity	Inactive	Not Classified
			FM/GP Practice	Medical Specialties	Surgical Specialties	Other Specialties				
Lanier	3	3	3							
Laurens	140	116	17	32	25	20	22	1	20	3
Lee	27	23	3	3	3	11	3	1	2	1
Liberty	55	48	3	14	5	10	16	3	3	1
Lincoln	10	5	2			1	2		5	
Lowndes	222	186	27	54	47	45	13	1	34	1
Lumpkin	26	25	6	4	6	6	3		1	
Macon	12	10	3	2	4	1			2	
Madison	7	6	5	1					1	
Marion	3	3	1			1	1			
Mc Duffie	18	18	7	6	3		2			
Mc Intosh	11	5		1		3	1		6	
Meriwether	20	15	6	5	1	1	2		5	
Miller	9	7	5				2		2	
Mitchell	16	14	6	4	2		2		2	
Monroe	20	15	7	3		1	4		5	
Montgomery	2	1					1		1	
Morgan	16	10	4	1	1	2	2		6	
Murray	10	7	2	3		1	1		2	1
Muscogee	627	507	94	111	114	93	95	17	81	22
Newton	73	61	6	27	13	11	4	1	11	
Oconee	82	70	9	23	6	24	8		12	
Oglethorpe	4	4	3				1			
Paulding	24	20	5	8	3	2	2	1	3	
Peach	18	16	6	5	3		2		2	
Pickens	43	31	7	7	7	8	2	1	11	
Pierce	14	10	8	1		1			4	
Pike	3	2	1	1					1	
Polk	24	16	7	2	2	2	3	1	7	
Pulaski	20	15	5	5	2	1	2	1	4	
Putnam	13	8	3	4			1		5	
Rabun	38	20	4	8	4	2	2	1	16	1
Randolph	3	2	2						1	
Richmond	1,172	925	41	213	190	148	333	85	110	52
Rockdale	145	136	17	57	30	21	11	3	3	3
Schley	1	1		1						
Screven	7	5	3				2		2	
Seminole	12	12	4	3	4		1			
Spalding	90	70	9	30	19	9	3		18	2
Stephens	45	33	5	13	12	2	1	1	10	1
Stewart	5	4	3	1					1	
Sumter	55	39	6	10	12	8	3		12	4
Talbot	2	1		1						1
Tattnall	11	6	4	1	1				5	
Taylor	1	1	1							
Telfair	8	6	4			1	1		2	
Terrell	8	4	1		1		2		4	
Thomas	170	134	12	37	31	38	16	6	29	1
Tift	111	100	11	40	24	21	4		11	
Toombs	62	57	7	21	17	6	6		4	1
Towns	18	13	5	4	1	2	1		5	
Treutlen	4	4	2				1	1		
Troup	121	103	6	41	25	27	4		15	3
Turner	10	5	1	1	1		2	1	4	
Union	32	22	9	5	4	2	2	1	9	
Upson	39	32	7	7	12	6			7	
Walker	35	25	9	5	5	5	1		9	1
Walton	76	65	14	26	11	10	4	1	6	4
Ware	102	85	7	35	19	15	9	2	10	5
Warren	3	1		1					1	1
Washington	26	20	6	8	3	1	2	1	4	1

Table 3.11

Physicians by State and County, 2006, continued

State / County	Total Physicians	Total Patient Care	FM/GP Practice	Medical Specialties	Surgical Specialties	Other Specialties	Hospital Based Practice	Other Professional Activity	Inactive	Not Classified
Wayne	33	26	7	7	7	3	2	1	5	1
Wheeler	1	1					1			
White	20	9	4	1		3	1	2	9	
Whitfield	191	167	19	56	52	32	8	1	21	2
Wilcox	2	1		1				1		
Wilkes	12	8	3	2	1	1	1		4	
Wilkinson	1	1	1							
Worth	12	8	3	2			3		4	
Hawaii	4,598	3,627	337	1,103	617	831	739	216	603	152
Hawaii	406	308	63	89	53	83	20	8	82	8
Honolulu	3,669	2,917	202	890	491	642	692	185	435	132
Kauai	168	128	26	31	22	39	10	10	26	4
Maui	355	274	46	93	51	67	17	13	60	8
Idaho	2,934	2,373	483	518	550	536	286	68	455	38
Ada	1,133	954	143	233	232	218	128	35	134	10
Adams	4	2		1			1		2	
Bannock	198	159	27	33	30	33	36	5	30	4
Bear Lake	6	6	3	1	2					
Benewah	9	7	3		2	1	1		1	1
Bingham	32	24	7	3	7	3	4	2	6	
Blaine	107	69	11	13	16	21	8	3	34	1
Boise	2	1	1						1	
Bonner	84	59	10	13	14	20	2	3	21	1
Bonneville	223	181	24	40	51	51	15	2	38	2
Boundary	13	8	6				2	1	3	1
Butte	3	3	1	1			1			
Canyon	186	148	33	32	37	31	15	3	33	2
Caribou	6	5	2		2	1			1	
Cassia	29	22	6	3	9	3	1		7	
Clearwater	17	12	6		2	1	3		5	
Custer	1	1		1						
Elmore	30	25	10	7	3		5	1	1	3
Franklin	4	4	3			1			1	
Fremont	5	1				1			4	
Gem	12	8	7				1	1	3	
Gooding	7	5	3	2					2	
Idaho	20	16	9		3	1	3		4	
Jefferson	2	2	1	1						
Jerome	14	14	9		2	1	2			
Kootenai	338	278	60	54	51	87	26	8	45	7
Latah	58	46	17	6	10	7	6	2	9	1
Lemhi	10	8	2	2	2	1	1		2	
Lewis	2	1		1					1	
Lincoln	1	1	1							
Madison	29	24	6	5	9	2	2		5	
Minidoka	9	7	3	2	2				2	
Nez Perce	107	84	15	23	20	18	8	1	21	1
Oneida	1	1	1							
Owyhee	1	1	1							
Payette	12	10	4	3	2	1			2	
Power	2	2	1				1			
Shoshone	14	11	6	2	1	1	1		3	
Teton	12	10	5	1	1	2	1		1	1
Twin Falls	159	132	23	35	40	24	10	1	24	2
Valley	29	19	11				6	2	9	1
Washington	3	2	2						1	
Illinois	39,240	31,367	3,004	9,172	5,014	6,205	7,972	1,699	3,929	2,245
Adams	180	137	23	38	24	27	25	5	31	7
Alexander	2	2	2							

Table 3.11

Physicians by State and County, 2006, continued

State County	Total Physicians	Total Patient Care	FM/GP Practice	Medical Specialties	Surgical Specialties	Other Specialties	Hospital Based Practice	Other Professional Activity	Inactive	Not Classified
Bond	15	11	6	1	1	1	2		4	
Boone	73	64	16	13	8	20	7	1	6	2
Brown	3	2	1				1		1	
Bureau	46	37	10	8	7	6	6	1	7	1
Calhoun	4	3	3						1	
Carroll	10	6	6						2	2
Cass	4	3	1	1			1		1	
Champaign	680	527	63	153	81	97	133	30	90	33
Christian	27	24	9	7	4	2	2		3	
Clark	8	6	3	1	1		1		2	
Clayx	10	8	3	3	1		1		2	
Clinton	27	22	9	6	5	1	1		4	1
Coles	87	73	15	14	15	12	17	1	11	2
Cook	21,969	17,341	1,162	4,901	2,389	3,145	5,744	1,100	1,824	1,704
Crawford	18	13	3	3	1	1	5		5	
Cumberland	3	2		2					1	
De Kalb	99	76	11	28	21	13	3	3	16	4
De Witt	13	11	3	2	3		3		2	
Douglas	14	11	9				2		3	
Du Page	4,297	3,607	328	1,173	633	893	580	133	413	144
Edgar	12	10	3	3		2	2		2	
Effingham	80	68	12	16	22	11	7	1	9	2
Fayette	11	7	2	1	2	1	1		4	
Ford	13	12	7	2	2	1			1	
Franklin	25	22	12	5	2	2	1		2	1
Fulton	28	21	8	3	5	3	2		7	
Gallatin	3	1	1						2	
Greene	8	5	3	1			1		3	
Grundy	52	45	4	12	13	9	7	1	6	
Hamilton	6	5	1	1	2		1		1	
Hancock	12	10	7		2		1		2	
Hardin	2	2	1	1						
Henderson	5	5	3		1	1				
Henry	34	27	8	9	4	1	5	1	6	
Iroquois	32	25	5	10	6	4		1	6	
Jackson	195	153	32	37	30	30	24	7	27	8
Jasper	3	3	2	1						
Jefferson	91	79	5	20	22	18	14	1	9	2
Jersey	21	16	6	4	3		3	1	4	
Jo Daviess	15	10	5	2		1	2	1	4	
Johnson	4	4	1	1			2			
Kane	743	600	76	196	141	155	32	26	100	17
Kankakee	179	145	15	52	39	22	17	4	25	5
Kendall	52	41	8	20	5	4	4	3	6	2
Knox	112	87	16	21	21	15	14	2	21	2
La Salle	133	100	20	23	30	14	13	1	30	2
Lake	2,537	1,997	169	678	337	489	324	141	304	95
Lawrence	13	13	5	2	1	4	1			
Lee	63	54	6	16	13	7	12	1	6	2
Livingston	31	28	10	7	8	2	1		2	1
Logan	20	15	11	2	1		1		5	
Macon	281	235	44	58	49	52	32	5	37	4
Macoupin	29	24	10	7	5		2		2	3
Madison	344	289	39	101	66	55	28	3	43	9
Marion	71	62	7	23	14	15	3		8	1
Marshall	8	4	1	1	1	1			4	
Mason	10	7	2	2	1	2		1	1	1
Massac	9	7	5	1		1		1	1	
Mc Donough	48	37	9	12	6	6	4		11	

Table 3.11

Physicians by State and County, 2006, continued

State County	Total Physicians	Total Patient Care	Office-Based Practice FM/GP Practice	Office-Based Practice Medical Specialties	Office-Based Practice Surgical Specialties	Office-Based Practice Other Specialties	Hospital Based Practice	Other Professional Activity	Inactive	Not Classified
Mc Henry	414	339	45	124	74	75	21	9	58	8
Mc Lean	349	296	34	87	78	79	18	8	41	4
Menard	9	4	1		1	1	1	1	4	
Mercer	6	6	2	1	1	2				
Monroe	23	21	8	1	5	3	4		2	
Montgomery	26	20	14	2	2	1	1		6	
Morgan	55	44	6	9	17	6	6	1	10	
Moultrie	6	5	3		1		1		1	
Ogle	38	30	20	3	3	3	1	4	4	
Peoria	963	780	79	187	135	175	204	50	93	40
Perry	21	17	9	3	2	1	2		4	
Piatt	11	7	3	3		1		1	3	
Pike	14	11	5	3	1	1	1		3	
Pope	2	2	1			1				
Putnam	1	1	1							
Randolph	38	28	15	5	4	1	3	2	6	2
Richland	37	29	3	11	8	5	2	1	7	
Rock Island	319	241	26	76	58	62	19	7	62	9
Saline	37	31	12	4	5	3	7		6	
Sangamon	1,060	866	64	234	146	189	233	51	102	41
Schuyler	3	2	2						1	
Scott	2	2	1	1						
Shelby	11	9	4	3		1	1	1	1	
St. Clair	545	444	80	105	83	86	90	17	67	17
Stark	2	1	1						1	
Stephenson	78	65	9	24	13	12	7	3	10	
Tazewell	166	125	22	31	14	25	33	5	29	7
Union	22	17	7	3	3	4		1	4	
Vermilion	149	114	20	26	20	21	27	5	27	3
Wabash	9	7	1	3	2	1			1	1
Warren	16	14	4	1		1	8		2	
Washington	8	7	1		1	3	2		1	
Wayne	11	10	4	3	3				1	
White	9	7	3	2		1	1		2	
Whiteside	80	64	17	19	10	13	5	2	13	1
Will	756	617	80	249	111	119	58	18	92	29
Williamson	157	133	24	37	28	19	25	2	16	6
Winnebago	826	655	98	197	136	139	85	33	118	20
Woodford	37	35	8	10	1	5	11	1	1	
Indiana	15,229	12,560	1,943	3,213	2,301	2,749	2,354	580	1,662	427
Adams	23	19	9	2	2	3	3		3	1
Allen	975	829	106	225	192	211	95	26	102	18
Bartholomew	194	169	28	46	46	42	7	3	19	3
Benton	6	4	3	1					2	
Blackford	11	9	7	1			1		2	
Boone	344	273	26	80	33	80	54	26	34	11
Brown	8	4	3	1				1	3	
Carroll	9	8	7			1			1	
Cass	63	55	11	5	14	14	11		7	1
Clark	182	163	26	47	34	40	16		18	1
Clay	20	14	8	4	1	1			6	
Clinton	25	21	5	4	3	3	6		4	
Crawford	2								1	1
Daviess	22	15	3	3	1	3	5		7	
De Kalb	47	37	16	4	4	7	6	1	9	
Dearborn	60	51	8	20	8	7	8		8	1
Decatur	22	17	4	5	3	4	1	1	3	1
Delaware	343	290	35	87	49	58	61	12	34	7
Dubois	75	66	12	14	17	12	11		7	2

Table 3.11

Physicians by State and County, 2006, continued

State County	Total Physicians	Total Patient Care	FM/GP Practice	Medical Specialties	Surgical Specialties	Other Specialties	Hospital Based Practice	Other Professional Activity	Inactive	Not Classified
Elkhart	297	231	53	47	55	48	28	7	52	7
Fayette	22	19	6	4	5	2	2		3	
Floyd	177	149	35	44	20	34	16	3	22	3
Fountain	9	7	3	2			2		2	
Franklin	6	5	2	1	2				1	
Fulton	18	13	3	2	1		7	1	4	
Gibson	23	21	8	5	2	2	4		2	
Grant	128	103	16	26	19	22	20	1	22	2
Greene	19	14	8		2	2	2		2	3
Hamilton	1,376	1,166	101	313	214	328	210	44	127	39
Hancock	124	107	28	24	15	28	12	3	11	3
Harrison	33	26	11	2	3	6	4	1	5	1
Hendricks	218	192	24	42	27	46	53	6	12	8
Henry	47	35	12	8	6	6	3	1	11	
Howard	158	129	26	41	28	25	9	2	27	
Huntington	43	36	13	10	5	6	2	1	6	
Jackson	52	46	20	5	9	9	3		6	
Jasper	28	23	14	2	2	2	3		5	
Jay	19	15	9	1	2	2	1		3	1
Jefferson	66	53	15	5	7	9	17		13	
Jennings	12	11	3	7	1				1	
Johnson	283	230	48	65	30	58	29	13	36	4
Knox	85	71	10	21	17	14	9	1	13	
Kosciusko	81	65	20	9	16	11	9		15	1
La Porte	187	147	32	35	36	29	15	3	36	1
Lagrange	13	10	8	1			1		3	
Lake	1,015	864	112	289	200	176	87	16	107	28
Lawrence	64	50	9	17	15	3	6	2	11	1
Madison	198	169	52	33	27	39	18	5	23	1
Marion	4,105	3,270	260	807	514	627	1,062	303	334	198
Marshall	48	37	20	4	3	4	6	1	10	
Martin	3	3	1	2						
Miami	29	21	5	4	5	4	3	1	5	2
Monroe	367	286	43	69	57	89	28	12	61	8
Montgomery	49	40	12	9	9	4	6	1	8	
Morgan	83	68	13	18	17	9	11	3	7	5
Newton	4	3	1	1		1			1	
Noble	32	31	15	5	4	3	4		1	
Ohio	1								1	
Orange	15	13	10	1		1	1		1	1
Owen	8	7	2	1		2	2		1	
Parke	10	7	7					2	1	
Perry	12	11	8	1	1		1	1		
Pike	3	3	2				1			
Porter	318	261	37	77	61	56	30	6	48	3
Posey	8	7	6				1		1	
Pulaski	7	6	5				1		1	
Putnam	28	24	9	4	2	3	6		2	2
Randolph	20	18	4	4	1	3	6		2	
Ripley	44	36	11	7	10	6	2	1	5	2
Rush	10	8	4	1	1	1	1		2	
Scott	18	16	9	2	2	1	2		1	1
Shelby	30	25	9	6	5	1	4	1	4	
Spencer	7	6	5				1	1		
St. Joseph	780	654	106	153	110	174	111	19	90	17
Starke	10	10	7		2	1				
Steuben	31	23	12	2	3	3	3		8	
Sullivan	9	7	4	2		1			1	1
Switzerland	2	1						1	1	
Tippecanoe	415	345	47	102	77	89	30	12	52	6

Table 3.11

Table 3.11

Physicians by State and County, 2006, continued

State County	Total Physicians	Total Patient Care	FM/GP Practice	Medical Specialties	Surgical Specialties	Other Specialties	Hospital Based Practice	Other Professional Activity	Inactive	Not Classified
			Major Professional Activity							
			Patient Care							
			Office-Based Practice							
Tipton	15	14	7	2	2	1	2		1	
Union	5	5	4	1						
Vanderburgh	603	501	100	122	101	117	61	16	77	9
Vermillion	7	3	1	1		1			3	1
Vigo	327	287	51	79	53	65	39	9	22	9
Wabash	32	26	11	2	3	6	4	2	4	
Warren	3	2	1				1			1
Warrick	227	198	22	57	42	48	29	3	17	9
Washington	21	19	7	5	1	2	4		2	
Wayne	161	133	15	40	26	27	25	5	21	2
Wells	47	40	14	11	10	3	2		7	
White	21	15	8		1	1	5		6	
Whitley	22	19	10	1	5	1	2	1	2	
Iowa	6,428	4,957	896	1,086	913	991	1,071	309	861	301
Adair	3	2	2						1	
Adams	5	5	2	1		2				
Allamakee	11	9	7	1		1			2	
Appanoose	13	11	8		1	1	1		2	
Audubon	1	1	1							
Benton	7	3	1	2					4	
Black Hawk	317	259	56	54	50	61	38	7	45	6
Boone	18	12	7	1		1	3		6	
Bremer	28	20	12		4	1	3		8	
Buchanan	14	13	3	2		1	7	1		
Buena Vista	15	10	8	1	1				5	
Butler	3	3	3							
Calhoun	11	6	3		2	1			5	
Carroll	34	26	8	6	6	1	5		7	1
Cass	14	10	8		1	1			4	
Cedar	8	4	3				1		3	1
Cerro Gordo	157	123	23	23	26	31	20	3	29	2
Cherokee	14	10	4	1		3	2	1	3	
Chickasaw	5	4	4						1	
Clarke	4	3	3						1	
Clay	29	28	10	1	13	3	1		1	
Clayton	13	11	8		3				2	
Clinton	73	67	13	17	14	14	9	1	4	1
Crawford	10	7	7						3	
Dallas	40	32	7	2	6	8	9	1	5	2
Davis	5	3	1		2				2	
Decatur	4	3	2	1					1	
Delaware	11	4	4						6	1
Des Moines	90	70	12	13	18	22	5		18	2
Dickinson	26	14	5		2	4	3		12	
Dubuque	248	208	16	79	56	45	12	4	31	5
Emmet	11	7	7						4	
Fayette	9	6	2	1	1	2			3	
Floyd	15	12	4	1	2	4	1	1	2	
Franklin	1	1	1							
Fremont	6	3	2			1			3	
Greene	8	5	3	1	1				3	
Grundy	9	5	3		1	1			4	
Guthrie	4	4	3				1			
Hamilton	10	8	5	1		1	1		1	1
Hancock	5	5	2	1			2			
Hardin	14	11	8		1	1	1		3	
Harrison	10	7	3	1	1		2		2	1
Henry	29	22	6	4	6	2	4		7	
Howard	9	8	6		1		1		1	

Table 3.11

Physicians by State and County, 2006, continued

State County	Total Physicians	Total Patient Care	Office-Based Practice FM/GP Practice	Medical Specialties	Surgical Specialties	Other Specialties	Hospital Based Practice	Other Professional Activity	Inactive	Not Classified
Humboldt	6	5	3	1		1			1	
Ida	2	1	1						1	
Iowa	13	11	5	2	1	1	2		2	
Jackson	18	13	7	1	2	2	1	1	4	
Jasper	19	16	11		3	1	1	1	1	1
Jefferson	22	14	6	1	1	5	1	5	3	
Johnson	1,840	1,307	67	234	157	239	610	184	133	216
Jones	10	7	6				1		3	
Keokuk	2	2			1		1			
Kossuth	9	9	3	2	2		2			
Lee	62	47	10	11	11	5	10	2	12	1
Linn	458	360	81	79	72	89	39	13	75	10
Louisa	2	2	1			1				
Lucas	3	3	3							
Lyon	2	2	2							
Madison	2	2	1			1				
Mahaska	25	22	12	1	6	1	2		3	
Marion	41	32	12	7	3	2	8	2	6	1
Marshall	61	45	12	11	16	6		1	15	
Mills	15	13	5	2		2	4	1	1	
Mitchell	5	2	1		1				3	
Monona	9	6	3		2	1			3	
Monroe	3	3	3							
Montgomery	10	7	2	2	2		1		3	
Muscatine	35	28	10	9	7		2	3	4	
O'Brien	9	8	5		2		1		1	
Osceola	2	2	2							
Page	23	15	7	1	2	3	2		7	1
Palo Alto	8	3	2			1			5	
Plymouth	18	13	9	1	1	1	1		5	
Pocahontas	3	3	2				1			
Polk	1,074	859	83	257	189	200	130	52	136	27
Pottawattamie	121	95	14	31	21	17	12	2	22	2
Poweshiek	37	29	13	1	4	5	6		8	
Ringgold	2	1	1						1	
Sac	8	4	3				1		3	1
Scott	396	323	50	80	81	80	32	13	53	7
Shelby	9	8	4	1			3		1	
Sioux	29	23	15	1	2	2	3		6	
Story	179	153	26	41	35	37	14	1	24	1
Tama	5	4	2	1			1		1	
Union	8	6	5		1				2	
Van Buren	2	2					2			
Wapello	73	65	6	28	12	16	3		7	1
Warren	23	18	4	4	3	3	4		5	
Washington	20	16	8	2	3		3		1	3
Wayne	3	3	1			1	1			
Webster	77	57	8	14	18	14	3		17	3
Winnebago	6	5	4	1					1	
Winneshiek	34	25	12	1	5	5	2	1	7	1
Woodbury	204	164	31	43	27	35	28	8	30	2
Worth	2	2	2							
Wright	8	7	4		1		2		1	
Kansas	7,079	5,602	888	1,371	1,037	1,178	1,128	259	975	243
Allen	4	2	1				1	1	1	
Anderson	8	4	3				1		4	
Atchison	19	16	8		4	2	2	1	2	
Barber	4	1	1						3	
Barton	41	34	8	7	10	6	3		5	2
Bourbon	26	17	8	2	3	3	1		9	
Brown	16	14	8	1		2	3		1	1

Table 3.11

Physicians by State and County, 2006, continued

State County	Total Physicians	Total Patient Care	Major Professional Activity							
			Patient Care				Hospital Based Practice	Other Professional Activity	Inactive	Not Classified
			Office-Based Practice							
			FM/GP Practice	Medical Specialties	Surgical Specialties	Other Specialties				
Butler	66	56	16	11	8	11	10	1	8	1
Chautauqua	1	1		1						
Cherokee	8	7	3	2			2		1	
Cheyenne	3	1	1						2	
Clark	4	3	3						1	
Clay	10	9	8				1			1
Cloud	13	6	1	1	3	1			6	1
Coffey	5	3			1		2			2
Cowley	41	30	13	6	4	3	4		10	1
Crawford	56	44	9	12	12	3	8	1	10	1
Decatur	6	6	4		1	1				
Dickinson	16	14	9		2	1	2		2	
Doniphan	4	2					2		2	
Douglas	240	181	36	48	35	38	24	5	49	5
Edwards	2	2	1	1						
Elk	1	1	1							
Ellis	78	60	3	11	20	19	7	3	13	2
Ellsworth	4	4	1	1		1	1			
Finney	40	33	8	9	8	3	5		6	1
Ford	55	48	11	17	12	8			6	1
Franklin	18	16	6	3	4	3			2	
Geary	29	24	4	5	3	2	10		3	2
Gove	7	4	4						2	1
Graham	3	3	1	1	1					
Grant	6	4	1	1			2		2	
Gray	2	2	2							
Greeley	2	2				1		1		
Greenwood	4	2	2						2	
Hamilton	3	2	1		1				1	
Harper	10	8	1	3		2	2	1	1	
Harvey	83	54	17	14	16	3	4	3	26	
Haskell	2	2	1	1						
Hodgeman	1	1	1							
Jackson	11	8	5				1	2	3	
Jefferson	9	6	3				2	1	2	1
Jewell	2	2				1		1		
Johnson	2,532	2,049	191	553	378	514	413	88	312	83
Kearny	3	3	1		1		1			
Kingman	1									
Kiowa	4	2				1	1		1	1
Labette	46	35	11	4	10	6	4	1	7	3
Lane	2	1					1		1	
Leavenworth	95	74	15	16	9	6	28	4	14	3
Lincoln	2	2	1	1						
Linn	3	3	1	1		1				
Logan	3	2		1			1		1	
Lyon	52	41	13	10	11	5	2	1	10	
Marion	10	6	5	1					4	
Marshall	9	8	5		1		2		1	
Mc Pherson	39	29	19		3	1	6		10	
Meade	5	3	2	1					2	
Miami	35	25	9	3		7	6	1	8	1
Mitchell	10	9	3	2	2	1	1		1	
Montgomery	40	34	7	10	9	6	2		6	
Morris	6	4	3				1		2	
Morton	8	7		1	3	1	2		1	
Nemaha	4	4	2				2			
Neosho	19	16	7	3	6			1	2	

Table 3.11

Physicians by State and County, 2006, continued

State County	Total Physicians	Total Patient Care	FM/GP Practice	Medical Specialties	Surgical Specialties	Other Specialties	Hospital Based Practice	Other Professional Activity	Inactive	Not Classified
				Major Professional Activity						
			Patient Care							
			Office-Based Practice							
Ness	1	1	1							
Norton	6	6	4	1	1					
Osage	7	4	3	1					3	
Osborne	2	2	1	1						
Ottawa	7	5	4			1			2	
Pawnee	12	9		1		4	4	1	1	1
Phillips	2	2	2							
Pottawatomie	20	15	10	1		1	3	1	4	
Pratt	13	13	4	3	2	1	3			
Rawlins	3	2	2						1	
Reno	145	120	21	41	30	20	8	1	22	2
Republic	6	5	4		1				1	
Rice	5	4	3				1		1	
Riley	147	119	16	32	36	25	10	2	21	5
Rooks	5	3	3						2	
Rush	3	2	1	1					1	
Russell	7	4	2		1	1			3	
Saline	149	117	19	23	30	31	14	4	24	4
Scott	6	4	3	1					1	1
Sedgwick	1,416	1,146	174	265	200	242	265	56	169	45
Seward	36	28	5	7	5	6	5		7	1
Shawnee	537	403	37	126	78	105	57	29	101	4
Sheridan	3	2	2						1	
Sherman	6	6	2		1		3			
Smith	4	3	1		1		1		1	
Stafford	1	1	1							
Stanton	2	1	1						1	
Stevens	1	1		1						
Sumner	10	8	4	1	1	1	1		1	1
Thomas	5	2	2						2	1
Trego	3	3	2	1						
Wabaunsee	2	2	1	1						
Wallace	1	1					1			
Washington	3	3	2				1			
Wichita	2	1	1						1	
Wilson	7	5	4			1			2	
Woodson	1	1					1			
Wyandotte	602	452	37	98	68	72	177	53	33	64
Kentucky	10,828	8,825	1,141	2,494	1,702	1,862	1,626	373	1,157	473
Adair	16	14	5	5		2	2		2	
Allen	6	5	3			2			1	
Anderson	16	13	3	5	3	2		1	2	
Ballard	2	2	2							
Barren	94	83	19	19	18	9	18	1	7	3
Bath	9	6	1	2		2	1		3	
Bell	56	43	6	14	11	4	8	3	10	
Boone	188	162	43	44	26	25	24	2	17	7
Bourbon	21	20	9	2	1	5	3		1	
Boyd	238	200	25	51	49	50	25	4	21	13
Boyle	103	88	9	27	24	20	8	3	10	2
Bracken	6	6	4			1	1			
Breathitt	20	18	5	8	3	1	1		2	
Breckinridge	8	7	5	1			1		1	
Bullitt	31	27	7	6	1	2	11	2		2
Butler	3	3	2	1						
Caldwell	12	12	3	3	2	1	3			
Calloway	67	56	8	18	18	12			9	2
Campbell	148	124	23	32	26	27	16	4	15	5
Carlisle	1	1	1							
Carroll	5	4	2		1		1		1	

Table 3.11

Physicians by State and County, 2006, continued

State County	Total Physicians	Total Patient Care	Patient Care — Office-Based Practice FM/GP Practice	Medical Specialties	Surgical Specialties	Other Specialties	Hospital Based Practice	Other Professional Activity	Inactive	Not Classified
Carter	12	10	6	3		1			2	
Casey	6	3	1	1	1				3	
Christian	126	104	11	26	24	31	12	3	13	6
Clark	57	52	9	17	9	11	6	1	2	2
Clay	15	11	3	3	3		2		3	1
Clinton	6	6	3	2	1					
Crittenden	5	5	3		1	1				
Cumberland	4	3	3						1	
Daviess	232	190	22	61	52	41	14	8	29	5
Edmonson	3	3	1			1	1			
Elliott	1								1	
Estill	8	7	3	2		2			1	
Fayette	2,104	1,644	92	409	290	351	502	116	189	155
Fleming	11	11	7	2		1	1			
Floyd	68	60	12	29	6	6	7		7	1
Franklin	83	60	8	22	16	7	7	3	17	3
Fulton	17	15	6	6	3				2	
Gallatin	2	2	1	1						
Garrard	10	8	4	1		2	1		2	
Grant	16	14	7	2	1		4		2	
Graves	42	33	7	8	9	6	3		8	1
Grayson	24	21	7	5	4	2	3		2	1
Green	6	6	5		1					
Greenup	41	34	10	14	1	6	3		5	2
Hancock	2	1				1			1	
Hardin	225	194	21	60	43	55	15	3	24	4
Harlan	43	31	8	11	9	2	1		11	1
Harrison	24	22	10	6	4	2			2	
Hart	9	8	3	3		1	1		1	
Henderson	70	58	11	19	14	11	3	2	9	1
Henry	13	11	4				3	4	2	
Hickman	2	1	1						1	
Hopkins	152	125	33	28	26	14	24	5	15	7
Jackson	4	3	1			1	1		1	
Jefferson	3,596	2,860	201	803	543	672	641	175	385	176
Jessamine	92	73	13	17	12	18	13	3	14	2
Johnson	35	27	6	9	6	4	2		8	
Kenton	448	390	51	105	74	91	69	10	39	9
Knott	7	4	2				2		2	1
Knox	18	13	6	1		3	3		4	1
Larue	4	4	2	1	1					
Laurel	82	74	13	35	9	10	7	1	2	5
Lawrence	16	14	3	3	3	3	2		1	1
Lee	4	4	3			1				
Leslie	6	6	2	2			2			
Letcher	37	31	6	13	3	4	5	1	4	1
Lewis	6	3	1	2					2	1
Lincoln	15	15	10	2		3				
Livingston	10	9	2	1	4	2			1	
Logan	23	20	4	6	4	4	2		2	1
Lyon	3	3	2	1						
Madison	121	95	16	32	26	14	7		18	8
Magoffin	4	3	2				1	1		
Marion	23	19	3	7	5	4			4	
Marshall	26	18	8	3	2	3	2		8	
Martin	6	5	5						1	
Mason	43	39	9	10	11	6	3		2	2
Mc Cracken	242	205	20	71	57	52	5	3	33	1
Mc Creary	6	6	4		1	1				
Mc Lean	2	1	1						1	
Meade	9	5	3			1	1		4	

Table 3.11

Physicians by State and County, 2006, continued

State County	Total Physicians	Total Patient Care	FM/GP Practice	Medical Specialties	Surgical Specialties	Other Specialties	Hospital Based Practice	Other Professional Activity	Inactive	Not Classified
				Major Professional Activity — Patient Care — Office-Based Practice						
Menifee	1	1	1							
Mercer	14	8	5	2		1		1	4	1
Metcalfe	3	3	3							
Monroe	9	7	3	2		1	1		2	
Montgomery	28	27	5	14	5	2	1		1	
Morgan	8	5	3	2					2	1
Muhlenberg	37	33	8	9	9	4	3	1	3	
Nelson	42	37	9	11	7	7	3		5	
Nicholas	5	3	1	1			1		2	
Ohio	12	10	4	2	1	2	1		2	
Oldham	106	88	8	29	10	30	11	3	10	5
Owen	7	6	4	1	1				1	
Owsley	2	2	1	1						
Pendleton	5	5	2	2		1				
Perry	108	94	14	41	10	16	13	2	7	5
Pike	149	126	13	41	32	24	16	1	17	5
Powell	8	8	4	1		1	2			
Pulaski	146	126	15	44	29	29	9	1	17	2
Robertson	1	1			1					
Rockcastle	15	11	6	1		1	3		2	2
Rowan	68	62	10	16	14	12	10		2	4
Russell	19	15	8	1	1	2	3		3	1
Scott	70	55	10	14	15	8	8	2	9	4
Shelby	52	39	10	8	9	8	4		9	4
Simpson	11	9	6	2		1			2	
Spencer	8	7	5	2					1	
Taylor	34	30	6	7	12	4	1	1	3	
Todd	2	2	2							
Trigg	8	6	3	1		2			2	
Trimble	2	2					2			
Union	7	6	3	1	1	1			1	
Warren	294	258	32	91	62	55	18		34	2
Washington	7	6	1	1		4			1	
Wayne	11	9	4	3		1	1		2	
Webster	4	3	1	1	1					1
Whitley	90	73	13	27	14	14	5	2	13	2
Wolfe	6	3		2		1		1	1	1
Woodford	52	43	12	10	6	10	5	3	6	
Louisiana	12,643	10,393	1,038	2,910	2,122	2,017	2,306	459	1,214	577
Acadia	55	44	15	9	10	6	4		7	4
Allen	19	16	7	4	2	1	2		2	1
Ascension	97	89	18	29	6	18	18	1	5	2
Assumption	9	7	5	1			1		1	1
Avoyelles	27	27	13	7	5	1	1			
Beauregard	31	29	7	9	8	1	4		1	1
Bienville	5	3	1		1		1		2	
Bossier	171	154	20	38	27	28	41	2	11	4
Caddo	1,611	1,310	79	325	254	215	437	66	131	104
Calcasieu	409	342	65	101	78	72	26	6	54	7
Caldwell	7	7	2	2	1	2				
Cameron	1							1		
Catahoula	5	3	3						2	
Claiborne	16	9	6	2		1			6	1
Concordia	23	19	8	6	4		1		2	2
De Soto	15	11	4	2	4	1			3	1
East Baton Rouge	1,602	1,324	119	410	300	290	205	50	184	44
East Carroll	9	6	1	2			3		3	
East Feliciana	22	18	4	2	1	4	7		4	
Evangeline	46	39	10	12	11	5	1		7	
Franklin	10	8	3	2	1	1	1		2	

Table 3.11

Physicians by State and County, 2006, continued

State County	Total Physicians	Total Patient Care	FM/GP Practice	Medical Specialties	Surgical Specialties	Other Specialties	Hospital Based Practice	Other Professional Activity	Inactive	Not Classified
				Major Professional Activity — Patient Care — Office-Based Practice						
Grant	6	5	2		1	1	1		1	
Iberia	128	101	21	30	25	12	13	1	22	4
Iberville	37	29	8	13	3	1	4	4	4	
Jackson	4	4	1	1	2					
Jefferson	1,963	1,675	91	501	330	317	436	59	138	91
Jefferson Davis	31	25	9	8	4	2	2		5	1
La Salle	12	11	8	2		1			1	
Lafayette	760	652	69	186	159	144	94	17	68	23
Lafourche	149	129	20	36	40	17	16	1	13	6
Lincoln	76	68	8	20	19	15	6		7	1
Livingston	36	31	14	6	2	5	4		4	1
Madison	8	8	3	3		1	1			
Morehouse	29	23	10	2	8	2	1	1	5	
Natchitoches	41	39	10	13	8	5	3		2	
Orleans	2,399	1,789	52	429	281	386	641	180	218	212
Ouachita	451	382	45	112	71	84	70	13	43	13
Plaquemines	19	11	2			3	6	3	3	2
Pointe Coupee	17	15	8	1	3		3		2	
Rapides	454	365	37	105	88	66	69	14	63	12
Red River	3	3	2			1				
Richland	26	23	11	6	3	2	1	1	2	
Sabine	15	11	5	4			2		2	2
St. Bernard	17	14	1	5	2	3	3		2	1
St. Charles	43	36	2	13	9	7	5		6	1
St. Helena	6	5	3	1	1				1	
St. James	20	18	7	4	4		3			2
St. John The Baptist	46	43	8	12	12	4	7		2	1
St. Landry	149	132	28	38	39	18	9		15	2
St. Martin	24	23	4	4	3	8	4			1
St. Mary	63	54	15	12	13	5	9	1	7	1
St. Tammany	811	696	45	230	155	187	79	20	79	16
Tangipahoa	137	118	19	42	31	13	13	5	13	1
Tensas	1								1	
Terrebonne	224	185	21	53	53	41	17	10	22	7
Union	11	9	4	4			1		2	
Vermilion	45	33	9	10	10	2	2	1	10	1
Vernon	64	58	8	16	14	6	14		4	2
Washington	44	36	9	10	5	4	8	1	6	1
Webster	41	34	17	7	5	4	1	1	6	
West Baton Rouge	8	8	3	1	1	1	2			
West Carroll	5	3		2			1		2	
West Feliciana	16	14	5	3	2	3	1		2	
Winn	14	10	4	2	3		1		4	
Maine	4,197	3,250	461	855	592	698	644	203	628	116
Androscoggin	292	233	32	67	49	49	36	17	30	12
Aroostook	173	143	31	27	36	25	24	4	18	8
Cumberland	1,564	1,247	107	352	207	288	293	90	177	50
Franklin	66	54	16	11	12	8	7	1	11	
Hancock	167	113	35	22	16	18	22	7	45	2
Kennebec	391	306	56	59	53	57	81	21	56	8
Knox	166	105	10	30	19	31	15	11	46	4
Lincoln	108	61	19	18	10	7	7	3	44	
Oxford	69	52	8	12	13	10	9	1	15	1
Penobscot	549	444	43	129	77	115	80	27	60	18
Piscataquis	34	28	7	4	7	2	8	1	4	1
Sagadahoc	71	45	8	13	7	10	7	4	20	2
Somerset	71	56	17	12	10	6	11	2	10	3
Waldo	84	66	12	14	14	17	9	3	14	1
Washington	69	51	13	15	11	7	5	1	14	3
York	323	246	47	70	51	48	30	10	64	3

Table 3.11

Physicians by State and County, 2006, continued

State County	Total Physicians	Total Patient Care	FM/GP Practice	Medical Specialties	Surgical Specialties	Other Specialties	Hospital Based Practice	Other Professional Activity	Inactive	Not Classified
				Office-Based Practice						
Maryland	25,969	19,205	1,060	5,893	3,066	4,036	5,150	2,458	2,638	1,668
Allegany	228	183	17	53	40	48	25	5	32	8
Anne Arundel	1,449	1,154	102	365	234	263	190	58	181	56
Baltimore	3,951	2,994	95	978	614	655	652	218	547	192
Baltimore (ic)	5,268	3,817	95	914	475	698	1,635	586	290	575
Calvert	156	130	13	50	33	22	12	4	14	8
Caroline	19	15	6	3	1	3	2	1	3	
Carroll	255	203	30	70	39	36	28	8	40	4
Cecil	131	90	20	13	16	26	15	8	26	7
Charles	153	128	13	63	23	13	16	3	17	5
Dorchester	59	46	5	16	7	7	11	2	7	4
Frederick	512	394	66	123	66	82	57	42	58	18
Garrett	34	24	10	3	4	6	1	1	7	2
Harford	458	366	34	133	69	69	61	22	55	15
Howard	1,865	1,479	81	499	166	372	361	125	117	144
Kent	85	47	11	14	9	7	6	3	34	1
Montgomery	8,535	5,862	247	1,798	824	1,323	1,670	1,268	886	519
Prince George's	1,658	1,377	125	487	243	205	317	69	122	90
Queen Anne's	41	28	7	8	1	8	4	1	11	1
Somerset	30	25	3	14	2	3	3	1	4	
St. Mary's	129	102	16	40	13	22	11	7	15	5
Talbot	213	147	11	45	42	36	13	16	49	1
Washington	326	262	27	85	67	52	31	7	50	7
Wicomico	327	271	13	101	71	64	22	3	48	5
Worcester	87	61	13	18	7	16	7		25	1
Massachusetts	32,574	24,657	1,065	7,636	3,363	5,227	7,366	2,319	2,818	2,780
Barnstable	840	562	46	201	116	138	61	38	230	10
Berkshire	590	447	27	144	69	112	95	27	82	34
Bristol	970	788	70	281	159	169	109	16	133	33
Dukes	67	38	6	8	4	8	12	6	23	
Essex	1,925	1,540	143	550	290	350	207	68	262	55
Franklin	138	103	25	36	14	20	8	3	28	4
Hampden	1,401	1,164	32	392	219	213	308	53	129	55
Hampshire	678	548	62	183	51	142	110	21	92	17
Middlesex	8,664	6,666	227	2,187	888	1,634	1,730	657	760	581
Nantucket	22	10	4	1	1	2	2	2	10	
Norfolk	4,212	3,231	102	1,033	474	736	886	275	371	335
Plymouth	974	791	58	302	147	164	120	25	124	34
Suffolk	9,211	6,494	77	1,582	623	1,142	3,070	973	319	1,425
Worcester	2,882	2,275	186	736	308	397	648	155	255	197
Michigan	27,877	22,003	2,156	6,129	3,593	4,233	5,892	1,235	3,135	1,504
Alcona	8	4	4						3	1
Alger	13	10	5	2	3			1	2	
Allegan	74	56	15	12	4	16	9	3	13	2
Alpena	80	71	13	19	12	23	4	1	8	
Antrim	29	13	5	3		4	1		16	
Arenac	10	7	1	3			3		3	
Baraga	8	6	3	1			2		2	
Barry	54	41	15	6	12	6	2		13	
Bay	167	134	15	43	33	30	13		29	4
Benzie	28	12	2	2	3	2	3	3	13	
Berrien	343	274	51	82	57	58	26	7	55	7
Branch	52	41	4	9	9	11	8	1	8	2
Calhoun	252	190	30	55	46	35	24	7	50	5
Cass	16	13	3	3	4	2	1		3	
Charlevoix	60	38	10	6	8	6	8		21	1
Cheboygan	26	19	5	3	1	4	6	1	5	1
Chippewa	48	41	13	8	8	4	8		5	2
Clare	21	18	4	4	4	2	4		3	
Clinton	46	35	6	12	3	5	9	3	6	2

Table 3.11

Physicians by State and County, 2006, continued

State County	Total Physicians	Total Patient Care	FM/GP Practice	Medical Specialties	Surgical Specialties	Other Specialties	Hospital Based Practice	Other Professional Activity	Inactive	Not Classified
				Office-Based Practice						
Crawford	19	16	3	5	5	1	2		2	1
Delta	58	41	13	8	9	5	6	4	12	1
Dickinson	79	66	16	11	15	10	14	3	9	1
Eaton	83	69	16	19	9	10	15	1	12	1
Emmet	188	131	12	45	38	32	4	7	48	2
Genesee	1,006	807	103	254	106	126	218	31	118	50
Gladwin	16	11	5	3	1		2		5	
Gogebic	26	25	11	6	3	3	2		1	
Grand Traverse	378	290	30	90	58	87	25	12	70	6
Gratiot	57	50	11	12	11	10	6		5	2
Hillsdale	33	28	9	9	4	2	4		2	3
Houghton	66	58	16	15	7	12	8		7	1
Huron	43	33	6	7	9	4	7	1	8	1
Ingham	993	739	74	197	129	156	183	90	127	37
Ionia	32	24	13	4	3	2	2	2	5	1
Iosco	28	22	3	5	6	5	3		6	
Iron	13	10	3	2	1	2	2	2	1	
Isabella	80	70	5	21	20	15	9		6	4
Jackson	215	173	26	63	41	23	20	4	37	1
Kalamazoo	984	760	66	215	133	156	190	66	128	30
Kalkaska	5	4	3				1	1		
Kent	1,863	1,569	150	403	315	343	358	50	193	51
Keweenaw	2								2	
Lake	3	2		1		1		1		
Lapeer	57	39	9	12	7	6	5	4	13	1
Leelanau	46	18	3	3	1	9	2		27	1
Lenawee	116	83	14	27	16	19	7		30	3
Livingston	178	138	23	42	21	33	19	9	27	4
Luce	12	9	1	3	1		4	1	2	
Mackinac	14	11	4	2		2	3		3	
Macomb	1,143	961	131	342	193	131	164	23	105	54
Manistee	38	25	6	6	6	4	3		13	
Marquette	259	215	35	50	42	42	46	11	27	6
Mason	34	30	7	5	7	8	3		4	
Mecosta	44	34	9	10	10	2	3	2	8	
Menominee	17	15	3	3	1	5	3		2	
Midland	221	181	33	33	39	38	38	10	28	2
Missaukee	5	3			3				2	
Monroe	162	131	25	33	24	25	24	7	18	6
Montcalm	35	25	9	3	3	5	5		10	
Montmorency	6	4	2	1	1			1	1	
Muskegon	302	232	41	70	47	51	23	8	60	2
Newaygo	43	33	17	9	4	2	1		10	
Oakland	6,833	5,552	350	1,718	916	1,122	1,446	233	668	380
Oceana	18	11	5	1	1	1	3		6	1
Ogemaw	26	24	4	7	7	5	1		2	
Ontonagon	7	4	3		1				3	
Osceola	13	10	4	2	3		1	1	2	
Oscoda	3							1	2	
Otsego	37	29	8	6	3	3	9		7	1
Ottawa	382	293	52	74	72	70	25	7	79	3
Presque Isle	4	3	1		1	1			1	
Roscommon	21	15	7	5	1	1	1		6	
Saginaw	580	487	78	118	85	83	123	20	58	15
Sanilac	30	25	7	5	6	3	4	1	3	1
Schoolcraft	8	6	3			1	2		2	
Shiawassee	61	48	8	15	12	8	5	1	11	1
St. Clair	235	191	35	56	45	41	14	2	38	4

Table 3.11

Physicians by State and County, 2006, continued

State County	Total Physicians	Total Patient Care	FM/GP Practice	Medical Specialties	Surgical Specialties	Other Specialties	Hospital Based Practice	Other Professional Activity	Inactive	Not Classified
				Major Professional Activity						
			Patient Care							
			Office-Based Practice							
St. Joseph	70	58	18	8	15	9	8		11	1
Tuscola	28	22	5	9	3	4	1		4	2
Van Buren	87	73	21	20	10	11	11	2	12	
Washtenaw	3,775	2,849	103	688	339	595	1,124	318	275	333
Wayne	5,250	4,039	257	1,057	509	672	1,544	269	480	462
Wexford	72	56	17	15	11	8	5	2	13	1
Minnesota	16,756	13,318	2,342	3,377	2,049	2,579	2,971	750	1,943	745
Aitkin	16	15	11		2	1	1		1	
Anoka	445	379	95	107	75	49	53	8	43	15
Becker	56	39	17	7	8	4	3	4	13	
Beltrami	87	73	21	19	17	9	7	3	11	
Benton	35	28	6	11	3	7	1		7	
Big Stone	7	6	6						1	
Blue Earth	180	147	23	43	39	35	7	5	26	2
Brown	45	41	18	6	10	2	5		4	
Carlton	36	29	18	3	3	2	3	1	6	
Carver	158	139	47	32	26	24	10	3	16	
Cass	22	14	10	1		1	2		8	
Chippewa	13	7	5		1		1	1	4	1
Chisago	46	40	20	10	3	4	3		4	2
Clay	35	24	7	5	2	6	4	1	10	
Clearwater	8	6	4	1			1		2	
Cook	11	5	4				1		6	
Cottonwood	12	9	7	1			1		3	
Crow Wing	167	127	32	26	32	25	12	2	34	4
Dakota	702	568	145	151	59	95	118	28	78	28
Dodge	14	12	5			1	6		1	1
Douglas	79	60	23	11	14	8	4	1	16	2
Faribault	9	5	3		1		1		4	
Fillmore	14	10	8	1		1			4	
Freeborn	54	41	10	8	9	9	5		13	
Goodhue	90	67	20	15	11	8	13	4	18	1
Grant	1									1
Hennepin	5,620	4,413	504	1,208	786	952	963	343	646	218
Houston	18	15	6	2		5	2	1	1	1
Hubbard	39	25	10	6	3	3	3	1	13	
Isanti	45	35	19	5	3	2	6	2	8	
Itasca	72	56	27	7	13	6	3	2	13	1
Jackson	4								4	
Kanabec	17	15	11		1		3		2	
Kandiyohi	133	96	30	23	20	20	3	6	29	2
Kittson	2	1	1						1	
Koochiching	19	13	7	2	1	1	2	1	5	
Lac Qui Parle	9	6	4	1			1		2	1
Lake	24	15	9	1	2	2	1	1	7	1
Lake Of The Woods	4	1	1						3	
Le Sueur	6	4	4						2	
Lincoln	8	7	3	2	1		1		1	
Lyon	26	21	10	2	6	1	2		5	
Mahnomen	1	1		1						
Marshall	2	2	1				1			
Martin	44	38	13	8	11	4	2	1	5	
Mc Leod	46	40	25	5	3	2	5	2	4	
Meeker	16	16	11	2	2		1			
Mille Lacs	38	31	15	2	3	3	8	4	2	1
Morrison	31	27	16	4	5	1	1	1	2	1
Mower	59	45	14	10	8	7	6	1	13	
Murray	7	6	2	2			1	1	1	
Nicollet	59	46	22	6	2	7	9	3	10	
Nobles	32	27	10	10	4		3		5	

Table 3.11

Physicians by State and County, 2006, continued

State County	Total Physicians	Total Patient Care	FM/GP Practice	Medical Specialties	Surgical Specialties	Other Specialties	Hospital Based Practice	Other Professional Activity	Inactive	Not Classified
					Major Professional Activity					
				Patient Care						
				Office-Based Practice						
Norman	5	3	2	1					2	
Olmsted	3,246	2,543	71	640	242	515	1,075	153	242	308
Otter Tail	78	59	18	12	11	13	5	2	17	
Pennington	25	19	5	6	7		1		4	2
Pine	15	15	11	3	1					
Pipestone	8	6	5		1				2	
Polk	22	18	8	4	3	1	2		3	1
Pope	12	9	9						3	
Ramsey	2,133	1,685	247	474	238	385	341	107	249	92
Red Lake	1								1	
Redwood	11	10	8		1		1		1	
Renville	9	7	6			1			2	
Rice	106	93	38	14	18	13	10		12	1
Rock	15	12	11		1				2	1
Roseau	15	11	9				2		4	
Scott	131	112	56	23	9	14	10	4	11	4
Sherburne	43	38	15	8	5	4	6	2		3
Sibley	5	4	2	1			1		1	
St. Louis	772	621	133	146	123	131	88	13	121	17
Stearns	453	388	75	119	79	79	36	11	48	6
Steele	57	47	23	10	12	1	1		10	
Stevens	11	9	5	1	2		1		2	
Swift	8	7	5	2						1
Todd	23	19	18	1					4	
Traverse	1								1	
Wabasha	32	26	14	3	3	3	3		6	
Wadena	14	10	9		1				4	
Waseca	12	10	9		1				2	
Washington	599	504	129	115	87	91	82	24	51	20
Watonwan	9	9	6		1	1	1			
Wilkin	4	3			1	1	1		1	
Winona	58	45	13	13	5	7	7		11	2
Wright	90	74	35	13	8	11	7	4	9	3
Yellow Medicine	10	9	7	1			1			1
Mississippi	5,890	4,782	659	1,252	1,024	886	961	191	741	176
Adams	79	65	11	19	17	14	4		13	1
Alcorn	58	51	8	15	14	11	3	1	3	3
Amite	3	2	1		1				1	
Attala	20	13	10	1	1	1			5	2
Benton	1	1					1			
Bolivar	43	33	8	8	10	3	4		9	1
Calhoun	4	4	3	1						
Carroll	6	5		2		1	2		1	
Chickasaw	11	11	1	4		1	5			
Choctaw	4	3	1	1			1		1	
Claiborne	4	4	2		1	1				
Clarke	6	4	3		1				2	
Clay	25	20	2	7	8		3		5	
Coahoma	51	44	5	16	12	4	7	2	4	1
Copiah	20	15	10	2		2	1	1	3	1
Covington	9	7	5			1	1		2	
De Soto	124	101	16	35	28	8	14	3	12	8
Forrest	429	377	49	113	96	84	35	9	37	6
Franklin	6	5	5						1	
George	16	12	2		4	1	5		3	1
Greene	5	2				2			2	1
Grenada	32	30	4	10	13	2	1		2	
Hancock	53	41	8	7	10	9	7		9	3
Harrison	467	385	23	113	92	79	78	13	60	9
Hinds	1,287	986	59	263	201	204	259	91	153	57

Table 3.11

Physicians by State and County, 2006, continued

State County	Total Physicians	Total Patient Care	Office-Based Practice				Hospital Based Practice	Other Professional Activity	Inactive	Not Classified
			FM/GP Practice	Medical Specialties	Surgical Specialties	Other Specialties				
Holmes	15	14	9	2	1		2		1	
Humphreys	6	5	3	2						1
Itawamba	10	8	5			1	2		1	1
Jackson	293	244	27	75	48	57	37	6	35	8
Jasper	3	3	2	1						
Jefferson	5	5	3	2						
Jefferson Davis	4	4	2	1			1			
Jones	110	90	14	23	29	14	10	3	15	2
Kemper	1	1	1							
Lafayette	115	91	11	30	25	13	12	1	23	
Lamar	14	11	7		1	1	2		2	1
Lauderdale	249	215	26	64	53	50	22	1	30	3
Lawrence	8	6	3				3		2	
Leake	8	8	3	1	1	1	2			
Lee	320	269	23	83	71	60	32	10	37	4
Leflore	59	47	2	16	15	8	6		12	
Lincoln	43	37	4	11	15	4	3		6	
Lowndes	133	114	15	38	29	23	9	1	16	2
Madison	491	402	47	85	46	88	136	27	41	21
Marion	24	16	5	5	1	2	3		7	1
Marshall	9	7	1	3	1	2			2	
Monroe	44	36	6	8	7	3	12		8	
Montgomery	11	9	7	1			1		2	
Neshoba	26	22	5	4	2	3	8		3	1
Newton	7	6	3	2			1		1	
Noxubee	6	3	2	1					2	1
Oktibbeha	50	41	15	6	10	7	3	1	6	2
Panola	21	18	7	4	3	2	2		3	
Pearl River	38	24	8	6	4	2	4		14	
Perry	7	4	4						1	2
Pike	86	72	9	17	24	14	8	2	11	1
Pontotoc	10	7	6			1		1	2	
Prentiss	19	17	5	5	5	1	1		2	
Quitman	5	4	2	1	1				1	
Rankin	450	382	33	46	67	72	164	10	41	17
Scott	11	6	3	2			1		5	
Sharkey	3	2	1	1					1	
Simpson	17	13	10	2		1			3	1
Smith	6	3	2				1		3	
Stone	15	10	2	4	1		3		5	
Sunflower	22	15	7		1	1	6	2	4	1
Tallahatchie	5	4	1	1		1	1		1	
Tate	12	8	3	3	1		1		4	
Tippah	10	6	5			1		1	3	
Tishomingo	12	10	8			1	1		2	
Tunica	6	4	1	1		1	1		1	1
Union	31	23	5	6	8	1	3	1	7	
Walthall	11	9	4	3	1	1			1	1
Warren	96	73	16	24	18	7	8	3	17	3
Washington	100	77	11	29	19	8	10	1	18	4
Wayne	11	10	4	4	2				1	
Webster	9	5	3	1	1				3	1
Wilkinson	10	10	2	4	2	1	1			
Winston	11	8	5		1		2		3	
Yalobusha	11	9	1	4		2	2		2	
Yazoo	18	14	4	3	1	3	3		2	2
Missouri	15,586	12,590	1,100	3,523	2,206	2,472	3,289	745	1,468	783
Adair	18	14	2	4	3	3	2	1	2	1
Andrew	5	2	1				1	1	2	

Table 3.11

Physicians by State and County, 2006, continued

State County	Total Physicians	Total Patient Care	FM/GP Practice	Medical Specialties	Surgical Specialties	Other Specialties	Hospital Based Practice	Other Professional Activity	Inactive	Not Classified
Atchison	4	3	2				1		1	
Audrain	43	37	7	9	10	6	5	2	4	
Barry	33	28	17	3	3		5	1	2	2
Barton	5	4				1	3		1	
Bates	5	4	3			1			1	
Benton	7	5	3	1			1		1	1
Bollinger	1	1					1			
Boone	1,208	967	59	203	144	189	372	59	93	89
Buchanan	195	158	16	46	35	37	24	7	25	5
Butler	137	122	22	40	26	17	17	2	13	
Caldwell	2								2	
Callaway	36	33	12	5	4	5	7		2	1
Camden	65	54	10	11	13	12	8	1	10	
Cape Girardeau	281	246	26	61	65	68	26	5	24	6
Carroll	5	3	1	1			1		2	
Carter	1								1	
Cass	49	36	15	5	1	9	6		12	1
Cedar	6	2	1				1		4	
Chariton	1								1	
Christian	82	74	14	12	15	26	7	2	6	
Clay	348	298	36	97	76	50	39	12	27	11
Clinton	12	11	6	2	2		1		1	
Cole	171	142	17	41	38	33	13	8	18	3
Cooper	11	9	4	2		2	1		2	
Crawford	4	3	1	1			1		1	
Dade	2	1	1						1	
Dallas	2	2	1			1				
Dent	8	6	3	2			1		2	
Douglas	4	3	1				2		1	
Dunklin	37	33	9	10	6	4	4	1	2	1
Franklin	116	103	25	28	25	16	9	3	9	1
Gasconade	9	4	1	1	1		1	2	2	1
Gentry	3	3		1	1		1			
Greene	913	769	90	219	172	190	98	22	111	11
Grundy	7	5	2	1	1		1		2	
Harrison	5	4	3			1			1	
Henry	17	15	8		2	2	3		2	
Hickory	3	2		2					1	
Holt	1	1	1							
Howard	8	5	4			1			2	1
Howell	66	59	16	11	10	12	10		5	2
Iron	9	8	3	2	1	2			1	
Jackson	1,828	1,491	115	423	250	282	421	98	172	67
Jasper	277	240	19	74	45	50	52	7	22	8
Jefferson	117	107	13	35	21	19	19	1	9	
Johnson	44	40	13	9	9	6	3	2	2	
Laclede	26	23	11	5	2	2	3		1	2
Lafayette	13	11	6	1	1	3			1	1
Lawrence	34	28	14	3		5	6	1	4	1
Lewis	1	1					1			
Lincoln	14	13	3	5	3	2			1	
Linn	6	5	2	3					1	
Livingston	11	7	1	3	2	1			4	
Macon	7	6	5				1		1	
Madison	9	9	2	3	3		1			
Maries	4	2				1	1		2	
Marion	59	50	6	21	12	8	3	1	7	1
Mc Donald	3	1	1						2	
Mercer	1	1	1							
Miller	11	9	7	1		1			2	

Table 3.11

Physicians by State and County, 2006, continued

State County	Total Physicians	Total Patient Care	FM/GP Practice	Medical Specialties	Surgical Specialties	Other Specialties	Hospital Based Practice	Other Professional Activity	Inactive	Not Classified
				Major Professional Activity						
			Patient Care							
			Office-Based Practice							
Mississippi	4	3	3						1	
Moniteau	4	2	2						2	
Monroe	1								1	
Montgomery	4	3		2		1		1		
Morgan	8	4	2	2					3	1
New Madrid	2	2	1	1						
Newton	22	14	5	2	4	1	2		8	
Nodaway	30	29	8	4	5	9	3		1	
Oregon	4	2				2			2	
Osage	1	1	1							
Ozark	1	1	1							
Pemiscot	15	12	1	5	3	1	2		3	
Perry	9	8	4		2		2		1	
Pettis	50	41	6	13	11	6	5	1	8	
Phelps	78	71	13	24	16	9	9	1	5	1
Pike	11	3	2				1	1	6	1
Platte	154	121	15	33	18	29	26	13	14	6
Polk	37	30	14	5	7		4		4	3
Pulaski	30	24	9	4	2	3	6	1	4	1
Ralls	1	1		1						
Randolph	16	12		2	6	2	2	1	3	
Ray	8	4	1	2	1				4	
Reynolds	4	3		2			1		1	
Ripley	10	8	3	2		2	1		1	1
Saint Louis City (ic)	2,457	1,835	48	346	213	285	943	260	94	268
Sainte Genevieve	12	11	2	3	1		5		1	
Saline	21	17	11	2	2	1	1		4	
Scotland	2	2	1		1					
Scott	69	58	11	16	9	10	12	1	9	1
Shannon	2	2	1			1				
Shelby	2	2	1			1				
St. Charles	387	324	42	128	70	45	39	10	45	8
St. Clair	9	8	5	1			2			1
St. Francois	60	46	7	17	7	8	7	2	10	2
St. Louis	5,448	4,397	167	1,458	807	961	1,004	213	568	270
Stoddard	17	16	7	6		1	2		1	
Stone	20	15	3	3	3	1	5		5	
Taney	69	61	15	21	8	10	7	1	7	
Texas	17	14	4	2	2	3	3		2	1
Vernon	26	21	4	3	2	6	6		5	
Warren	6	5	1		2		2		1	
Washington	6	5	2	2				1	1	
Wayne	7	5	4	1					2	
Webster	26	16	3	3	2	4	4		10	
Worth	1	1	1							
Wright	8	7	7							1
Montana	2,548	1,991	365	460	443	460	263	66	462	29
Beaverhead	16	14	3	4	2	3	2		2	
Big Horn	19	17	10			1	6	1	1	
Blaine	7	6	2	2			2			1
Broadwater	6	4	2		1	1			2	
Carbon	17	13	7		3	3		1	3	
Carter	1								1	
Cascade	238	190	28	53	46	53	10	6	40	2
Chouteau	4	4	2				2			
Custer	25	20	2	8	7		3		5	
Daniels	2	1			1				1	

Table 3.11

Physicians by State and County, 2006, continued

State County	Total Physicians	Total Patient Care	Office-Based Practice FM/GP Practice	Medical Specialties	Surgical Specialties	Other Specialties	Hospital Based Practice	Other Professional Activity	Inactive	Not Classified
Dawson	11	9	4	1	3	1			2	
Deer Lodge	17	16	3	2	2	4	5		1	
Fergus	19	17	7	4	2		4	1	1	
Flathead	284	220	33	48	60	65	14	3	59	2
Gallatin	263	184	41	36	39	46	22	6	68	5
Glacier	13	9	4	1		1	3		3	1
Golden Valley	1	1		1						
Granite	2								2	
Hill	25	20	4	5	5	2	4	1	3	1
Jefferson	27	19	5	3	2	7	2	1	7	
Lake	56	33	18	1	7	1	6		22	1
Lewis And Clark	187	148	19	36	25	32	36	12	25	2
Liberty	4	3	3					1		
Lincoln	30	22	9	4	4	1	4		8	
Madison	13	7	4	1			2		6	
Mc Cone	1								1	
Meagher	3	3	1				2			
Mineral	4	2	1			1			2	
Missoula	414	321	30	87	77	89	38	10	78	5
Musselshell	3	2	1				1		1	
Park	32	23	8	1	6	3	5		8	1
Phillips	1	1	1							
Pondera	7	6	5		1				1	
Powell	11	9	5	1		1	2	1	1	
Prairie	1	1	1							
Ravalli	78	56	16	13	8	12	7	6	16	
Richland	18	14	3	3	6	2			4	
Roosevelt	5	4	3			1			1	
Rosebud	8	7	5				2		1	
Sanders	11	10	7		2	1			1	
Sheridan	2	2	2							
Silver Bow	78	64	11	20	21	10	2		14	
Stillwater	7	6	3		2	1			1	
Sweet Grass	5	2	1				1	1	2	
Teton	2	2	2							
Toole	7	6	4				2		1	
Treasure	1								1	
Valley	10	8	1	1	4	1	1	1	1	
Wheatland	2	2					2			
Yellowstone	550	463	44	124	107	117	71	14	65	8
Nebraska	4,852	3,874	689	873	714	716	882	209	579	190
Adams	90	71	15	15	22	14	5	2	14	3
Antelope	5	4	2	1			1		1	
Boone	8	8	4	1			3			
Box Butte	7	5	3			1	1		2	
Boyd	5	4	4						1	
Brown	4	3		1		1	1		1	
Buffalo	132	118	22	33	37	23	3		12	2
Burt	4	3	1	1			1		1	
Butler	6	4	4						2	
Cass	20	15	5	2	1	6	1		4	1
Cedar	6	6	3			1	2			
Chase	4	3	3						1	
Cherry	6	6	2	1		1	2			
Cheyenne	10	6	4		1	1			3	1
Clay	2	1				1				1
Colfax	3	2	1				1		1	
Cuming	5	5	4		1					
Custer	10	8	7				1		1	1
Dakota	5	3	2				1		2	
Dawes	12	8	6		1		1		4	

Table 3.11

Physicians by State and County, 2006, continued

State County	Total Physicians	Total Patient Care	FM/GP Practice	Medical Specialties	Surgical Specialties	Other Specialties	Hospital Based Practice	Other Professional Activity	Inactive	Not Classified
Dawson	23	22	16	1	1	2	2		1	
Deuel	2	2			1		1			
Dixon	2	1	1							1
Dodge	56	43	12	10	14	6	1	1	11	1
Douglas	2,661	2,098	191	507	367	399	634	161	270	132
Dundy	2	1	1						1	
Fillmore	6	6	6							
Franklin	3	2	1				1		1	
Furnas	3	2	2						1	
Gage	23	16	11	2	1		2	2	5	
Garden	3								2	1
Garfield	2	1	1						1	
Hall	118	100	19	21	28	21	11	2	16	
Hamilton	12	10	3		1	2	4		2	
Harlan	4	3	1		1	1			1	
Holt	15	12	9	2			1	1	2	
Hooker	2	2	2							
Howard	4	1	1						1	2
Jefferson	6	5	5						1	
Johnson	4	4	3	1						
Kearney	6	4	2				2		2	
Keith	10	8	7		1				2	
Keya Paha	1								1	
Kimball	1	1		1						
Knox	7	5	3				2		2	
Lancaster	780	618	100	182	126	134	76	23	116	23
Lincoln	84	65	16	12	16	20	1		15	4
Madison	80	73	17	12	19	14	11	1	4	2
Merrick	3	3	3							
Morrill	5	3	1				2		2	
Nance	1								1	
Nemaha	7	5	5						2	
Nuckolls	6	5	4				1		1	
Otoe	15	10	8			1	1		4	1
Pawnee	2	2	2							
Perkins	2	2	2							
Phelps	10	9	6	2	1				1	
Pierce	7	7	4	2		1				
Platte	32	25	11	3	9	1	1		7	
Polk	3	2	1	1					1	
Red Willow	16	12	7	1	3		1		4	
Richardson	5	2	2						3	
Rock	3	2		1	1				1	
Saline	12	8	7				1	1	2	1
Sarpy	260	227	34	43	32	35	83	11	11	11
Saunders	14	11	7			2	2	1	2	
Scotts Bluff	100	84	19	10	25	22	8	1	15	
Seward	12	9	8				1		3	
Sheridan	5	4	3				1		1	
Sherman	1	1	1							
Sioux	1								1	
Stanton	1	1				1				
Thayer	5	4	3				1		1	
Thurston	9	8	4	3	1				1	
Valley	7	5	2			2	1		1	1
Washington	19	16	6	1	2	3	4		3	
Wayne	6	4	4						1	1
Webster	3	3	3							
York	16	12	10			1		1	2	2

Table 3.11

Physicians by State and County, 2006, continued

State County	Total Physicians	Total Patient Care	FM/GP Practice	Medical Specialties	Surgical Specialties	Other Specialties	Hospital Based Practice	Other Professional Activity	Inactive	Not Classified
				Major Professional Activity						
				Patient Care						
				Office-Based Practice						
Nevada	5,383	4,306	485	1,359	822	1,093	547	131	773	173
Carson City	160	136	20	38	32	34	12	2	19	3
Churchill	33	31	7	9	8	1	6		2	
Clark	3,685	2,955	296	1,022	542	745	350	75	525	130
Douglas	104	74	14	16	10	25	9	4	24	2
Elko	48	40	5	13	12	5	5	1	7	
Eureka	1	1	1							
Humboldt	11	10	4	3		1	2			1
Lander	6	6	2	2			2			
Lincoln	1	1	1							
Lyon	21	13	7	3			3		7	1
Mineral	4	3	1	1			1		1	
Nye	32	21	5	9	2	3	2	1	9	1
Pershing	2	1			1				1	
Washoe	1,261	1,001	117	241	213	277	153	48	177	35
White Pine	14	13	5	2	2	2	2		1	
New Hampshire	4,079	3,176	392	887	605	677	615	161	616	126
Belknap	157	114	9	31	33	30	11	5	37	1
Carroll	122	76	9	15	19	17	16	4	41	1
Cheshire	186	116	26	32	23	23	12	5	63	2
Coos	84	66	16	13	8	15	14	2	14	2
Grafton	995	747	46	165	107	134	295	78	102	68
Hillsborough	1,013	833	101	287	168	189	88	28	131	21
Merrimack	500	388	60	95	81	90	62	22	72	18
Rockingham	633	517	77	167	106	111	56	10	97	9
Strafford	268	223	32	63	48	51	29	5	37	3
Sullivan	121	96	16	19	12	17	32	2	22	1
New Jersey	30,182	24,127	1,222	8,440	4,358	4,853	5,254	1,520	3,092	1,443
Atlantic	676	535	28	162	131	113	101	21	95	25
Bergen	5,130	4,128	114	1,477	754	948	835	242	559	201
Burlington	1,313	1,082	98	350	184	271	179	50	128	53
Camden	1,810	1,467	105	452	257	294	359	83	167	93
Cape May	156	95	12	26	20	21	16	5	52	4
Cumberland	215	185	21	73	46	28	17	6	20	4
Essex	3,753	2,913	88	918	532	537	838	251	379	210
Gloucester	349	282	38	89	41	47	67	14	30	23
Hudson	1,273	1,014	62	354	162	145	291	30	111	118
Hunterdon	463	359	72	101	51	80	55	32	59	13
Mercer	1,549	1,158	50	407	228	272	201	144	178	69
Middlesex	3,014	2,436	105	885	355	405	686	164	201	213
Monmouth	2,595	2,141	81	772	414	477	397	82	267	105
Morris	2,129	1,693	69	606	300	379	339	127	213	96
Ocean	953	758	38	346	177	121	76	27	143	25
Passaic	1,163	951	49	392	173	138	199	33	110	69
Salem	74	56	12	16	11	10	7	4	13	1
Somerset	1,548	1,262	89	408	205	271	289	103	129	54
Sussex	232	184	13	63	45	45	18	4	39	5
Union	1,592	1,280	57	503	242	224	254	92	162	58
Warren	195	148	21	40	30	27	30	6	37	4
New Mexico	5,424	4,162	617	1,052	646	895	952	280	743	239
Bernalillo	2,940	2,261	207	563	317	510	664	194	316	169
Catron	4	4	2		1	1				
Chaves	130	105	20	33	24	16	12	1	15	9
Cibola	23	19	9	5	2		3		3	1
Colfax	27	16	5	4	4	2	1	1	10	
Curry	63	51	4	19	12	9	7	2	8	2
De Baca	2	2	1	1						
Dona Ana	342	271	52	75	49	59	36	14	45	12
Eddy	80	59	10	11	16	11	11	1	17	3
Grant	80	65	16	15	15	12	7	1	14	

Table 3.11

Physicians by State and County, 2006, continued

State County	Total Physicians	Total Patient Care	FM/GP Practice	Medical Specialties	Surgical Specialties	Other Specialties	Hospital Based Practice	Other Professional Activity	Inactive	Not Classified
					Major Professional Activity					
				Patient Care						
				Office-Based Practice						
Guadalupe	2	2	1	1						
Hidalgo	1								1	
Lea	65	52	5	17	13	8	9		11	2
Lincoln	36	28	8	4	6	5	5	1	7	
Los Alamos	61	47	10	21	6	6	4	3	9	2
Luna	29	22	5	7	3	2	5		5	2
Mc Kinley	177	148	32	31	17	15	53	7	20	2
Mora	2	1		1					1	
Otero	80	60	15	14	15	9	7	1	14	5
Quay	8	8	4	2	1	1				
Rio Arriba	43	36	11	6	9	5	5		5	2
Roosevelt	10	8	3	4	1				2	
San Juan	200	165	37	40	29	26	33	2	29	4
San Miguel	56	51	13	12	5	13	8		4	1
Sandoval	196	146	36	39	15	41	15	12	32	6
Santa Fe	594	404	74	98	67	120	45	35	141	14
Sierra	16	9	1	5	1	1	1		6	1
Socorro	17	16	6	2	1	4	3		1	
Taos	95	72	16	14	14	14	14	3	19	1
Torrance	1	1	1							
Union	3	3	1	1	1					
Valencia	41	30	12	7	2	5	4	2	8	1
New York	83,826	65,224	2,875	18,880	9,951	12,283	21,235	4,507	8,083	6,012
Albany	1,703	1,347	61	373	282	267	364	115	158	83
Allegany	48	36	8	9	8	5	6		11	1
Bronx	3,553	2,684	88	634	242	320	1,400	240	203	426
Broome	651	506	42	142	113	102	107	29	97	19
Cattaraugus	134	106	19	39	19	19	10	2	22	4
Cayuga	102	72	2	32	22	9	7	2	28	
Chautauqua	217	171	22	57	42	42	8	2	41	3
Chemung	264	206	17	79	39	45	26	11	43	4
Chenango	68	51	13	6	14	7	11	5	11	1
Clinton	219	173	16	60	33	42	22	4	35	7
Columbia	124	86	14	25	16	20	11	10	25	3
Cortland	74	56	13	17	9	16	1	3	13	2
Delaware	55	42	8	10	5	6	13	1	11	1
Dutchess	867	701	54	234	145	169	99	30	110	26
Erie	3,826	2,962	178	803	487	541	953	236	396	232
Essex	47	33	10	7	5	6	5	2	11	1
Franklin	104	81	12	25	15	16	13	3	17	3
Fulton	72	50	12	16	9	8	5	3	18	1
Genesee	90	68	6	21	15	13	13	1	21	
Greene	47	33	7	9	5	6	6	1	12	1
Hamilton	3	2	1	1					1	
Herkimer	54	37	10	13	4	4	6		13	4
Jefferson	246	195	17	50	45	53	30	3	44	4
Kings	7,736	6,102	180	1,644	604	734	2,940	305	446	883
Lewis	31	26	9	4	6	2	5		4	1
Livingston	70	57	17	17	11	4	8	4	9	
Madison	113	101	28	19	22	22	10	3	8	1
Monroe	3,720	2,827	134	850	411	488	944	262	394	237
Montgomery	89	71	10	22	15	14	10	3	15	
Nassau	9,042	7,384	200	2,529	1,287	1,420	1,948	346	875	437
New York	20,593	15,538	235	3,674	2,277	3,299	6,053	1,558	1,552	1,945
Niagara	334	252	43	72	61	38	38	6	66	10
Oneida	603	484	59	137	98	98	92	14	91	14
Onondaga	2,308	1,813	152	422	324	350	565	124	240	131
Ontario	310	229	20	72	49	52	36	9	63	9
Orange	867	733	49	302	134	157	91	25	81	28
Orleans	33	26	3	10	6	4	3		7	

Table 3.11

Physicians by State and County, 2006, continued

State County	Total Physicians	Total Patient Care	Office-Based Practice FM/GP Practice	Medical Specialties	Surgical Specialties	Other Specialties	Hospital Based Practice	Other Professional Activity	Inactive	Not Classified
Oswego	119	98	21	33	20	15	9	3	17	1
Otsego	327	272	8	80	66	44	74	12	34	9
Putnam	215	170	7	64	38	41	20	8	33	4
Queens	6,414	4,956	190	1,611	547	712	1,896	220	636	602
Rensselaer	324	256	32	82	42	44	56	17	40	11
Richmond	1,810	1,481	35	524	210	245	467	66	138	125
Rockland	1,310	1,033	38	394	172	249	180	66	167	44
Saratoga	455	383	69	99	68	93	54	16	44	12
Schenectady	554	419	53	108	86	92	80	22	103	10
Schoharie	21	14	5	5	1	2	1	1	6	
Schuyler	20	13	4	4	2	2	1		6	1
Seneca	21	15	7	2	1	5		1	4	1
St. Lawrence	179	140	20	42	29	30	19	6	25	8
Steuben	177	144	20	44	26	26	28	6	25	2
Suffolk	4,910	3,865	222	1,202	680	845	916	203	615	227
Sullivan	119	93	11	31	13	19	19	2	20	4
Tioga	39	29	11	3	3	6	6	2	6	2
Tompkins	304	240	39	69	37	53	42	11	49	4
Ulster	399	329	78	82	51	78	40	12	49	9
Warren	260	214	27	65	54	48	20	10	33	3
Washington	38	28	9	8	3	2	6		10	
Wayne	89	68	9	27	13	10	9	1	19	1
Westchester	7,229	5,561	174	1,846	898	1,214	1,429	460	799	409
Wyoming	46	40	10	14	10	4	2		5	1
Yates	30	22	7	5	2	6	2		8	
North Carolina	25,383	20,013	2,334	5,678	3,784	4,079	4,138	1,256	2,979	1,135
Alamance	246	193	26	71	38	35	23	6	40	7
Alexander	20	18	9	2	2	3	2		2	
Alleghany	22	15	9	3		1	2		7	
Anson	14	11	5	4	1	1			2	1
Ashe	40	25	13	1	6	4	1		14	1
Avery	43	27	9	5	4	3	6	1	15	
Beaufort	93	67	11	17	16	15	8	2	23	1
Bertie	7	6	3	1			2		1	
Bladen	24	18	7	5	4	1	1	2	4	
Brunswick	126	86	17	21	21	14	13	5	34	1
Buncombe	1,153	884	126	247	179	205	127	35	220	14
Burke	192	157	32	31	33	41	20	5	27	3
Cabarrus	378	327	49	110	65	60	43	8	32	11
Caldwell	94	77	25	14	15	15	8	2	12	3
Camden	8	5	1			3	1		3	
Carteret	130	104	13	26	27	22	16	1	24	1
Caswell	10	7	2	1		3	1		3	
Catawba	419	363	57	91	91	96	28	5	46	5
Chatham	97	61	14	16	8	11	12	5	27	4
Cherokee	39	32	5	11	6	4	6		7	
Chowan	30	26	7	4	9	3	3		4	
Clay	12	11	3		2	4	2		1	
Cleveland	171	136	25	44	30	27	10	2	32	1
Columbus	57	50	9	19	13	6	3		6	1
Craven	275	230	17	82	55	54	22	3	38	4
Cumberland	771	654	84	179	117	111	163	17	63	37
Currituck	10	5	3	1			1	1	4	
Dare	64	51	14	10	11	7	9	1	12	
Davidson	121	99	21	29	30	12	7	1	18	3
Davie	68	44	10	12	5	9	8	3	18	3
Duplin	31	26	8	9	4	1	4	1	4	
Durham	2,981	2,181	76	449	259	382	1,015	275	168	357
Edgecombe	41	31	6	12	9	2	2	2	8	

Table 3.11

Physicians by State and County, 2006, continued

State County	Total Physicians	Total Patient Care	Office-Based Practice FM/GP Practice	Medical Specialties	Surgical Specialties	Other Specialties	Hospital Based Practice	Other Professional Activity	Inactive	Not Classified
Forsyth	2,108	1,683	111	410	249	342	571	128	174	123
Franklin	27	19	5	9	4		1	2	5	1
Gaston	375	324	50	101	84	65	24	2	38	11
Gates	3	1		1					1	1
Graham	7	3	2	1				1	3	
Granville	64	44	19	4	6	5	10	5	11	4
Greene	4	3	2	1					1	
Guilford	1,340	1,112	125	370	261	230	126	40	158	30
Halifax	82	70	12	24	16	10	8	2	10	
Harnett	67	59	12	19	12	11	5		8	
Haywood	141	108	23	28	23	24	10	2	29	2
Henderson	302	226	37	64	49	52	24	8	67	1
Hertford	38	31	7	6	8	2	8	1	3	3
Hoke	11	6	1		1		4	1	2	2
Hyde	1								1	
Iredell	308	265	34	87	69	60	15	2	35	6
Jackson	112	81	19	21	17	12	12	1	30	
Johnston	100	86	28	26	16	6	10	2	10	2
Jones	14	12	1	9		1	1			2
Lee	95	74	13	24	15	13	9	5	16	
Lenoir	112	82	9	31	21	16	5	2	26	2
Lincoln	62	52	17	14	13	5	3	1	7	2
Macon	102	75	15	15	18	21	6	1	26	
Madison	19	13	6	4		1	2	1	5	
Martin	19	17	6	6	3	1	1		2	
Mc Dowell	34	28	9	7	8	2	2	1	5	
Mecklenburg	2,727	2,278	203	726	473	499	377	101	265	83
Mitchell	27	19	9	3	4		3	1	5	2
Montgomery	14	10	4	5			1	1	2	1
Moore	377	284	16	84	71	73	40	15	76	2
Nash	180	153	24	44	39	32	14	4	20	3
New Hanover	831	650	51	222	146	146	85	25	133	23
Northampton	7	4	2	1		1			3	
Onslow	254	201	29	38	48	28	58	5	27	21
Orange	2,058	1,405	78	340	170	365	452	289	192	172
Pamlico	12	9	4	2	1	2			3	
Pasquotank	113	97	7	32	28	21	9	1	13	2
Pender	32	26	9	5	2	5	5		5	1
Perquimans	7	5	1	1		1	2		2	
Person	38	28	5	8	4	8	3	3	7	
Pitt	1,023	813	51	209	122	150	281	81	59	70
Polk	54	30	4	7	6	12	1		24	
Randolph	147	126	34	42	18	21	11	3	16	2
Richmond	48	38	12	12	8	5	1	1	9	
Robeson	136	113	22	33	28	15	15	2	16	5
Rockingham	103	91	17	26	22	15	11		12	
Rowan	229	168	24	46	37	27	34	7	47	7
Rutherford	104	85	16	30	15	18	6	2	17	
Sampson	53	44	18	9	11	5	1	1	7	1
Scotland	63	54	13	20	12	6	3		7	2
Stanly	72	54	7	17	18	8	4		17	1
Stokes	16	13	5	2	2	4			1	2
Surry	93	78	21	24	18	4	11	1	13	1
Swain	15	14	8	4			2	1		
Transylvania	81	52	12	16	14	7	3	2	27	
Union	200	170	39	63	27	27	14	4	22	4
Vance	68	58	15	17	13	10	3		10	
Wake	2,285	1,864	195	632	377	433	227	108	245	68
Warren	5	3	2		1				2	
Washington	9	7	4	1	1		1	1	1	

Table 3.11

Physicians by State and County, 2006, continued

State County	Total Physicians	Total Patient Care	Office-Based Practice FM/GP Practice	Medical Specialties	Surgical Specialties	Other Specialties	Hospital Based Practice	Other Professional Activity	Inactive	Not Classified
Watauga	126	103	16	30	29	24	4		22	1
Wayne	209	169	37	47	28	43	14	3	28	9
Wilkes	71	61	14	24	14	6	3	1	9	
Wilson	120	102	12	37	23	20	10	1	15	2
Yadkin	19	16	8	3	1	3	1		3	
Yancey	23	17	7	7		1	2	1	5	
North Dakota	1,745	1,437	278	342	243	280	294	62	201	45
Adams	17	16	7	4	1	2	2	1		
Barnes	15	10	4	2	3		1		5	
Benson	4	4					4			
Bottineau	6	5	2	2			1		1	
Bowman	4	3	3						1	
Burke	1								1	
Burleigh	337	281	29	73	56	73	50	11	39	6
Cass	633	522	68	156	92	109	97	24	63	24
Cavalier	6	5	3	1			1		1	
Dickey	5	4	1	2	1			1		
Emmons	3	3	3							
Foster	6	5	5						1	
Golden Valley	2	1	1						1	
Grand Forks	263	221	44	39	28	52	58	15	19	8
Grant	3	3	1	1			1			
Griggs	3	2	1	1					1	
Kidder	2	1			1					1
Mc Henry	1	1					1			
Mc Intosh	4	3	1	1	1				1	
Mc Kenzie	2	2	1				1			
Mc Lean	5	2					2		2	1
Mercer	6	6	4		2					
Morton	16	11	4		4	1	2	1	4	
Mountrail	7	6	4	1			1	1		
Nelson	2	2	1	1						
Pembina	6	5	2	1	1		1		1	
Pierce	8	8	5	2	1					
Ramsey	25	20	8	8	2	2			5	
Ransom	8	5	3				2		3	
Renville	2	1	1						1	
Richland	21	14	7	2	3		2	2	4	1
Rolette	12	9	2	2	3	1	1	1	2	
Sioux	4	4	1		1	1	1			
Stark	39	33	9	5	5	4	10		6	
Stutsman	36	32	11	6	5	4	6		4	
Towner	4	1	1					1	2	
Traill	12	10	7	1			2		2	
Walsh	13	9	6		1	1	1		4	
Ward	155	129	15	27	24	21	42	4	18	4
Wells	3	3	1	1	1					
Williams	44	35	12	3	7	9	4		9	
Ohio	34,090	26,843	2,742	7,320	4,496	5,307	6,978	1,392	3,770	2,085
Adams	20	15	4	4	1	2	4	1	4	
Allen	284	232	36	60	53	64	19	5	42	5
Ashland	62	50	11	14	11	9	5		12	
Ashtabula	88	65	16	24	14	9	2		21	2
Athens	58	43	7	12	6	8	10	2	10	3
Auglaize	65	54	15	17	6	10	6	2	7	2
Belmont	91	71	16	20	15	11	9	5	15	
Brown	34	24	12	4	3		5	1	7	2
Butler	543	455	73	140	85	90	67	6	68	14
Carroll	12	9	4	2		2	1		3	

Table 3.11

Physicians by State and County, 2006, continued

State County	Total Physicians	Total Patient Care	FM/GP Practice	Medical Specialties	Surgical Specialties	Other Specialties	Hospital Based Practice	Other Professional Activity	Inactive	Not Classified
Champaign	21	16	9	4		2	1		4	1
Clark	247	201	28	62	43	49	19	9	35	2
Clermont	311	254	42	77	37	39	59	12	36	9
Clinton	86	74	17	15	10	12	20	3	7	2
Columbiana	119	96	19	32	22	12	11	1	21	1
Coshocton	29	23	4	8	8	2	1		5	1
Crawford	41	25	6	4	10	3	2	2	14	
Cuyahoga	8,530	6,419	254	1,715	929	1,183	2,338	392	779	940
Darke	44	35	17	6	5	2	5	1	8	
Defiance	60	52	16	11	13	8	4	1	7	
Delaware	510	421	62	109	71	112	67	15	49	25
Erie	149	120	9	41	22	34	14	3	25	1
Fairfield	215	184	43	43	29	45	24	5	22	4
Fayette	21	16	6	5	3	1	1		5	
Franklin	4,383	3,487	353	908	585	676	965	240	385	271
Fulton	40	30	15	7	1	6	1	1	8	1
Gallia	101	84	7	38	17	16	6	4	11	2
Geauga	229	179	16	46	35	54	28	4	38	8
Greene	477	398	55	67	39	73	164	13	41	25
Guernsey	67	51	4	15	13	9	10	3	10	3
Hamilton	4,656	3,613	228	994	606	747	1,038	273	466	304
Hancock	141	117	12	39	35	25	6	2	20	2
Hardin	19	14	4	4		4	2	1	3	1
Harrison	13	11	4	3	2		2		2	
Henry	18	15	8	2	2	2	1		2	1
Highland	35	27	15	4	3	2	3		6	2
Hocking	20	16	6	4	2	3	1		4	
Holmes	33	28	13	5	3	6	1	1	4	
Huron	84	65	23	9	17	12	4	2	16	1
Jackson	21	17	4	6	4		3		4	
Jefferson	106	88	10	29	22	17	10		15	3
Knox	84	62	17	16	15	9	5	2	20	
Lake	362	288	25	102	65	62	34	4	58	12
Lawrence	59	52	10	10	6	6	20	1	5	1
Licking	165	129	32	27	25	27	18	5	29	2
Logan	49	37	11	6	10	2	8	4	6	2
Lorain	527	410	46	131	81	88	64	5	89	23
Lucas	1,854	1,471	147	362	263	324	375	71	211	101
Madison	43	36	9	8	6	4	9	1	6	
Mahoning	807	634	45	193	115	105	176	34	84	55
Marion	130	108	9	36	34	18	11	2	18	2
Medina	266	220	44	61	46	37	32	7	33	6
Meigs	5	3	3						2	
Mercer	42	31	9	9	7	2	4	1	9	1
Miami	131	105	22	25	20	23	15	3	20	3
Monroe	6	4	3				1		2	
Montgomery	1,968	1,581	179	450	253	312	387	94	230	63
Morgan	1	1	1							
Morrow	11	8	4		1	2	1		3	
Muskingum	159	125	19	38	34	29	5	1	28	5
Noble	3	1	1						2	
Ottawa	55	37	18	4	3	10	2	3	15	
Paulding	9	8	3	1			4		1	
Perry	9	7	3	2		1	1	1		1
Pickaway	42	35	12	6	5	8	4	1	6	
Pike	27	18	6	3	1	4	4		9	
Portage	194	153	25	30	27	34	37	4	33	4
Preble	12	9	5	3			1		3	
Putnam	18	16	13	1		1	1		2	
Richland	248	199	24	68	49	44	14	1	46	2

Table 3.11

Physicians by State and County, 2006, continued

State County	Total Physicians	Total Patient Care	Major Professional Activity							
			Patient Care				Hospital Based Practice	Other Professional Activity	Inactive	Not Classified
			Office-Based Practice							
			FM/GP Practice	Medical Specialties	Surgical Specialties	Other Specialties				
Ross	135	113	20	27	25	20	21	3	14	5
Sandusky	57	43	14	10	6	9	4	1	12	1
Scioto	126	101	12	40	18	21	10	2	18	5
Seneca	70	63	10	18	17	14	4		6	1
Shelby	48	43	12	8	10	7	6	1	4	
Stark	946	782	83	269	137	157	136	24	114	26
Summit	1,808	1,471	126	382	235	292	436	64	191	82
Trumbull	302	231	19	83	51	56	22	10	58	3
Tuscarawas	113	88	18	21	19	18	12	3	19	3
Union	39	34	9	9	8	6	2		5	
Van Wert	28	25	11	4	6	4			3	
Warren	460	397	55	133	35	94	80	13	27	23
Washington	94	75	14	19	17	19	6		17	2
Wayne	169	139	29	43	30	22	15	2	25	3
Williams	46	38	14	8	7	2	7		6	2
Wood	263	205	42	44	24	52	43	14	36	8
Wyandot	17	13	6	1	3	1	2		4	
Oklahoma	7,111	5,667	800	1,455	1,101	1,186	1,125	272	947	225
Adair	13	13	5	2	1	1	4			
Beaver	2	2	2							
Beckham	30	28	8	5	7	3	5		2	
Blaine	8	7	5		1		1		1	
Bryan	33	27	2	11	10	3	1		6	
Caddo	11	7	5	1			1	1	3	
Canadian	89	68	25	13	7	6	17	2	1/	2
Carter	86	68	7	22	21	9	9	2	12	4
Cherokee	54	46	8	11	8	5	14	3	4	1
Choctaw	7	5	3		2				2	
Cimarron	3	1	1						2	
Cleveland	409	338	45	77	45	83	88	10	49	12
Coal	1								1	
Comanche	247	214	25	40	40	44	65	4	20	9
Cotton	3	3	2		1					
Craig	19	11	6				5	1	6	1
Creek	31	24	14	5	2	3			7	
Custer	27	22	8	6	4		4		5	
Delaware	33	29	16	3	5	2	3	1	3	
Dewey	2	2	2							
Ellis	6	4	4						1	1
Garfield	132	102	14	22	29	24	13	2	26	2
Garvin	12	10	7	1	2				2	
Grady	40	31	6	9	7	5	4		8	1
Grant	1								1	
Greer	6	4	3				1		2	
Harmon	2	1	1						1	
Harper	1	1	1							
Haskell	4	4	1	2	1					
Hughes	4	1					1		3	
Jackson	42	36	9	6	9	5	7	1	5	
Jefferson	1	1	1							
Johnston	7	3	2	1					3	1
Kay	58	45	11	9	11	10	4	4	9	
Kingfisher	11	9	3	1	1	1	3		2	
Kiowa	8	8	5		1	2				
Latimer	17	15	3	3	5	1	3		1	1
Le Flore	10	5	1		2	1	1		5	
Lincoln	11	10	7				1	2	1	
Logan	16	13	1	4		5	3		3	
Love	4	2	2						2	

Table 3.11

Physicians by State and County, 2006, continued

State County	Total Physicians	Total Patient Care	FM/GP Practice	Medical Specialties	Surgical Specialties	Other Specialties	Hospital Based Practice	Other Professional Activity	Inactive	Not Classified
Major	2	2	2							
Marshall	4	3	2	1					1	
Mayes	21	16	7	4	2	1	2		5	
Mc Clain	15	13	9			2	2	1	1	
Mc Curtain	14	13	4	5	4				1	
Mc Intosh	7	7	2	2	1	1	1			
Murray	10	7	4	2	1			1	2	
Muskogee	139	95	10	35	21	13	16	6	35	3
Noble	9	3	3						4	2
Nowata	3	3	2	1						
Okfuskee	5	4	4						1	
Oklahoma	2,886	2,298	201	576	433	540	548	170	300	118
Okmulgee	21	18	5	6	4	1	2		3	
Osage	6	2	1				1		4	
Ottawa	28	20	3	2	5	3	7		8	
Pawnee	6	5	3	1			1			1
Payne	107	89	13	32	25	16	3	1	17	
Pittsburg	69	56	9	17	14	12	4	1	11	1
Pontotoc	82	69	8	20	20	10	11	1	11	1
Pottawatomie	74	56	11	18	13	9	5		17	1
Pushmataha	4	3	3						1	
Roger Mills	5	2	1				1		2	1
Rogers	61	51	11	12	12	4	12		8	2
Seminole	7	5	4	1					1	
Sequoyah	11	8	4	1		1	2	1	1	1
Stephens	41	34	17	2	8	3	4		7	
Texas	11	10	2	4	4				1	
Tillman	5	4	1		1		2		1	
Tulsa	1,823	1,444	159	436	287	335	227	56	265	58
Wagoner	16	12	4	2		3	3	1	3	
Washington	89	70	11	16	20	15	8	1	17	1
Washita	2	2	1	1						
Woods	4	4	2	1		1				
Woodward	23	19	6	3	4		2	4		4
Oregon	11,741	9,036	1,192	2,534	1,728	2,084	1,498	510	1,737	458
Baker	23	20	9	2	4	4	1		3	
Benton	292	219	27	73	35	60	24	11	59	3
Clackamas	1,020	774	72	226	159	218	99	41	179	26
Clatsop	65	56	16	10	12	10	8	1	8	
Columbia	21	14	4	6	1	1	2		6	1
Coos	175	141	22	42	31	27	19	1	28	5
Crook	19	15	10		3	1	1	2	2	
Curry	37	19	10	3	1	4	1	2	16	
Deschutes	514	373	58	94	95	104	22	19	106	16
Douglas	228	171	27	52	33	35	24	4	51	2
Grant	8	8	5		2		1			
Harney	9	6	3		1		2		3	
Hood River	97	77	28	11	13	20	5	5	11	4
Jackson	641	479	73	154	98	110	44	21	127	14
Jefferson	21	15	6	1	2		6		3	3
Josephine	151	123	33	34	28	20	8	2	23	3
Klamath	158	121	27	20	25	25	24	6	24	7
Lake	6	5	3				2		1	
Lane	990	770	139	220	164	200	47	26	182	12
Lincoln	87	51	9	11	13	12	6	1	34	1
Linn	156	124	47	25	26	14	12	2	27	3
Malheur	51	41	6	8	12	9	6		9	1
Marion	673	533	114	131	115	119	54	23	111	6

Table 3.11

Physicians by State and County, 2006, continued

State County	Total Physicians	Total Patient Care	FM/GP Practice	Medical Specialties	Surgical Specialties	Other Specialties	Hospital Based Practice	Other Professional Activity	Inactive	Not Classified
				Major Professional Activity						
				Patient Care						
				Office-Based Practice						
Morrow	3	3				1	2			
Multnomah	4,120	3,160	205	899	522	714	820	275	406	279
Polk	98	68	21	16	9	13	9	3	25	2
Sherman	1	1	1							
Tillamook	52	37	12	4	6	11	4	2	12	1
Umatilla	94	74	14	15	22	18	5	1	19	
Union	51	44	8	10	11	12	3	1	6	
Wallowa	13	12	7	2	2	1			1	
Wasco	57	43	7	8	14	12	2	2	10	2
Washington	1,629	1,304	138	421	244	281	220	57	202	66
Wheeler	1	1				1				
Yamhill	180	134	31	36	24	28	15	2	43	1
Pennsylvania	42,204	32,324	2,808	8,754	5,283	6,498	8,981	2,343	5,248	2,289
Adams	115	91	26	22	17	18	8	2	17	5
Allegheny	7,594	5,829	329	1,524	930	1,154	1,892	436	789	540
Armstrong	66	51	6	25	8	9	3		15	
Beaver	255	199	29	58	40	53	19	8	43	5
Bedford	29	22	6	5	5	3	3		7	
Berks	796	617	90	175	129	113	110	25	133	21
Blair	341	275	36	84	58	56	41	7	53	6
Bradford	264	225	22	53	48	34	68	4	27	8
Bucks	1,644	1,293	119	452	238	279	205	91	216	44
Butler	309	235	23	75	38	51	48	12	47	15
Cambria	435	353	51	73	63	53	113	13	49	20
Cameron	5	2		2					2	1
Carbon	52	39	7	14	11	6	1		13	
Centre	337	280	37	75	45	72	51	11	40	6
Chester	1,434	1,033	95	368	173	243	154	80	275	46
Clarion	26	19	4	6		4	5	2	3	2
Clearfield	132	104	8	25	25	21	25	6	22	
Clinton	43	34	9	8	9	5	3		8	1
Columbia	107	86	14	23	16	16	17	1	18	2
Crawford	136	114	22	30	30	22	10	2	20	
Cumberland	714	555	71	157	119	123	85	25	125	9
Dauphin	1,331	1,037	65	215	140	188	429	94	89	111
Delaware	2,844	2,138	120	711	330	506	471	196	376	134
Elk	51	40	11	7	11	6	5		11	
Erie	610	472	75	107	111	90	89	21	106	11
Fayette	178	145	28	46	30	26	15	2	31	
Franklin	229	174	44	42	42	34	12	2	47	6
Fulton	5	5	4		1					
Greene	30	23	7	11	4	1			6	1
Huntingdon	52	41	11	7	6	11	6		11	
Indiana	125	103	15	32	21	24	11	3	19	
Jefferson	51	38	10	9	12	2	5	1	12	
Juniata	9	8	5	1			2		1	
Lackawanna	592	474	27	174	100	99	74	19	89	10
Lancaster	1,003	766	186	183	141	159	97	30	183	24
Lawrence	129	101	18	32	20	17	14	4	21	3
Lebanon	339	250	40	48	39	43	80	9	62	18
Lehigh	1,069	884	93	237	191	183	180	24	122	39
Luzerne	782	626	80	167	122	114	143	21	114	21
Lycoming	261	200	45	39	35	42	39	9	47	5
Mc Kean	68	55	10	16	12	8	9	1	10	2
Mercer	216	157	19	44	36	39	19	3	51	5
Mifflin	73	58	12	22	10	9	5	2	13	
Monroe	237	190	24	71	35	40	20	9	34	4
Montgomery	5,216	3,834	220	1,175	596	962	881	391	762	229
Montour	498	407	7	97	50	54	199	26	29	36

Table 3.11

Physicians by State and County, 2006, continued

State County	Total Physicians	Total Patient Care	FM/GP Practice	Medical Specialties	Surgical Specialties	Other Specialties	Hospital Based Practice	Other Professional Activity	Inactive	Not Classified
Northampton	807	660	46	181	138	129	166	33	89	25
Northumberland	90	61	17	18	5	16	5	2	23	4
Perry	22	14	8	3		2	1	1	7	
Philadelphia	7,608	5,697	159	1,194	649	907	2,788	622	485	804
Pike	60	46	9	16	8	5	8		14	
Potter	31	24	3	8	8	1	4		3	4
Schuylkill	185	138	16	51	26	32	13	3	40	4
Snyder	38	28	8	6	4	4	6	1	8	1
Somerset	108	82	20	20	15	13	14	4	21	1
Sullivan	5	1		1					4	
Susquehanna	41	25	2	7	3	6	7	1	13	2
Tioga	51	39	15	6	4	8	6		12	
Union	131	102	10	23	28	26	15	4	19	6
Venango	105	86	11	29	19	16	11	3	14	2
Warren	85	60	10	8	9	13	20	2	21	2
Washington	396	312	58	89	52	61	52	17	61	6
Wayne	70	53	9	17	9	9	9	2	14	1
Westmoreland	711	567	106	156	97	127	81	21	111	12
Wyoming	23	19	9	5	2	2	1		4	
York	805	628	112	169	110	129	108	35	117	25
Puerto Rico	11,900	9,173	1,742	2,281	1,180	2,115	1,855	428	805	1,494
Adjuntas	17	14	4	3		3	4		1	2
Aguada	76	56	18	19		9	10	1	3	16
Aguadilla	178	149	35	32	17	38	27	3	7	19
Aguas Buenas	23	17	5	2	1	5	4	2		4
Aibonito	72	61	16	17	14	4	10	4	1	6
Anasco	52	36	11	8	3	12	2	1	4	11
Arecibo	372	282	69	54	30	73	56	7	28	55
Arroyo	28	25	8	4		7	6			3
Barceloneta	27	17	6	2	1	6	2	1		9
Barranquitas	29	20	4	6	2	3	5	1	1	7
Bayamon	904	724	136	190	99	151	148	27	33	120
Cabo Rojo	125	98	33	15	12	23	15	2	11	14
Caguas	563	467	103	145	55	103	61	13	27	56
Camuy	39	25	12	3		6	4		3	11
Canovanas	50	37	20	5	1	5	6		1	12
Carolina	453	341	77	76	26	95	67	15	23	74
Catano	27	23	9	1		7	6	1	3	
Cayey	104	92	21	26	10	19	16	1	7	4
Ceiba	17	14	6	4	1	2	1			3
Ciales	21	17	12	2	1	1	1		1	3
Cidra	47	37	6	9	4	15	3		3	7
Coamo	38	30	7	9	1	6	7	2		6
Comerio	15	10	7			2	1		1	4
Corozal	41	27	10	6	2	7	2	1	2	11
Culebra	2	2	1			1				
Dorado	100	82	10	24	8	24	16	2	6	10
Fajardo	119	93	18	19	14	25	17	4	10	12
Florida	9	5	2			1	2			4
Guanica	28	23	5	5	2	3	8		1	4
Guayama	98	70	13	14	9	19	15	2	7	19
Guayanilla	66	51	16	10	5	8	12	1	2	12
Guaynabo	797	610	73	157	92	157	131	41	69	77
Gurabo	86	68	18	20	5	14	11	2	4	12
Hatillo	51	37	15	4	3	9	6	1	3	10
Hormigueros	31	24	3	5	5	7	4	1		6
Humacao	171	136	23	39	19	32	23	6	10	19
Isabela	64	42	21	6	1	12	2		6	16
Jayuya	19	17	7	4	1	2	3			2

Table 3.11

Physicians by State and County, 2006, continued

State County	Total Physicians	Total Patient Care	FM/GP Practice	Medical Specialties	Surgical Specialties	Other Specialties	Hospital Based Practice	Other Professional Activity	Inactive	Not Classified
Juana Diaz	46	32	7	10	3	8	4		1	13
Juncos	51	40	10	11	2	12	5	1		10
Lajas	33	20	6	7	1	2	4	1	5	7
Lares	59	38	20	6	1	5	6		3	18
Las Marias	4	3	2				1			1
Las Piedras	52	41	10	11	2	8	10	3		8
Loiza	6	5	1	1		3			1	
Luquillo	33	24	4	6	2	8	4	1	2	6
Manati	138	111	25	22	24	23	17	5	6	16
Maricao	5	4	1				3		1	
Maunabo	12	8	3	3			2		1	3
Mayaguez	559	445	75	117	80	96	77	9	42	63
Moca	54	38	13	9	2	7	7	2	3	11
Morovis	27	19	5	7	2	3	2		2	6
Naguabo	15	11	4	2		2	3			4
Naranjito	23	16	6	4		5	1		1	6
Orocovis	18	15	5	2	1	6	1	1		2
Patillas	29	23	6	6	1	3	7		2	4
Penuelas	26	22	4	8		5	5			4
Ponce	949	745	90	214	98	151	192	25	55	124
Quebradillas	38	24	6	6	2	4	6	1	3	10
Rincon	14	13	5	3		5			1	
Rio Grande	36	27	8	6	1	10	2	1	3	5
Sabana Grande	49	38	12	11	3	4	8	1	3	7
Salinas	24	14	6	2		3	3	1	1	8
San German	127	102	17	34	13	14	24	2	10	13
San Juan	3,699	2,805	348	703	461	654	639	209	345	340
San Lorenzo	35	26	9	7	1	5	4	3	3	3
San Sebastian	71	46	10	14	2	15	5		6	19
Santa Isabel	21	14	5	1	1	3	4		1	6
Toa Alta	72	57	16	13		18	10	1	1	13
Toa Baja	145	122	37	23	10	28	24	6	2	15
Trujillo Alto	157	115	21	27	11	27	29	6	6	30
Utuado	34	27	11	5		7	4	2	2	3
Vega Alta	31	25	10	6	1	3	5	1	1	4
Vega Baja	106	79	33	8	6	23	9	1	6	20
Vieques	7	3	1		1	1		1	2	1
Villalba	13	9	1	2	2	1	3	1		3
Yabucoa	20	14	3	4		6	1		2	4
Yauco	103	74	26	15	2	21	10	1	4	24
Rhode Island	4,368	3,458	173	1,088	544	614	1,039	209	457	244
Bristol	295	233	9	96	32	61	35	12	42	8
Kent	542	437	26	140	85	98	88	20	68	17
Newport	267	193	16	56	34	43	44	8	59	7
Providence	2,887	2,301	96	680	336	349	840	157	223	206
Washington	377	294	26	116	57	63	32	12	65	6
South Carolina	11,241	9,155	1,224	2,338	1,798	1,907	1,888	401	1,354	331
Abbeville	22	17	7	2	4	3	1	1	4	
Aiken	245	190	27	38	41	41	43	2	45	8
Allendale	10	9	6		1	1	1		1	
Anderson	386	321	57	66	59	80	59	10	40	15
Bamberg	12	11	8		1	1	1		1	
Barnwell	13	10	3	3	3	1			1	2
Beaufort	592	335	35	92	92	78	38	12	231	14
Berkeley	125	117	23	30	13	30	21	1	4	3
Calhoun	6	6	3	1		2				
Charleston	2,621	2,099	126	470	362	482	659	157	233	132
Cherokee	52	44	9	8	12	7	8		8	
Chester	28	22	6	5	4	3	4	1	4	1

Table 3.11
Physicians by State and County, 2006, continued

State County	Total Physicians	Total Patient Care	Office-Based Practice FM/GP Practice	Office-Based Practice Medical Specialties	Office-Based Practice Surgical Specialties	Office-Based Practice Other Specialties	Hospital Based Practice	Other Professional Activity	Inactive	Not Classified
Chesterfield	34	27	15	4	3	2	3		6	1
Clarendon	35	31	12	6	7	2	4		4	
Colleton	57	47	8	14	15	6	4		10	
Darlington	81	68	27	24	9	7	1	3	9	1
Dillon	25	23	7	7	3		6	1	1	
Dorchester	115	93	32	18	16	11	16	3	15	4
Edgefield	15	11	6		1	1	3		4	
Fairfield	15	15	7	3	1	2	2			
Florence	420	366	51	100	87	83	45	14	32	8
Georgetown	133	99	21	27	22	26	3	4	29	1
Greenville	1,397	1,178	133	335	231	214	265	39	151	29
Greenwood	245	210	43	44	39	42	42	8	25	2
Hampton	10	8	6	1	1				2	
Horry	464	391	40	121	94	109	27	7	58	8
Jasper	20	15	5	3	3	1	3		4	1
Kershaw	92	79	10	25	17	16	11	1	10	2
Lancaster	62	53	12	12	16	12	1	2	7	
Laurens	63	53	21	10	12	6	4	1	9	
Lee	4	2	2						2	
Lexington	446	388	71	95	60	86	76	10	37	11
Marion	39	34	7	10	10	3	4		5	
Marlboro	25	20	7	5	2	2	4		4	1
Mc Cormick	6	4	3			1			2	
Newberry	39	36	19	5	5	4	3		2	1
Oconee	156	123	27	23	25	35	13	1	29	3
Orangeburg	150	126	23	47	25	21	10	3	16	5
Pickens	179	150	42	36	24	25	23	1	28	
Richland	1,599	1,304	100	372	249	259	324	93	163	39
Saluda	4	2	2						2	
Spartanburg	672	566	87	127	134	105	113	21	62	23
Sumter	173	144	19	42	31	34	18	2	18	9
Union	29	25	7	8	4	3	3		4	
Williamsburg	13	11	4	2	3	2				2
York	312	272	38	97	57	60	20	3	32	5
South Dakota	1,975	1,627	302	382	351	307	285	53	256	39
Aurora	1	1					1			
Beadle	25	20	4	5	7	2	2		5	
Bon Homme	5	4	3		1				1	
Brookings	30	24	9	4	8		3		5	1
Brown	90	72	14	13	22	15	8	4	13	1
Brule	10	7	4	1	1		1		3	
Buffalo	1	1	1							
Butte	6	5	4				1		1	
Charles Mix	6	4	1	1			2		1	1
Clay	19	17	6	3		4	4		1	1
Codington	62	53	14	13	14	8	4		9	
Custer	14	12	7	1	1	2	1		2	
Davison	44	40	8	11	12	9			4	
Day	5	4	4						1	
Deuel	2	2	1	1						
Dewey	3	3	2				1			
Douglas	2	1	1						1	
Edmunds	4	4			2	1	1			
Fall River	27	16	3	1	4	1	7	1	10	
Faulk	1									1
Grant	7	6	3		1		2		1	
Gregory	7	6	4		1		1			1
Haakon	3	2	1			1			1	

Table 3.11

Physicians by State and County, 2006, continued

State County	Total Physicians	Total Patient Care	FM/GP Practice	Medical Specialties	Surgical Specialties	Other Specialties	Hospital Based Practice	Other Professional Activity	Inactive	Not Classified
Hamlin	1	1					1			
Hand	3	3	3							
Hanson	2	2	1				1			
Hughes	29	24	5	9	6	1	3		5	
Hutchinson	12	8	7	1					4	
Jerauld	4	3	2			1			1	
Kingsbury	6	4	2	2					2	
Lake	9	7	5	2					2	
Lawrence	57	34	14	6	10	1	3	2	20	1
Lincoln	203	181	25	52	41	35	28	2	14	6
Marshall	2	2	1	1						
Mc Cook	4	2	2						2	
Mc Pherson	3	2	2						1	
Meade	39	31	7	5		3	16	2	5	1
Minnehaha	644	541	67	135	98	118	123	28	58	17
Moody	2	1					1		1	
Pennington	360	287	39	77	62	65	44	12	56	5
Potter	2	2		1			1			
Roberts	12	11	6	2	2	1			1	
Sanborn	1								1	
Shannon	11	10		3	1		6		1	
Spink	9	5	1	2			2		4	
Stanley	1								1	
Todd	9	8		3		2	3	1		
Tripp	7	7	5		2					
Turner	6	5		2		2	1		1	
Union	67	63	3	6	33	17	4		2	2
Walworth	7	5	3	1			1		1	1
Yankton	89	74	8	18	22	18	8	1	14	
Tennessee	17,791	14,557	1,629	4,305	2,867	2,872	2,884	730	1,866	638
Anderson	210	177	32	47	41	44	13	7	24	2
Bedford	35	28	10	8	6	2	2		6	1
Benton	6	4	3		1				2	
Bledsoe	6	4	1	1			2	1	1	
Blount	239	192	24	67	36	40	25	2	43	2
Bradley	155	131	23	42	32	22	12	4	20	
Campbell	36	31	8	13	3	4	3		5	
Cannon	8	4	3			1			4	
Carroll	27	23	11	4	4	3	1		3	1
Carter	50	37	12	7	10	4	4	2	10	1
Cheatham	21	19	8	4	2	1	4	1	1	
Chester	5	5	4	1						
Claiborne	26	21	7	7	5	2			2	3
Clay	4	3	2	1					1	
Cocke	22	20	13	5	1		1	1	1	
Coffee	105	95	16	28	29	17	5		8	2
Crockett	5	4	1	1		1	1		1	
Cumberland	115	81	14	28	21	13	5	3	29	2
Davidson	3,802	3,032	106	811	578	617	920	241	320	209
De Kalb	18	12	10		1	1			6	
Decatur	8	8	6	1	1					
Dickson	59	51	17	15	10	5	4		5	3
Dyer	74	59	6	27	14	6	6	1	13	1
Fayette	15	15	8	2	1	1	3			
Fentress	13	10	4	3	2		1		3	
Franklin	54	44	13	12	10	4	5	1	5	4
Gibson	43	37	19	7	7	2	2		6	
Giles	31	25	9	9	5	2			5	1
Grainger	8	3		2			1		5	

Table 3.11

Physicians by State and County, 2006, continued

State County	Total Physicians	Total Patient Care	FM/GP Practice	Medical Specialties	Surgical Specialties	Other Specialties	Hospital Based Practice	Other Professional Activity	Inactive	Not Classified
				Major Professional Activity						
			Patient Care							
			Office-Based Practice							
Greene	112	93	26	21	19	16	11	4	13	2
Grundy	7	5	1	3		1			2	
Hamblen	139	117	14	44	30	23	6	1	20	1
Hamilton	1,361	1,105	95	334	235	235	206	52	178	26
Hancock	3	1	1						2	
Hardeman	15	6	2	1		2	1		7	2
Hardin	19	17	7	4	3	2	1		1	1
Hawkins	36	29	11	9	2	2	5	1	6	
Haywood	11	8	3	3		1	1		3	
Henderson	16	14	7	3	2	1	1		1	1
Henry	53	38	6	12	12	8			15	
Hickman	7	7	2	1		2	2			
Houston	4	4	3		1					
Humphreys	11	9	4	3	2				2	
Jackson	4	3		1	1		1		1	
Jefferson	49	36	12	15	2	4	3		12	1
Johnson	12	9	7	1		1			3	
Knox	1,940	1,631	170	526	341	367	227	50	225	34
Lake	3	2	1				1		1	
Lauderdale	8	6	3	1	2				1	1
Lawrence	32	25	9	7	5	2	2		6	1
Lewis	6	5	2	1	2				1	
Lincoln	34	29	18	3	3	2	3		5	
Loudon	57	39	10	10	4	8	7		18	
Macon	8	5	2	3					3	
Madison	444	370	34	127	102	69	38	13	48	13
Marion	20	16	6	5	3	1	1	1	3	
Marshall	20	19	6	4	4	4	1		1	
Maury	211	181	25	56	45	40	15	4	21	5
Mc Minn	66	56	18	11	16	7	4	2	8	
Mc Nairy	17	15	8	3	3		1		1	1
Meigs	4	2	1	1					2	
Monroe	27	22	8	5	4	2	3		5	
Montgomery	227	195	23	58	50	36	28	2	27	3
Moore	2	2	1				1			
Morgan	4	3	3						1	
Obion	47	37	9	7	13	7	1	1	9	
Overton	24	20	5	6	3	4	2		3	1
Perry	3	3	1	1		1				
Pickett	1	1		1						
Polk	18	17	4	6		3	4		1	
Putnam	185	161	19	52	39	39	12	2	20	2
Rhea	15	12	5	4	1	1	1	1	2	
Roane	39	31	14	10	3	2	2	1	7	
Robertson	59	51	17	12	14	4	4		8	
Rutherford	389	329	36	102	74	63	54	14	40	6
Scott	22	19	4	9	3	3		2		1
Sequatchie	8	6	4	1			1		2	
Sevier	85	72	32	12	12	9	7		12	1
Shelby	3,588	2,927	201	912	523	565	726	165	314	182
Smith	14	12	8		4				1	1
Stewart	3	2	2						1	
Sullivan	671	549	87	167	125	110	60	27	82	13
Sumner	234	202	42	64	44	35	17	6	22	4
Tipton	49	42	9	14	8	6	5	2	3	2
Trousdale	4	3	2			1			1	
Unicoi	15	13	7	4	1	1			2	
Union	8	7	1	5			1			1

Table 3.11

Physicians by State and County, 2006, continued

State County	Total Physicians	Total Patient Care	Office-Based Practice				Hospital Based Practice	Other Professional Activity	Inactive	Not Classified
			FM/GP Practice	Medical Specialties	Surgical Specialties	Other Specialties				
Van Buren	3	1	1						2	
Warren	40	32	10	7	9	3	3		8	
Washington	905	736	65	180	118	104	269	45	69	55
Wayne	7	7	4	2			1			
Weakley	41	34	7	14	7	4	2		5	2
White	25	19	9	3	4		3		5	1
Williamson	978	806	70	251	120	253	112	67	66	39
Wilson	122	107	15	30	29	25	8	2	9	4
Texas	54,971	44,813	5,233	12,456	8,478	9,526	9,120	2,229	5,231	2,698
Anderson	69	57	8	19	14	12	4		12	
Andrews	9	8	3	2	2		1		1	
Angelina	154	130	19	47	27	24	13	1	20	3
Aransas	37	19	5	6	2	6			18	
Archer	4	4	1	2		1				
Atascosa	24	24	7	7	4	4	2			
Austin	17	9	3	2	1	2	1		7	1
Bailey	5	5	4		1					
Bandera	20	15	1	4	1	6	3		4	1
Bastrop	37	28	9	8	4	4	3	2	7	
Baylor	2	2					2			
Bee	21	18	7	4	5	1	1		3	
Bell	1,120	909	70	215	123	148	353	49	116	46
Bexar	5,919	4,830	422	1,177	771	981	1,479	316	497	276
Blanco	10	7	3	1		3		1	2	
Bosque	20	11	5	2	2	1	1		9	
Bowie	295	243	39	63	67	58	16	2	44	6
Brazoria	757	628	67	189	56	97	219	13	38	78
Brazos	449	371	69	93	77	81	51	20	36	22
Brewster	15	9	2	1	3	2	1	1	5	
Brooks	3	1					1		2	
Brown	67	56	12	16	16	10	2	2	7	2
Burleson	6	4	2	1		1			2	
Burnet	53	40	11	10	4	8	7	3	10	
Caldwell	22	19	8	6	2	3			3	
Calhoun	21	17	5	6	2	1	3		3	1
Callahan	3	2	1			1			1	
Cameron	567	477	65	183	101	71	57	11	62	17
Camp	13	11	7	3			1		2	
Cass	17	15	11		1		3		1	1
Castro	3	3	2		1					
Chambers	7	5	3	1			1		2	
Cherokee	69	57	7	11	11	19	9	2	10	
Childress	10	9	7		2				1	
Clay	7	5	3			1	1		2	
Cochran	1							1		
Coke	3	3		1		2				
Coleman	7	4	4						3	
Collin	1,684	1,469	168	494	281	373	153	31	98	86
Colorado	31	22	11	3	7		1	1	8	
Comal	208	166	38	33	34	40	21	10	29	3
Comanche	12	9	4	1	1	1	2		3	
Concho	1	1				1				
Cooke	26	21	5	6	7	3			5	
Coryell	23	21	9	2	2	4	4	1	1	
Crane	4	3		1	1		1		1	
Crosby	1	1	1							
Culberson	1	1		1						
Dallam	6	6	4		1		1			
Dallas	7,391	5,950	382	1,647	1,137	1,391	1,393	374	629	438
Dawson	10	8	5	2			1		2	

Table 3.11

Physicians by State and County, 2006, continued

State County	Total Physicians	Total Patient Care	FM/GP Practice	Medical Specialties	Surgical Specialties	Other Specialties	Hospital Based Practice	Other Professional Activity	Inactive	Not Classified
			Major Professional Activity							
			Patient Care							
			Office-Based Practice							
De Witt	10	8	5	1	2				2	
Deaf Smith	8	6	3	1	2				2	
Denton	940	802	115	268	166	164	89	25	81	32
Dimmit	10	7	2	2	2	1		1	2	
Donley	1	1	1							
Eastland	10	7	7						3	
Ector	272	222	19	67	50	29	57	11	19	20
Edwards	3	1	1					1	1	
El Paso	1,405	1,150	89	324	228	204	305	56	128	71
Ellis	127	114	25	35	31	9	14	1	12	
Erath	39	35	11	8	11	5			4	
Falls	14	13	2		2	4	5		1	
Fannin	20	17	2	2	1	2	10		3	
Fayette	20	14	4	1	5		4		6	
Fisher	3	2		2				1		
Floyd	6	6	5	1						
Fort Bend	1,031	862	140	265	127	196	134	26	81	62
Franklin	7	6	4	1			1		1	
Freestone	5	4	3		1				1	
Frio	8	7	5	1			1		1	
Gaines	7	7	4	1	2					
Galveston	1,473	1,138	71	198	126	197	546	121	94	120
Garza	1	1	1							
Gillespie	103	76	16	18	21	15	6	2	25	
Goliad	2	2		1	1					
Gonzales	14	11	4	4		3			3	
Gray	26	23	5	10	5	1	2		3	
Grayson	241	194	24	61	48	46	15	2	42	3
Gregg	314	265	35	87	68	61	14	3	38	8
Grimes	14	8	2	3		2	1		5	1
Guadalupe	129	102	18	15	18	12	39	8	13	6
Hale	28	22	5	7	6	4		1	5	
Hall	2	1	1						1	
Hamilton	10	10	5	1	1	2	1			
Hansford	1	1	1							
Hardeman	4	3		2		1			1	
Hardin	25	21	7	5	5	4			4	
Harris	11,973	9,487	784	2,644	1,714	2,028	2,317	626	942	918
Harrison	50	41	8	13	8	8	4		9	
Haskell	2	1	1						1	
Hays	180	140	30	37	28	31	14	4	34	2
Hemphill	4	4	3	1						
Henderson	71	61	20	12	15	12	2		9	1
Hidalgo	851	759	142	295	151	112	59	12	53	27
Hill	27	16	9	2	4	1			10	1
Hockley	17	17	8	5	2		2			
Hood	66	48	9	12	12	7	8	2	13	3
Hopkins	38	34	11	9	7	5	2		4	
Houston	10	9	6		1	1	1		1	
Howard	64	51	7	10	11	9	14	1	9	3
Hudspeth	1	1	1							
Hunt	66	53	15	13	14	10	1	1	11	1
Hutchinson	19	16	6	3	5	1	1		3	
Irion	1	1	1							
Jack	4	4	2	1	1					
Jackson	4	4		1	1		2			
Jasper	34	31	16	5	8	1	1		3	
Jeff Davis	3	1	1						2	

Table 3.11

Physicians by State and County, 2006, continued

State County	Total Physicians	Total Patient Care	FM/GP Practice	Medical Specialties	Surgical Specialties	Other Specialties	Hospital Based Practice	Other Professional Activity	Inactive	Not Classified
Jefferson	606	510	62	164	122	142	20	9	81	6
Jim Hogg	2	2	2							
Jim Wells	33	29	7	12	6	2	2		3	1
Johnson	135	100	23	24	19	19	15	6	23	6
Jones	6	4	2	1	1				2	
Karnes	6	5	4				1		1	
Kaufman	72	59	16	12	10	8	13		10	3
Kendall	183	145	14	28	19	54	30	7	29	2
Kent	1							1		
Kerr	202	133	13	40	31	30	19	6	60	3
Kimble	4	2	2						2	
Kinney	1								1	
Kleberg	34	27	9	8	3	2	5		7	
Knox	1	1					1			
Lamar	123	100	7	31	33	26	3	4	19	
Lamb	6	3	3						3	
Lampasas	18	16	9			4	3		2	
Lavaca	19	16	9	2	1	3	1		2	1
Lee	3	3	2	1						
Leon	7	3	2			1		1	3	
Liberty	41	32	10	11	8	3		1	7	1
Limestone	12	10	5	2		1	2		1	1
Live Oak	1	1	1							
Llano	42	27	18	2	5	2		3	12	
Lubbock	1,091	895	84	229	167	186	229	46	98	52
Lynn	3	3	2		1					
Madison	5	4	3			1			1	
Marion	4	2			1		1		2	
Martin	2	2	2							
Mason	1	1					1			
Matagorda	37	32	9	9	10	2	2	3	2	
Maverick	39	32	5	12	8	4	3		3	4
Mc Culloch	5	4	3				1		1	
Mc Lennan	529	430	78	80	88	98	86	24	63	12
Medina	31	23	12	2	2	4	3		6	2
Menard	2	2	1				1			
Midland	233	210	17	66	48	56	23	6	13	4
Milam	18	14	5	2	1	4	2	2	2	
Mills	3								3	
Mitchell	4	3	1				2		1	
Montague	16	10	8	1	1			1	5	
Montgomery	758	641	115	200	134	138	54	16	79	22
Moore	13	10	5	1	1	2	1	1		2
Morris	5	4	2	1		1			1	
Nacogdoches	131	117	23	32	33	25	4		13	1
Navarro	62	44	11	15	12	4	2	1	16	1
Newton	8	4	3		1				4	
Nolan	8	6	2	1	1	2			2	
Nueces	964	783	96	238	162	167	120	21	115	45
Ochiltree	4	3	3						1	
Orange	47	36	12	8	8	7	1	2	8	1
Palo Pinto	24	22	6	5	8	3			2	
Panola	9	8	5	2	1				1	
Parker	87	67	14	15	12	19	7	3	14	3
Parmer	5	4	3				1		1	
Pecos	8	8	4	2	1		1			
Polk	58	36	9	14	6	2	5	6	14	2
Potter	446	377	29	109	95	73	71	19	38	12
Presidio	5	5	3			2				
Rains	3	3	1	2						

Table 3.11

Physicians by State and County, 2006, continued

State County	Total Physicians	Total Patient Care	FM/GP Practice	Medical Specialties	Surgical Specialties	Other Specialties	Hospital Based Practice	Other Professional Activity	Inactive	Not Classified
Randall	239	195	29	58	30	42	36	8	24	12
Reagan	2	1	1						1	
Real	1	1				1				
Red River	9	6	1	1	1	1	2	1	2	
Reeves	7	6	1	3	1		1		1	
Refugio	2	2	2							
Robertson	3	2		1		1			1	
Rockwall	119	103	19	15	22	27	20	2	9	5
Runnels	8	7	5				2		1	
Rusk	39	31	14	4	5	7	1	1	7	
Sabine	5	4	1	2		1			1	
San Augustine	5	4	3	1					1	
San Jacinto	6	4	1	2			1		2	
San Patricio	34	30	7	9	2	6	6		4	
Schleicher	4	3	2				1		1	
Scurry	13	13	8	2		1	2			
Shackelford	3	2	2						1	
Shelby	13	11	7	2	2				2	
Smith	777	645	75	197	144	145	84	31	93	8
Somervell	9	8	6	2					1	
Starr	18	15	7	6	1		1	1	1	1
Stephens	6	5	5					1		
Stonewall	1	1		1						
Sutton	2	2	2							
Swisher	5	3	1				2		2	
Tarrant	3,027	2,563	303	773	594	609	284	83	299	82
Taylor	313	267	38	81	66	57	25	7	37	2
Terry	8	5	4	1					3	
Throckmorton	1	1					1			
Titus	44	39	5	7	14	12	1		4	1
Tom Green	239	204	20	54	58	51	21	1	29	5
Travis	2,921	2,416	284	722	503	671	236	123	293	89
Trinity	5	5	1	4						
Tyler	14	10	5	1		2	2		3	1
Upshur	18	11	8	1		2		2	5	
Upton	2	1	1						1	
Uvalde	31	26	10	6	5	1	4		4	1
Val Verde	50	42	9	11	11	4	7	2	3	3
Van Zandt	16	11	5		1	3	2		5	
Victoria	213	183	25	58	43	43	14	6	22	2
Walker	62	51	15	12	12	10	2	2	8	1
Waller	8	5	2	1			2		3	
Ward	5	5	3	1			1			
Washington	51	38	8	12	12	4	2	1	12	
Webb	251	211	38	70	46	35	22	2	28	10
Wharton	57	46	11	17	13	3	2		11	
Wheeler	6	4	3	1					2	
Wichita	345	289	51	74	56	64	44	8	39	9
Wilbarger	18	16	4	2	2	4	4		2	
Willacy	6	6	4	1			1			
Williamson	497	394	96	108	75	65	50	10	76	17
Wilson	25	19	8	3		2	6	1	5	
Winkler	3	2		2						1
Wise	38	32	10	7	9	3	3		5	1
Wood	31	24	11	7	4	2			7	
Yoakum	5	4	2	1			1	1		
Young	16	15	9	1	3		2		1	
Zapata	4	4	1	1		1	1			
Zavala	6	6	3	1	1		1			

Table 3.11

Physicians by State and County, 2006, continued

State County	Total Physicians	Total Patient Care	FM/GP Practice	Medical Specialties	Surgical Specialties	Other Specialties	Hospital Based Practice	Other Professional Activity	Inactive	Not Classified
Utah	6,093	4,862	621	1,202	955	1,105	979	286	692	253
Beaver	8	5	5						2	1
Box Elder	37	29	12	5	8	4		1	6	1
Cache	181	149	20	35	42	31	21	2	28	2
Carbon	27	25	5	5	10	4	1	1	1	
Davis	467	383	69	80	80	87	67	8	59	17
Duchesne	23	18	3	6	6	1	2		1	4
Emery	1									1
Garfield	1	1	1							
Grand	21	16	7	2	2	3	2		5	
Iron	43	34	6	9	10	7	2	1	7	1
Juab	8	8	5		2		1			
Kane	6	4	2	1			1		2	
Millard	9	8	7				1	1		
Morgan	9	9	3	1		4	1			
Piute	1	1			1					
Rich	1								1	
Salt Lake	3,622	2,849	235	751	501	666	696	235	341	197
San Juan	4	3	3						1	
Sanpete	27	24	17	1	1	2	3	1	2	
Sevier	9	9	6	1	1	1				
Summit	176	134	15	29	18	49	23	5	29	8
Tooele	33	29	9	6	7	4	3		4	
Uintah	24	24	7	5	5	3	4			
Utah	679	573	102	136	127	119	89	12	82	12
Wasatch	25	20	7	4	3	6			5	
Washington	251	190	30	47	51	46	16	4	53	4
Wayne	3	2			1	1		1		
Weber	397	315	45	78	79	67	46	14	63	5
Vermont	2,659	1,980	259	472	309	378	562	155	396	128
Addison	99	75	18	20	18	8	11	2	21	1
Bennington	150	107	16	27	25	24	15	12	29	2
Caledonia	66	52	16	10	11	7	8	2	12	
Chittenden	1,274	945	82	207	124	180	352	92	137	100
Essex	4	4	2	1		1				
Franklin	70	55	7	18	14	10	6	2	12	1
Grand Isle	19	15	1	4	1	9		1	2	1
Lamoille	70	48	17	6	6	10	9	1	20	1
Orange	70	48	6	15	10	7	10	5	16	1
Orleans	60	49	8	11	9	10	11	1	10	
Rutland	179	131	23	37	27	21	23	6	36	6
Washington	172	134	21	37	26	29	21	7	28	3
Windham	143	113	23	30	19	28	13	4	23	3
Windsor	283	204	19	49	19	34	83	20	50	9
Virginia	23,545	18,538	2,097	5,216	3,281	3,712	4,232	1,019	2,914	1,074
Accomack	34	21	3	4	3	5	6	1	11	1
Albemarle	755	566	50	140	67	112	197	43	93	53
Alexandria (ic)	539	426	34	109	87	90	106	28	54	31
Alleghany	25	19	3	5	5	1	5		6	
Amelia	3	2					2		1	
Amherst	15	10	8			1	1		5	
Appomattox	4	4	3	1						
Arlington	854	655	30	170	103	127	225	49	73	77
Augusta	105	89	22	17	25	18	7	1	14	1
Bath	7	3	2		1				4	
Bedford	102	69	27	9	12	13	8	2	30	1
Bland	3	3	1	1		1				
Botetourt	39	27	11	2	3	5	6		9	3
Bristol (ic)	11	6		2		3	1		5	

Table 3.11

Physicians by State and County, 2006, continued

State County	Total Physicians	Total Patient Care	FM/GP Practice	Medical Specialties	Surgical Specialties	Other Specialties	Hospital Based Practice	Other Professional Activity	Inactive	Not Classified
				Office-Based Practice						
Brunswick	7	5	2	2		1			2	
Buchanan	22	14	2	8	1	1	2		7	1
Buckingham	5	3	2	1					1	1
Buena Vista (ic)	3	3	2	1						
Campbell	13	10	10						3	
Caroline	7	5	2	2		1			2	
Carroll	14	10	8	2					4	
Charles City	3	2		2					1	
Charlotte	7	7	4	1		1	1			
Charlottesville (ic)	1,201	864	27	149	92	152	444	113	73	151
Chesapeake	617	547	73	137	100	81	156	18	36	16
Chesterfield	915	751	106	215	105	170	155	30	94	40
Clarke	29	22	4	8	1	5	4	2	5	
Clifton Forge (ic)	4	4		1		2	1			
Colonial Heights	65	49	5	23	11	6	4	4	12	
Covington (ic)	10	7		1	3	2	1		3	
Culpeper	52	40	6	13	13	6	2	1	10	1
Cumberland	5	3	2			1			2	
Danville (ic)	176	148	12	55	38	30	13		24	4
Dickenson	12	11	4	5	1		1		1	
Dinwiddie	10	6	4	1	1				4	
Essex	21	17	2	5	4	3	3	1	3	
Fairfax	4,082	3,283	261	1,122	578	751	571	205	416	178
Fairfax (ic)	129	99	9	39	16	25	10	3	14	13
Falls Church (ic)	100	83	6	32	15	17	13	4	10	3
Fauquier	114	92	14	27	19	27	5	4	18	
Floyd	13	9	3	1	1	3	1		4	
Fluvanna	49	44	4	11		4	25	2	2	1
Franklin	60	47	17	11	5	8	6	1	10	2
Franklin (ic)	31	27	9	6	5	6	1		4	
Frederick	113	94	11	24	16	36	7		14	5
Fredericksburg (ic)	181	160	10	60	43	32	15	4	14	3
Galax (ic)	46	40	7	13	10	5	5	1	4	1
Giles	20	13	6	2	4		1		6	1
Gloucester	67	49	6	16	12	11	4	3	14	1
Goochland	63	46	10	7	6	13	10	5	12	
Grayson	5	5	1	1	1	1	1			
Greene	15	12	2	2		3	5	1	1	1
Greensville	19	18	6	7	3		2			1
Halifax	72	60	5	24	17	12	2	3	9	
Hampton City (ic)	237	192	33	47	32	36	44	9	33	3
Hanover	179	148	26	50	21	28	23	3	20	8
Harrisonburg (ic)	212	170	27	46	42	40	15	4	36	2
Henrico	1,743	1,278	111	375	273	255	264	75	317	73
Henry	10	8	4		2	1	1		2	
Highland	5	3	2	1					2	
Hopewell (ic)	39	36	8	14	7	5	2		3	
Isle Of Wight	55	47	9	10	5	13	10	1	7	
James City	372	282	33	68	53	72	56	14	70	6
King And Queen	6	4	1	1			1	1	2	
King George	9	6	3		2	1			2	
King William	11	8	7				1		3	
Lancaster	61	40	10	11	9	4	6	2	18	1
Lee	32	26	5	9	7	3	2	1	2	3
Lexington (ic)	47	37	10	12	6	4	5		10	
Loudoun	579	456	55	162	81	87	71	33	60	30
Louisa	23	8	4	2	1	1		1	13	1
Lunenburg	6	5	5						1	
Lynchburg (ic)	398	315	33	96	74	67	45	13	67	3
Madison	15	10	3	2	1	1	3		4	1

Table 3.11

Physicians by State and County, 2006, continued

State County	Total Physicians	Total Patient Care	FM/GP Practice	Medical Specialties	Surgical Specialties	Other Specialties	Hospital Based Practice	Other Professional Activity	Inactive	Not Classified
				Major Professional Activity						
				Patient Care						
				Office-Based Practice						
Manassas (ic)	138	117	21	36	31	17	12	3	15	3
Martinsville (ic)	100	76	10	27	19	16	4	1	23	
Mathews	11	3	1	1		1		1	7	
Mecklenburg	51	36	11	7	6	4	8	4	9	2
Middlesex	17	12	6	1	1	1	3		5	
Montgomery	173	143	22	36	34	30	21	4	21	5
Nelson	39	23	6	4	1	7	5	5	11	
New Kent	13	7	4	1			2	2	3	1
Newport News (ic)	476	389	53	106	92	58	80	13	62	12
Norfolk (ic)	1,145	931	39	287	181	139	285	50	105	59
Northampton	51	39	5	15	10	5	4	1	11	
Northumberland	22	12	6	2	1	1	2		9	1
Norton (ic)	47	43	7	13	18	4	1		3	1
Nottoway	26	18	13	1		1	3	1	5	2
Orange	46	34	14	7	3	3	7	3	7	2
Page	18	12	5	3	2	1	1	2	4	
Patrick	14	7	4	2	1				6	1
Petersburg (ic)	80	55	8	13	12	13	9		24	1
Pittsylvania	8	5	4			1			3	
Poquoson (ic)	40	30	1	5	5	9	10	4	5	1
Portsmouth (ic)	328	252	19	43	36	39	115	17	40	19
Powhatan	21	18	10	2	1	1	4		2	1
Prince Edward	42	37	5	12	9	6	5		5	
Prince George	13	10	3	3	1	1	2		2	1
Prince William	394	322	56	114	56	51	45	7	50	15
Pulaski	50	40	11	11	6	7	5		10	
Radford (ic)	59	48	7	12	8	16	5	1	10	
Rappahannock	8	6	2	1		2	1		2	
Richmond	2								2	
Richmond (ic)	1,122	821	46	184	94	146	351	98	91	112
Roanoke	433	349	42	60	58	85	104	10	54	20
Roanoke (ic)	471	374	14	104	72	69	115	27	54	16
Rockbridge	6	3		1			2	1	2	
Rockingham	56	37	14	5	4	11	3	1	18	
Russell	20	18	4	8		2	4		2	
Salem (ic)	185	144	15	42	25	21	41	5	29	7
Scott	10	8	8						2	
Shenandoah	42	35	10	9	5	6	5	1	6	
Smyth	68	53	9	10	13	10	11	1	13	1
Southampton	6	2		1			1	1	3	
Spotsylvania	154	130	22	38	17	43	10	4	14	6
Stafford	99	72	14	26	12	13	7	2	20	5
Staunton (ic)	87	62	7	13	13	19	10	3	21	1
Suffolk (ic)	290	250	24	69	41	45	71	3	23	14
Surry	2	1	1							1
Sussex	3	3	3							
Tazewell	130	118	15	45	18	23	17		8	4
Virginia Beach (ic)	1,234	993	139	257	192	252	153	45	171	25
Warren	41	33	8	7	8	3	7		6	2
Washington	122	103	17	26	25	20	15		19	
Waynesboro (ic)	67	39	9	10	5	8	7		24	4
Westmoreland	8	4	2			2			4	
Williamsburg (ic)	11	9	1	1		4	3		2	
Winchester (ic)	245	208	15	73	71	32	17	5	28	4
Wise	49	43	10	15	5	6	7		3	3
Wythe	52	45	14	7	6	10	8	1	6	
York	188	168	34	37	19	38	40	5	15	

Table 3.11

Physicians by State and County, 2006, continued

State County	Total Physicians	Total Patient Care	FM/GP Practice	Medical Specialties	Surgical Specialties	Other Specialties	Hospital Based Practice	Other Professional Activity	Inactive	Not Classified
Major Professional Activity										
Patient Care										
Office-Based Practice										
Virgin Islands	200	167	17	35	45	27	43	2	23	8
St. Croix	91	75	7	16	19	10	23	2	12	2
St. John	6	6	2	1	1		2			
St. Thomas	103	86	8	18	25	17	18		11	6
Washington	19,864	15,168	2,448	3,941	2,558	3,513	2,708	1,066	2,899	731
Adams	15	11	8	1	2				3	1
Asotin	43	35	10	7	7	8	3		8	
Benton	359	294	44	88	56	67	39	9	49	7
Chelan	254	208	39	57	43	54	15	9	35	2
Clallam	215	132	40	33	21	23	15	15	66	2
Clark	772	612	108	194	120	129	61	23	111	26
Columbia	4	3	2	1					1	
Cowlitz	212	172	29	49	38	46	10	2	36	2
Douglas	33	20	9	8	1	1	1	1	12	
Ferry	5	4	1			1	2		1	
Franklin	60	54	12	17	12	7	6	1	4	1
Garfield	2	1		1					1	
Grant	76	64	25	17	11	6	5	2	10	
Grays Harbor	75	57	13	19	12	12	1	1	14	3
Island	178	127	24	17	20	25	41	9	42	
Jefferson	93	50	18	10	6	11	5	10	32	1
King	9,378	7,042	869	1,871	1,077	1,661	1,564	696	1,113	527
Kitsap	662	488	77	107	78	122	104	34	124	16
Kittitas	48	37	18	5	8	3	3		11	
Klickitat	24	17	14	1		1	1	1	4	2
Lewis	101	78	20	19	21	14	4	4	18	1
Lincoln	8	5	3			1	1	2	1	
Mason	54	30	8	4	9	6	3	3	19	2
Okanogan	63	47	26	6	3	8	4		15	1
Pacific	24	14	3	2	3	4	2		10	
Pend Oreille	11	7	3		1		3		4	
Pierce	1,994	1,625	215	408	291	349	362	60	261	48
San Juan	64	32	9	7	3	9	4	3	29	
Skagit	330	255	74	51	50	66	14	6	66	3
Skamania	6	4	2		1	1			2	
Snohomish	1,157	892	186	244	158	221	83	40	195	30
Spokane	1,456	1,129	182	285	229	285	148	59	244	24
Stevens	49	42	19	8	3	3	9	1	6	
Thurston	707	558	116	132	87	141	82	33	105	11
Wahkiakum	4	2	1			1		1	1	
Walla Walla	233	174	32	47	35	40	20	3	55	1
Whatcom	565	431	97	110	71	108	45	22	105	7
Whitman	72	53	15	15	9	9	5		18	1
Yakima	458	362	77	100	72	70	43	16	68	12
West Virginia	4,710	3,762	505	922	667	708	960	189	544	215
Barbour	9	7	2	3			2		2	
Berkeley	160	126	20	34	21	15	36	5	27	2
Boone	9	7	3	2	1	1			1	1
Braxton	7	6	3	2	1				1	
Brooke	6	5	4				1		1	
Cabell	608	488	44	119	87	97	141	34	44	42
Calhoun	1								1	
Clay	5	3	2	1					2	
Doddridge	2	1		1					1	
Fayette	48	38	10	11	4	4	9		9	1
Gilmer	2	2	2							
Grant	16	13	3	1	1	4	4	2	1	
Greenbrier	86	64	5	27	15	10	7		21	1
Hampshire	13	12	3	3	1	1	4		1	
Hancock	69	58	8	18	10	15	7	2	7	2

Table 3.11

Physicians by State and County, 2006, continued

State / County	Total Physicians	Total Patient Care	Office-Based Practice FM/GP Practice	Medical Specialties	Surgical Specialties	Other Specialties	Hospital Based Practice	Other Professional Activity	Inactive	Not Classified
Hardy	10	7	2	2	1	2		1	2	
Harrison	196	160	30	43	27	18	42	7	25	4
Jackson	17	11	2	3	2	2	2		6	
Jefferson	75	48	15	8	5	7	13	6	14	7
Kanawha	898	736	70	195	156	151	164	34	95	33
Lewis	23	18	1	6	5	3	3	1	4	
Lincoln	6	4	3				1		1	1
Logan	54	47	11	11	10	5	10	1	3	3
Marion	99	77	10	27	14	10	16		19	3
Marshall	34	29	4	8	6	6	5		4	1
Mason	29	26	5	8	8	2	3		2	1
Mc Dowell	16	13	7	2		2	2		2	1
Mercer	155	134	14	39	25	37	19	2	19	
Mineral	24	19	4	3	2	5	5		5	
Mingo	27	20	5	8	3	3	1		5	2
Monongalia	893	693	37	119	99	129	309	64	49	87
Monroe	5	3	2			1		1	1	
Morgan	12	7	4	2			1		4	1
Nicholas	33	31	10	6	5	3	7	1		1
Ohio	270	218	26	47	43	49	53	5	44	3
Pendleton	5	4	2	1		1				1
Pleasants	3	3	1	1			1			
Pocahontas	10	4	2			1	1	1	5	
Preston	29	18	8	1	3	3	3	4	7	
Putnam	81	71	20	21	8	15	7	1	4	5
Raleigh	212	174	12	59	42	36	25	6	28	4
Randolph	62	52	13	11	12	6	10		8	2
Ritchie	3	2	2						1	
Roane	22	16	6	4	3	2	1	1	3	2
Summers	12	9	3	5		1			3	
Taylor	13	9	6	1	1		1	1	2	1
Tucker	9	5	4				1		3	1
Tyler	5	4	1	1			2		1	
Upshur	30	21	6	3	5	2	5		9	
Wayne	51	39	8	8	3	6	14	5	6	1
Webster	3	2					2		1	
Wetzel	18	15	5	4	1	2	3		3	
Wirt	2	2		1			1			
Wood	215	175	33	41	36	50	15	4	35	1
Wyoming	8	6	2	1	1	1	1		2	
Wisconsin	16,154	13,126	1,994	3,443	2,253	2,921	2,515	677	1,897	454
Adams	6	5	1	1		1	2		1	
Ashland	60	55	16	9	16	11	3		5	
Barron	90	79	35	11	15	14	4		11	
Bayfield	20	11	6		1	3	1	1	8	
Brown	650	566	63	167	142	144	50	11	69	4
Buffalo	7	5	4			1			2	
Burnett	9	6	5				1		3	
Calumet	17	13	7	1	1	3	1		3	1
Chippewa	85	68	23	17	14	8	6	3	13	1
Clark	20	14	6	2	2	1	3	1	5	
Columbia	67	56	22	14	7	5	8	1	10	
Crawford	25	16	11	1	2	1	1	1	8	
Dane	2,845	2,200	234	504	301	463	698	227	296	122
Dodge	111	99	36	15	24	15	9		10	2
Door	84	43	10	10	3	11	9	2	39	
Douglas	36	32	13	7	3	3	6	2	2	
Dunn	41	32	11	9	6	1	5	1	8	
Eau Claire	435	375	51	112	86	90	36	9	41	10

Table 3.11

Physicians by State and County, 2006, continued

State County	Total Physicians	Total Patient Care	FM/GP Practice	Medical Specialties	Surgical Specialties	Other Specialties	Hospital Based Practice	Other Professional Activity	Inactive	Not Classified
			Office-Based Practice							

Major Professional Activity — Patient Care

State County	Total Physicians	Total Patient Care	FM/GP Practice	Medical Specialties	Surgical Specialties	Other Specialties	Hospital Based Practice	Other Professional Activity	Inactive	Not Classified
Florence	5	3		2	1				2	
Fond Du Lac	197	168	29	51	30	37	21	3	24	2
Forest	4	4	2	2						
Grant	46	35	18	4	4	3	6	2	8	1
Green	80	57	7	22	10	12	6	2	21	
Green Lake	29	21	6	2	6	3	4	1	6	1
Iowa	22	17	9	1	4	1	2	1	4	
Iron	5	3		2	1				2	
Jackson	28	24	19	1	1	2	1	1	2	1
Jefferson	74	63	20	14	13	4	12	1	9	1
Juneau	24	22	13		3		5	1	2	
Kenosha	243	201	31	54	40	50	26	6	30	6
Kewaunee	16	8	4	2		1	1	1	6	1
La Crosse	611	517	58	146	88	126	99	13	67	14
Lafayette	10	6	5			1		1	2	1
Langlade	29	21	7	3	3	4	4		8	
Lincoln	36	29	16	4	2	4	3		6	1
Manitowoc	160	132	21	42	32	19	18		27	1
Marathon	380	307	61	84	60	76	26	19	46	8
Marinette	75	61	10	22	12	10	7	2	12	
Marquette	5	4	2				2		1	
Menominee	4	4	3				1			
Milwaukee	3,603	2,920	242	784	495	602	797	195	326	162
Monroe	56	47	24	5	3	3	12	3	6	
Oconto	29	23	11	5	2	3	2		5	1
Oneida	169	141	13	44	39	31	14	2	26	
Outagamie	410	346	65	92	77	74	38	11	46	7
Ozaukee	434	368	39	114	57	124	34	19	46	1
Pepin	5	4	2	1	1				1	
Pierce	35	23	18	2	1	2		1	11	
Polk	65	50	31	6	6	3	4	3	11	1
Portage	129	107	17	26	22	21	21	4	17	1
Price	15	12	7	2		1	2		3	
Racine	367	313	57	81	62	74	39	6	41	7
Richland	29	22	12	3	3	3	1		6	1
Rock	344	279	39	86	44	55	55	13	44	8
Rusk	14	11	3	6	1		1		3	
Sauk	96	86	41	14	16	7	8	4	6	
Sawyer	28	22	13	1	1	5	2	1	5	
Shawano	37	29	20		3	1	5		8	
Sheboygan	203	169	36	43	45	39	6		32	2
St. Croix	90	65	27	8	11	13	6	4	16	5
Taylor	12	10	3	4	1		2		2	
Trempealeau	35	27	9	6	3	5	4	1	6	1
Vernon	38	33	16	3	5	5	4		5	
Vilas	33	18	11		1	3	3		13	2
Walworth	111	82	26	15	17	16	8	2	27	
Washburn	22	16	12	1	2		1		5	1
Washington	173	138	32	39	22	32	13	6	23	6
Waukesha	1,782	1,478	155	438	217	431	237	55	198	51
Waupaca	66	48	29	3	4	7	5		17	1
Waushara	16	13	6	1	2	4			3	
Winnebago	470	397	49	111	80	120	37	11	61	1
Wood	547	447	34	161	77	102	73	24	59	17
Wyoming	1,132	903	185	175	215	205	123	38	182	9
Albany	84	74	10	9	20	20	15		10	
Big Horn	10	7	6				1		3	
Campbell	58	54	10	13	14	12	5		3	
Carbon	16	13	6		2	3	2	1	2	

Table 3.11

Physicians by State and County, 2006, continued

State County	Total Physicians	Total Patient Care	Major Professional Activity — Patient Care — Office-Based Practice				Hospital Based Practice	Other Professional Activity	Inactive	Not Classified
			FM/GP Practice	Medical Specialties	Surgical Specialties	Other Specialties				
Converse	19	15	5	2	4	1	3		4	
Crook	4	3	2				1		1	
Fremont	99	81	20	11	15	23	12	1	17	
Goshen	14	10	6	1	2		1		4	
Hot Springs	7	7	2		3		2			
Johnson	14	11	7	1	1	2			3	
Laramie	254	197	30	50	48	40	29	13	41	3
Lincoln	10	9	5		1		3		1	
Natrona	188	151	25	38	38	33	17	6	27	4
Niobrara	1	1					1			
Park	71	62	16	9	12	14	11	1	8	
Platte	9	8	3	1	1	2	1		1	
Sheridan	71	51	6	11	13	13	8	3	16	1
Sublette	11	7	3	1		1	2	2	2	
Sweetwater	38	32	9	7	7	8	1	1	5	
Teton	104	69	3	15	25	22	4	7	27	1
Uinta	33	28	4	6	4	11	3	2	3	
Washakie	9	8	4		3		1		1	
Weston	8	5	3		2				3	
Pacific Islands	238	193	42	50	31	20	50	11	18	16
American Samoa	13	5	1	1	1		2	2	4	2
Fed States Of Micronesia	4	3	1	1			1	1		
Guam	216	181	38	47	29	20	47	8	14	13
Marshall Islands	1	1	1							
Palau	4	3	1	1	1					1
APO SF	1,029	898	116	104	108	118	452	52	19	60
APO SF	1,029	898	116	104	108	118	452	52	19	60

Note: Does not include 9 physicians whose county could not be determined.

Table 3.12

Physicians in Metropolitan Areas by Self-Designated Specialty and Activity, 2006

Specialty	Total Physicians	Major Professional Activity								
		Patient Care					Other Professional Activity			
					Hospital Based					
		Total Patient Care	Office Based	Locum Tenens	Resid./ Fellows	Phys. Staff	Admin.	Med. Teach.	Research	Other
Total Physicians	709,321	558,108	427,019	996	80,436	49,657	11,376	8,235	11,403	3,499
GP/FM Prac	62,968	60,334	49,314	187	6,653	4,180	1,092	1,146	186	210
FM	56,221	53,876	43,710	156	6,653	3,357	929	1,126	155	135
GP	6,747	6,458	5,604	31		823	163	20	31	75
Med. Spec.	230,614	215,752	162,555	280	34,981	17,936	3,990	3,436	6,561	875
AI	3,441	3,085	2,741	1	205	138	47	35	256	18
CD	17,676	16,620	13,745	10	1,696	1,169	194	258	539	65
D	8,605	8,424	7,139	6	916	363	30	62	77	12
GE	9,795	9,293	7,882	3	851	557	85	131	266	20
IM	123,186	114,647	83,665	130	21,004	9,848	2,427	1,804	3,826	482
PD	58,240	54,811	40,538	124	9,188	4,961	1,026	946	1,204	253
PDC	1,556	1,443	1,027		222	194	24	23	63	3
PUD	8,115	7,429	5,818	6	899	706	157	177	330	22
Sur. Spec.	124,670	121,283	97,266	90	16,543	7,384	1,060	1,211	733	383
CRS	1,083	1,059	944		55	60	7	11	3	3
GS	28,285	27,328	18,659	25	6,443	2,201	356	306	186	109
NS	4,319	4,198	3,262	5	628	303	30	37	31	23
OBG	33,015	31,979	26,476	31	3,495	1,977	340	434	200	62
OPH	14,252	13,959	12,411	3	941	604	72	94	103	24
ORS	18,467	18,092	14,477	11	2,687	917	80	116	69	110
OTO	7,681	7,534	6,287	4	863	380	48	64	25	10
PS	5,786	5,689	4,928		538	223	19	43	16	19
TS	3,857	3,707	3,199	3	208	297	43	41	58	8
U	7,925	7,738	6,623	8	685	422	65	65	42	15
Oth. Spec.	174,369	160,739	117,884	439	22,259	20,157	5,234	2,442	3,923	2,031
AM	316	199	118		5	76	87	2	18	10
AN	32,549	31,675	24,965	81	3,812	2,817	218	399	192	65
CHP	5,905	5,495	4,348	11	477	659	161	113	101	35
DR	19,014	18,425	13,257	76	3,318	1,774	113	195	96	185
EM	23,163	22,314	15,430	40	3,401	3,443	504	224	63	58
FOP	548	381	332		23	26	37	7	5	118
GPM	1,686	1,318	947	3	181	187	171	31	119	47
MG	421	316	192		62	62	19	22	60	4
N	11,326	10,337	8,059	15	1,321	942	146	200	580	63
NM	1,200	1,085	775	1	98	211	31	21	44	19
OM	2,124	1,525	1,243	12	28	242	401	32	72	94
P	33,738	31,180	22,204	108	3,769	5,099	1,144	470	701	243
PHP	1,142	240	173	3	1	63	538	56	240	68
PM	6,210	5,959	4,477	4	729	749	140	40	38	33
PTH	15,084	12,962	8,920	29	2,048	1,965	553	324	617	628
R	6,945	6,575	5,388	37	334	816	69	131	77	93
RO	3,479	3,388	2,645	15	417	311	34	23	30	4
TTS	118	109	88			21		3	6	
OTH	4,050	2,120	1,739	1	34	346	817	121	775	217
UNSP	5,335	5,121	2,570	3	2,201	347	51	28	88	47
VM	16	15	14			1			1	
Not Class	80,071									
Inactive	36,629									

Note: Above excludes Address Unknown.

Subspecialties in this table are condensed into major specialties. See Appendix A.

Table 3.13

Physicians in Rural Areas by Self-Designated Specialty and Activity, 2006

		Major Professional Activity								
		Patient Care					Other Professional Activity			
					Hospital Based					
Specialty	Total Physicians	Total Patient Care	Office Based	Locum Tenens	Resid./ Fellows	Phys. Staff	Admin.	Med. Teach.	Research	Other
Total Physicians	211,908	164,873	132,284	16,664	15,925	3,194	2,034	3,071	896	
GP/FM Prac	30,363	29,513	25,378	1,613	2,522	401	321	56	72	
FM	26,622	25,877	22,146	1,613	2,118	350	309	45	41	
GP	3,741	3,636	3,232		404	51	12	11	31	
Med. Spec.	59,992	56,261	44,432	6,817	5,012	1,032	778	1,707	214	
AI	755	650	568	43	39	15	6	81	3	
CD	4,748	4,460	3,723	394	343	63	61	150	14	
D	2,138	2,063	1,774	184	105	19	16	35	5	
GE	2,471	2,339	1,994	207	138	30	33	66	3	
IM	32,489	30,371	23,464	4,055	2,852	622	381	989	126	
PD	14,953	14,161	11,140	1,704	1,317	242	232	264	54	
PDC	321	296	216	38	42	2	7	15	1	
PUD	2,117	1,921	1,553	192	176	39	42	107	8	
Sur. Spec.	36,677	35,763	29,750	3,565	2,448	302	315	201	96	
CRS	257	249	220	12	17	1	3	3	1	
GS	9,334	9,079	6,972	1,309	798	101	72	57	25	
NS	1,106	1,076	836	173	67	5	12	10	3	
OBG	9,310	9,050	7,714	709	627	79	113	54	14	
OPH	3,802	3,701	3,347	184	170	26	29	37	9	
ORS	5,824	5,721	4,730	639	352	32	33	12	26	
OTO	2,291	2,243	1,908	219	116	18	24	3	3	
PS	1,210	1,191	1,022	113	56	6	5	5	3	
TS	950	917	782	42	93	14	8	7	4	
U	2,593	2,536	2,219	165	152	20	16	13	8	
Oth. Spec.	47,036	43,336	32,724	4,669	5,943	1,459	620	1,107	514	
AM	157	95	52		43	49	5	5	3	
AN	8,644	8,398	6,700	849	849	74	105	52	15	
CHP	1,355	1,260	986	106	168	43	25	24	3	
DR	5,604	5,455	4,238	652	565	31	45	21	52	
EM	6,815	6,540	4,579	628	1,333	171	69	19	16	
FOP	109	87	77	3	7		3	4	15	
GPM	473	362	267	45	50	54	11	32	14	
MG	112	69	41	15	13	5	2	35	1	
N	3,224	2,904	2,345	301	258	43	57	204	16	
NM	277	238	177	23	38	13	7	16	3	
OM	517	366	295	4	67	119	7	10	15	
P	7,636	7,034	5,064	693	1,277	282	109	149	62	
PHP	290	57	42		15	140	12	58	23	
PM	1,526	1,487	1,153	165	169	21	5	10	3	
PTH	4,085	3,500	2,515	469	516	160	73	182	170	
R	1,939	1,830	1,528	81	221	16	35	18	40	
RO	944	925	758	89	78	5	4	9	1	
TTS	33	28	26		2	2		2	1	
OTH	1,115	581	494	5	82	216	38	230	50	
UNSP	2,173	2,112	1,379	541	192	15	8	27	11	
VM	8	8	8							
Not Class	28,221									
Inactive	9,619									

Does not include 195 physicians whose counties could not be determined as rural or metropolitan.

Note: Above excludes Address Unknown.

Subspecialties in this table are condensed into major specialties. See Appendix A.

Table 3.14

Physicians by Metropolitan Area, 2006

Metropolitan Areas	Total Physicians	Major Professional Activity								
		Patient Care					Hospital Based Practice	Other Professional Activity	Inactive	Not Classified
		Total Patient Care	Office-Based Practice							
			FM/GP Practice	Medical Specialties	Surgical Specialties	Other Specialties				
Total Metros	709,096	557,949	49,475	162,799	97,330	118280	130,065	34,504	80,019	36,624
Abilene TX	312	266	38	81	66	57	24	7	37	2
Aguadilla PR	132	116	26	27	13	28	22	3	3	10
Albany GA	222	194	14	70	55	33	22	6	19	3
Albany NY*	2,735	2,159	191	598	429	435	506	153	318	105
Albuquerque NM	2,481	1,903	201	522	267	440	473	151	315	112
Alexandria LA	425	345	35	99	85	65	61	14	55	11
Allentown PA*	1,747	1,433	135	378	308	305	307	52	205	57
Altoona PA	328	263	32	82	53	55	41	7	52	6
Amarillo TX	685	572	58	167	125	115	107	27	62	24
Anchorage AK	1,016	852	122	193	177	200	160	54	88	22
Anniston AL	224	197	27	56	55	30	29	1	24	2
Appleton WI*	870	736	114	202	155	191	74	21	105	8
Asheville NC	775	607	89	176	106	147	89	22	137	9
Athens GA	376	320	22	88	90	79	41	9	43	4
Atlanta GA	11,554	9,324	691	3,025	1,876	2,059	1,673	684	1,046	500
Auburn AL*	114	101	12	31	34	14	10	3	8	2
Augusta GA*	1,996	1,589	112	362	273	286	556	109	209	89
Austin TX*	3,351	2,753	401	816	560	693	283	122	377	99
Bakersfield CA	1,162	979	135	316	173	193	162	34	120	29
Bangor ME	526	426	41	125	74	109	77	27	56	17
Barnstable MA*	780	525	45	190	106	128	56	34	214	7
Baton Rouge LA*	1,700	1,415	140	441	306	307	221	51	188	46
Beaumont TX*	638	533	73	169	124	147	20	10	89	6
Bellingham WA	483	376	86	94	67	89	40	18	82	7
Benton Harbor MI	295	237	43	73	52	48	21	6	47	5
Billings MT	549	462	44	124	107	117	70	14	65	8
Biloxi MS*	726	603	49	182	131	133	108	18	88	17
Binghamton NY	688	533	53	145	115	107	113	31	103	21
Birmingham AL	2,718	2,210	138	633	451	365	623	143	221	144
Bismarck ND	337	281	29	73	56	73	50	11	39	6
Bloomington IL*	343	290	32	84	78	79	17	8	41	4
Bloomington IN	367	286	43	69	57	89	28	12	61	8
Boise City ID	1,229	1,031	163	251	259	228	130	33	153	12
Boston MA*	30,425	23,148	1,170	7,104	3,237	4,898	6,739	2,132	2,581	2,564
Brownsville TX*	555	470	64	183	99	67	57	11	57	17
Bryan TX*	191	159	31	36	38	35	19	5	21	6
Buffalo NY*	3,424	2,687	194	764	489	511	729	183	396	158
Burlington VT	635	466	58	106	71	116	115	55	88	26
Canton OH*	617	507	75	161	73	97	101	12	76	22
Casper WY	188	151	25	38	38	33	17	6	27	4
Cedar Rapids IA	430	338	79	70	68	86	35	13	72	7
Champaign IL*	680	527	63	153	81	97	133	30	90	33
Charleston SC*	2,766	2,244	170	506	385	507	676	157	230	135
Charleston WV	868	707	75	188	141	145	158	33	94	34
Charlotte NC*	4,182	3,507	399	1,124	752	725	507	125	430	120
Charlottesville VA	594	436	38	110	43	96	149	38	79	41
Chattanooga TN	1,215	1,002	102	297	222	197	184	45	146	22
Cheyenne WY	168	128	22	35	31	26	14	8	30	2
Chicago IL*	29,838	23,816	1,843	7,085	3,602	4,671	6,615	1,379	2,682	1,961
Chico CA*	532	418	69	117	94	106	32	10	96	8
Cincinnati OH*	5,448	4,357	405	1,254	710	915	1,073	244	569	278
Clarksville TN*	353	299	34	84	74	67	40	5	40	9
Cleveland OH*	6,596	5,168	389	1,467	818	960	1,534	246	785	397
Colorado Springs CO	491	408	38	100	64	122	84	13	66	4

† Does not include 199 physicians whose MSA could not be determined.

* The metropolitan statistical area name is abbreviated.

Table 3.14

Physicians by Metropolitan Area, 2006, continued

Metropolitan Areas	Total Physicians	Major Professional Activity								
		Patient Care					Hospital Based Practice	Other Professional Activity	Inactive	Not Classified
		Total Patient Care	Office-Based Practice							
			FM/GP Practice	Medical Specialties	Surgical Specialties	Other Specialties				
Columbia MO	935	749	51	163	121	151	263	43	88	55
Columbia SC	2,017	1,672	165	464	307	344	392	97	198	50
Columbus GA	485	383	79	77	82	69	76	16	66	20
Columbus OH	4,625	3,724	457	981	628	766	892	237	400	264
Corpus Christi TX	116	97	12	31	18	23	13	2	17	
Corvalis OR	292	219	27	73	35	60	24	11	59	3
Cumberland MD	228	183	17	53	40	48	25	5	32	8
Dallas TX*	12,721	10,577	1,035	3,124	2,169	2,489	1,760	421	1,133	590
Danville VA	184	153	16	55	38	31	13		27	4
Davenport IA*	686	547	72	155	132	139	49	19	105	15
Daytona Beach FL	880	691	108	208	131	156	88	24	151	14
Dayton OH	2,402	1,939	254	500	308	370	507	102	281	80
Decatur AL	222	192	33	58	50	41	10	2	26	2
Decatur IL	281	235	44	58	49	52	32	5	37	4
Denver CO*	7,548	5,961	649	1,716	1,019	1,386	1,191	437	868	282
Des Moines IA	843	681	60	204	157	151	109	42	96	24
Detroit MI*	16,925	13,295	914	3,728	1,953	2,504	4,196	849	1,584	1,197
Dothan AL	350	307	25	98	84	84	16	3	37	3
Dover DE	214	175	17	60	39	44	15	8	24	7
Dubuque IA	248	208	16	79	56	45	12	4	31	5
Duluth MN*	770	619	133	145	122	131	88	13	121	17
Eau Claire WI	461	396	64	114	89	90	39	9	46	10
Elkhart IN*	297	231	53	47	55	48	28	7	52	7
Elmira NY	264	206	17	79	39	45	26	11	43	4
El Paso TX	1,405	1,150	89	324	228	204	305	56	128	71
Enid OK	132	102	14	22	29	24	13	2	26	2
Erie PA	609	472	75	107	111	90	89	20	106	11
Eugene OR*	959	749	131	214	163	195	46	26	172	12
Evansville IN*	797	671	120	172	142	158	79	16	94	16
Fargo ND*	423	349	56	96	68	76	53	16	47	11
Fayetteville AR*	685	565	108	144	126	96	91	15	93	12
Fayetteville NC	687	583	76	168	110	92	137	17	58	29
Flagstaff AZ	176	143	25	28	30	33	27	5	23	5
Florence AL	284	235	26	86	64	46	13	4	44	1
Florence SC	420	366	51	100	87	83	45	14	32	8
Fort Collins CO*	730	591	131	140	122	131	67	19	108	12
Fort Myers FL*	1,338	925	75	316	225	215	94	39	351	23
Fort Pierce FL*	711	504	37	161	130	123	53	14	182	11
Fort Smith AR	468	368	78	106	75	60	49	14	71	15
Fort Wayne IN	972	826	106	225	191	209	95	26	102	18
Fresno CA	1,909	1,508	199	462	288	299	260	71	244	86
Ft Walton Beach FL	366	312	49	74	62	50	77	9	38	7
Gadsden AL	209	181	29	61	48	35	8	3	21	4
Gainsesville FL	2,107	1,624	109	373	206	297	639	168	179	136
Glens Falls NY	292	239	36	72	57	48	26	10	40	3
Goldsboro NC	201	162	34	46	27	43	12	3	28	8
Grand Forks ND	259	217	43	39	27	52	56	15	19	8
Grand Junction CO	230	179	26	31	38	54	30	11	36	4
Grand Rapids MI*	1,452	1,167	189	326	196	298	158	28	237	20
Great Falls MT	235	188	27	53	45	53	10	6	40	1
Green Bay WI	649	565	62	167	142	144	50	11	69	4
Greensboro NC*	3,575	2,936	307	838	542	568	681	114	395	130
Greenville NC	1,023	813	51	209	122	150	281	81	59	70
Greenville SC*	2,588	2,178	303	562	448	421	444	71	274	65
Harrisburg PA*	2,075	1,604	143	355	260	305	541	112	226	133
Hartford CT	4,379	3,382	233	1,123	564	694	768	243	582	172
Hattiesburg MS	429	377	49	113	96	84	35	9	37	6

* The metropolitan statistical area name is abbreviated.

Table 3.14

Physicians by Metropolitan Area, 2006, continued

Metropolitan Areas	Total Physicians	Total Patient Care	FM/GP Practice	Medical Specialties	Surgical Specialties	Other Specialties	Hospital Based Practice	Other Professional Activity	Inactive	Not Classified
Hickory NC*	695	590	112	134	137	151	56	12	82	11
Honolulu HI	3,552	2,818	195	871	475	627	650	181	432	121
Houma LA	373	314	41	89	93	58	33	11	35	13
Houston TX*	14,397	11,465	1,090	3,162	1,923	2,390	2,900	691	1,136	1,105
Huntington WV*	570	451	47	102	88	90	124	39	46	34
Huntsville AL	952	804	131	221	168	180	104	21	97	30
Indianapolis IN	6,029	4,921	487	1,229	803	1,057	1,345	341	525	242
Iowa City IA	1,840	1,307	67	234	157	239	610	184	133	216
Jackson MI	215	173	26	63	41	23	20	4	37	1
Jackson MS	2,228	1,770	139	394	314	364	559	128	235	95
Jackson TN	444	370	34	127	102	69	38	13	48	13
Jacksonville FL	3,729	2,982	342	879	519	631	611	154	447	146
Jacksonville NC	241	193	25	38	46	27	57	5	26	17
Jamestown NY	217	171	22	57	42	42	8	2	41	3
Janesville WI*	304	245	38	78	35	48	46	11	40	8
Johnson City TN*	1,499	1,236	145	329	243	191	328	63	131	69
Johnstown PA	541	434	71	93	78	66	126	17	69	21
Jonesboro AR	306	261	39	70	65	55	32	11	33	1
Joplin MO	164	141	15	40	27	33	26	3	18	2
Kalamazoo MI*	1,320	1,021	117	288	189	202	225	75	189	35
Kansas City MO	3,573	2,846	262	784	479	585	736	155	427	145
Kileen-Temple TX	657	521	34	108	52	65	262	24	84	28
Knoxville TN	1,770	1,467	200	446	312	317	192	39	239	25
Kokomo IN	158	129	26	41	28	25	9	2	27	
La Crosse WI	612	518	58	146	88	126	100	13	67	14
Lafayette IN	415	345	47	102	77	89	30	12	52	6
Lafayette LA	964	828	112	233	208	168	107	17	90	29
Lake Charles LA	409	342	65	101	78	72	26	6	54	7
Lakeland FL*	990	754	84	275	179	156	60	16	192	28
Lancaster PA	994	760	184	181	140	158	97	29	181	24
Lansing MI*	1,120	842	96	228	141	170	207	93	145	40
Laredo TX	251	211	38	70	46	35	22	2	28	10
Las Cruces NM	311	246	44	67	47	53	35	14	41	10
Las Vegas NV	3,632	2,911	289	999	551	741	331	77	515	129
Lawrence KS	230	173	32	47	35	36	23	4	48	5
Lawton OK	247	214	25	40	40	44	65	4	20	9
Lewiston ME*	289	230	29	67	49	49	36	17	30	12
Lexington KY	1,853	1,470	101	380	272	322	395	77	196	110
Lima OH	284	232	36	60	53	64	19	5	42	5
Lincoln NE	780	618	100	182	126	134	76	23	116	23
Little Rock AR*	2,813	2,338	210	548	384	522	674	149	227	99
Longview TX*	363	306	43	100	76	69	18	3	46	8
Los Angeles CA*	41,594	32,307	3,461	10,008	6,110	7,230	5,498	1,736	5,473	2,078
Louisville KY	3,686	2,950	238	841	548	698	625	172	405	159
Lubbock TX	759	636	68	183	128	140	117	20	77	26
Lynchburg VA	488	376	62	102	82	79	51	15	93	4
Macon GA	987	803	67	250	182	155	149	29	122	33
Madison WI	2,370	1,824	233	449	239	393	510	168	278	100
Mansfield OH	248	199	24	68	49	44	14	1	46	2
Mayaguez PR	308	257	43	68	55	57	34	6	28	17
McAllen TX	762	674	132	259	131	100	52	12	50	26
Medford OR	638	478	73	153	98	110	44	21	125	14
Melbourne FL*	937	757	91	259	172	173	62	16	141	23
Memphis TN	3,505	2,877	214	931	533	565	634	154	319	155
Merced CA	259	220	60	55	45	24	36	6	26	7
Miami FL*	9,147	6,785	577	2,156	1,251	1,410	1,391	360	1,451	551
Milwaukee WI*	5,768	4,698	476	1,291	771	1,183	977	261	602	207

* The metropolitan statistical area name is abbreviated.

Table 3.14

Physicians by Metropolitan Area, 2006, continued

Metropolitan Areas	Total Physicians	Major Professional Activity								
		Patient Care					Hospital Based Practice	Other Professional Activity	Inactive	Not Classified
		Total Patient Care	Office-Based Practice							
			FM/GP Practice	Medical Specialties	Surgical Specialties	Other Specialties				
Minneapolis MN*	7,720	6,181	955	1,673	1,063	1,228	1,262	430	812	297
Missoula MT	409	317	26	87	77	89	38	10	77	5
Mobile AL	1,528	1,267	134	359	294	228	252	47	165	49
Modesto CA	914	750	153	238	157	144	58	19	115	30
Monroe LA	450	381	44	112	71	84	70	13	43	13
Montgomery AL	716	606	63	192	137	111	103	22	72	16
Muncie IN	340	288	34	86	49	58	61	12	33	7
Mytle Beach SC	372	321	25	102	87	83	24	5	40	6
Naples FL	1,180	654	48	225	160	170	51	33	472	21
Nashville TN	4,854	3,955	259	1,109	758	893	936	233	438	228
New London CT*	240	180	17	69	35	35	24	7	51	2
New Orleans LA	5,187	4,172	189	1,165	767	892	1,159	259	437	319
New York NY*	89,457	69,853	2,277	21,484	10,817	13,336	21,939	4,984	8,201	6,419
Norfolk VA*	3,429	2,849	305	766	524	460	794	123	336	121
Ocala FL	583	473	55	181	104	113	20	5	97	8
Odessa TX*	505	432	36	133	98	85	80	17	32	24
Oklahoma City OK	3,092	2,477	268	603	413	585	608	160	329	126
Omaha NE	2,661	2,140	227	515	382	398	618	111	292	118
Orlando FL	4,168	3,398	400	1,126	651	751	470	112	544	114
Owensboro KY	232	190	22	61	52	41	14	8	29	5
Panama City FL	271	239	28	73	60	57	21	3	22	7
Parkersburg WV*	257	212	38	51	51	53	19	3	39	3
Pensacola FL	1,132	944	129	237	152	219	207	42	124	22
Peoria IL*	970	791	95	191	140	165	200	40	103	36
Philadelphia PA*	20,044	15,259	964	4,420	2,373	3,143	4,359	1,257	2,301	1,227
Phoenix AZ*	9,123	7,121	730	2,189	1,342	1,710	1,150	315	1,316	371
Pine Bluff AR	188	161	35	44	33	22	27	4	16	7
Pittsburgh PA	8,368	6,475	482	1,684	1,029	1,330	1,950	445	916	532
Pittsfield MA	547	415	24	137	64	99	91	25	73	34
Pocatello ID	184	151	26	33	30	33	29	3	28	2
Ponce PR	343	269	36	79	35	44	75	13	22	39
Portland ME	1,181	941	83	253	153	213	239	69	130	41
Portland OR*	7,130	5,606	624	1,660	1,016	1,313	993	298	960	266
Providence RI*	2,924	2,295	109	667	366	389	764	146	296	187
Provo UT*	628	533	90	124	121	113	85	12	74	9
Pueblo CO	375	308	49	75	53	86	45	8	56	3
Punta Gorda FL	191	109	9	30	23	37	10	5	71	6
Raleigh NC*	6,023	4,589	347	1,204	651	975	1,412	442	570	422
Rapid City SD	358	285	38	76	62	65	44	12	56	5
Reading PA	669	516	69	151	110	95	91	21	118	14
Redding CA	489	387	63	87	87	109	41	17	74	11
Reno NV	1,033	832	83	208	193	232	116	35	147	19
Richland WA*	320	275	39	87	52	60	37	6	33	6
Richmond VA*	3,708	2,815	266	767	463	558	761	186	483	224
Roanoke VA	870	695	50	157	127	151	210	37	104	34
Rochester MN	1,775	1,374	47	290	103	247	687	49	146	206
Rochester NY	3,180	2,455	170	783	368	423	711	157	429	139
Rockford IL	718	569	102	160	126	109	72	28	103	18
Rocky Mount NC	112	91	21	27	16	19	8	3	16	2
Sacramento CA*	6,005	4,719	578	1,374	844	1,107	816	290	741	255
Saginaw MI*	899	752	115	190	147	143	157	25	106	16
Saint Cloud MN	465	398	78	123	79	82	36	11	50	6
Saint Joseph MO	58	45	5	14	8	10	8	3	8	2
Saint Louis MO	7,510	5,996	323	1,728	1,041	1,174	1,730	412	648	454
Salinas CA	923	681	110	193	147	152	79	35	192	15
Salt Lake City UT*	1,829	1,456	204	373	313	366	200	73	245	55

The metropolitan statistical area name is abbreviated.

Table 3.14

Physicians by Metropolitan Area, 2006, continued

Metropolitan Areas	Total Physicians	Total Patient Care	FM/GP Practice	Medical Specialties	Surgical Specialties	Other Specialties	Hospital Based Practice	Other Professional Activity	Inactive	Not Classified
				Major Professional Activity						
				Patient Care						
				Office-Based Practice						
San Angelo TX	208	180	16	51	52	44	17	1	24	3
San Antonio TX	5,196	4,243	404	1,061	735	855	1,188	272	456	225
San Diego CA	10,361	7,769	796	2,123	1,375	1,848	1,627	622	1,499	471
San Francisco CA*	28,083	21,243	1,770	6,968	3,630	5,082	3,793	1,490	3,687	1,663
San Juan PR*	3,803	2,976	470	764	436	704	602	179	321	327
San Luis Obispo CA*	568	432	69	91	66	151	55	16	110	10
Santa Barbara CA*	1,361	1,004	130	315	197	255	107	39	292	26
Santa Fe NM	504	356	65	87	61	104	39	27	108	13
Sarasota FL*	2,205	1,428	139	512	354	337	86	50	712	15
Savannah GA	901	717	53	198	145	167	154	29	128	27
Scranton PA*	1,064	858	89	266	167	163	173	36	152	18
Seattle WA*	13,287	10,173	1,415	2,655	1,634	2,366	2,103	764	1,757	593
Sharon PA	190	139	15	40	33	35	16	3	43	5
Sheboygan WI	197	165	35	42	45	37	6		31	1
Sherman TX*	241	194	24	61	48	46	15	2	42	3
Shreveport LA*	1,782	1,464	99	363	281	243	478	68	142	108
Sioux City IA	200	160	28	42	27	35	28	8	30	2
Sioux Falls SD	824	701	82	186	137	150	146	30	70	23
South Bend IN	780	654	106	153	110	174	111	19	90	17
Spokane WA	1,327	1,030	156	258	211	269	136	56	219	22
Springfield IL	1,022	835	63	230	144	168	230	47	100	40
Springfield MA	723	576	74	191	59	147	105	18	111	18
Springfield MO	906	763	87	219	170	190	97	22	110	11
State College PA	327	271	34	74	44	71	48	10	40	6
Steubenville OH*	102	85	8	29	22	16	10		14	3
Stockton CA*	1,102	921	136	297	186	177	125	19	121	41
Sumter SC	173	144	19	42	31	34	18	2	18	9
Syracuse NY	2,607	2,052	197	492	382	394	587	131	291	133
Tallahassee FL	808	615	108	148	113	130	116	48	122	23
Tampa FL*	5,930	4,681	383	1,609	829	1,062	798	239	791	219
Terre Haute IN	326	286	51	79	53	65	38	9	22	9
Texarkana TX-AR	271	222	32	60	63	54	13	2	43	4
Toledo OH	1,540	1,220	140	282	181	275	342	70	157	93
Topeka KS	525	394	37	126	78	104	49	28	99	4
Tucson AZ	3,026	2,315	214	641	397	617	446	124	478	109
Tulsa OK	1,902	1,506	182	448	300	339	237	57	280	59
Tuscaloosa AL	472	389	46	107	75	90	71	17	57	9
Tyler TX	758	635	69	197	144	142	83	30	85	8
Utica NY*	647	513	66	148	102	100	97	14	102	18
Victoria TX	213	183	25	58	43	43	14	6	22	2
Visalia CA*	509	421	75	142	90	78	36	6	75	7
Waco TX	528	429	77	80	88	98	86	24	63	12
Washington DC*	30,573	23,269	1,363	7,077	3,618	4,844	6,367	2,422	2,946	1,936
Waterloo IA*	314	256	53	54	50	61	38	7	45	6
Wausau WI	380	307	61	84	60	76	26	19	46	8
West Palm Beach FL*	2,902	2,047	133	795	470	473	176	77	710	68
Wheeling WV	56	46	10	14	10	5	7	1	9	
Wichita Falls TX	345	289	51	74	56	64	44	8	39	9
Wichita KS	1,480	1,201	190	276	208	253	274	57	176	46
Williamsport PA	257	196	42	38	35	42	39	9	47	5
Wilmington NC	894	697	61	233	160	151	92	28	145	24
Yakima WA	458	362	77	100	72	70	43	16	68	12
York PA	773	600	104	163	108	123	102	34	115	24
Youngstown OH*	1,195	936	82	294	184	170	206	45	155	59
Yuba City CA	263	216	50	71	37	42	16	2	41	4
Yuma AZ	235	202	19	83	47	38	15	1	21	11

† Does not include 199 physicians whose MSA could not be determined.

* MSA name is abbreviated.

Chapter 4
Primary Care Specialties

Chapter 4 provides data for two groups of physicians: (1) physicians in general primary care specialties and (2) physicians in primary care subspecialties. Information is provided on major professional activity, age, sex, board certification, school and year of graduation, and state of location. Data are also presented for International Medical Graduates (IMGs) in primary care and the number of primary care physicians located in metropolitan areas.

General primary care specialties are defined as Family Medicine, General Practice, Internal Medicine, Obstetrics/Gynecology, and Pediatrics, excluding the subspecialties within these general specialties. The primary care subspecialties, which include only the subspecialties of the mentioned groups, are listed in the "Definitions" section of the Introduction and in the footnotes to Tables 4.5, 4.7-4.9, 4.11-4.13, and 4.15.

The statistics in this chapter focus on the general primary care specialties and primary care subspecialties, but also provide information on the total active physician population, the number of physicians in all other specialties, physicians Not Classified by major professional activity, and Inactive physicians.

Trends in Primary Care

Table 4.1

From 1975 to 2006, the total number of physicians more than doubled, whereas the percentage of primary care physicians increased by 107.7%. During this same period, the proportion in the pri-

mary care subspecialties increased by 695.5%. The largest percentage increase in the primary care specialties was in Family Medicine (572.1%), followed by Pediatrics (163.0%). At the same time, physicians in General Practice decreased 75.2%. Among the primary care subspecialties, the highest increase (1661.2%) was in the Pediatric subspecialties. Figure 5 displays the trends of the total physician population in comparison with the general primary care specialties and the primary care subspecialties.

Primary care physicians and their subspecialties comprised 41.9% of all active physicians in 1975 and 45.3% in 2006. The largest component, Internal Medicine and subspecialties, represented 14.8% of all active physicians in 1975 and 19.5% in 2006. Figure 6 illustrates the percentage of physicians practicing in the general primary care specialties and subspecialties.

Activity and Sex

Table 4.2

Office-Based practice represented a higher percentage of primary care physicians (74.8%) than physicians in the primary care subspecialties (67.0%), with All Other Specialties in between (72.5%). By contrast, Research activities included a higher percentage of the subspecialties (6.2%) compared with the primary care specialties (0.9%). Among the primary care specialties, 77.2% of male physicians were in Office-Based practice; for the subspecialties, 6.9% of male physicians were in Research.

Figure 5

Trends in Self-Designated Primary Care With and Without Subspecialties, 1975–2006

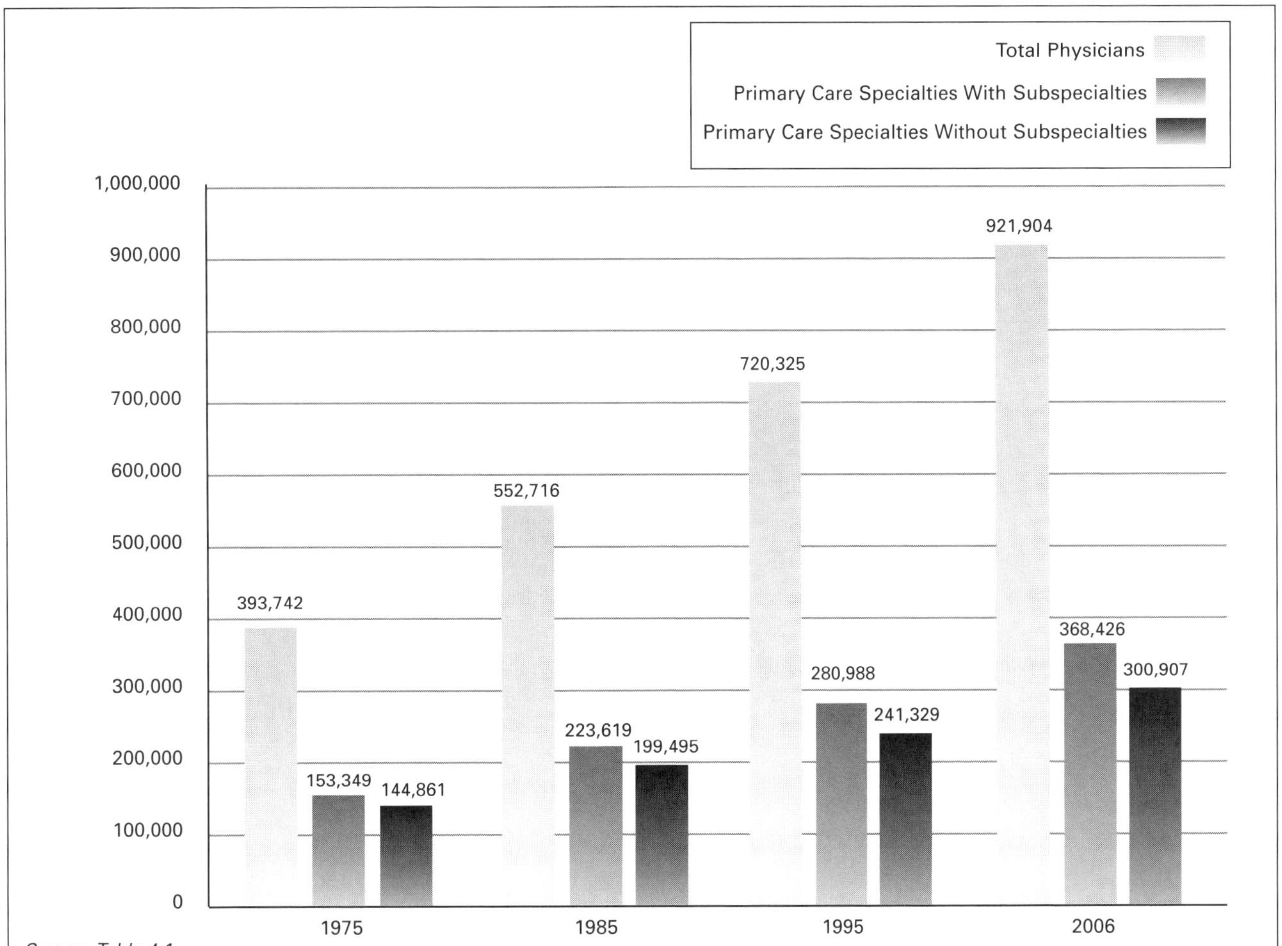

Legend:
- Total Physicians
- Primary Care Specialties With Subspecialties
- Primary Care Specialties Without Subspecialties

	1975	1985	1995	2006
Total Physicians	393,742	552,716	720,325	921,904
Primary Care Specialties With Subspecialties	153,349	223,619	280,988	368,426
Primary Care Specialties Without Subspecialties	144,861	199,495	241,329	300,907

Source: Table 4.1.

Figure 6

Distribution of Self-Designated Primary Care Specialties and Subspecialties, 2006

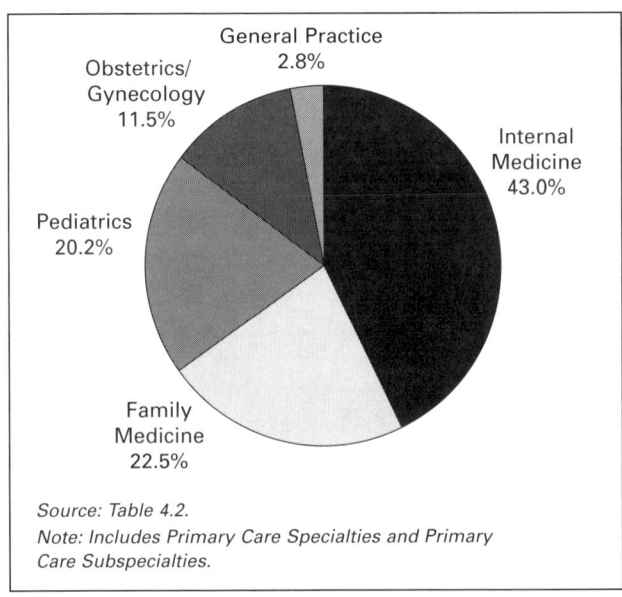

- General Practice 2.8%
- Obstetrics/Gynecology 11.5%
- Internal Medicine 43.0%
- Pediatrics 20.2%
- Family Medicine 22.5%

Source: Table 4.2.
Note: Includes Primary Care Specialties and Primary Care Subspecialties.

However, a larger percentage of female physicians compared with male physicians were in primary care (45.8% and 27.6%, respectively). In each of the primary care specialties except General Practice, the percentages of female physicians surpassed those of male physicians. This difference was especially apparent for Pediatrics, which represented 12.6% of all female physicians but only 3.8% of male physicians.

Age and Sex

Table 4.3

The largest percentage of active physicians was in the age group 45 to 54 years (27.0%), with the age groups 35 to 44 years and 55 to 64 years having the next largest percentages (26.1% and 19.2%, respectively).

Among primary care physicians, the largest percentage (27.3%) was in the age group 45 to 54 years, whereas the next largest group was 35 to 44 (26.7%). The age group 55 to 64 years included only 18.2% of primary care physicians. Among General Practice physicians, the largest percentage was found in the group 65 years and older (46.7%); the group 35 to 44 years represented only 3.2% of General Practice physicians.

Primary care accounted for nearly half (49.0%) of female physicians in the age group younger than 35 years. The comparable percentage for male physicians was 33.2%. A similar gender gap existed for the age group 35 to 44 years. In the older age groups, the gender gap is less because of the relatively small female physician population in these groups. For example, in the age group 65 years and older, primary care included 16.1% of male physicians and 21.1% of female physicians.

Board Certification and Sex

Table 4.4

Among all active physicians, 70.6% were board certified and 29.4% were not board certified. Of the primary care physician population, 67.4% were board certified; in comparison, the proportions were 87.0% for the primary care subspecialties and 74.1% for all other specialties.

Among female physicians in primary care specialties, the highest board certification occurred for Family Medicine, in which 73.4% were certified. The lowest percentage, excluding General Practice, was in Internal Medicine (61.1%). A different pattern was observed for male physicians; the highest percentage (79.5%) of board certification was in Obstetrics/Gynecology, and the lowest percentage, excluding General Practice, occurred in Internal Medicine (64.9%).

Primary care specialties with the highest incidence of no board certification were General Practice (89.7%) and Internal Medicine (36.4%). The high percentage for General Practice occurred because

this specialty does not have a board that grants certification.

School and Year of Graduation

Tables 4.5 and 4.6

Table 7 shows the top 10 schools with the largest numbers of total graduates with the number and percentage of their graduates practicing in the primary care specialties. Four schools had 50% or more of their graduates practicing in primary care: University of Minnesota-Duluth (59.3%), Mercer University (56.6%), Morehouse University (54.9%), and Wright State University (51.0%).

More than three fifths (71.1%) of primary care physicians and 68.4% of all active physicians have graduated since 1980. However, great differences exist with respect to sex. Among primary care physicians, 62.0% of males and 85.3% of females graduated since 1980. This difference reflects the great increase in numbers of female physicians in recent years. Similarly, for all active physicians, 61.9% of male physicians and 83.7% of female physicians graduated since 1980.

Among female physicians, the highest percentage of graduates since 1980 occurred in Family Medicine (89.7%), followed by Obstetrics/Gynecology (88.3%). For male physicians, the highest percentages were in Internal Medicine (67.4%), and Family Medicine (67.3%).

Mini-Table 7			
Top 10 Schools in Number of Graduates and Self-Designated Primary Care Specialists, 2006			
School	Total Graduates	Primary Care Graduates	Primary Care Graduates (%)
U of Illinois	13,768	4,319	31.4%
Jefferson Med Coll	12,688	3,584	28.2%
Indiana U	12,241	3,889	31.8%
U of Minnesota	10,748	3,913	36.4%
U of Michigan	10,468	2,350	22.4%
Med Coll of PA	10,373	3,040	29.3%
SUNY (Brooklyn)	10,300	2,682	26.0%
Wayne State U	10,009	3,187	31.8%
Ohio State U	9,866	3,068	31.1%
New York Med Coll	9,191	2,589	28.2%
Source: Table 4.5.			

Mini-Table 8

Top 10 States With Largest Number and Percentage of Primary Care Physicians Compared to Total Physicians in State, 2006

State	Total Physicians	Primary Care Physicians	Primary Care Physicians (%)
CA	110,406	35,917	32.5%
NY	83,826	26,580	31.7%
TX	54,971	18,178	33.1%
FL	53,566	15,618	29.2%
PA	42,204	12,435	29.5%
IL	39,240	13,738	35.0%
OH	34,091	11,018	32.3%
MA	32,575	9,344	28.7%
NJ	30,183	10,062	33.3%
MI	27,877	9,419	33.8%

Source: Table 4.7.

State of Location and Sex

Tables 4.7, 4.8, and 4.9

The 10 states with the largest number of total physicians are shown in Table 8, along with the number and percentage of primary care physicians in those states.

Among male physicians in 26 states and the District of Columbia, Internal Medicine was the primary care specialty with the largest number of physicians. In the remaining 24 states, the number of physicians in Family Medicine exceeded that in Internal Medicine. In the Possessions, General Practice represented the largest number of primary care physicians.

Among female physicians in primary care, Family Medicine was the specialty with the largest number of primary care physicians in 24 states. In the remaining 26 states, Internal Medicine had the largest number of physicians in 20 states and the District of Columbia and Pediatrics in 6.

Country of Graduation

Tables 4.10, 4.11, 4.12, and 4.13

Table 9 shows that a higher percentage (37.0%) of IMGs, compared with US Medical Graduates (USMGs) and Canadian Medical Graduates (CMGs), were in the primary care specialties

Mini-Table 9

Country of Graduation of Active Physicians, 2006

Country	Total Physicians	Primary Care Physicians	Primary Care Physicians (%)
Total	**921,904**	**300,907**	**32.6**
USMGs	673,081	210,361	31.3
IMGs	236,669	87,494	37.0
CMGs	12,154	3,052	25.1

Source: Tables 4.5, 4.11, 4.12, and 4.13.

(31.3% and 25.1%, respectively). Among all IMGs, the largest number (41,787) were in Internal Medicine, which represented 48.9% of IMGs in primary care.

Nearly half (45.6%) of female IMGs were in primary care, compared with one third (33.2%) of male IMGs. For female IMGs, Internal Medicine was the specialty representing the largest number of primary care physicians (42.9%), followed by Pediatrics (27.1%). Among male IMGs in primary care, Internal Medicine accounted for the largest number of physicians (52.4%), followed by Family Medicine (19.4%).

The age group with the highest number of IMG primary care physicians was 45 to 54 years, which comprised 24.5% of these physicians. Among IMG male primary care physicians, this age group represented 25.8% of these physicians; for female IMGs, this age group was 22.2% of these physicians.

Graduates of US medical schools (USMGs) have a smaller percentage in primary care compared with IMGs (31.3% and 37.0%, respectively). Moreover, USMGs were found in higher proportions in Family/General Practice (10.2%) compared with IMGs (9.3%); conversely, IMGs were represented in a higher proportion in Internal Medicine (18.1%) compared with USMGs (10.4%). The states with the highest percentages of USMGs in primary care were Alaska (41.7%), North Dakota (38.1%), and South Dakota (37.3%). Lowest percentages were found in Florida (25.9%) and New York (27.5%). Among graduates of Canadian medical schools, only 25.1% were in primary care, and the highest percentage of these was in Family Medicine (12.3%).

Metropolitan Areas

Tables 4.14 and 4.15

Of all active physicians practicing in metropolitan areas, 44.6% were in primary care or primary care subspecialties, mostly Internal Medicine and its subspecialties (19.9%). Among active male physicians, 39.1% were in primary care or primary care subspecialties; for active female physicians, the percentage was 57.0%.

Of the five specialties comprising the primary care physicians in metropolitan areas (226,489), Internal Medicine represented the largest proportion (39.4%), followed by Family Medicine (24.5%) and Pediatrics (20.0%). Internal Medicine represented 43.8% of male physicians in primary care but only 33.2% of female physicians. Although

Family Medicine was the second highest specialty of male physicians, it was Pediatrics for female physicians, representing 28.1% of this population.

Of the 280 metropolitan areas listed in Table 4.15, seven recorded more than 20,000 physicians within their boundaries: New York (89,457), Los Angeles (41,594), Washington, DC (30,573), Boston (30,425), Chicago (29,837), San Francisco (28,083), and Philadelphia (20,044). The percentage of primary care physicians in these metropolitan areas ranged from 28.6 (Philadelphia) to 34.4% (Chicago). Although Internal Medicine comprised the primary care specialty with the largest number of physicians in each of these metropolitan areas, the percentage in Internal Medicine of total primary care physicians varied from 52.3% in New York to 36.4% in Los Angeles.

Table 4.1

Primary Care Physicians by Self-Designated Specialty for Selected Years, 1975–2006

	1975	1980	1985	1990	1995	2000	2006
				Number			
Total Physicians*	393,742	467,679	552,716	615,421	720,325	813,770	921,904
Active Physicians	366,425	435,545	511,090	559,988	646,022	737,504	813,088
Primary Care	144,861	170,705	199,495	213,514	241,329	274,653	300,907
Family Medicine	12,183	27,530	40,021	47,639	59,109	71,102	81,878
General Practice	42,374	32,519	27,030	22,841	16,867	15,210	10,493
Internal Medicine	47,761	58,462	70,691	76,295	88,240	101,353	113,340
Obstetrics/Gynecology	20,797	24,612	28,754	30,220	33,519	35,922	37,996
Pediatrics	21,746	27,582	32,999	36,519	43,594	51,066	57,200
Prim. Care Subspec.	8,488	16,642	24,124	30,911	39,659	52,294	67,519
FM Subspecialties	0	0	0	0	236	483	938
IM Subspecialties	6,570	13,069	18,171	22,054	26,928	34,831	44,914
OBG Subspecialties	934	1,693	2,113	3,477	4,133	4,319	4,337
PD Subspecialties	984	1,880	3,840	5,380	8,362	12,661	17,330
All Other Specialties	186,931	227,569	273,521	302,885	344,455	365,421	398,410
Inactive	21,449	25,744	38,646	52,653	72,326	75,168	108,344
Not Classified	26,145	20,629	13,950	12,678	20,579	45,136	46,252
Address Unknown	5,868	6,390	2,980	2,780	1,977	1,098	472
				Percent Distribution			
Total Physicians*	100.0	100.0	100.0	100.0	100.0	100.0	100.0
Active Physicians	93.1	93.1	92.5	91.0	89.7	90.6	88.2
Primary Care	36.8	36.5	36.1	34.7	33.5	33.8	32.6
Family Medicine	3.1	5.9	7.2	7.7	8.2	8.7	8.9
General Practice	10.8	7.0	4.9	3.7	2.3	1.9	1.1
Internal Medicine	12.1	12.5	12.8	12.4	12.3	12.5	12.3
Obstetrics/Gynecology	5.3	5.3	5.2	4.9	4.7	4.4	4.1
Pediatrics	5.5	5.9	6.0	5.9	6.1	6.3	6.2
Prim. Care Subspec.	2.2	3.6	4.4	5.0	5.5	6.4	7.3
FM Subspecialties	0.0	0.0	0.0	0.0	0.0	0.1	0.1
IM Subspecialties	1.7	2.8	3.3	3.6	3.7	4.3	4.9
OBG Subspecialties	0.2	0.4	0.4	0.6	0.6	0.5	0.5
PD Subspecialties	0.2	0.4	0.7	0.9	1.2	1.6	1.9
All Other Specialties	47.5	48.7	49.5	49.2	47.8	44.9	43.2
Inactive	5.4	5.5	7.0	8.6	10.0	9.2	11.8
Not Classified	6.6	4.4	2.5	2.1	2.9	5.5	5.0
Address Unknown	1.5	1.4	0.5	0.5	0.3	0.1	0.1

	1975-2006	1975-1985	1985-1995	1975-1980	1980-1985	1985-1990	1990-2006
				Percent Change			
Total Physicians*	134.1	40.4	30.3	18.8	18.2	11.3	49.8
Active Physicians	121.9	39.5	26.4	18.9	17.3	9.6	45.2
Primary Care	107.7	37.7	21.0	17.8	16.9	7.0	40.9
Family Medicine	572.1	228.5	47.7	126.0	45.4	19.0	71.9
General Practice	-75.2	-36.2	-37.6	-23.3	16.9	-15.5	-54.1
Internal Medicine	137.3	48.0	24.8	22.4	20.9	7.9	48.6
Obstetrics/Gynecology	82.7	38.3	16.6	18.3	16.8	5.1	25.7
Pediatrics	163.0	51.7	32.1	26.8	19.6	10.7	56.6
Prim. Care Subspec.	695.5	184.2	64.4	96.1	45.0	28.1	118.4
FM Subspecialties	0.0	0.0	0.0	0.0	0.0	0.0	0.0
IM Subspecialties	583.6	176.6	48.2	98.9	39.0	21.4	103.7
OBG Subspecialties	364.3	126.2	95.6	81.3	24.8	64.6	24.7
PD Subspecialties	1661.2	290.2	117.8	91.1	104.3	40.1	222.1
All Other Specialties	113.1	46.3	25.9	21.7	20.2	10.7	31.5
Inactive	405.1	80.2	87.2	20.0	50.1	36.2	105.8
Not Classified	76.9	-46.6	47.5	-21.1	-32.4	-9.1	264.8
Address Unknown	-92.0	-49.2	-33.7	8.9	-53.4	-6.7	-83.0

Note: Data for 1990 are as of January 1; all others are as of December 31.

*Includes Active, Inactive, and Address Unknown.

Table 4.2

Physicians by Self-Designated Primary Care Specialty, Activity, and Sex, 2006

Specialty	Total Physicians	Patient Care					Other Professional Activity			
		Total Patient Care	Office Based	Locum Tenens	Hospital Based Resid./ Fellows	Hospital Based Phys. Staff	Admin.	Med. Teach.	Research	Other
Both Sexes										
Total Physicians	921,904	723,118	558,950	1,461	97,102	65,605	14,575	10,273	14,475	4,395
Active Physicians	813,088	723,118	558,950	1461	97,102	65,605	14,575	10,273	14,475	4,395
Primary Care	300,907	288,336	225,011	609	40,285	22,431	4,839	3,958	2,748	1,026
Family Medicine	81,878	78,835	65,106	218	8,091	5,420	1,256	1,417	197	173
General Practice	10,493	10,099	8,827	45		1,227	214	32	42	106
Internal Medicine	113,340	108,054	78,136	153	20,688	9,077	2,020	1,250	1,581	435
Obstetrics/Gynecology	37,996	37,022	30,574	52	4,205	2,191	324	414	176	60
Pediatrics	57,200	54,326	42,368	141	7,301	4,516	1,025	845	752	252
Prim. Care Subspec.	67,519	60,219	45,221	60	8,709	6,229	1,421	1,460	4,164	255
FM Subspecialties	938	890	703	1	125	61	23	19	3	3
IM Subspecialties	44,914	39,455	30,709	32	4,930	3,784	1,037	956	3,289	177
OBG Subspecialties	4,337	4,014	3,595	4		415	96	133	78	16
PD Subspecialties	17,330	15,860	10,214	23	3,654	1,969	265	352	794	59
All Other Specialties	398,410	374,563	288,718	792	48,108	36,945	8,315	4,855	7,563	3,114
Inactive	108,344									
Not Classified	46,252									
Address Unknown	472									
Male										
Total Physicians	665,647	509,474	406,958	949	55,078	46,489	11,817	7,618	11,394	3,188
Active Physicians	570,849	509,474	406,958	949	55,078	46,489	11,817	7,618	11,394	3,188
Primary Care	183,608	174,670	141,783	322	18,659	13,906	3,676	2,617	1,995	650
Family Medicine	53,736	51,455	43,853	119	3,801	3,682	1,013	1,017	132	119
General Practice	8,438	8,149	7,232	32		885	159	21	34	75
Internal Medicine	75,721	71,713	53,798	82	11,776	6,057	1,608	857	1,237	306
Obstetrics/Gynecology	20,690	19,975	17,597	40	1,006	1,332	261	289	128	37
Pediatrics	25,023	23,378	19,303	49	2,076	1,950	635	433	464	113
Prim. Care Subspec.	45,806	40,220	31,429	38	4,640	4,113	1,158	1,088	3,169	171
FM Subspecialties	680	645	510	1	92	42	17	15	1	2
IM Subspecialties	32,261	27,952	22,400	22	2,900	2,630	851	743	2,592	123
OBG Subspecialties	3,123	2,863	2,571	3		289	80	105	63	12
PD Subspecialties	9,742	8,760	5,948	12	1,648	1,152	210	225	513	34
All Other Specialties	314,077	294,584	233,746	589	31,779	28,470	6,983	3,913	6,230	2,367
Inactive	94,469									
Not Classified	27,358									
Address Unknown	329									
Female										
Total Physicians	256,257	213,644	151,992	512	42,024	19,116	2,758	2,655	3,081	1,207
Active Physicians	242,239	213,644	151,992	512	42,024	19,116	2,758	2,655	3,081	1,207
Primary Care	117,299	113,666	83,228	287	21,626	8,525	1,163	1,341	753	376
Family Medicine	28,142	27,380	21,253	99	4,290	1,738	243	400	65	54
General Practice	2,055	1,950	1,595	13		342	55	11	8	31
Internal Medicine	37,619	36,341	24,338	71	8,912	3,020	412	393	344	129
Obstetrics/Gynecology	17,306	17,047	12,977	12	3,199	859	63	125	48	23
Pediatrics	32,177	30,948	23,065	92	5,225	2,566	390	412	288	139
Prim. Care Subspec.	21,713	19,999	13,792	22	4,069	2,116	263	372	995	84
FM Subspecialties	258	245	193		33	19	6	4	2	1
IM Subspecialties	12,653	11,503	8,309	10	2,030	1,154	186	213	697	54
OBG Subspecialties	1,214	1,151	1,024	1		126	16	28	15	4
PD Subspecialties	7,588	7,100	4,266	11	2,006	817	55	127	281	25
All Other Specialties	84,333	79,979	54,972	203	16,329	8,475	1,332	942	1,333	747
Inactive	13,875									
Not Classified	18,894									
Address Unknown	143									

Table 4.3

Physicians by Self-Designated Primary Care Specialty, Age, and Sex, 2006

Specialty	Total Physicians	< 35	35-44	45-54	55-64	≥ 65
			Both Sexes			
Total Physicians	921,904	141,492	213,311	223,864	166,005	177,232
Active Physicians	813,088	141,410	211,968	219,152	155,747	84,811
Primary Care	300,907	55,680	80,417	82,051	54,779	27,980
Family Medicine	81,878	12,597	24,208	25,197	14,529	5,347
General Practice	10,493	72	333	1,798	3,391	4,899
Internal Medicine	113,340	25,290	29,961	30,513	18,845	8,731
Obstetrics/Gynecology	37,996	6,136	10,583	9,943	7,484	3,850
Pediatrics	57,200	11,585	15,332	14,600	10,530	5,153
Prim. Care Subspec.	67,519	10,000	20,484	18,651	13,022	5,362
FM Subspecialties	938	261	363	169	91	54
IM Subspecialties	44,914	5,621	13,948	12,738	9,130	3,477
OBG Subspecialties	4,337	30	318	1,403	1,483	1,103
PD Subspecialties	17,330	4,088	5,855	4,341	2,318	728
All Other Specialties	398,410	54,923	93,963	113,301	85,932	50,291
Inactive	108,344	79	1,342	4,711	10,157	92,055
Not Classified	46,252	20,807	17,104	5,149	2,014	1,178
Address Unknown	472	3	1	1	101	366
			Male			
Total Physicians	657,140	77,699	134,871	161,211	130,416	152,943
Active Physicians	569,415	77,668	134,184	158,545	123,386	75,632
Primary Care	185,583	25,833	41,492	53,700	39,882	24,676
Family Medicine	53,673	6,154	13,602	18,054	10,921	4,942
General Practice	8,950	38	222	1,376	2,648	4,666
Internal Medicine	76,200	14,832	17,959	21,440	14,164	7,805
Obstetrics/Gynecology	21,338	1,437	4,481	5,970	5,964	3,486
Pediatrics	25,422	3,372	5,228	6,860	6,185	3,777
Prim. Care Subspec.	44,859	5,288	12,371	12,703	9,898	4,599
FM Subspecialties	593	151	207	119	71	45
IM Subspecialties	31,581	3,253	8,952	9,140	7,229	3,007
OBG Subspecialties	3,169	11	192	847	1,117	1,002
PD Subspecialties	9,516	1,873	3,020	2,597	1,481	545
All Other Specialties	315,137	36,763	71,338	89,200	72,316	45,520
Inactive	87,383	27	687	2,662	6,942	77,065
Not Classified	23,836	9,784	8,983	2,942	1,290	837
Address Unknown	342	4		4	88	246
			Female			
Total Physicians	256,257	64,324	79,796	63,611	30,215	18,311
Active Physicians	242,239	64,283	79,130	61,606	27,808	9,412
Primary Care	117,299	31,506	39,874	29,560	12,494	3,865
Family Medicine	28,142	6,888	10,720	7,539	2,457	538
General Practice	2,055	31	113	552	790	569
Internal Medicine	37,619	11,248	12,480	9,386	3,602	903
Obstetrics/Gynecology	17,306	4,810	6,383	4,159	1,508	446
Pediatrics	32,177	8,529	10,178	7,924	4,137	1,409
Prim. Care Subspec.	21,713	4,819	7,802	5,952	2,547	593
FM Subspecialties	258	77	119	42	12	8
IM Subspecialties	12,653	2,448	4,759	3,629	1,513	304
OBG Subspecialties	1,214	22	140	598	326	128
PD Subspecialties	7,588	2,272	2,784	1,683	696	153
All Other Specialties	84,333	18,299	24,855	24,358	12,156	4,665
Inactive	13,875	41	665	2,005	2,386	8,778
Not Classified	18,894	9,659	6,599	1,736	611	289
Address Unknown	143		1		21	121

Table 4.4

Physicians by Self-Designated Primary Care Specialty and Corresponding Board Certification, 2006

Activity	Total Physicians	Total Certified	By Corresponding Board Only	By Corresponding Boards and Other Boards	By Non-corresponding Board	Not Board Certified
Both Sexes						
Total Physicians	921,904	638,987	496,475	23,588	118,924	282,917
Active Physicians	813,088	574,765	496,475	23,588	54,702	238,323
Primary Care	300,907	202,950	195,226	3,748	3,976	97,957
Family Medicine	81,878	59,862	58,185	693	984	22,016
General Practice	10,493	1,080			1,080	9,413
Internal Medicine	113,340	72,129	68,864	1,906	1,359	41,211
Obstetrics/Gynecology	37,996	27,439	27,018	249	172	10,557
Pediatrics	57,200	42,440	41,159	900	381	14,760
Prim. Care Subspec.	67,519	58,766	44,412	852	13,502	8,753
FM Subspecialties	938	786	684	5	97	152
IM Subspecialties	44,914	39,854	30,708	540	8,606	5,060
OBG Subspecialties	4,337	3,877	1,540	44	2,293	460
PD Subspecialties	17,330	14,249	11,480	263	2,506	3,081
All Other Specialties	398,410	295,340	256,837	18,988	19,515	103,070
Inactive	108,344	64,186			64,186	44,158
Not Classified	46,252	17,709			17,709	28,543
Address Unknown	472	36			36	436
Male						
Total Physicians	665,647	473,134	358,886	18,873	95,375	192,513
Active Physicians	570,849	415,568	358,886	18,873	37,809	155,281
Primary Care	183,608	125,259	119,612	2,666	2,981	58,349
Family Medicine	53,736	39,213	37,853	558	802	14,523
General Practice	8,438	873			873	7,565
Internal Medicine	75,721	49,155	46,791	1,387	977	26,566
Obstetrics/Gynecology	20,690	16,441	16,179	166	96	4,249
Pediatrics	25,023	19,577	18,789	555	233	5,446
Prim. Care Subspec.	45,806	40,331	30,438	612	9,281	5,475
FM Subspecialties	680	565	501	5	59	115
IM Subspecialties	32,261	28,749	22,082	404	6,263	3,512
OBG Subspecialties	3,123	2,820	1,188	31	1,601	303
PD Subspecialties	9,742	8,197	6,667	172	1,358	1,545
All Other Specialties	314,077	240,013	208,836	15,595	15,582	74,064
Inactive	94,469	57,543			57,543	36,926
Not Classified	27,358	9,965			9,965	17,393
Address Unknown	329	23			23	306
Female						
Total Physicians	256,257	165,853	137,589	4,715	23,549	90,404
Active Physicians	242,239	159,197	137,589	4,715	16,893	83,042
Primary Care	117,299	77,691	75,614	1,082	995	39,608
Family Medicine	28,142	20,649	20,332	135	182	7,493
General Practice	2,055	207			207	1,848
Internal Medicine	37,619	22,974	22,073	519	382	14,645
Obstetrics/Gynecology	17,306	10,998	10,839	83	76	6,308
Pediatrics	32,177	22,863	22,370	345	148	9,314
Prim. Care Subspec.	21,713	18,435	13,974	240	4,221	3,278
FM Subspecialties	258	221	183		38	37
IM Subspecialties	12,653	11,105	8,626	136	2,343	1,548
OBG Subspecialties	1,214	1,057	352	13	692	157
PD Subspecialties	7,588	6,052	4,813	91	1,148	1,536
All Other Specialties	84,333	55,327	48,001	3,393	3,933	29,006
Inactive	13,875	6,643			6,643	7,232
Not Classified	18,894	7,744			7,744	11,150
Address Unknown	143	13			13	130

Table 4.5
Physicians by Self-Designated Primary Care Specialty and School of Graduation, 2006

School	Total Physicians	Total Primary Care	Family Medicine	General Practice	Internal Medicine	OB/Gyn	Pediatrics	Subspec- ialties	All Other Special- ties	Not Class- ified	Inactive/ Address Un- known
Total Physicians	921,904	300,907	81,878	10,493	113340	37,996	57,200	67,519	398,410	46,252	108816
AL-U Of Alabama	6,334	2,210	626	58	715	379	432	411	2,894	207	612
" -U Of So Alabama	1,833	791	267	15	248	112	149	150	802	55	35
AZ-U Of Arizona	2,973	1,172	422	11	309	168	262	158	1,453	123	67
AR-U Of Arkansas	5,823	2,092	1,056	103	401	236	296	310	2,468	111	842
CA-Loma Linda U	6,834	2,226	964	145	533	328	256	204	2,948	266	1,190
" -Stanford U	4,120	914	185	25	411	79	214	368	1,855	228	755
" -U Of Cal (Davis)	3,038	1,399	569	21	409	166	234	145	1,317	115	62
" -U Of Cal (Irvine)	4,659	1,585	574	154	397	218	242	194	1,768	132	980
" -U Of Cal (La)	6,540	2,229	717	46	717	308	441	426	3,303	238	344
" -U Of Cal (San Diego)	3,612	1,382	397	14	441	188	342	288	1,696	191	55
" -U Of Cal (Sf)	7,071	2,225	588	54	853	270	460	395	3,142	294	1,015
" -U Of So Cal (La)	6,286	1,984	538	62	724	339	321	375	2,903	228	796
CO-U Of Colorado	5,814	1,950	763	70	575	238	304	314	2,477	169	904
CT-U Of Connecticut	2,558	961	204	3	375	156	223	232	1,182	139	44
" -Yale U	4,972	1,011	92	12	491	153	263	493	2,477	210	781
DC-George Wash U	6,928	2,025	452	50	802	321	400	453	3,124	258	1,068
" -Georgetown U	8,539	2,240	449	50	888	401	452	569	4,340	303	1,087
" -Howard U	4,845	1,876	427	85	613	399	352	245	1,866	182	676
FL-U Of Florida	4,238	1,430	428	27	395	257	323	284	2,124	174	226
" -U Of Miami	6,164	1,850	396	57	752	352	293	420	3,282	178	434
" -U Of So Florida	2,702	977	302	9	284	164	218	214	1,346	121	44
GA-Emory U	5,171	1,320	218	31	552	206	313	313	2,580	152	806
" -Med Coll Of Georgia	7,429	2,561	738	98	765	454	506	402	3,331	192	943
" -Morehouse U	678	372	134	2	92	68	76	23	219	59	5
" -Mercer U	858	486	179	1	152	75	79	44	273	47	8
HI-U Of Hawaii	1,850	843	192	26	348	111	166	146	743	80	38
IL-Chgo Med School	6,440	1,992	462	28	777	407	318	367	3,177	240	664
" -Loyola U/Stritch	6,120	1,818	448	56	663	281	370	459	2,746	154	943
" -Northwestern U	8,803	1,987	356	33	852	323	423	578	4,179	303	1,756
" -Rush Med Coll	3,831	1,353	459	6	505	171	212	307	1,812	175	184
" -Southern Illinois U	2,040	919	418	6	239	111	145	145	876	73	27
" -U Of Chgo/Pritzker	4,950	1,077	119	19	515	126	298	528	2,426	203	716
" -U Of Illinois	13,768	4,319	1,276	96	1,604	598	745	895	5,932	401	2,221
IN-Indiana U	12,241	3,889	1,697	112	915	505	660	697	5,690	303	1,662
IA-U Of Iowa	7,762	2,526	1,267	69	517	321	352	369	3,319	220	1,328
KS-U Of Kansas	7,946	2,712	1,179	68	740	340	385	553	3,300	184	1,197
KY-U Of Kentucky	3,660	1,420	545	34	366	240	235	219	1,714	151	156
" -U Of Louisville	6,197	2,007	630	101	621	267	388	332	2,645	156	1,057
LA-Lsu (New Orleans)	7,782	2,387	620	119	687	470	491	449	3,686	231	1,029
" -Lsu (Shreveport)	2,863	1,102	369	30	280	233	190	207	1,392	107	55
" -Tulane U	7,696	1,802	371	67	609	354	401	421	3,798	251	1,424
MD-Johns Hopkins	5,767	1,154	97	18	564	108	367	656	2,765	277	915
" -U Of Maryland	7,491	2,204	556	42	920	262	424	483	3,309	245	1,250
" -Uniformed Services U	3,897	1,166	595	22	171	167	211	190	2,328	190	23

Notes:

Total Physicians include Active, Inactive, and Address Unknown.

FM subspecialties include FPG and FSM.

IM subspecialties include AMI, CCM, DIA, END, HEM, HEP, HO, ICE, ID, ILI, IMG, ISM, NEP, NTR, ON, PCC, and RHU.

OBG Subspecialties include: GO, GYN, MFM, OBS, OCC, and REN.

PD subspecialties include ADL, CCP, MPD, NPM, PDA, PDC, PDE, PDI, PDP, PDT, PEM, PG, PHO, PLI, PN, PPR, and PSM.

Table 4.5

Physicians by Self-Designated Primary Care Specialty and School of Graduation, 2006, continued

School	Total Physicians	Total Primary Care	Family Medicine	General Practice	Internal Medicine	OB/Gyn	Pediatrics	Subspec- ialties	All Other Special- ties	Not Class- ified	Inactive/ Address Un- known
MA-Boston U	6,287	1,785	287	33	813	266	386	437	2,984	301	780
" -Harvard U	8,995	1,826	200	27	1,016	162	421	946	4,195	398	1,630
" -Tufts U	7,733	2,175	347	37	1,016	290	485	590	3,437	289	1,242
" -U Of Massachusetts	2,866	1,214	343	5	510	100	256	242	1,220	147	43
MI-Michigan State U	3,316	1,543	649	24	395	218	257	240	1,340	117	76
" -U Of Michigan	10,468	2,350	667	64	770	384	465	597	5,239	280	2,002
" -Wayne State U	10,009	3,187	961	54	1,127	587	458	663	4,793	373	993
MN-Mayo Medical School	1,211	395	178	3	102	49	63	80	649	62	25
" -U Of Minnesota	10,748	3,913	1,944	104	1,029	351	485	617	4,179	208	1,831
" -U Of Minnesota-Duluth	644	382	272		57	29	24	38	170	51	3
MS-U Of Mississippi	4,515	1,702	669	69	460	240	264	291	2,100	90	332
MO-St Louis U	7,171	2,140	503	56	720	346	515	499	3,044	196	1,292
" -U Of Mo (Columbia)	4,351	1,617	638	39	434	227	279	329	1,943	111	351
" -U Of Mo (Kansas City)	2,516	925	299	7	322	138	159	203	1,228	117	43
" -Washington U	6,147	1,390	222	26	589	170	383	536	2,873	203	1,145
NE-Creighton U	5,155	1,693	539	64	494	332	264	275	2,296	117	774
" -U Of Nebraska	6,151	1,932	896	61	436	213	326	323	2,643	144	1,109
NV-U Of Nevada	1,282	543	222	5	155	98	63	56	617	50	16
NH-Dartmouth Med School	2,110	732	213	5	267	91	156	163	1,073	125	17
NJ-N Jersey Med Sch (Newark)	5,931	1,925	360	19	735	368	443	470	2,984	285	267
" -N Jersey Med Sch (Rutgers)	3,960	1,401	365	5	508	220	303	337	1,933	236	53
NM-U Of New Mexico	2,391	987	427	20	276	97	167	136	1,103	83	82
NY-Albany Med Coll	5,374	1,595	447	31	553	233	331	433	2,578	196	572
" -Albert Einstein Coll Of Med	6,863	1,972	205	20	946	249	552	694	3,606	319	272
" -Columbia U	7,735	1,448	135	23	740	196	354	685	4,001	321	1,280
" -Cornell U	5,463	1,063	83	10	575	158	237	522	2,705	208	965
" -Mt Sinai School Of Med	3,950	1,171	104	7	531	234	295	385	2,113	230	51
" -New York Med Coll	9,191	2,589	325	50	1,171	512	531	624	4,375	284	1,319
" -New York U	8,562	1,938	129	19	1,043	272	475	779	4,071	307	1,467
" -Suny (Brooklyn)	10,300	2,682	267	50	1,241	440	684	833	5,031	378	1,376
" -Suny (Buffalo)	6,523	1,955	456	30	696	277	496	487	2,952	233	896
" -Suny (Stony Brook)	2,809	1,029	197	4	446	181	201	241	1,368	142	29
" -Suny (Syracuse)	6,506	1,974	595	25	639	239	476	509	3,051	221	751
" -U Of Rochester	4,822	1,327	233	14	604	151	325	391	2,142	173	789
NC-Bowman Gray	4,377	1,411	476	29	413	194	299	267	2,006	132	561
" -Duke University	5,296	1,119	205	21	470	149	274	485	2,539	189	964
" -East Carolina U	1,617	779	348	3	148	130	150	113	615	91	19
" -U Of No Carolina	5,910	2,128	658	39	629	324	478	509	2,573	227	473
ND-U Of No Dakota	1,518	723	360	6	138	131	88	53	687	39	16
OH-Case Western Res	6,593	1,810	438	30	707	232	403	529	2,970	260	1,024
" -Med Coll Of Ohio	3,872	1,566	603	9	490	209	255	262	1,797	191	56
" -Northeastern Ohio U	2,351	858	297	1	277	137	146	190	1,161	114	28

Notes:

Total Physicians include Active, Inactive, and Address Unknown.

FM subspecialties include FPG and FSM.

IM subspecialties include AMI, CCM, DIA, END, HEM, HEP, HO, ICE, ID, ILI, IMG, ISM, NEP, NTR, ON, PCC, and RHU.

OBG Subspecialties include: GO, GYN, MFM, OBS, OCC, and REN.

PD subspecialties include ADL, CCP, MPD, NPM, PDA, PDC, PDE, PDI, PDP, PDT, PEM, PG, PHO, PLI, PN, PPR, and PSM.

Table 4.5

Physicians by Self-Designated Primary Care Specialty and School of Graduation, 2006, continued

School	Total Physicians	Total Primary Care	Family Medicine	General Practice	Internal Medicine	OB/Gyn	Pediatrics	Subspec-ialties	All Other Special-ties	Not Class-ified	Inactive/ Address Un-known
" -Ohio State U	9,866	3,068	1,124	63	903	459	519	699	4,384	297	1,418
" -U Of Cincinnati	7,278	2,297	699	51	751	304	492	472	3,251	179	1,079
" -Wright State U	2,217	1,130	536	5	294	123	172	137	822	95	33
OK-U Of Oklahoma	6,611	2,067	819	94	562	284	308	383	3,089	156	916
OR-U Of Oregon	4,882	1,570	555	72	504	187	252	228	2,006	126	952
PA-Med Coll Of Penn	10,373	3,040	789	90	1,224	431	506	736	4,598	101	1,898
" -Jefferson Med Coll	12,688	3,584	1,251	74	1,190	493	576	809	5,756	598	1,941
" -Pennsylvania State U	3,246	1,208	418	10	355	164	261	260	1,589	132	57
" -Temple U	8,815	2,552	778	77	889	359	449	555	3,785	315	1,608
" -U Of Pennsylvania	8,199	1,824	280	41	765	254	484	647	3,759	316	1,653
" -U Of Pittsburgh	6,386	1,790	430	36	616	264	444	479	2,797	220	1,100
PR-Ponce Med Sch	1,317	513	109	2	197	106	99	95	588	112	9
" -U Central Del Caribe	1,903	772	148	24	297	139	164	180	755	155	41
" -U Of Puerto Rico	4,762	1,464	248	42	417	287	470	452	2,388	210	248
RI-Brown U	2,126	750	187	3	311	99	150	195	1,022	125	34
SC-Med Coll Of So Carolina	6,135	2,104	772	88	513	329	402	343	2,773	169	746
" -U Of So Carolina	1,518	720	257	2	197	91	173	87	631	70	10
SD-U Of So Dakota	1,414	652	318	11	153	103	67	65	636	45	16
TN-East Tennessee State U	1,322	612	239	5	185	86	97	81	545	65	19
" -Meharry Med Coll	3,742	1,591	441	76	459	384	231	136	1,316	171	528
" -U Of Tennessee	8,933	2,750	780	175	861	441	493	493	3,739	206	1,745
" -Vanderbilt U	4,350	1,001	112	20	413	164	292	377	2,180	154	638
TX-Baylor Coll Of Med	7,013	1,924	471	63	573	341	476	551	3,431	272	835
" -Texas A&M U	1,267	511	183	5	103	110	110	73	586	90	7
" -Texas Tech U	2,779	1,168	424	17	276	250	201	123	1,306	141	41
" -U Of Tx (Dallas)	8,031	2,412	630	52	830	456	444	545	3,944	307	823
" -U Of Tx (Galveston)	8,834	2,791	955	132	777	443	484	437	4,078	257	1,271
" -U Of Tx (Houston)	5,153	1,963	790	14	496	278	385	384	2,483	266	57
" -U Of Tx (San Antonio)	5,919	2,316	934	40	558	346	438	287	2,907	302	107
UT-U Of Utah	4,277	1,248	494	35	249	205	265	178	2,180	131	540
VT-U Of Vermont	3,925	1,315	361	17	408	201	328	243	1,682	149	536
VA-Eastern Virginia Med Sch	2,584	1,140	389	12	331	162	246	158	1,130	124	32
" -Med Coll Of Va	7,425	2,535	989	72	689	348	437	477	2,965	247	1,201
" -U Of Virginia	5,956	1,761	555	32	521	242	411	409	2,705	210	871
WA-U Of Washington	6,679	2,615	1,241	55	708	257	354	390	2,723	252	699
WV-Marshall U	1,091	508	234	4	107	62	101	64	431	78	10
" -West Virginia U	3,264	1,074	399	24	318	146	187	273	1,641	109	167
WI-Med Coll Of Wisconsin	7,893	2,404	822	65	778	296	443	445	3,645	235	1,164
" -U Of Wisconsin	6,669	2,116	805	48	607	217	439	344	2,960	200	1,049
INA-Inactive Schools	1,527	662	263	148	135	29	87	51	400	95	319
CAN-Canadian Schools	12,154	3,052	1,490	312	600	322	328	775	5,329	961	2,037
IMG-Internat"L Schools	236,669	87,494	17,056	4,982	42,745	6,680	16,031	20,913	84,084	21,255	22,923

Notes:

Total Physicians include Active, Inactive, and Address Unknown.

FM subspecialties include FPG and FSM.

IM subspecialties include AMI, CCM, DIA, END, HEM, HEP, HO, ICE, ID, ILI, IMG, ISM, NEP, NTR, ON, PCC, and RHU.

OBG Subspecialties include: GO, GYN, MFM, OBS, OCC, and REN.

PD subspecialties include ADL, CCP, MPD, NPM, PDA, PDC, PDE, PDI, PDP, PDT, PEM, PG, PHO, PLI, PN, PPR, and PSM.

Table 4.6

Physicians by Self-Designated Primary Care Specialty, Year of Graduation, and Sex, 2006

Specialty	Total Physicians	Prior 1950	1950-1959	1960-1969	1970-1979	1980-1989	1990-1999	2000-Present
Both Sexes								
Total Physicians	921,904	30,253	62,466	105,547	161,230	219,789	208,039	134,580
Active Physicians	813,088	4,496	21,871	77,744	152,543	215,138	206,777	134,519
Primary Care	300,907	1,551	7,500	23,853	54,115	79,629	82,191	52,068
Family Medicine	81,878	168	1,425	4,233	14,609	22,906	25,778	12,759
General Practice	10,493	470	1,535	3,176	3,059	1,815	345	93
Internal Medicine	113,340	542	2,426	7,465	18,907	30,916	30,064	23,020
Obstetrics/Gynecology	37,996	138	863	3,734	7,136	9,537	10,838	5,750
Pediatrics	57,200	233	1,251	5,245	10,404	14,455	15,166	10,446
Prim. Care Subspec.	67,519	229	1,327	5,518	13,562	19,150	19,680	8,053
FM Subspecialties	938	4	13	36	98	168	386	233
IM Subspecialties	44,914	143	797	3,747	9,467	13,327	13,267	4,166
OBG Subspecialties	4,337	52	344	930	1,448	1,280	275	8
PD Subspecialties	17,330	30	173	805	2,549	4,375	5,752	3,646
All Other Specialties	398,410	2,509	12,799	47,480	82,914	110,590	87,972	54,146
Inactive	108,344	25,597	40,495	27,678	8,604	4,651	1,259	60
Not Classified	46,252	207	245	893	1,952	5,769	16,934	20,252
Address Unknown	472	160	100	125	83		3	1
Male								
Total Physicians	665,647	27,254	56,682	92,603	132,215	155,688	126,418	74,787
Active Physicians	570,849	3,976	19,712	67,885	125,659	153,077	125,784	74,756
Primary Care	183,608	1,384	6,673	19,603	42,168	50,215	40,133	23,432
Family Medicine	53,736	156	1,321	3,718	12,353	16,001	13,944	6,243
General Practice	8,438	421	1,387	2,670	2,403	1,275	228	54
Internal Medicine	75,721	506	2,223	6,592	15,389	20,990	17,046	12,975
Obstetrics/Gynecology	20,690	127	780	3,137	5,796	5,484	4,095	1,271
Pediatrics	25,023	174	962	3,486	6,227	6,465	4,820	2,889
Prim. Care Subspec.	45,806	199	1,201	4,858	10,783	12,825	11,767	4,173
FM Subspecialties	680	3	12	29	85	130	258	163
IM Subspecialties	32,261	127	744	3,408	7,835	9,327	8,446	2,374
OBG Subspecialties	3,123	46	310	800	1,094	720	151	2
PD Subspecialties	9,742	23	135	621	1,769	2,648	2,912	1,634
All Other Specialties	314,077	2,233	11,645	42,806	71,344	86,180	63,678	36,191
Inactive	94,469	23,166	36,911	24,629	6,490	2,611	632	30
Not Classified	27,358	160	193	618	1,364	3,857	10,206	10,960
Address Unknown	329	112	59	89	66		2	1
Female								
Total Physicians	256,257	2,999	5,784	12,944	29,015	64,101	81,621	59,793
Active Physicians	242,239	520	2,159	9,859	26,884	62,061	80,993	59,763
Primary Care	117,299	167	827	4,250	11,947	29,414	42,058	28,636
Family Medicine	28,142	12	104	515	2,256	6,905	11,834	6,516
General Practice	2,055	49	148	506	656	540	117	39
Internal Medicine	37,619	36	203	873	3,518	9,926	13,018	10,045
Obstetrics/Gynecology	17,306	11	83	597	1,340	4,053	6,743	4,479
Pediatrics	32,177	59	289	1,759	4,177	7,990	10,346	7,557
Prim. Care Subspec.	21,713	30	126	660	2,779	6,325	7,913	3,880
FM Subspecialties	258	1	1	7	13	38	128	70
IM Subspecialties	12,653	16	53	339	1,632	4,000	4,821	1,792
OBG Subspecialties	1,214	6	34	130	354	560	124	6
PD Subspecialties	7,588	7	38	184	780	1,727	2,840	2,012
All Other Specialties	84,333	276	1,154	4,674	11,570	24,410	24,294	17,955
Inactive	13,875	2,431	3,584	3,049	2,114	2,040	627	30
Not Classified	18,894	47	52	275	588	1,912	6,728	9,292
Address Unknown	143	48	41	36	17		1	

Table 4.7

Total Physicians by Self-Designated Primary Care Specialty and State of Location, 2006

State	Total Physicians	Total Primary Care	Family Medicine	General Practice	Internal Medicine	OB/Gyn	Pediatrics	Subspec-ialties	All Other Special-ties	Not Class-ified	Inactive/ Address Un-known
Totals	921,904	300,907	81,878	10,493	113340	37,996	57,200	67,519	398,410	46,252	108,816
AL	10,994	3,855	1,196	128	1,394	480	657	768	4,865	405	1,101
AK	1,697	707	362	30	138	75	102	69	734	37	150
AZ	15,127	4,687	1,344	154	1,697	606	886	983	6,532	595	2,330
AR	6,464	2,315	1,121	109	485	239	361	472	2,753	163	761
CA	110,406	35,917	9,002	1,763	13,521	4,527	7,104	7,012	47,259	5,488	14,730
CO	14,175	4,589	1,682	95	1,422	598	792	971	6,300	436	1,879
CT	14,488	4,477	540	57	2,328	646	906	1,176	6,465	783	1,587
DE	2,414	747	229	16	249	90	163	221	1,054	111	281
DC	5,023	1,421	182	33	676	206	324	506	2,296	423	377
FL	53,566	15,618	3,885	964	5,776	1,903	3,090	3,715	22,686	1,865	9,682
GA	22,805	8,030	2,104	232	2,851	1,231	1,612	1,585	9,858	877	2,455
HI	4,599	1,601	333	78	629	226	335	288	1,955	152	603
ID	2,934	1,018	518	38	227	129	106	144	1,279	38	455
IL	39,240	13,738	3,439	401	5,789	1,698	2,411	2,855	16,473	2,245	3,929
IN	15,229	5,292	2,225	177	1,447	647	796	1,196	6,652	427	1,662
IA	6,428	2,107	1,088	53	472	195	299	397	2,762	301	861
KS	7,079	2,366	1,036	66	658	267	339	431	3,064	243	975
KY	10,828	3,630	1,196	139	1,194	459	642	770	4,798	473	1,157
LA	12,643	4,186	1,136	187	1,420	635	808	942	5,724	577	1,214
ME	4,197	1,429	571	21	462	156	219	238	1,786	116	628
MD	25,969	7,690	1,178	162	3,604	980	1,766	2,415	11,558	1,668	2,638
MA	32,575	9,344	1,182	132	5,028	991	2,011	3,025	14,607	2,780	2,819
MI	27,877	9,419	2,561	220	3,782	1,259	1,597	2,107	11,712	1,504	3,135
MN	16,756	5,840	2,681	80	1,726	552	801	1,336	6,892	745	1,943
MS	5,890	2,011	698	105	589	304	315	375	2,587	176	741
MO	15,586	4,901	1,226	122	1,970	643	940	1,390	7,044	783	1,468
MT	2,548	865	420	21	227	103	94	117	1,075	29	462
NE	4,852	1,737	847	33	436	174	247	322	2,024	190	579
NV	5,384	1,816	505	56	743	231	281	323	2,299	173	773
NH	4,079	1,363	455	27	458	179	244	263	1,711	126	616
NJ	30,183	10,062	1,344	229	4,640	1,350	2,499	2,453	13,133	1,443	3,092
NM	5,424	1,891	725	63	578	201	324	328	2,223	239	743
NY	83,826	26,580	3,412	432	13,343	3,409	5,984	6,586	36,565	6,012	8,083
NC	25,385	8,311	2,675	161	2,802	1,141	1,532	1,987	10,973	1,135	2,979
ND	1,745	675	343	27	186	49	70	106	718	45	201
OH	34,091	11,018	3,136	276	4,124	1,355	2,127	2,684	14,534	2,085	3,770
OK	7,111	2,418	938	106	718	296	360	451	3,070	225	947
OR	11,741	3,949	1,268	123	1,512	464	582	674	4,923	458	1,737
PA	42,204	12,435	3,371	304	5,067	1,472	2,221	3,381	18,851	2,289	5,248
RI	4,368	1,426	211	18	693	180	324	374	1,867	244	457
SC	11,241	3,897	1,441	120	1,081	555	700	709	4,950	331	1,354
SD	1,975	735	357	30	204	75	69	115	830	39	256
TN	17,791	5,996	1,731	196	2,182	795	1,092	1,508	7,783	638	1,866
TX	54,971	18,178	5,678	620	5,562	2,690	3,628	4,293	24,571	2,698	5,231
UT	6,093	1,951	698	39	522	267	425	394	2,803	253	692
VT	2,659	884	296	18	307	103	160	157	1,094	128	396
VA	23,545	7,986	2,422	246	2,655	1,081	1,582	1,574	9,997	1,074	2,914
WA	19,864	6,687	2,754	202	1,995	677	1,059	1,299	8,248	731	2,899
WV	4,710	1,623	579	86	533	184	241	312	2,016	215	544
WI	16,154	5,640	2,281	116	1,806	586	851	1,083	7,080	454	1,897
WY	1,132	430	227	22	90	48	43	35	476	9	182
POSS.	13,367	5,419	1,049	1,360	1,342	589	1,079	604	4,901	1,578	865
UNK.	472										472

Notes:

Total Physicians include Active, Inactive, and Address Unknown.

FM subspecialties include FPG and FSM.

IM subspecialties include AMI, CCM, DIA, END, HEM, HEP, HO, ICE, ID, ILI, IMG, ISM, NEP, NTR, ON, PCC, and RHU.

OBG subspecialties include GO, GYN, MFM, OBS, OCC, and REN.

PD subspecialties include ADL, CCP, MPD, NPM, PDA, PDC, PDE, PDI, PDP, PDT, PEM, PG, PHO, PLI, PN, PPR, and PSM.

Table 4.8

Male Physicians by Self-Designated Primary Care Specialty and State of Location, 2006

State	Total Physicians	Total Primary Care	Family Medicine	General Practice	Internal Medicine	OB/Gyn	Pediatrics	Subspec-ialties	All Other Special-ties	Not Class-ified	Inactive/Address Un-known
Totals	665,647	183,608	53,736	8,438	75,721	20,690	25,023	45,806	314,077	27,358	94,798
AL	8,563	2,644	862	113	1,024	327	318	591	4,084	255	989
AK	1,187	400	198	25	88	36	53	48	591	22	126
AZ	11,331	2,922	876	130	1,154	336	426	706	5,273	351	2,079
AR	5,073	1,665	862	100	371	163	169	347	2,264	105	692
CA	79,323	21,424	5,690	1,422	8,843	2,417	3,052	4,791	37,128	3,173	12,807
CO	10,079	2,614	1,020	82	904	267	341	624	4,960	240	1,641
CT	10,252	2,669	360	43	1,514	328	424	782	4,977	438	1,386
DE	1,690	420	123	14	166	38	79	137	827	69	237
DC	3,177	747	103	28	419	89	108	287	1,611	237	295
FL	41,965	10,397	2,705	780	4,220	1,220	1,472	2,777	18,904	1,203	8,684
GA	16,699	4,933	1,399	193	1,913	707	721	1,102	7,953	518	2,193
HI	3,338	980	192	65	441	114	168	193	1,586	82	497
ID	2,387	704	374	34	149	82	65	109	1,129	23	422
IL	26,735	7,810	2,094	298	3,638	830	950	1,885	12,425	1,290	3,325
IN	11,417	3,396	1,545	158	1,009	361	323	828	5,472	260	1,461
IA	4,957	1,382	760	43	342	104	133	292	2,303	190	790
KS	5,318	1,504	720	53	455	135	141	298	2,484	147	885
KY	8,145	2,402	859	115	852	261	315	554	3,886	291	1,012
LA	9,586	2,839	832	165	1,056	408	378	641	4,679	357	1,070
ME	3,069	878	355	19	318	75	111	152	1,422	68	549
MD	17,589	4,283	662	124	2,277	508	712	1,554	8,614	932	2,206
MA	21,520	4,962	621	98	3,012	406	825	1,839	10,686	1,664	2,369
MI	19,780	5,565	1,539	173	2,518	664	671	1,436	9,164	878	2,737
MN	12,003	3,519	1,703	65	1,157	261	333	914	5,385	452	1,733
MS	4,732	1,455	543	91	455	213	153	292	2,210	104	671
MO	11,427	3,056	790	106	1,387	357	416	963	5,627	482	1,299
MT	2,017	579	287	18	167	64	43	77	919	20	422
NE	3,659	1,161	632	30	290	98	111	231	1,622	106	539
NV	4,179	1,200	351	47	518	151	133	242	1,952	105	680
NH	3,010	821	300	24	307	80	110	175	1,403	64	547
NJ	20,742	5,749	787	165	3,037	732	1,028	1,574	10,093	795	2,531
NM	3,742	1,090	424	48	370	99	149	204	1,683	128	637
NY	57,063	15,572	2,137	348	8,758	1,788	2,541	4,077	27,285	3,491	6,638
NC	18,612	5,107	1,737	138	1,924	634	674	1,379	8,820	656	2,650
ND	1,379	465	238	23	138	27	39	87	601	33	193
OH	24,675	6,694	2,031	210	2,818	748	887	1,852	11,476	1,348	3,305
OK	5,527	1,671	704	87	536	180	164	315	2,552	141	848
OR	8,471	2,282	790	108	936	198	250	462	3,874	284	1,569
PA	30,364	7,497	2,174	240	3,379	770	934	2,243	14,778	1,367	4,479
RI	2,968	779	102	15	448	79	135	256	1,414	124	395
SC	8,669	2,561	1,034	100	760	323	344	527	4,104	218	1,259
SD	1,546	485	243	28	146	35	33	97	710	19	235
TN	13,666	3,980	1,279	174	1,560	449	518	1,103	6,507	401	1,675
TX	40,296	11,358	3,925	525	3,779	1,537	1,592	2,984	19,709	1,632	4,613
UT	4,870	1,404	555	36	382	183	248	283	2,365	169	649
VT	1,856	498	167	16	199	44	72	97	838	74	349
VA	16,756	4,702	1,605	183	1,744	536	634	1,068	7,816	657	2,513
WA	14,285	3,913	1,701	161	1,204	342	505	888	6,540	410	2,534
WV	3,659	1,103	403	75	397	125	103	234	1,704	135	483
WI	11,914	3,498	1,493	97	1,234	283	391	786	5,678	261	1,691
WY	915	301	163	18	65	31	24	25	418	3	168
POSS.	9,136	3,568	687	987	943	447	504	398	3,572	886	712
UNK.	329										329

Notes:

Total Physicians include Active, Inactive, and Address Unknown.

FM subspecialties include FPG and FSM.

IM subspecialties include AMI, CCM, DIA, END, HEM, HEP, HO, ICE, ID, ILI, IMG, ISM, NEP, NTR, ON, PCC, and RHU.

OBG subspecialties include GO, GYN, MFM, OBS, OCC, and REN.

PD subspecialties include ADL, CCP, MPD, NPM, PDA, PDC, PDE, PDI, PDP, PDT, PEM, PG, PHO, PLI, PN, PPR, and PSM.

Table 4.9

Female Physicians by Self-Designated Primary Care Specialty and State of Location, 2006

State	Total Physicians	Total Primary Care	Family Medicine	General Practice	Internal Medicine	OB/Gyn	Pediatrics	Subspec-ialties	All Other Special-ties	Not Class-ified	Inactive/ Address Un-known
Totals	256,257	117,299	28,142	2,055	37,619	17,306	32,177	21,713	84,333	18,894	14,018
AL	2,431	1,211	334	15	370	153	339	177	781	150	112
AK	510	307	164	5	50	39	49	21	143	15	24
AZ	3,796	1,765	468	24	543	270	460	277	1,259	244	251
AR	1,391	650	259	9	114	76	192	125	489	58	69
CA	31,083	14,493	3,312	341	4,678	2,110	4,052	2,221	10,131	2,315	1,923
CO	4,096	1,975	662	13	518	331	451	347	1,340	196	238
CT	4,236	1,808	180	14	814	318	482	394	1,488	345	201
DE	724	327	106	2	83	52	84	84	227	42	44
DC	1,846	674	79	5	257	117	216	219	685	186	82
FL	11,601	5,221	1,180	184	1,556	683	1,618	938	3,782	662	998
GA	6,106	3,097	705	39	938	524	891	483	1,905	359	262
HI	1,261	621	141	13	188	112	167	95	369	70	106
ID	547	314	144	4	78	47	41	35	150	15	33
IL	12,505	5,928	1,345	103	2,151	868	1,461	970	4,048	955	604
IN	3,812	1,896	680	19	438	286	473	368	1,180	167	201
IA	1,471	725	328	10	130	91	166	105	459	111	71
KS	1,761	862	316	13	203	132	198	133	580	96	90
KY	2,683	1,228	337	24	342	198	327	216	912	182	145
LA	3,057	1,347	304	22	364	227	430	301	1,045	220	144
ME	1,128	551	216	2	144	81	108	86	364	48	79
MD	8,380	3,407	516	38	1,327	472	1,054	861	2,944	736	432
MA	11,055	4,382	561	34	2,016	585	1,186	1,186	3,921	1,116	450
MI	8,097	3,854	1,022	47	1,264	595	926	671	2,548	626	398
MN	4,753	2,321	978	15	569	291	468	422	1,507	293	210
MS	1,158	556	155	14	134	91	162	83	377	72	70
MO	4,159	1,845	436	16	583	286	524	427	1,417	301	169
MT	531	286	133	3	60	39	51	40	156	9	40
NE	1,193	576	215	3	146	76	136	91	402	84	40
NV	1,205	616	154	9	225	80	148	81	347	68	93
NH	1,069	542	155	3	151	99	134	88	308	62	69
NJ	9,441	4,313	557	64	1,603	618	1,471	879	3,040	648	561
NM	1,682	801	301	15	208	102	175	124	540	111	106
NY	26,763	11,008	1,275	84	4,585	1,621	3,443	2,509	9,280	2,521	1,445
NC	6,773	3,204	938	23	878	507	858	608	2,153	479	329
ND	366	210	105	4	48	22	31	19	117	12	8
OH	9,416	4,324	1,105	66	1,306	607	1,240	832	3,058	737	465
OK	1,584	747	234	19	182	116	196	136	518	84	99
OR	3,270	1,667	478	15	576	266	332	212	1,049	174	168
PA	11,840	4,938	1,197	64	1,688	702	1,287	1,138	4,073	922	769
RI	1,400	647	109	3	245	101	189	118	453	120	62
SC	2,572	1,336	407	20	321	232	356	182	846	113	95
SD	429	250	114	2	58	40	36	18	120	20	21
TN	4,125	2,016	452	22	622	346	574	405	1,276	237	191
TX	14,675	6,820	1,753	95	1,783	1,153	2,036	1,309	4,862	1,066	618
UT	1,223	547	143	3	140	84	177	111	438	84	43
VT	803	386	129	2	108	59	88	60	256	54	47
VA	6,789	3,284	817	63	911	545	948	506	2,181	417	401
WA	5,579	2,774	1,053	41	791	335	554	411	1,708	321	365
WV	1,051	520	176	11	136	59	138	78	312	80	61
WI	4,240	2,142	788	19	572	303	460	297	1,402	193	206
WY	217	129	64	4	25	17	19	10	58	6	14
POSS.	4,231	1,851	362	373	399	142	575	206	1,329	692	153
UNK.	143										143

Notes:

Total Physicians include Active, Inactive, and Address Unknown.

FM subspecialties include FPG and FSM.

IM subspecialties include AMI, CCM, DIA, END, HEM, HEP, HO, ICE, ID, ILI, IMG, ISM, NEP, NTR, ON, PCC, and RHU.

OBG subspecialties include GO, GYN, MFM, OBS, OCC, and REN.

PD subspecialties include ADL, CCP, MPD, NPM, PDA, PDC, PDE, PDI, PDP, PDT, PEM, PG, PHO, PLI, PN, PPR, and PSM.

Table 4.10

International Medical Graduates by Self-Designated Primary Care Specialty, Age, and Sex, 2006

Specialty	Total Physicians	< 35	35-44	45-54	55-64	≥ 65
			Both Sexes			
Total Physicians	236,669	31,451	55,767	52,657	47,656	49,138
Active Physicians	213,746	31,430	55,556	51,807	45,129	29,824
Primary Care	87,494	16,395	21,269	21,398	17,432	11,000
Family Medicine	17,056	3,216	4,591	4,451	3,055	1,743
General Practice	4,982	32	111	801	1,811	2,227
Internal Medicine	42,745	10,506	12,186	10,449	6,288	3,316
Obstetrics/Gynecology	6,680	768	870	1,188	2,293	1,561
Pediatrics	16,031	1,873	3,511	4,509	3,985	2,153
Prim. Care Subspec.	20,913	2,762	7,782	5,689	3,286	1,394
FM Subspecialties	207	35	90	47	25	10
IM Subspecialties	15,364	2,074	6,123	4,125	2,191	851
OBG Subspecialties	766	1	15	120	337	293
PD Subspecialties	4,576	652	1,554	1,397	733	240
All Other Specialties	84,084	6,253	17,382	21,074	22,846	16,529
Inactive	22,838	19	211	850	2,517	19,241
Not Classified	21,255	6,020	9,123	3,646	1,565	901
Address Unknown	85	2			10	73
			Male			
Total Physicians	165,377	17,695	34,391	37,589	35,650	40,052
Active Physicians	147,228	17,682	34,279	37,028	33,971	24,268
Primary Care	54,984	8,567	11,562	14,172	12,180	8,503
Family Medicine	10,655	1,533	2,414	2,975	2,315	1,418
General Practice	3,746	15	71	556	1,279	1,825
Internal Medicine	28,813	6,136	7,314	7,607	4,982	2,774
Obstetrics/Gynecology	4,547	321	444	858	1,715	1,209
Pediatrics	7,223	562	1,319	2,176	1,889	1,277
Prim. Care Subspec.	14,487	1,586	5,103	4,151	2,510	1,137
FM Subspecialties	135	23	50	34	22	6
IM Subspecialties	11,074	1,241	4,204	3,120	1,781	728
OBG Subspecialties	551		10	91	234	216
PD Subspecialties	2,727	322	839	906	473	187
All Other Specialties	64,574	4,220	12,000	16,199	18,197	13,958
Inactive	18,086	11	112	561	1,672	15,730
Not Classified	13,183	3,309	5,614	2,506	1,084	670
Address Unknown	63	2			7	54
			Female			
Total Physicians	71,292	13,756	21,376	15,068	12,006	9,086
Active Physicians	66,518	13,748	21,277	14,779	11,158	5,556
Primary Care	32,510	7,828	9,707	7,226	5,252	2,497
Family Medicine	6,401	1,683	2,177	1,476	740	325
General Practice	1,236	17	40	245	532	402
Internal Medicine	13,932	4,370	4,872	2,842	1,306	542
Obstetrics/Gynecology	2,133	447	426	330	578	352
Pediatrics	8,808	1,311	2,192	2,333	2,096	876
Prim. Care Subspec.	6,426	1,176	2,679	1,538	776	257
FM Subspecialties	72	12	40	13	3	4
IM Subspecialties	4,290	833	1,919	1,005	410	123
OBG Subspecialties	215	1	5	29	103	77
PD Subspecialties	1,849	330	715	491	260	53
All Other Specialties	19,510	2,033	5,382	4,875	4,649	2,571
Inactive	4,752	8	99	289	845	3,511
Not Classified	8,072	2,711	3,509	1,140	481	231
Address Unknown	22				3	19

Table 4.11

International Medical Graduates by Self-Designated Primary Care Specialty and State of Location, 2006

State	Total Physicians	Total Primary Care	Family Medicine	General Practice	Internal Medicine	OB/Gyn	Pediatrics	Subspec-ialties	All Other Special-ties	Not Class-ified	Inactive/ Address Un-known
Totals	236,669	87,494	17,056	4,982	42,745	6,680	16,031	20,913	84,084	21,255	22,923
AL	1,754	725	217	20	360	20	108	158	630	170	71
AK	118	46	19	1	18	3	5	9	41	7	15
AZ	3,215	1,224	240	37	681	67	199	336	1,074	228	353
AR	1,017	357	153	16	130	7	51	145	398	89	28
CA	25,408	10,021	2,214	771	4,122	913	2,001	1,906	8,810	2,030	2,641
CO	1,053	309	85	9	144	23	48	112	407	94	131
CT	4,192	1,514	144	31	1,020	146	173	349	1,552	403	374
DE	753	234	64	10	92	23	45	78	292	58	91
DC	1,075	313	30	13	179	30	61	127	381	171	83
FL	19,536	6,859	1,444	686	2,922	414	1,393	1,691	6,722	1,106	3,158
GA	4,438	1,868	473	67	865	130	333	494	1,417	307	352
HI	708	254	32	14	129	23	56	49	266	34	105
ID	105	42	18	3	18	3		15	30	2	16
IL	13,439	5,462	1,252	286	2,629	400	895	1,047	4,474	1,083	1,373
IN	3,157	1,135	377	41	489	80	148	385	1,207	162	268
IA	1,252	363	128	10	140	17	68	133	501	152	103
KS	1,314	385	88	21	192	20	64	120	600	101	108
KY	2,272	732	163	28	379	40	122	262	906	200	172
LA	2,285	881	222	32	395	59	173	290	790	227	97
ME	592	183	63	3	81	17	19	52	231	48	78
MD	7,106	2,463	269	73	1,431	224	466	638	2,573	644	788
MA	7,106	1,878	196	54	1,206	125	297	629	2,919	1,166	514
MI	9,459	3,867	832	125	1,957	291	662	900	3,136	828	728
MN	2,482	730	257	14	334	34	91	307	936	316	193
MS	780	277	60	16	135	14	52	89	321	66	27
MO	3,431	1,101	152	43	705	79	122	414	1,340	324	252
MT	116	47	18	4	15	5	5	11	37	2	19
NE	678	199	91	5	74	6	23	92	281	73	33
NV	1,580	695	142	20	369	36	128	136	449	93	207
NH	577	193	56	9	93	12	23	59	198	40	87
NJ	13,617	5,491	591	168	2,868	476	1,388	1,132	4,923	874	1,197
NM	936	327	125	16	123	17	46	81	357	82	89
NY	35,180	13,317	1,448	262	7,455	1,231	2,921	2,730	12,391	3,473	3,269
NC	3,221	1,166	257	31	660	42	176	317	1,141	327	270
ND	459	188	62	10	101	3	12	52	157	29	33
OH	9,911	3,357	620	140	1,847	270	480	852	3,572	1,140	990
OK	1,351	498	149	34	211	20	84	144	519	102	88
OR	1,034	337	90	12	173	26	36	90	340	137	130
PA	10,920	3,690	760	120	2,030	300	480	925	4,341	1,025	939
RI	1,177	388	35	12	256	32	53	123	408	97	161
SC	1,427	499	152	15	237	26	69	185	529	97	117
SD	270	104	21	6	65	5	7	35	95	12	24
TN	2,930	1,119	272	37	613	45	152	379	1,018	259	155
TX	13,250	4,935	1,326	209	1,981	346	1,073	1,484	4,687	1,172	972
UT	510	157	44	6	70	10	27	75	206	39	33
VT	244	45	12	2	25	2	4	22	90	45	42
VA	4,981	1,801	386	101	820	158	336	372	1,743	432	633
WA	2,448	860	289	52	370	57	92	224	818	224	322
WV	1,711	621	121	55	293	56	96	142	670	108	170
WI	2,948	1,077	312	37	552	53	123	314	1,118	204	235
WY	109	59	30	5	18	3	3	6	30	4	10
POSS.	6,833	3,045	440	1,184	656	233	532	192	1,963	1,146	487
APO/FPO	119	56	15	6	17	8	10	4	49	3	7
UNK.	85										85

Notes:

Total Physicians include Active, Inactive, and Address Unknown.

FM subspecialties include FPG and FSM.

IM subspecialties include AMI, CCM, DIA, END, HEM, HEP, HO, ICE, ID, ILI, IMG, ISM, NEP, NTR, ON, PCC, and RHU.

OBG subspecialties include GO, GYN, MFM, OBS, OCC, and REN.

PD subspecialties include ADL, CCP, MPD, NPM, PDA, PDC, PDE, PDI, PDP, PDT, PEM, PG, PHO, PLI, PN, PPR, and PSM.

Table 4.12

Graduates of US Medical Schools by Self-Designated Primary Care Specialty and State of Location, 2006

State	Total Physicians	Total Primary Care	Family Medicine	General Practice	Internal Medicine	OB/Gyn	Pediatrics	Subspec-ialties	All Other Special-ties	Not Class-ified	Inactive/ Address Un-known
Totals	673,081	210,361	63,332	5,199	69,995	30,994	40,841	45,831	308,997	24,036	83,856
AL	9,121	3,078	946	98	1,029	457	548	601	4,190	230	1,022
AK	1,567	654	339	26	120	72	97	60	689	30	134
AZ	11,571	3,377	1,052	108	1,001	533	683	629	5,303	356	1,906
AR	5,401	1,939	954	92	354	230	309	325	2,337	73	727
CA	83,026	25,459	6,606	939	9,295	3,570	5,049	4,989	37,589	3,328	11,661
CO	12,957	4,239	1,573	83	1,273	572	738	848	5,811	332	1,727
CT	10,093	2,917	381	23	1,301	494	718	815	4,824	361	1,176
DE	1,639	509	163	6	156	67	117	141	752	51	186
DC	3,896	1,103	151	20	494	176	262	377	1,880	247	289
FL	33,411	8,642	2,383	258	2,837	1,474	1,690	1,996	15,673	735	6,365
GA	18,159	6,097	1,599	160	1,977	1,093	1,268	1,074	8,345	562	2,081
HI	3,817	1,325	293	61	495	199	277	232	1,655	116	489
ID	2,775	951	485	31	203	126	106	128	1,232	34	430
IL	25,481	8,194	2,146	109	3,141	1,295	1,503	1,786	11,870	1,110	2,521
IN	11,890	4,085	1,801	120	951	565	648	803	5,385	250	1,367
IA	5,091	1,723	944	42	329	177	231	257	2,224	141	746
KS	5,695	1,963	939	42	465	244	273	307	2,428	140	857
KY	8,423	2,854	1,010	102	812	412	518	504	3,825	265	975
LA	10,275	3,284	903	155	1,021	572	633	648	4,888	346	1,109
ME	3,436	1,188	475	15	372	135	191	181	1,495	67	505
MD	18,611	5,181	897	87	2,158	751	1,288	1,757	8,863	984	1,826
MA	24,656	7,275	941	73	3,748	838	1,675	2,310	11,372	1,468	2,231
MI	18,033	5,487	1,708	91	1,803	958	927	1,182	8,398	652	2,314
MN	13,861	5,021	2,380	62	1,368	509	702	999	5,748	394	1,699
MS	5,066	1,716	624	88	453	288	263	285	2,247	109	709
MO	12,049	3,780	1,065	76	1,261	563	815	967	5,656	443	1,203
MT	2,406	808	396	16	209	98	89	106	1,028	26	438
NE	4,129	1,529	748	27	362	168	224	223	1,719	115	543
NV	3,733	1,098	352	33	373	191	149	184	1,819	78	554
NH	3,335	1,109	358	17	356	161	217	197	1,449	82	498
NJ	16,410	4,540	740	60	1,765	870	1,105	1,307	8,143	550	1,870
NM	4,426	1,547	590	45	453	183	276	243	1,843	153	640
NY	47,598	13,066	1,898	157	5,834	2,145	3,032	3,780	23,671	2,439	4,642
NC	21,912	7,067	2,376	123	2,128	1,090	1,350	1,651	9,738	784	2,672
ND	1,183	451	256	12	82	44	57	54	512	12	154
OH	23,773	7,567	2,471	123	2,257	1,075	1,641	1,806	10,795	883	2,722
OK	5,709	1,900	775	70	505	274	276	307	2,528	121	853
OR	10,466	3,528	1,124	101	1,326	432	545	573	4,489	306	1,570
PA	30,895	8,678	2,589	180	3,010	1,165	1,734	2,428	14,312	1,228	4,249
RI	3,109	1,014	170	5	431	143	265	244	1,422	144	285
SC	9,751	3,381	1,280	105	841	525	630	523	4,394	232	1,221
SD	1,687	629	335	23	139	70	62	80	728	26	224
TN	14,667	4,802	1,416	148	1,561	742	935	1,112	6,685	374	1,694
TX	41,014	13,013	4,213	378	3,556	2,329	2,537	2,764	19,591	1,484	4,162
UT	5,498	1,774	641	31	451	256	395	310	2,561	206	647
VT	2,318	810	269	16	280	93	152	130	960	82	336
VA	18,351	6,118	2,002	137	1,829	912	1,238	1,196	8,164	626	2,247
WA	16,923	5,701	2,399	137	1,597	611	957	1,044	7,214	478	2,486
WV	2,958	990	454	29	239	124	144	169	1,328	106	365
WI	13,065	4,516	1,934	74	1,253	530	725	762	5,900	245	1,642
WY	1,013	369	197	15	72	45	40	29	440	5	170
POSS.	5,495	1,931	391	161	609	304	466	377	2,461	371	355
APO/FPO	907	384	200	9	60	44	71	31	424	56	12
UNK.	350										350

Notes:

Total Physicians include Active, Inactive, and Address Unknown.

FM subspecialties include FPG and FSM.

IM subspecialties include AMI, CCM, DIA, END, HEM, HEP, HO, ICE, ID, ILI, IMG, ISM, NEP, NTR, ON, PCC, and RHU.

OBG subspecialties include GO, GYN, MFM, OBS, OCC, and REN.

PD subspecialties include ADL, CCP, MPD, NPM, PDA, PDC, PDE, PDI, PDP, PDT, PEM, PG, PHO, PLI, PN, PPR, and PSM.

Table 4.13

Graduates of Canadian Medical Schools by Self-Designated Primary Care Specialty and State of Location, 2006

State	Total Physicians	Total Primary Care	Family Medicine	General Practice	Internal Medicine	OB/Gyn	Pediatrics	Subspecialties	All Other Specialties	Not Classified	Inactive/ Address Unknown
Totals	12,154	3,052	1,490	312	600	322	328	775	5,329	961	2,037
AL	119	52	33	10	5	3	1	9	45	5	8
AK	12	7	4	3					4		1
AZ	341	86	52	9	15	6	4	18	155	11	71
AR	46	19	14	1	1	2	1	2	18	1	6
CA	1,972	437	182	53	104	44	54	117	860	130	428
CO	165	41	24	3	5	3	6	11	82	10	21
CT	203	46	15	3	7	6	15	12	89	19	37
DE	22	4	2		1		1	2	10	2	4
DC	52	5	1		3		1	2	35	5	5
FL	619	117	58	20	17	15	7	28	291	24	159
GA	208	65	32	5	9	8	11	17	96	8	22
HI	74	22	8	3	5	4	2	7	34	2	9
ID	54	25	15	4	6			1	17	2	9
IL	320	82	41	6	19	3	13	22	129	52	35
IN	182	72	47	16	7	2		8	60	15	27
IA	85	21	16	1	3	1		7	37	8	12
KS	70	18	9	3	1	3	2	4	36	2	10
KY	133	44	23	9	3	7	2	4	67	8	10
LA	83	21	11		4	4	2	4	46	4	8
ME	169	58	33	3	9	4	9	5	60	1	45
MD	252	46	12	2	15	5	12	20	122	40	24
MA	813	191	45	5	74	28	39	86	316	146	74
MI	385	65	21	4	22	10	8	25	178	24	93
MN	413	89	44	4	24	9	8	30	208	35	51
MS	44	18	14	1	1	2		1	19	1	5
MO	106	20	9	3	4	1	3	9	48	16	13
MT	26	10	6	1	3				10	1	5
NE	45	9	8	1				7	24	2	3
NV	71	23	11	3	1	4	4	3	31	2	12
NH	167	61	41	1	9	6	4	7	64	4	31
NJ	156	31	13	1	7	4	6	14	67	19	25
NM	62	17	10	2	2	1	2	4	23	4	14
NY	1,048	197	66	13	54	33	31	76	503	100	172
NC	252	78	42	7	14	9	6	19	94	24	37
ND	103	36	25	5	3	2	1		49	4	14
OH	407	94	45	13	20	10	6	26	167	62	58
OK	51	20	14	2	2	2			23	2	6
OR	241	84	54	10	13	6	1	11	94	15	37
PA	389	67	22	4	27	7	7	28	198	36	60
RI	82	24	6	1	6	5	6	7	37	3	11
SC	63	17	9		3	4	1	1	27	2	16
SD	18	2	1	1					7	1	8
TN	194	75	43	11	8	8	5	17	80	5	17
TX	707	230	139	33	25	15	18	45	293	42	97
UT	85	20	13	2	1	1	3	9	36	8	12
VT	97	29	15		2	8	4	5	44	1	18
VA	213	67	34	8	6	11	8	6	90	16	34
WA	493	126	66	13	28	9	10	31	216	29	91
WV	41	12	4	2	1	4	1	1	18	1	9
WI	141	47	35	5	1	3	3	7	62	5	20
WY	10	2		2					6		2
POSS.	10	2	2						3	1	4
APO/FPO	3	1	1						1	1	
UNK.	37										37

Notes:

Total Physicians include Active, Inactive, and Address Unknown.

FM subspecialties include FPG and FSM.

IM subspecialties include AMI, CCM, DIA, END, HEM, HEP, HO, ICE, ID, ILI, IMG, ISM, NEP, NTR, ON, PCC, and RHU.

OBG subspecialties include GO, GYN, MFM, OBS, OCC, and REN.

PD subspecialties include ADL, CCP, MPD, NPM, PDA, PDC, PDE, PDI, PDP, PDT, PEM, PG, PHO, PLI, PN, PPR, and PSM.

Table 4.14

Metropolitan Physicans by Self-Designated Primary Care Specialty and Activity, 2006

Specialty	Total Physicians	Patient Care				Other Professional Activity			
		Total Patient Care	Office Based	Hospital Based		Admin.	Med. Teach.	Research	Other
				Resid./ Fellows	Phys. Staff				
Both Sexes									
Total Physicians	709,345	558,124	428,028	80,437	49,659	11,376	8,235	11,403	3,499
Active Physicians	629,269	558,124	428,028	80,437	49,659	11,376	8,235	11,403	3,499
Primary Care	226,489	216,490	166,614	33,596	16,280	3,794	3,169	2,224	812
Family Medicine	55,487	53,176	43,336	6,521	3,319	919	1,108	152	132
General Practice	6,748	6,459	5,636		823	163	20	31	75
Internal Medicine	89,345	85,075	60,686	17,421	6,968	1,619	1,040	1,262	349
Obstetrics/Gynecology	29,575	28,788	23,652	3,495	1,641	258	334	145	50
Pediatrics	45,334	42,992	33,304	6,159	3,529	835	667	634	206
Prim. Care Subspec.	53,982	48,181	35,996	7,213	4,972	1,118	1,186	3,294	203
FM Subspecialties	699	665	530	96	39	10	18	3	3
IM Subspecialties	35,849	31,516	24,482	4,036	2,998	815	777	2,603	138
OBG Subspecialties	3,441	3,192	2,856		336	82	100	55	12
PD Subspecialties	13,993	12,808	8,128	3,081	1,599	211	291	633	50
All Other Specialties	312,166	293,453	225,418	39,628	28,407	6,464	3,880	5,885	2,484
Inactive	80,076								
Not Classified	36,632								
Male									
Total Physicians	505,937	388,601	308,407	45,389	34,805	9,184	6,078	8,882	2,504
Active Physicians	436,766	388,601	308,407	45,389	34,805	9,184	6,078	8,882	2,504
Primary Care	134,447	127,385	102,042	15,514	9,829	2,878	2,086	1,594	504
Family Medicine	35,118	33,393	28,142	3,031	2,220	746	794	95	90
General Practice	5,335	5,124	4,547		577	119	15	24	53
Internal Medicine	58,832	55,622	41,143	9,895	4,584	1,278	705	983	244
Obstetrics/Gynecology	15,703	15,124	13,327	839	958	209	235	105	30
Pediatrics	19,459	18,122	14,883	1,749	1,490	526	337	387	87
Prim. Care Subspec.	36,365	31,960	24,880	3,794	3,286	909	882	2,478	136
FM Subspecialties	497	473	382	66	25	7	14	1	2
IM Subspecialties	25,563	22,163	17,750	2,346	2,067	668	607	2,029	96
OBG Subspecialties	2,473	2,274	2,041		233	68	78	44	9
PD Subspecialties	7,832	7,050	4,707	1,382	961	166	183	404	29
All Other Specialties	244,437	229,256	181,485	26,081	21,690	5,397	3,110	4,810	1,864
Inactive	69,171								
Not Classified	21,517								
Female									
Total Physicians	203,408	169,523	119,621	35,048	14,854	2,192	2,157	2,521	995
Active Physicians	192,503	169,523	119,621	35,048	14,854	2,192	2,157	2,521	995
Primary Care	92,042	89,105	64,572	18,082	6,451	916	1,083	630	308
Family Medicine	20,369	19,783	15,194	3,490	1,099	173	314	57	42
General Practice	1,413	1,335	1,089		246	44	5	7	22
Internal Medicine	30,513	29,453	19,543	7,526	2,384	341	335	279	105
Obstetrics/Gynecology	13,872	13,664	10,325	2,656	683	49	99	40	20
Pediatrics	25,875	24,870	18,421	4,410	2,039	309	330	247	119
Prim. Care Subspec.	17,617	16,221	11,116	3,419	1,686	209	304	816	67
FM Subspecialties	202	192	148	30	14	3	4	2	1
IM Subspecialties	10,286	9,353	6,732	1,690	931	147	170	574	42
OBG Subspecialties	968	918	815		103	14	22	11	3
PD Subspecialties	6,161	5,758	3,421	1,699	638	45	108	229	21
All Other Specialties	67,729	64,197	43,933	13,547	6,717	1,067	770	1,075	620
Inactive	10,905								
Not Classified	15,115								

Table 4.15

Metropolitan Physicians by Self-Designated Primary Care Specialty, 2006

State	Total Physicians	Total Primary Care	Family Medicine	General Practice	Internal Medicine	OB/Gyn	Pediatrics	Subspec- ialties	All Other Special- ties	Not Classified/ Inactive
Total Metros	709,095	226,419	55,460	6,743	89,325	29,568	45,323	53,973	312,060	116,643
Abilene TX	312	108	37	7	25	21	18	23	142	39
Aguadilla PR	132	63	8	19	18	9	9	3	53	13
Albany GA	222	87	28		26	18	15	19	94	22
Albany NY*	2,735	805	238	25	285	106	151	206	1,301	423
Albuquerque NM	2,481	794	238	18	290	84	164	170	1,090	427
Alexandria LA	425	144	47	5	48	20	24	25	190	66
Allentown PA*	1,747	564	180	12	194	92	86	121	800	262
Altoona PA	328	110	38	2	36	16	18	16	144	58
Amarillo TX	685	260	80	6	92	39	43	50	289	86
Anchorage AK	1,016	363	159	12	76	49	67	60	483	110
Anniston AL	224	95	38	2	27	16	12	11	92	26
Appleton WI*	870	310	135	4	93	36	42	45	402	113
Asheville NC	775	239	102	4	73	40	20	62	328	146
Athens GA	376	109	24	5	35	29	16	26	194	47
Atlanta GA	11,554	3,963	747	85	1,566	651	914	859	5,186	1,546
Auburn AL*	114	41	9	4	14	7	7	11	52	10
Augusta GA*	1,996	576	164	11	189	92	120	165	957	298
Austin TX*	3,351	1,207	410	34	335	173	255	193	1,475	476
Bakersfield CA	1,162	508	142	21	182	79	84	52	453	149
Bangor ME	526	161	61	3	59	12	26	42	250	73
Barnstable MA*	780	217	42	6	112	21	36	28	314	221
Baton Rouge LA*	1,700	572	155	17	192	84	124	132	762	234
Beaumont TX*	638	214	71	10	66	35	32	36	293	95
Bellingham WA	483	176	94	5	35	16	26	23	195	89
Benton Harbor MI	295	115	41	6	33	17	18	13	115	52
Billings MT	549	157	67	1	47	21	21	39	280	73
Biloxi MS*	726	218	49	12	80	37	40	40	363	105
Binghamton NY	688	249	82	1	106	32	28	29	286	124
Birmingham AL	2,718	869	172	12	367	120	198	235	1,249	365
Bismarck ND	337	91	48	1	20	11	11	24	177	45
Bloomington IL*	343	105	35	1	29	19	21	15	178	45
Bloomington IN	367	109	43	6	30	18	12	13	176	69
Boise City ID	1,229	423	188	9	102	72	52	88	553	165
Boston MA*	30,425	8,860	1,307	135	4,509	975	1,934	2,831	13,589	5,145
Brownsville TX*	555	241	70	8	64	34	65	43	197	74
Bryan TX*	191	79	39	4	18	11	7	8	77	27
Buffalo NY*	3,424	1,088	218	17	476	146	231	256	1,526	554
Burlington VT	635	172	62	4	62	16	28	54	295	114
Canton OH*	617	257	100	3	92	23	39	37	225	98
Casper WY	188	61	36	1	11	6	7	8	88	31
Cedar Rapids IA	430	143	99	4	14	9	17	22	186	79
Champaign IL*	680	254	74	7	126	18	29	57	246	123
Charleston SC*	2,766	748	201	17	250	121	159	235	1,418	365
Charleston WV	868	284	85	9	100	40	50	71	385	128
Charlotte NC*	4,182	1,491	457	18	515	214	287	307	1,834	550
Charlottesville VA	594	163	44	2	60	15	42	55	256	120
Chattanooga TN	1,215	426	114	10	143	64	95	93	528	168

† Does not include 220 physicians whose MSA could not be determined.

* MSA name is abbreviated.

Notes:

FM subspecialties include FPG and FSM.

IM subspecialties include AMI, CCM, DIA, END, HEM, HEP, HO, ICE, ID, ILI, IMG, ISM, NEP, NTR, ON, PCC, and RHU.

OBG subspecialties include GO, GYN, MFM, OBS, OCC, and REN.

PD subspecialties include ADL, CCP, MPD, NPM, PDA, PDC, PDE, PDI, PDP, PDT, PEM, PG, PHO, PLI, PN, PPR, and PSM.

Table 4.15

Metropolitan Physicians by Self-Designated Primary Care Specialty, 2006, continued

State	Total Physicians	Total Primary Care	Family Medicine	General Practice	Internal Medicine	OB/Gyn	Pediatrics	Subspec- ialties	All Other Special- ties	Not Classified/ Inactive
Cheyenne WY	168	53	26	1	13	5	8	11	72	32
Chicago IL*	29,837	10,274	2,045	301	4,679	1,300	1,949	2,252	12,668	4,643
Chico CA*	532	168	59	13	50	23	23	25	235	104
Cincinnati OH*	5,448	1,764	432	39	630	221	442	535	2,302	847
Clarksville TN*	353	131	40	3	33	23	32	15	158	49
Cleveland OH*	6,596	2,138	457	66	929	270	416	512	2,764	1,182
Colorado Springs CO	491	138	50	3	31	17	37	30	253	70
Columbia MO	935	217	68	4	74	30	41	103	472	143
Columbia SC	2,017	675	201	22	209	98	145	134	960	248
Columbus GA	485	187	118	6	30	16	17	26	186	86
Columbus OH	4,625	1,534	533	34	469	207	291	418	2,009	664
Corpus Christi TX	116	43	13	5	13	5	7	3	53	17
Corvalis OR	292	98	28	6	36	12	16	14	118	62
Cumberland MD	228	63	17	5	23	8	10	14	111	40
Dallas TX*	12,721	4,081	1,073	111	1,377	704	816	995	5,922	1,723
Danville VA	184	57	18		21	9	9	13	83	31
Davenport IA*	686	211	97	2	52	29	31	36	319	120
Dayton OH	880	305	128	14	98	29	36	54	356	165
Daytona Beach FL	2,402	856	299	14	306	98	139	158	1,027	361
Decatur AL	222	89	34	1	25	16	13	12	93	28
Decatur IL	281	107	61	1	26	10	9	14	119	41
Denver CO*	7,548	2,492	750	48	860	333	501	612	3,294	1,150
Des Moines IA	843	264	97	4	79	30	54	65	394	120
Detroit MI*	16,925	5,461	1,144	116	2,449	762	990	1,413	7,270	2,781
Dothan AL	350	91	24	1	33	15	18	22	197	40
Dover DE	214	73	24		25	9	15	15	95	31
Dubuque IA	248	83	19	1	35	12	16	14	115	36
Duluth MN*	770	277	160	6	63	26	22	41	314	138
Eau Claire WI	461	156	76	2	48	15	15	35	214	56
El Paso TX	297	105	58	2	20	10	15	14	119	59
Elkhart IN*	264	77	20	3	35	9	10	23	117	47
Elmira NY	1,405	494	111	12	177	73	121	103	609	199
Enid OK	132	40	20	1	5	6	8	2	62	28
Erie PA	609	167	92	2	33	19	21	42	283	117
Eugene OR*	959	325	120	19	98	39	49	51	399	184
Evansville IN*	797	277	149	4	57	34	33	51	359	110
Fargo ND*	423	162	60	1	67	12	22	24	179	58
Fayetteville AR*	685	271	136	8	51	35	41	43	266	105
Fayetteville NC	687	278	109	5	83	37	44	42	280	87
Flagstaff AZ	176	72	28	2	15	14	13	4	72	28
Florence AL	284	90	24	3	36	12	15	16	133	45
Florence SC	420	156	75	8	37	22	14	35	189	40
Fort Collins CO*	730	263	153	4	41	27	38	45	302	120
Fort Myers FL*	1,338	338	68	17	125	50	78	76	550	374
Fort Pierce FL*	711	175	36	5	72	35	27	39	304	193
Fort Smith AR	468	186	103	8	38	17	20	30	166	86
Fort Wayne IN	972	268	130	5	60	40	33	79	505	120
Fresno CA	1,909	735	217	32	234	84	168	94	750	330
Ft Walton Beach FL	366	147	62	9	37	15	24	14	160	45
Gadsden AL	209	74	28	3	21	6	16	8	102	25

† Does not include 220 physicians whose MSA could not be determined.

* MSA name is abbreviated.

Notes:

FM subspecialties include FPG and FSM.

IM subspecialties include AMI, CCM, DIA, END, HEM, HEP, HO, ICE, ID, ILI, IMG, ISM, NEP, NTR, ON, PCC, and RHU.

OBG subspecialties include GO, GYN, MFM, OBS, OCC, and REN.

PD subspecialties include ADL, CCP, MPD, NPM, PDA, PDC, PDE, PDI, PDP, PDT, PEM, PG, PHO, PLI, PN, PPR, and PSM.

Table 4.15

Metropolitan Physicians by Self-Designated Primary Care Specialty, 2006, continued

State	Total Physicians	Total Primary Care	Family Medicine	General Practice	Internal Medicine	OB/Gyn	Pediatrics	Subspec-ialties	All Other Special-ties	Not Classified/Inactive
Gainsesville FL	2,107	568	134	17	224	49	144	216	1,008	315
Glens Falls NY	292	105	41	1	24	15	24	15	129	43
Goldsboro NC	201	72	27	7	19	7	12	14	79	36
Grand Forks ND	259	101	65	2	21	4	9	18	113	27
Grand Junction CO	230	63	36	2	13	9	3	14	113	40
Grand Rapids MI*	1,452	526	221	9	156	54	86	96	573	257
Great Falls MT	235	71	26	1	22	11	11	14	109	41
Green Bay WI	649	203	68	7	62	36	30	50	323	73
Greensboro NC*	3,575	1,186	354	25	426	156	225	249	1,615	525
Greenville NC	1,023	307	83	3	104	43	74	118	469	129
Greenville SC*	2,588	1,013	389	23	267	145	189	154	1,082	339
Harrisburg PA*	2,075	582	176	9	224	75	98	156	978	359
Hartford CT	4,379	1,432	263	21	670	189	289	332	1,861	754
Hattiesburg MS	429	131	50	3	33	22	23	32	223	43
Hickory NC*	695	239	123	4	55	34	23	30	333	93
Honolulu HI	3,552	1,205	208	49	516	177	255	259	1,535	553
Houma LA	373	126	37	7	25	31	26	18	181	48
Houston TX*	14,397	4,311	1,162	156	1,371	632	990	1,373	6,472	2,241
Huntington WV*	570	210	59	7	75	29	40	36	244	80
Huntsville AL	952	352	156	11	83	45	57	51	422	127
Indianapolis IN	6,029	1,864	607	41	609	258	349	640	2,758	767
Iowa City IA	1,840	390	97	4	143	50	96	176	925	349
Jackson MI	215	73	26	1	27	8	11	17	87	38
Jackson MS	2,228	637	177	17	211	102	130	185	1,076	330
Jackson TN	444	162	56	1	54	30	21	29	192	61
Jacksonville FL	3,729	1,192	392	47	371	140	242	281	1,663	593
Jacksonville NC	241	97	44	2	14	18	19	8	93	43
Jamestown NY	217	85	22	4	38	11	10	6	82	44
Janesville WI*	304	123	56	2	38	13	14	11	122	48
Johnson City TN*	1,499	561	204	9	217	64	67	114	624	200
Johnstown PA	541	196	89	6	69	17	15	17	238	90
Jonesboro AR	306	114	61	1	20	16	16	16	142	34
Joplin MO	164	44	15	2	12	7	8	12	88	20
Kalamazoo MI*	1,320	450	146	7	173	43	81	100	546	224
Kansas City MO	3,573	1,094	337	14	356	137	250	296	1,611	572
Kileen-Temple TX	657	202	51	5	88	28	30	35	308	112
Knoxville TN	1,770	580	208	20	156	96	100	132	794	264
Kokomo IN	158	61	25	2	16	8	10	8	62	27
La Crosse WI	612	211	78	2	85	19	27	45	275	81
Lafayette IN	415	133	47	4	40	19	23	31	193	58
Lafayette LA	964	382	126	18	121	56	61	48	415	119
Lake Charles LA	409	157	72	6	33	24	22	21	170	61
Lakeland FL*	990	307	71	21	122	37	56	64	399	220
Lancaster PA	994	359	227	3	56	38	35	55	375	205
Lansing MI*	1,120	404	122	9	140	50	83	82	449	185
Laredo TX	251	101	37	7	21	16	20	14	98	38
Las Cruces NM	311	114	52	9	28	11	14	14	132	51
Las Vegas NV	3,632	1,240	281	43	539	175	202	218	1,530	644
Lawrence KS	230	80	32	3	27	9	9	9	88	53

† Does not include 220 physicians whose MSA could not be determined.

* MSA name is abbreviated.

Notes:

FM subspecialties include FPG and FSM.

IM subspecialties include AMI, CCM, DIA, END, HEM, HEP, HO, ICE, ID, ILI, IMG, ISM, NEP, NTR, ON, PCC, and RHU.

OBG subspecialties include GO, GYN, MFM, OBS, OCC, and REN.

PD subspecialties include ADL, CCP, MPD, NPM, PDA, PDC, PDE, PDI, PDP, PDT, PEM, PG, PHO, PLI, PN, PPR, and PSM.

Table 4.15

Metropolitan Physicians by Self-Designated Primary Care Specialty, 2006, continued

State	Total Physicians	Total Primary Care	Family Medicine	General Practice	Internal Medicine	OB/Gyn	Pediatrics	Subspec-ialties	All Other Special-ties	Not Classified/ Inactive
Lawton OK	247	100	40	6	26	17	11	7	111	29
Lewiston ME*	289	91	41		34	10	6	20	136	42
Lexington KY	1,853	487	110	11	200	80	86	150	910	306
Lima OH	284	80	42	3	14	12	9	22	135	47
Lincoln NE	780	261	129	3	62	27	40	47	333	139
Little Rock AR*	2,813	738	237	24	197	92	188	295	1,454	326
Longview TX*	363	118	42	3	37	19	17	27	164	54
Los Angeles CA*	41,594	13,473	3,245	834	4,908	1,760	2,726	2,776	17,794	7,551
Louisville KY	3,686	1,033	234	31	387	134	247	309	1,780	564
Lubbock TX	759	240	81	12	70	29	48	47	369	103
Lynchburg VA	488	164	84	7	34	16	23	29	198	97
Macon GA	987	353	91	4	136	69	53	72	407	155
Madison WI	2,370	752	287	13	257	67	128	173	1,067	378
Mansfield OH	248	78	23	3	32	9	11	17	105	48
Mayaguez PR	308	124	15	34	33	24	18	17	122	45
McAllen TX	762	366	147	9	83	43	84	66	254	76
Medford OR	638	185	72	8	58	25	22	45	269	139
Melbourne FL*	937	281	82	14	111	35	39	56	436	164
Memphis TN	3,505	1,099	211	37	429	171	251	377	1,555	474
Merced CA	259	135	75	6	26	15	13	11	80	33
Miami FL*	9,147	2,521	385	277	945	297	617	703	3,921	2,002
Milwaukee WI*	5,768	1,826	568	35	645	234	344	425	2,708	809
Minneapolis MN*	7,720	2,733	1,125	29	791	322	466	686	3,192	1,109
Missoula MT	409	97	32	1	35	15	14	27	203	82
Mobile AL	1,528	511	136	18	173	80	104	98	705	214
Modesto CA	914	369	161	8	111	39	50	44	356	145
Monroe LA	450	162	68	13	35	21	25	28	204	56
Montgomery AL	716	271	79	4	116	32	40	51	306	88
Muncie IN	340	136	54	5	53	9	15	23	141	40
Mytle Beach SC	372	118	24	3	44	28	19	23	185	46
Naples FL	1,180	211	42	12	91	33	33	53	423	493
Nashville TN	4,854	1,428	265	39	624	210	290	416	2,344	666
New London CT*	240	83	19	1	31	10	22	8	96	53
New Orleans LA	5,187	1,423	219	40	595	230	339	446	2,562	756
New York NY*	89,457	28,445	2,578	471	14,881	3,756	6,759	7,247	39,145	14,620
Norfolk VA*	3,429	1,226	388	43	337	181	277	237	1,509	457
Ocala FL	583	178	49	8	79	13	29	41	259	105
Odessa TX*	505	202	48	6	84	36	28	41	206	56
Oklahoma City OK	3,092	896	339	33	270	100	154	243	1,498	455
Omaha NE	2,661	889	314	12	291	110	162	188	1,174	410
Orlando FL	4,168	1,446	415	72	465	193	301	299	1,765	658
Owensboro KY	232	68	23	1	25	9	10	12	118	34
Panama City FL	271	88	28	6	35	10	9	18	136	29
Parkersburg WV*	257	80	38	3	24	9	6	14	121	42
Pensacola FL	1,132	360	165	11	70	42	72	79	547	146
Peoria IL*	970	328	135	3	98	36	56	93	410	139
Philadelphia PA*	20,044	5,733	1,072	143	2,499	722	1,297	1,787	8,996	3,528
Phoenix AZ*	9,123	2,867	801	77	1,042	386	561	647	3,922	1,687
Pine Bluff AR	188	89	56	2	13	7	11	9	67	23

† Does not include 220 physicians whose MSA could not be determined.

* MSA name is abbreviated.

Notes:

FM subspecialties include FPG and FSM.

IM subspecialties include AMI, CCM, DIA, END, HEM, HEP, HO, ICE, ID, ILI, IMG, ISM, NEP, NTR, ON, PCC, and RHU.

OBG subspecialties include GO, GYN, MFM, OBS, OCC, and REN.

PD subspecialties include ADL, CCP, MPD, NPM, PDA, PDC, PDE, PDI, PDP, PDT, PEM, PG, PHO, PLI, PN, PPR, and PSM.

Table 4.15

Metropolitan Physicians by Self-Designated Primary Care Specialty, 2006, continued

State	Total Physicians	Total Primary Care	Family Medicine	General Practice	Internal Medicine	OB/Gyn	Pediatrics	Subspec-ialties	All Other Special-ties	Not Classified/ Inactive
Pittsburgh PA	8,368	2,314	639	55	953	272	395	718	3,888	1,448
Pittsfield MA	547	173	25	1	111	11	25	22	245	107
Pocatello ID	184	68	35	2	16	7	8	7	79	30
Ponce PR	343	151	20	26	55	23	27	21	110	61
Portland ME	1,181	366	106	2	134	48	76	89	555	171
Portland OR*	7,130	2,477	680	56	1,048	294	399	414	3,013	1,226
Providence RI*	2,924	937	141	11	454	126	205	258	1,246	483
Provo UT*	628	236	101	8	41	36	50	22	287	83
Pueblo CO	375	122	64	2	29	11	16	18	176	59
Punta Gorda FL	191	34	10	2	15	3	4	4	76	77
Raleigh NC*	6,023	1,756	407	14	684	231	420	578	2,697	992
Rapid City SD	358	106	52	6	24	12	12	22	169	61
Reading PA	669	211	79	5	70	30	27	36	290	132
Redding CA	489	147	75	7	40	13	12	24	233	85
Reno NV	1,033	275	89	7	101	41	37	70	522	166
Richland WA*	320	119	38	4	35	20	22	23	139	39
Richmond VA*	3,708	1,114	303	27	391	156	237	282	1,605	707
Roanoke VA	870	268	82	3	108	42	33	59	405	138
Rochester MN	1,775	346	64	3	207	28	44	172	905	352
Rochester NY	3,180	1,174	218	8	566	147	235	209	1,229	568
Rockford IL	718	276	139	3	65	37	32	47	274	121
Rocky Mount NC	112	54	22	1	17	10	4	6	34	18
Sacramento CA*	6,005	2,072	612	75	766	251	368	346	2,591	996
Saginaw MI*	899	340	141	10	112	43	34	46	391	122
Saint Cloud MN	465	189	91	2	50	18	28	28	192	56
Saint Joseph MO	58	14	7	1	4		2	6	28	10
Saint Louis MO	7,510	2,264	382	32	1,058	305	487	671	3,473	1,102
Salinas CA	923	297	133	15	73	38	38	45	374	207
Salt Lake City UT*	1,829	601	236	9	133	89	134	109	819	300
San Angelo TX	208	67	16	2	26	13	10	8	106	27
San Antonio TX	5,196	1,558	475	40	485	233	325	467	2,490	681
San Diego CA	10,361	2,950	824	124	1,036	386	580	712	4,729	1,970
San Francisco CA*	28,083	9,087	1,733	309	3,934	1,123	1,988	1,730	11,916	5,350
San Juan PR*	3,803	1,436	211	383	362	163	317	197	1,522	648
San Luis Obispo CA*	568	166	74	7	52	12	21	8	274	120
Santa Barbara CA*	1,361	416	109	26	180	41	60	62	565	318
Santa Fe NM	504	156	75	5	41	12	23	28	199	121
Sarasota FL*	2,205	474	120	26	185	73	70	111	893	727
Savannah GA	901	293	74	8	95	52	64	53	400	155
Scranton PA*	1,064	375	97	17	184	36	41	64	455	170
Seattle WA*	13,287	4,304	1,631	123	1,384	440	726	971	5,662	2,350
Sharon PA	190	46	14	1	20	6	5	10	86	48
Sheboygan WI	197	72	33	3	15	11	10	10	83	32
Sherman TX*	241	73	24	2	22	13	12	13	110	45
Shreveport LA*	1,782	533	134	11	203	87	98	171	828	250
Sioux City IA	200	72	50		8	6	8	14	82	32
Sioux Falls SD	824	266	111	3	97	31	24	76	389	93
South Bend IN	780	278	156	3	50	33	36	52	343	107
Spokane WA	1,327	399	181	13	127	41	37	85	602	241

† Does not include 220 physicians whose MSA could not be determined.

* MSA name is abbreviated.

Notes:

FM subspecialties include FPG and FSM.

IM subspecialties include AMI, CCM, DIA, END, HEM, HEP, HO, ICE, ID, ILI, IMG, ISM, NEP, NTR, ON, PCC, and RHU.

OBG subspecialties include GO, GYN, MFM, OBS, OCC, and REN.

PD subspecialties include ADL, CCP, MPD, NPM, PDA, PDC, PDE, PDI, PDP, PDT, PEM, PG, PHO, PLI, PN, PPR, and PSM.

Table 4.15

Metropolitan Physicians by Self-Designated Primary Care Specialty, 2006, continued

State	Total Physicians	Total Primary Care	Family Medicine†	General Practice	Internal Medicine	OB/Gyn	Pediatrics‖	Subspec-ialties	All Other Special-ties	Not Classified/ Inactive
Springfield IL	1,022	303	91	3	118	42	49	83	496	140
Springfield MA	723	286	73	8	118	28	59	44	264	129
Springfield MO	906	291	109	9	95	39	39	63	431	121
State College PA	327	108	34	5	34	15	20	19	154	46
Steubenville OH*	102	36	5	4	16	5	6	4	45	17
Stockton CA*	1,102	460	142	26	150	59	83	47	433	162
Sumter SC	173	66	19	3	20	10	14	8	72	27
Syracuse NY	2,607	784	234	11	279	101	159	198	1,201	424
Tallahassee FL	808	295	157	8	60	28	42	46	322	145
Tampa FL*	5,930	1,802	389	74	770	207	362	466	2,652	1,010
Terre Haute IN	326	133	72	2	36	14	9	15	147	31
Texarkana TX-AR	271	84	29	5	24	17	9	12	128	47
Toledo OH	1,540	546	205	14	151	63	113	95	649	250
Topeka KS	525	139	42	6	57	14	20	34	249	103
Tucson AZ	3,026	859	233	21	316	106	183	173	1,407	587
Tulsa OK	1,902	656	229	11	230	80	106	124	783	339
Tuscaloosa AL	472	162	64	6	54	19	19	25	219	66
Tyler TX	758	226	86	8	71	31	30	66	373	93
Utica NY*	647	233	99	5	78	22	29	38	256	120
Victoria TX	213	80	26	2	26	12	14	10	99	24
Visalia CA*	509	229	69	11	68	36	45	26	172	82
Waco TX	528	206	120	5	33	27	21	19	228	75
Washington DC*	30,573	9,562	1,555	205	4,337	1,275	2,190	2,723	13,406	4,882
Waterloo IA*	314	117	73	1	22	12	9	16	130	51
Wausau WI	380	130	73	2	31	5	19	21	175	54
West Palm Beach FL*	2,902	707	112	34	349	97	115	183	1,234	778
Wheeling WV	56	25	9	2	10	2	2	4	18	9
Wichita Falls TX	345	130	74	3	21	14	18	15	152	48
Wichita KS	1,480	531	261	4	138	54	74	97	630	222
Williamsport PA	257	90	61	4	17	5	3	12	103	52
Wilmington NC	894	285	71	5	116	57	36	70	370	169
Yakima WA	458	192	93	8	46	21	24	20	166	80
York PA	773	270	130	9	75	24	32	54	310	139
Youngstown OH*	1,195	443	107	8	204	49	75	65	473	214
Yuba City CA	263	109	45	5	25	11	23	8	101	45
Yuma AZ	235	89	18	4	34	14	19	21	93	32

† Does not include 220 physicians whose MSA could not be determined.

* MSA name is abbreviated.

Notes:

FM subspecialties include FPG and FSM.

IM subspecialties include AMI, CCM, DIA, END, HEM, HEP, HO, ICE, ID, ILI, IMG, ISM, NEP, NTR, ON, PCC, and RHU.

OBG subspecialties include GO, GYN, MFM, OBS, OCC, and REN.

PD subspecialties include ADL, CCP, MPD, NPM, PDA, PDC, PDE, PDI, PDP, PDT, PEM, PG, PHO, PLI, PN, PPR, and PSM.

Chapter 5
Osteopathic Physicians

Activity by Age and Sex

Table 5.1 indicates that in 2006, nearly half of osteopathic physicians (DOs) were younger than 45 years (48.3%). The 35- to 44-year age interval accounted for the highest percentage of total DOs (28.1%). The DOs 65 and older numbered 7,353, or 12.3% of the DOs in the US. In general, the DO population trends young, especially so when compared with the MD population, as in Figure 7.

The youth trend among DOs is especially prevalent among females. Of total female DOs (16,108), the highest percentage (33.3%) was 35 to 44 years old, with 64.4% younger than 45 years. It is no surprise, then, that a mere 5.6% were 65 years or older. Although male DOs have a higher ratio of DOs younger than 45 years than the overall MD population (42.4% vs 38.5%), they are still clearly outpaced by their female counterparts in this category.

Self-Designated Specialty by Age and Sex

An analysis of Table 5.2 indicates that at the end of 2006, more than three fifths (65.5%) of all DOs (59,560) were in the following ten specialty fields:

Family Medicine (14,553)

Internal Medicine (6,813)

Emergency Medicine (3,416)

General Practice (3,177)

Pediatrics (2,636)

Anesthesiology (2,560)

Obstetrics/Gynecology (2,133)

Psychiatry (1,473)

Orthopedic Surgery (1,163)

General Surgery (1,114)

These same specialties were also highest for all male DOs (Table 5.3), representing 64.2% of the male population. The five disciplines with the most male DOs younger than 35 years were Family Medicine (17.0% of males younger than 35 years), Internal Medicine (15.2%), Anesthesiology (6.4%), Emergency Medicine (5.2%), and Pediatrics (4.7%).

For female DOs, the specialties demonstrating the highest numbers differed from the male and overall DO populations. The top 10 disciplines for female DOs (Table 5.4) consisted of the following:

Family Medicine (4,351)

Internal Medicine (1,998)

Pediatrics (1,451)

Obstetrics/Gynecology (920)

Emergency Medicine (708)

Psychiatry (522)

General Practice (481)

Anesthesiology (469)

Physical Medicine & Rehabilitation (281)

Neurology (183)

These 10 specialties accounted for 70.5% of the female DO population, and among female DOs younger than 35 years, the highest percentages were found in Family Medicine (22.4% of females younger than 35 years), Internal Medicine (12.5%), Pediatrics (12.0%), Obstetrics/Gynecology (6.1%), and Emergency Medicine (3.6%).

Figure 7

Percent Distribution of Total US Physicians by Age and Degree, 2006

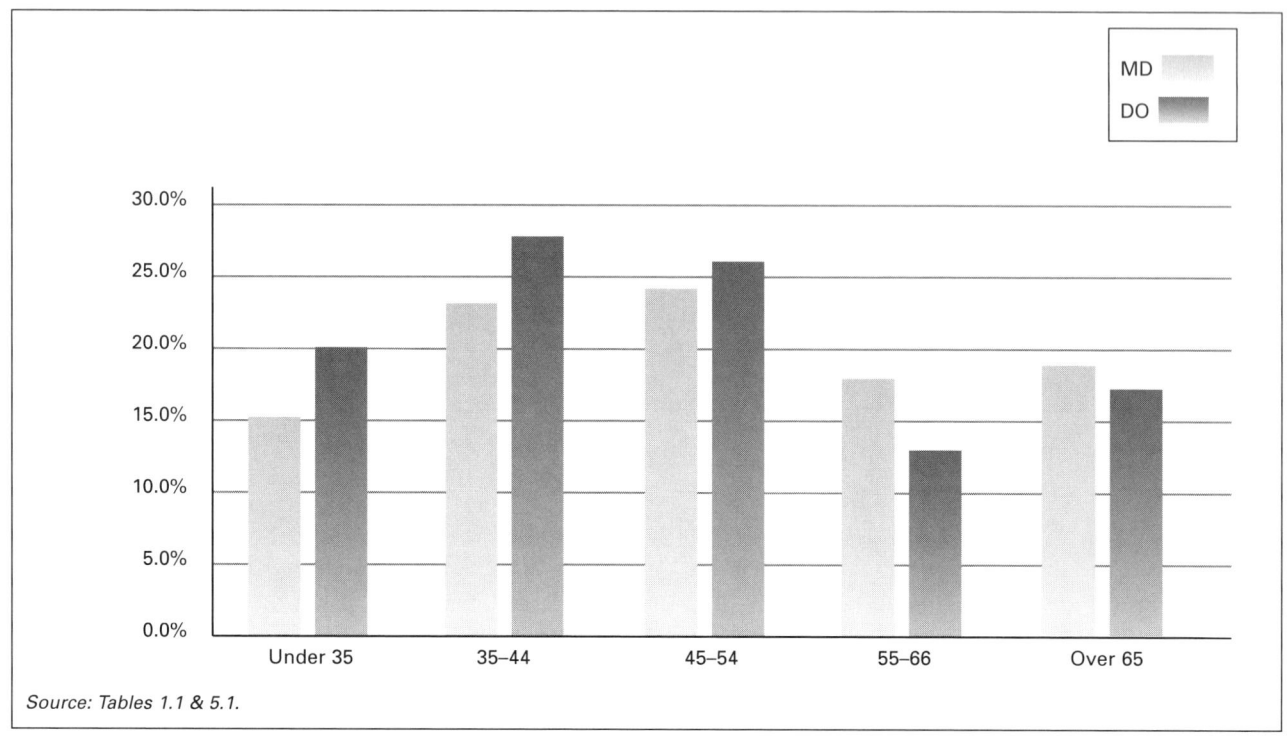

Source: Tables 1.1 & 5.1.

Distribution of Detail Specialties by Activity

The 10 specialties showing highest counts of DOs in 2006, in the detail specialties in Table 5.6, included the following: Family Medicine (14,373), Internal Medicine (5,524), Emergency Medicine (3,374), General Practice (3,177), Anesthesiology (2,391), Pediatrics (2,116), Obstetrics/Gynecology (2,025), Psychiatry (1,427), Physical Medicine and Rehabilitation (1,050), and General Surgery (962). Of these ten specialties, eight were among those in the top 10 for MDs, with General Practice and Physical Medicine and Rehabilitation for the DO population taking the place of Diagnostic Radiology and Cardiovascular Disease among the MD population.

Mean Age by Detail Specialty and Activity

Table 5.5 shows the mean age of DOs in the detail specialties. The 10 specialties with the highest mean ages include the following:

Legal Medicine (89.6)

Nutrition (73.0)

Pediatric Psychiatry/Child Psychiatry (69.5)

Psychoanalysis (65.0)

Head and Neck Surgery (62.0)

Anatomic Pathology (61.9)

Allergy (61.7)

Otology/Neurotology (61.0)

Proctology (59.7)

Addiction Medicine (59.1)

MDs and DOs shared only three specialties—Legal Medicine, Psychoanalysis, and Allergy—among the ten specialties with the highest average ages.

DOs by Self-Designated Specialty and Activity

Patient Care accounted for 86.9% of all DOs in 2006 (Table 5.7), significantly higher than the 78.4% of MDs in that category. Of the total number of DOs in Patient Care (51,765), more than

Mini-Table 10

Percent Distribution of DOs by Age and Sex, 2006

Sex	Total	< 35	35–44	45–54	55–64	≥ 65
Both	100.0	20.2	28.1	25.9	13.4	12.3
Male	100.0	16.2	26.2	26.7	16.0	14.8
Female	100.0	31.1	33.3	23.7	6.3	5.6

Source: Tables 5.13, 5.14, and 5.15.

three fourths (76.3%) were in Office-Based practice. Of a total of 7,783 Residents/Fellows, more than one half (58.2%) were specialists in the disciplines of Internal Medicine, Family Medicine, Pediatrics, Anesthesiology, and Emergency Medicine. Percentages of total DOs in residency/fellowship training in these specialties are as follows: Internal Medicine, 19.0%; Family Medicine, 17.7%; Pediatrics, 9.5%; Anesthesiology, 6.8%; and Emergency Medicine, 5.3%.

State of Location, Age, and Activity by Sex

Table 5.13 demonstrates that of the total 2006 US DO population (59,560), more than three fifths (64.9%) were located in 10 states, a much higher concentration than the 55.2% of MDs in the top 10 most MD-populated states. The 10 leading states for DOs were Pennsylvania (6,177), Michigan (5,740), Florida (4,288), Ohio (4,273), Texas (3,625), California (3,604), New York (3,431), New Jersey (2,961), Illinois (2,469), and Missouri (2,098).

Table 5.15 indicates that there were more female DOs in Pennsylvania in 2006 than in any other state (1,675, or 10.4% of total female DOs). Michigan followed with 1,446 female DOs and New York with 1,243. These three states, in addition to California (1,136), Ohio (1,043), Florida (978), and Texas (916), accounted for more than half (52.4%) of all female DOs in 2006.

The distribution of DOs by age categories reveals a higher proportion of female DOs than male DOs younger than 35 years. Table 10 demonstrates the percent distributions by age groups and sex.

Male DOs younger than 35 years (Table 5.14) showed the highest concentrations in Pennsylvania (772), Ohio (651), Michigan (555), New York (554), and California (499). More than two fifths (43.0%) of all male DOs younger than 35 years were located in these states. Table 5.15 reveals that female DOs younger than 35 years had the highest counts in Pennsylvania (598), Ohio (428), New York (426), California (373), and Michigan (366). Cumulatively, these five states accounted for 43.7% of all female DOs younger than 35 years.

State of Location and Activity

Tables 5.16 through 5.18 show the distribution of total DOs, male DOs, and female DOs among the states and major professional activity. Patient Care DOs were in largest number in Pennsylvania (5,282), followed by Michigan (4,849), Ohio (3,637), Florida (3,627), and California (3,183). Together, these states represented almost two fifths (39.8%) of all Patient-Care DOs.

For male DOs, Table 5.17 shows that Patient Care had the highest percentage representation in Alaska (95.2%), followed by Arkansas (93.2%), Minnesota (92.9%), and Alabama (92.6%). Lowest representation among male DOs in Patient Care was in Wyoming (80.3%) and Vermont (81.3%). Among female DOs (Table 5.18), Patient Care had highest proportional representation in Idaho (97.5%) and South Carolina (94.9%). The lowest was Wyoming (73.3%).

Metropolitan Data

Table 5.20 illustrates that of the total number of DOs in metropolitan areas, 86.7% were in Patient Care. Office-Based practice accounted for three fourths (75.1%) of these Patient Care DOs in 2006. The specialties showing the largest numbers of DOs in Office-Based practice were Family Medicine, Internal Medicine, General Practice, Emergency Medicine, and Pediatrics. These disciplines represented more than half (57.9%) of all Office-Based DOs in metropolitan areas.

In 2006, the 280 metropolitan statistical areas (MSAs) listed in Table 5.22 included 70.7% of the total DO population of 59,560. In those MSAs, Office-Based medical specialties represented 69.7% of the medical specialties Patient Care population, whereas the same category in the Surgical Specialties was 77.0%, Other Specialties was 71.0%, and Family/General Practice was 82.8% (Table 5.20).

Activity and Sex for Primary Care DOs

Office-Based practice represented a higher percentage of primary care DOs (77.6%) than DOs in the primary care subspecialties (65.8%), with All Other Specialties in between (71.9%).

A larger percentage of female DOs compared with male DOs was in primary care (53.0% vs 43.0%, respectively). In each of the primary care specialties except General Practice, the percentages of female DOs surpassed those of male DOs. This difference was especially apparent for Pediatrics, which represented 7.6% of all female DOs but only 2.0% of male DOs.

Age and Sex for Primary Care DOs

The largest percentage of active DOs was in the age group 35 to 44 years (29.5%), with the age groups 45 to 54 years and younger than 35 years having the next largest percentages (26.8% and 21.4%, respectively).

Among primary care DOs, the largest percentage (29.3%) was in the age group 35 to 44 years, whereas the next largest group was 45 to 54 years (29.1%). The age group 55 to 64 years included only 14.8% of primary care DOs.

Primary care accounted for nearly half (48.5%) of female DOs in the age group younger than 35 years. The comparable percentage for male DOs was 34.4%. A similar gender gap existed for the age group 35 to 44 years. In the older age groups, the gender gap is less because of the relatively small female DO population in these groups. For example, in the age group 65 years and older, primary care included 32.3% of male DOs and 37.3% of female DOs.

Table 5.1

DOs by Age, Activity, and Sex, 2006

Activity	Total Physicians	< 35	35-44	45-54	55-64	≥ 65
			Both Sexes			
Total Physicians	59,560	12,060	16,736	15,436	7,975	7,353
Patient Care	51,765	10,167	15,545	14,501	7,179	4,373
Office-Based Practice	39,515	4,330	12,951	12,756	6,387	3,091
Hospital-Based Practice	12,250	5,837	2,594	1,745	792	1,282
Residents	7,783	5,598	1,041	141	18	985
Full-Time Staff	4,467	239	1,553	1,604	774	297
Other Professional Activity	1,110	36	144	418	341	171
Administration	447	2	31	169	160	85
Medical Teaching	406	23	70	173	89	51
Research	132	3	17	47	57	8
Other	125	8	26	29	35	27
Inactive	3,129	3	83	309	397	2,337
Not Classified	3,556	1,854	964	208	58	472
			Male			
Total Physicians	43,452	7,048	11,380	11,613	6,963	6,448
Patient Care	37,504	5,916	10,617	10,953	6,277	3,741
Office-Based Practice	29,519	2,588	8,780	9,658	5,600	2,893
Hospital-Based Practice	7,985	3,328	1,837	1,295	677	848
Residents	4,537	3,190	696	66	8	577
Full-Time Staff	3,448	138	1,141	1,229	669	271
Other Professional Activity	884	13	93	319	298	161
Administration	378	1	21	135	139	82
Medical Teaching	306	6	44	129	80	47
Research	104	2	10	35	49	8
Other	96	4	18	20	30	24
Inactive	2,819	2	46	222	345	2,204
Not Classified	2,245	1,117	624	119	43	342
			Female			
Total Physicians	16,108	5,012	5,356	3,823	1,012	905
Patient Care	14,261	4,251	4,928	3,548	902	632
Office-Based Practice	9,996	1,742	4,171	3,098	787	198
Hospital-Based Practice	4,265	2,509	757	450	115	434
Residents	3,246	2,408	345	75	10	408
Full-Time Staff	1,019	101	412	375	105	26
Other Professional Activity	226	23	51	99	43	10
Administration	69	1	10	34	21	3
Medical Teaching	100	17	26	44	9	4
Research	28	1	7	12	8	
Other	29	4	8	9	5	3
Inactive	310	1	37	87	52	133
Not Classified	1,311	737	340	89	15	130

Table 5.2

DOs by Age and Self-Designated Specialty, 2006

Activity	Total Physicians	< 35	35-44	45-54	55-64	≥ 65
Total Physicians	59,560	12,060	16,736	15,436	7,975	7,353
Aerospace Medicine	98	7	5	32	33	21
Allergy/Immunology	113	15	26	39	23	10
Anesthesiology	2,560	587	742	828	270	133
Cardiovascular Disease	701	90	204	264	123	20
Child Psychiatry	263	33	89	83	46	12
Colon/Rectal Surgery	23	4	6	5	4	4
Dermatology	423	57	127	137	69	33
Diagnostic Radiology	746	137	253	194	110	52
Emergency Medicine	3,416	542	1,084	1,130	533	127
Family Medicine	14,553	2,321	4,599	4,441	2,014	1,178
Forensic Pathology	20	1	12	5	1	1
Gastroenterology	386	52	129	136	60	9
General Practice	3,177	8	260	1,140	1,063	706
General Preventive Medicine	211	11	62	76	42	20
General Surgery	1,114	229	400	271	116	98
Internal Medicine	6,813	1,697	2,275	1,799	675	367
Medical Genetics	6	3	2	1		
Neurological Surgery	75	8	26	26	10	5
Neurology	632	123	194	204	96	15
Nuclear Medicine	49	8	5	11	13	12
Obstetrics/Gynecology	2,133	437	714	577	294	111
Occupational Medicine	241	2	27	122	71	19
Ophthalmology	383	29	132	129	71	22
Orthopedic Surgery	1,163	90	372	401	207	93
Otolaryngology	357	21	118	132	61	25
Pathology-Anatomic/Clinical	437	93	91	110	88	55
Pediatric Cardiology	17	6	5	5	1	
Pediatrics	2,636	931	847	492	232	134
Physical Medicine & Rehabilitation	1,057	295	360	281	75	46
Plastic Surgery	79	4	28	24	21	2
Psychiatry	1,473	284	311	455	264	159
Public Health & General Preventive Medicine	37	1	7	13	8	8
Pulmonary Diseases	415	75	120	143	71	6
Radiation Oncology	76	8	20	32	15	1
Radiology	407	30	98	89	102	88
Thoracic Surgery	68	2	18	25	19	4
Urological Surgery	193	14	42	77	44	16
Vascular Medicine	6		3	3		
Other Specialty	315	8	50	120	78	59
Unspecified	6,003	1,940	1,826	867	497	873
Inactive	3,129	3	83	309	397	2,337
Not Classified	3,556	1,854	964	208	58	472

Table 5.3

Male DOs by Age and Self-Designated Specialty, 2006

Activity	Total Physicians	< 35	35-44	45-54	55-64	≥ 65
Total Physicians	43,452	7,048	11,380	11,613	6,963	6,448
Aerospace Medicine	91	6	5	30	29	21
Allergy/Immunology	87	12	18	25	22	10
Anesthesiology	2,091	449	584	686	250	122
Cardiovascular Disease	614	77	168	233	116	20
Child Psychiatry	155	16	49	52	30	8
Colon/Rectal Surgery	21	2	6	5	4	4
Dermatology	313	35	77	104	64	33
Diagnostic Radiology	590	99	192	147	101	51
Emergency Medicine	2,708	363	848	921	480	96
Family Medicine	10,202	1,196	2,982	3,262	1,724	1,038
Forensic Pathology	15	1	7	5	1	1
Gastroenterology	350	44	118	122	58	8
General Practice	2,696	2	194	884	945	671
General Preventive Medicine	153	7	42	51	35	18
General Surgery	954	188	330	237	107	92
Internal Medicine	4,815	1,071	1,528	1,336	593	287
Medical Genetics	3	2	1			
Neurological Surgery	70	8	24	24	9	5
Neurology	449	75	127	155	81	11
Nuclear Medicine	42	7	4	8	11	12
Obstetrics/Gynecology	1,213	130	364	385	254	80
Occupational Medicine	193	1	21	97	58	16
Ophthalmology	329	24	106	107	70	22
Orthopedic Surgery	1,080	77	341	375	195	92
Otolaryngology	325	17	104	121	58	25
Pathology-Anatomic/Clinical	314	48	68	74	77	47
Pediatric Cardiology	13	5	4	3	1	
Pediatrics	1,185	332	348	243	188	74
Physical Medicine & Rehabilitation	776	198	266	212	64	36
Plastic Surgery	71	4	24	20	21	2
Psychiatry	951	151	192	293	189	126
Public Health & General Preventive Medicine	23		3	7	5	8
Pulmonary Diseases	349	54	92	129	68	6
Radiation Oncology	63	6	15	28	14	
Radiology	360	20	82	78	92	88
Thoracic Surgery	65	2	15	25	19	4
Urological Surgery	177	11	38	68	44	16
Vascular Medicine	6		3	3		
Other Specialty	255	6	36	91	69	53
Unspecified	4,221	1,183	1,284	626	429	699
Inactive	2,819	2	46	222	345	2,204
Not Classified	2,245	1,117	624	119	43	342

Table 5.4

Female DOs by Age and Self-Designated Specialty, 2006

Activity	Total Physicians	< 35	35-44	45-54	55-64	≥ 65
Total Physicians	16,108	5,012	5,356	3,823	1,012	905
Aerospace Medicine	7	1		2	4	
Allergy/Immunology	26	3	8	14	1	
Anesthesiology	469	138	158	142	20	11
Cardiovascular Disease	87	13	36	31	7	
Child Psychiatry	108	17	40	31	16	4
Colon/Rectal Surgery	2	2				
Dermatology	110	22	50	33	5	
Diagnostic Radiology	156	38	61	47	9	1
Emergency Medicine	708	179	236	209	53	31
Family Medicine	4,351	1,125	1,617	1,179	290	140
Forensic Pathology	5		5			
Gastroenterology	36	8	11	14	2	1
General Practice	481	6	66	256	118	35
General Preventive Medicine	58	4	20	25	7	2
General Surgery	160	41	70	34	9	6
Internal Medicine	1,998	626	747	463	82	80
Medical Genetics	3	1	1	1		
Neurological Surgery	5		2	2	1	
Neurology	183	48	67	49	15	4
Nuclear Medicine	7	1	1	3	2	
Obstetrics/Gynecology	920	307	350	192	40	31
Occupational Medicine	48	1	6	25	13	3
Ophthalmology	54	5	26	22	1	
Orthopedic Surgery	83	13	31	26	12	1
Otolaryngology	32	4	14	11	3	
Pathology-Anatomic/Clinical	123	45	23	36	11	8
Pediatric Cardiology	4	1	1	2		
Pediatrics	1,451	599	499	249	44	60
Physical Medicine & Rehabilitation	281	97	94	69	11	10
Plastic Surgery	8		4	4		
Psychiatry	522	133	119	162	75	33
Public Health & General Preventive Medicine	14	1	4	6	3	
Pulmonary Diseases	66	21	28	14	3	
Radiation Oncology	13	2	5	4	1	1
Radiology	47	10	16	11	10	
Thoracic Surgery	3		3			
Urological Surgery	16	3	4	9		
Vascular Medicine	60	2	14	29	9	6
Other Specialty	1,782	757	542	241	68	174
Unspecified	310	1	37	87	52	133
Inactive	1,311	737	340	89	15	130
Not Classified						

Table 5.5

DOs' Mean Age by Self-Designated Specialty and Activity (166 Specialties), 2006

Specialty	Total Physicians	Patient Care		Hospital Based		Other Professional Activity			
		Total Patient Care	Office Based	Resid./Fellows	Phys. Staff	Admin.	Med. Teach.	Research	Other
Total Physicians	48.2	46.8	47.8	40.9	48.6	56.8	51.9	53.7	55.2
A	61.7	61.7	61.7			64.0			
ADL	45.0	46.1	45.0		49.0	58.5	54.0		49.0
ADM	59.1	59.0	59.1		58.0		50.0	51.0	
ADP	48.0	43.8	48.0	34.0		53.0			
AI	49.9	48.4	49.9	33.5	51.3	53.0	52.0		
ALI	49.0	47.0	49.0		45.0				
AM	57.7	56.5	57.7	33.5	55.9	59.5	50.0	52.0	57.0
AN	46.7	45.0	46.7	37.2	49.9	55.6	55.8	50.5	85.0
APM	44.8	43.4	44.8	35.8	42.6		106.0		
AR	35.5	35.5	35.5						
AS	56.7	56.3	56.7		55.0				
ATP	61.9	61.9	61.9				55.0		55.0
BBK	50.0	48.6	50.0		43.0				
CCA	43.9	40.8	43.9	33.3	37.0				
CCM	45.2	43.6	45.2	33.8	47.0	49.0		47.0	
CCP	44.1	39.9	44.1	33.1	48.0				
CCS	45.1	41.9	45.1	34.7	41.3				
CD	48.2	46.3	48.2	33.7	47.4	60.8	61.4	56.2	59.5
CHN	47.2	42.7	47.2	36.2	43.0			53.5	
CHP	48.5	45.9	48.5	33.7	48.3	57.5	49.3	49.5	
CLP	44.5	44.5			44.5				
CN	39.7	37.7	39.7	34.1			35.0		
CPP	69.5	69.5		69.5					
CRS	52.1	48.2	52.1	34.3	47.5				
CS	43.0	43.0	43.0						
D	48.4	47.5	48.4	43.4	42.4	56.0	56.0	33.0	46.0
DBP	33.7	33.7		33.7					
DIA	51.0	51.0	51.0			54.0	39.0		
DMP	47.8	45.2	47.8	35.3	52.0				
DR	47.8	45.8	47.8	36.0	50.8	64.5	54.7		52.7
DS	40.3	38.8	40.3		34.0		47.0		
EM	46.2	46.2	46.2	43.6	47.8	52.0	49.4	54.9	58.0
EMP	33.5	33.5		33.5					
END	43.8	40.2	43.8	33.2	41.3		54.0		
EP	49.0							49.0	
ESM	44.3	44.3	44.3						
ETX	36.0	34.6	36.0	34.2					
FM	47.6	46.9	47.6	40.4	47.3	53.9	50.3	52.9	60.6
FOP	42.5	41.6	42.5	36.0	42.5	52.0			53.0
FPG	53.0	52.0	53.0	34.2	57.8	61.0	59.0		
FPP	35.6	35.6		35.6					
FPS	55.0	55.0	55.0						

A	Allergy		CN	Clinical Neurophysiology
ADL	Adolescent Medicine (Pediatrics)		CPP	Pediatric Psychiatry/Child Psychiatry
ADM	Addiction Medicine		CRS	Colon & Rectal Surgery
ADP	Addiction Psychiatry		CS	Cosmetic Surgery
AI	Allergy & Immunology		D	Dermatology
ALI	Clinical Laboratory Immunology (Allergy & Immunology)		DBP	Developmental-Behavioral Pediatrics
AM	Aerospace Medicine		DIA	Diabetes
AN	Anesthesiology		DMP	Dermatopathology
APM	Pain Management		DR	Diagnostic Radiology
AR	Abdominal Radiology		DS	Dermatologic Surgery
AS	Abdominal Surgery		EM	Emergency Medicine
ATP	Anatomic Pathology		EMP	Pediatrics/Emergency Medicine
BBK	Blood Banking/Transfusion Medicine		END	Endocrinology, Diabetes and Metabolism
CCA	Critical Care Medicine (Anesthesiology)		EP	Epidemiology
CCM	Critical Care Medicine (Internal Medicine)		ESM	Sports Medicine (Emergency Medicine)
CCP	Pediatric Critical Care Medicine		ETX	Medical Toxicology (Emergency Medicine)
CCS	Surgical Critical Care (Surgery)		FM	Family Medicine
CD	Cardiovascular Disease		FOP	Forensic Pathology
CHN	Child Neurology		FPG	Geriatric Medicine (Family Practice)
CHP	Child and Adolescent Psychiatry		FPP	Family Practice/Psychiatry
CLP	Clinical Pathology		FPS	Facial Plastic Surgery

Table 5.5

DOs' Mean Age by Self-Designated Specialty and Activity (166 Specialties), 2006, continued

| Specialty | Total Physicians | Patient Care | | | | Other Professional Activity | | | |
| | | Total Patient Care | Office Based | Hospital Based | | Admin. | Med. Teach. | Research | Other |
				Resid./ Fellows	Phys. Staff				
FSM	40.9	39.3	40.9	31.0	39.3	51.0	37.0		
GE	47.5	45.4	47.5	32.8	47.0	54.5	51.0	59.7	
GO	47.8	50.0	47.8		53.3				
GP	58.0	57.7	58.0		55.4	62.2	58.2	66.0	70.3
GPM	51.5	49.9	51.5	36.4	49.7	54.8	41.0	48.0	46.5
GS	47.4	45.0	47.4	36.8	47.1	70.0	59.3		
GYN	58.0	58.3	58.0		65.0	67.3		69.0	60.5
HEM	52.6	51.3	52.6	33.0	55.0	61.5		55.0	
HMP	42.1	39.4	42.1	33.0					
HNS	62.0	62.0	62.0						
HO	41.9	39.5	41.9	34.2	43.0	53.0		50.0	
HOS	40.8	41.0	40.8		41.2				
HS	45.9	46.2	45.9		49.0				
HSO	35.7	35.7		35.7					
IC	42.1	41.5	42.1	39.4					
ICE	43.4	41.8	43.4	35.0			49.0	48.0	
ID	44.4	42.7	44.4	33.2	51.3	47.3	60.5	54.0	
IEC	31.0	31.0		31.0					
IFP	45.2	45.2		45.2					
IG	56.0	57.0			57.0		56.0		
IM	45.2	44.5	45.2	42.1	45.4	53.9	50.5	52.3	48.3
IMG	43.7	42.9	43.7	31.5	46.5	54.0	39.0	43.5	
IPM	31.0	31.0		31.0					
ISM	35.3	36.8	35.3		41.0				
LM	89.6	89.6	89.6			89.0			55.0
MDM	57.0	52.3	57.0		43.0	57.0			
MEM	38.4	38.4		38.4					
MFM	49.7	50.3	49.7		51.4				
MG	39.0	37.3	39.0	34.0					
MM	58.0	47.5	58.0		37.0				
MN	31.0	31.0		31.0					
MP	43.9	43.9		43.9					
MPD	39.2	40.1	39.2	41.5	38.1		42.0		
MSR	34.5	33.3	34.5	31.0					
N	47.4	45.5	47.4	34.5	48.6	53.0	61.4	51.0	49.0
NEP	44.2	42.2	44.2	33.7	46.4	60.5	54.5	52.0	
NM	55.8	53.3	55.8	31.2	57.1	55.0	50.0	59.0	55.0
NO	61.0						61.0		
NP	49.0	49.0	49.0						
NPM	46.2	43.1	46.2	32.9	50.4	52.0	57.0		
NR	44.7	43.1	44.7	30.0	42.0				
NRN	50.0	50.0	50.0						

FSM	Sports Medicine (Family Practice)	IMG	Geriatric Medicine (Internal Medicine)
GE	Gastroenterology	IPM	Internal Medicine (Preventive Medicine)
GO	Gynecological Oncology	ISM	Sports Medicine (Internal Medicine)
GP	General Practice	LM	Legal Medicine
GPM	General Preventive Medicine	MDM	Medical Management
GS	General Surgery	MEM	Internal Medicine/Emergency Medicine
GYN	Gynecology	MFM	Maternal & Fetal Medicine
HEM	Hematology (Internal Medicine)	MG	Medical Genetics
HMP	Hematology (Pathology)	MM	Medical Microbiology
HNS	Head & Neck Surgery	MN	Internal Medicine/Neurology
HO	Hematology/Oncology	MP	Internal Medicine/Psychiatry
HOS	Hospitalist	MPD	Internal Medicine/Pediatrics
HS	Hand Surgery	MSR	Musculoskeletal Radiology
HSO	Hand Surgery (Orthopedics)	N	Neurology
IC	Interventional Cardiology	NEP	Nephrology
ICE	Clinical Cardiac Electrophysiology	NM	Nuclear Medicine
ID	Infectious Disease	NO	Otology/Neurotology
IEC	Internal Medicine/Emergency Medicine/Critical Care Medicine	NP	Neuropathology
IFP	Internal Medicine/Family Practice	NPM	Neonatal-Perinatal Medicine
IG	Immunology	NR	Nuclear Radiology
IM	Internal Medicine	NRN	Neurology/Diagnostic Radiology/Neuroradiology

Table 5.5

DOs' Mean Age by Self-Designated Specialty and Activity (166 Specialties), 2006, continued

Specialty	Total Physicians	Patient Care				Other Professional Activity			
		Total Patient Care	Office Based	Hospital Based		Admin.	Med. Teach.	Research	Other
				Resid./ Fellows	Phys. Staff				
NS	49.2	47.4	49.2	32.0	43.6		35.0		
NSP	56.0	56.0	56.0						
NTR	73.0	73.0	73.0						
OAR	47.7	46.8	47.7		37.0				
OBG	45.8	44.8	45.8	39.8	46.6	55.7	52.6	57.0	57.0
OBS	49.2	48.6	49.2		47.0		46.0		
OCC	52.3	52.3	52.3						
OFA	44.3	44.3	44.3						
OM	53.5	53.0	53.5	35.0	51.9	55.4	55.8	53.5	63.7
OMM	52.5	52.0	52.5		42.3	42.0	50.9		36.0
OMO	56.0	45.0	56.0	34.0					
ON	52.3	50.2	52.3	32.3	52.0	69.0		57.3	46.0
OP	45.6	45.7	45.6		48.0				
OPH	48.4	47.9	48.4	32.3	50.8		64.5	56.0	
ORS	49.3	49.0	49.3	34.3	51.7	55.3	46.6	60.0	66.0
OS	52.7	52.2	52.7		48.0	59.9	58.4	42.0	55.5
OSM	41.3	40.5	41.3	31.5	42.7	82.0			
OSS	42.5	42.5	42.5						
OTO	49.6	48.5	49.6	34.0	43.0	40.0	52.5		68.0
OTR	50.5	47.0	50.5		33.0				
P	50.6	48.9	50.6	42.0	53.8	59.1	53.3	55.8	46.0
PA	50.0					61.0	64.0	50.0	
PAN	40.9	38.9	40.9	35.0	34.3		36.0		
PCC	40.6	37.9	40.6	32.9	42.4	53.0	29.0	38.0	
PCH	54.0	54.0	54.0						66.0
PCP	44.5	41.9	44.5	33.5	42.0				
PD	43.2	42.5	43.2	40.1	45.3	60.4	50.2	57.0	42.0
PDA	55.5	58.0	55.5		63.0				
PDC	42.7	40.2	42.7	34.0	43.0				
PDE	48.7	41.3	48.7	32.7	45.0			57.0	
PDI	34.0	33.8	34.0	32.8	39.0			44.0	
PDO	48.0	45.2	48.0	31.0			39.0		
PDP	46.3	41.1	46.3	32.3	47.7			50.0	
PDR	45.5	43.3	45.5	32.0	48.7				43.5
PDS	52.0	52.0	52.0						
PE	38.3	35.7	38.3	33.8					
PEM	45.8	39.5	45.8	32.6	43.8			35.0	
PFP	42.8	42.2	42.8	35.0	42.7				
PG	41.2	36.0	41.2	32.4	41.0				
PHL	51.0	51.0	51.0						
PHM	47.5	47.0			47.0			47.5	
PHO	43.5	38.1	43.5	31.8				44.0	

NS	Neurological Surgery	PA	Clinical Pharmacology
NSP	Pediatric Surgery (Neurology)	PAN	Pediatric Anesthesiology
NTR	Nutrition	PCC	Pulmonary Critical Care Medicine
OAR	Adult Reconstructive Orthopedics	PCH	Chemical Pathology
OBG	Obstetrics & Gynecology	PCP	Cytopathology
OBS	Obstetrics	PD	Pediatrics
OCC	Critical Care Medicine (Obstetrics & Gynecology)	PDA	Pediatric Allergy
OFA	Foot and Ankle, Orthopedics	PDC	Pediatric Cardiology
OM	Occupational Medicine	PDE	Pediatric Endocrinology
OMM	Osteopathic Manipulative Medicine	PDI	Pediatric Infectious Disease
OMO	Musculoskeletal Oncology	PDO	Pediatric Otolaryngology
ON	Medical Oncology	PDP	Pediatric Pulmonology
OP	Pediatric Orthopedics	PDR	Pediatric Radiology
OPH	Ophthalmology	PDS	Pediatric Surgery (Surgery)
ORS	Orthopedic Surgery	PE	Pediatric Emergency Medicine (Emergency Medicine)
OS	Other (i.e., a specialty other than those appearing above)	PEM	Pediatric Emergency Medicine (Pediatrics)
OSM	Sports Medicine (Orthopedic Surgery)	PFP	Forensic Psychiatry
OSS	Orthopedic Surgery of the Spine	PG	Pediatric Gastroenterology
OTO	Otolaryngology	PHL	Phlebology
OTR	Orthopedic Trauma	PHM	Pharmaceutical Medicine
P	Psychiatry	PHO	Pediatric Hematology/Oncology

Table 5.5

DOs' Mean Age by Self-Designated Specialty and Activity (166 Specialties), 2006, continued

Specialty	Total Physicians	Patient Care		Hospital Based		Other Professional Activity			
		Total Patient Care	Office Based	Resid./ Fellows	Phys. Staff	Admin.	Med. Teach.	Research	Other
PHP	50.1	51.3	50.1		53.8	61.4		47.5	41.0
PLM	46.5	46.5	46.5			60.0	35.0		
PM	45.1	42.7	45.1	34.7	50.9	55.5	47.0	55.0	59.0
PMD	49.1	50.4	49.1		58.8				
PMM	41.0	40.3	41.0	38.0					
PMP	32.7	32.7		32.7					
PN	43.0	40.8	43.0	33.0	42.0				
PO	41.7	41.7	41.7						
PP	45.0	41.5	45.0	31.0					
PPM	29.0	29.0		29.0					
PPR	34.5	34.5		34.5					
PRO	59.7	59.7	59.7						
PS	48.8	48.0	48.8	32.0	33.0	58.0		62.0	
PSM	36.0	34.7	36.0	32.0					
PTH	52.3	50.6	52.3	46.6	53.7	59.8	59.3	67.5	59.0
PTX	38.0	36.3	38.0	34.0	37.0				
PUD	51.4	51.4	51.4	33.7	55.0	57.0	58.0	58.7	
PYA	65.0	65.0	65.0						
PYG	45.8	42.4	45.8	34.0	42.0		41.0		
PYN	32.0	32.0		32.0					
R	57.8	59.4	57.8		65.9	66.2	58.0		66.0
REN	56.0	56.5	56.0		59.0				
RHU	45.5	43.4	45.5	33.0	48.1	66.0	55.5	46.5	47.0
RNR	41.4	40.2	41.4	33.8	40.5				
RO	48.0	47.1	48.0	33.2	50.3	64.0	45.0		
SCI	39.5	40.7	39.5	43.0					
SME	52.6	50.8	52.6	36.0					
SO	55.7	52.0	55.7		41.0				
SP	40.3	36.1	40.3	33.0					
TRS	48.7	47.1	48.7	42.0	41.5				
TS	51.5	50.3	51.5	37.4	50.0	63.0		66.0	
U	50.8	49.5	50.8	32.5	48.9	73.0	50.0	35.0	63.5
UCM	48.2	48.5	48.2	50.7					
UM	45.8	45.7	45.8	45.5					
UP	37.0	37.0	37.0						
US	46.2	46.9	46.2	49.6	46.1	66.4	43.7	106.0	44.6
VIR	41.9	42.4	41.9	34.3	48.7				
VM	44.8	44.8	44.8						
VN	32.0	32.0		32.0					
VS	47.7	46.3	47.7	37.3	35.0		45.0		38.0
Inactive	43.9								
Not Class	72.8								

PHP	Public Health and General Preventive Medicine	R	Radiology
PLM	Palliative Medicine	REN	Reproductive Endocrinology
PM	Physical Medicine & Rehabilitation	RHU	Rheumatology
PMD	Pain Medicine	RNR	Neuroradiology
PMM	Sports Medicine (Physical Medicine & Rehabilitation)	RO	Radiation Oncology
PMP	Pain Management (Physical Medicine & Rehabilitation)	SCI	Spinal Cord Injury Medicine
PN	Pediatric Nephrology	SME	Sleep Medicine
PO	Pediatric Ophthalmology	SO	Surgical Oncology
PP	Pediatric Pathology	SP	Selective Pathology
PPM	Pediatrics/Physical Medicine & Rehabilitation	TRS	Trauma Surgery
PPR	Pediatric Rheumatology	TS	Thoracic Surgery
PRO	Proctology	U	Urology
PS	Plastic Surgery	UCM	Urgent Care Medicine
PSM	Sports Medicine (Pediatrics)	UM	Underseas Medicine (Preventive Medicine)
PTH	Anatomic/Clinical Pathology	UP	Pediatric Urology
PTX	Medical Toxicology (Preventive Medicine)	US	Unspecified
PUD	Pulmonary Disease	VIR	Vascular and Interventional Radiology
PYA	Psychoanalysis	VM	Vascular Medicine
PYG	Geriatric Psychiatry	VN	Vascular Neurology
PYN	Psychiatry/Neurology	VS	Vascular Surgery

Table 5.6
DOs by Self-Designated Specialty and Activity (166 Specialties), 2006

Specialty	Total Physicians	Patient Care				Other Professional Activity			
		Total Patient Care	Office Based	Hospital Based		Admin.	Med. Teach.	Research	Other
				Resid./ Fellows	Phys. Staff				
Total Physicians	59,560	51,765	39,515	7,783	4,467	447	406	132	125
A	7	6	6			1			
ADL	11	7	5		2	2	1		1
ADM	19	17	15		2		1	1	
ADP	11	10	7	3		1			
AI	102	100	84	10	6	1	1		
ALI	2	2	1		1				
AM	98	83	53	2	28	10	1	3	1
AN	2,391	2,364	1,650	501	213	10	12	4	1
APM	153	152	122	22	8		1		
AR	2	2	2						
AS	4	4	3		1				
ATP	10	7	7				2		1
BBK	5	5	4		1				
CCA	16	16	11	4	1				
CCM	67	65	48	10	7	1		1	
CCP	38	38	18	16	4				
CCS	23	23	14	6	3				
CD	701	676	552	90	34	4	8	11	2
CHN	26	24	13	9	2			2	
CHP	263	254	190	43	21	4	3	2	
CLP	2	2			2				
CN	47	46	30	16			1		
CPP	2	2		2					
CRS	16	16	11	3	2				
CS	10	10	10						
D	423	418	351	42	25	1	2	1	1
DBP	6	6		6					
DIA	4	2	2			1	1		
DMP	11	11	6	3	2				
DR	746	727	486	149	92	2	7		10
DS	5	4	3		1		1		
EM	3,374	3,287	2,231	403	653	49	25	9	4
EMP	2	2		2					
END	95	94	60	31	3		1		
EP	2							2	
ESM	4	4	4						
ETX	8	8	2	6					
FM	14,373	14,090	11,597	1,350	1,143	102	137	14	30
FOP	20	15	11	2	2	1			4
FPG	77	73	64	5	4	3	1		
FPP	5	5		5					
FPS	3	3	3						

A	Allergy		CN	Clinical Neurophysiology
ADL	Adolescent Medicine (Pediatrics)		CPP	Pediatric Psychiatry/Child Psychiatry
ADM	Addiction Medicine		CRS	Colon & Rectal Surgery
ADP	Addiction Psychiatry		CS	Cosmetic Surgery
AI	Allergy & Immunology		D	Dermatology
ALI	Clinical Laboratory Immunology (Allergy & Immunology)		DBP	Developmental-Behavioral Pediatrics
AM	Aerospace Medicine		DIA	Diabetes
AN	Anesthesiology		DMP	Dermatopathology
APM	Pain Management		DR	Diagnostic Radiology
AR	Abdominal Radiology		DS	Dermatologic Surgery
AS	Abdominal Surgery		EM	Emergency Medicine
ATP	Anatomic Pathology		EMP	Pediatrics/Emergency Medicine
BBK	Blood Banking/Transfusion Medicine		END	Endocrinology, Diabetes and Metabolism
CCA	Critical Care Medicine (Anesthesiology)		EP	Epidemiology
CCM	Critical Care Medicine (Internal Medicine)		ESM	Sports Medicine (Emergency Medicine)
CCP	Pediatric Critical Care Medicine		ETX	Medical Toxicology (Emergency Medicine)
CCS	Surgical Critical Care (Surgery)		FM	Family Medicine
CD	Cardiovascular Disease		FOP	Forensic Pathology
CHN	Child Neurology		FPG	Geriatric Medicine (Family Practice)
CHP	Child and Adolescent Psychiatry		FPP	Family Practice/Psychiatry
CLP	Clinical Pathology		FPS	Facial Plastic Surgery

Table 5.6

DOs by Self-Designated Specialty and Activity (166 Specialties), 2006, continued

Specialty	Total Physicians	Patient Care				Other Professional Activity			
		Total Patient Care	Office Based	Hospital Based		Admin.	Med. Teach.	Research	Other
				Resid./ Fellows	Phys. Staff				
FSM	93	91	73	14	4	1	1		
GE	386	379	303	52	24	2	2	3	
GO	10	10	6		4				
GP	3,177	3,131	2,849		282	32	10	1	3
GPM	201	184	139	16	29	11	2	2	2
GS	962	947	641	210	96	5	10		
GYN	53	47	45		2	3		1	2
HEM	31	26	22	2	2	2		3	
HMP	10	10	7	3					
HNS	1	1	1						
HO	162	159	97	51	11	1		2	
HOS	9	9	4		5				
HS	29	29	26		3				
HSO	6	6		6					
IC	35	35	27	8					
ICE	22	20	16	4			1	1	
ID	170	161	111	34	16	3	2	4	
IEC	1	1		1					
IFP	5	5		5					
IG	2	1			1		1		
IM	5,524	5,448	3,841	1,211	396	28	32	10	6
IMG	88	83	73	6	4	2	1	2	
IPM	1	1		1					
ISM	4	4	3		1				
LM	18	14	14			1			3
MDM	13	3	2		1	10			
MEM	10	10		10					
MFM	21	21	14		7				
MG	6	6	4	2					
MM	2	2	1		1				
MN	1	1		1					
MP	7	7		7					
MPD	195	193	110	76	7		2		
MSR	3	3	2	1					
N	558	545	430	84	31	1	7	3	2
NEP	275	269	205	53	11	2	2	2	
NM	49	44	29	5	10	1	2	1	1
NO	1						1		
NP	2	2	2						
NPM	119	116	73	31	12	1	2		
NR	11	11	9	1	1				
NRN	1	1	1						

FSM	Sports Medicine (Family Practice)		IMG	Geriatric Medicine (Internal Medicine)
GE	Gastroenterology		IPM	Internal Medicine (Preventive Medicine)
GO	Gynecological Oncology		ISM	Sports Medicine (Internal Medicine)
GP	General Practice		LM	Legal Medicine
GPM	General Preventive Medicine		MDM	Medical Management
GS	General Surgery		MEM	Internal Medicine/Emergency Medicine
GYN	Gynecology		MFM	Maternal & Fetal Medicine
HEM	Hematology (Internal Medicine)		MG	Medical Genetics
HMP	Hematology (Pathology)		MM	Medical Microbiology
HNS	Head & Neck Surgery		MN	Internal Medicine/Neurology
HO	Hematology/Oncology		MP	Internal Medicine/Psychiatry
HOS	Hospitalist		MPD	Internal Medicine/Pediatrics
HS	Hand Surgery		MSR	Musculoskeletal Radiology
HSO	Hand Surgery (Orthopedics)		N	Neurology
IC	Interventional Cardiology		NEP	Nephrology
ICE	Clinical Cardiac Electrophysiology		NM	Nuclear Medicine
ID	Infectious Disease		NO	Otology/Neurotology
IEC	Internal Medicine/Emergency Medicine/Critical Care Medicine		NP	Neuropathology
IFP	Internal Medicine/Family Practice		NPM	Neonatal-Perinatal Medicine
IG	Immunology		NR	Nuclear Radiology
IM	Internal Medicine		NRN	Neurology/Diagnostic Radiology/Neuroradiology

Table 5.6

DOs by Self-Designated Specialty and Activity (166 Specialties), 2006, continued

Specialty	Total Physicians	Patient Care		Hospital Based		Other Professional Activity			
		Total Patient Care	Office Based	Resid./ Fellows	Phys. Staff	Admin.	Med. Teach.	Research	Other
NS	73	72	59	5	8		1		
NSP	1	1	1						
NTR	2	2	2						
OAR	12	12	11		1				
OBG	2,025	2,006	1,492	348	166	7	9	1	2
OBS	8	7	5		2		1		
OCC	3	3	3						
OFA	3	3	3						
OM	241	200	157	2	41	29	4	2	6
OMM	170	160	152		8	2	7		1
OMO	2	2	1	1					
ON	120	114	89	12	13	1		4	1
OP	19	19	18		1				
OPH	380	377	337	15	25		2	1	
ORS	880	865	717	36	112	4	8	1	2
OS	278	245	160	68	17	18	12	1	2
OSM	46	45	38	4	3	1			
OSS	20	20	20						
OTO	349	345	311	17	17	1	2		1
OTR	5	5	4		1				
P	1,427	1,384	890	330	164	25	13	4	1
PA	3					1	1	1	
PAN	28	27	18	6	3		1		
PCC	197	194	112	71	11	1	1	1	
PCH	2	1	1						1
PCP	18	18	13	4	1				
PD	2,116	2,068	1,393	542	133	14	22	8	4
PDA	3	3	2		1				
PDC	17	17	9	5	3				
PDE	8	7	3	3	1			1	
PDI	10	8	1	6	1			2	
PDO	7	6	5	1			1		
PDP	11	10	3	4	3			1	
PDR	22	20	13	4	3				2
PDS	1	1	1						
PE	7	7	3	4					
PEM	26	25	8	11	6			1	
PFP	14	14	10	1	3				
PG	17	17	5	10	2				
PHL	3	3	3						
PHM	3	1			1			2	
PHO	25	24	13	11				1	

NS	Neurological Surgery	PA	Clinical Pharmacology
NSP	Pediatric Surgery (Neurology)	PAN	Pediatric Anesthesiology
NTR	Nutrition	PCC	Pulmonary Critical Care Medicine
OAR	Adult Reconstructive Orthopedics	PCH	Chemical Pathology
OBG	Obstetrics & Gynecology	PCP	Cytopathology
OBS	Obstetrics	PD	Pediatrics
OCC	Critical Care Medicine (Obstetrics & Gynecology)	PDA	Pediatric Allergy
OFA	Foot and Ankle, Orthopedics	PDC	Pediatric Cardiology
OM	Occupational Medicine	PDE	Pediatric Endocrinology
OMM	Osteopathic Manipulative Medicine	PDI	Pediatric Infectious Disease
OMO	Musculoskeletal Oncology	PDO	Pediatric Otolaryngology
ON	Medical Oncology	PDP	Pediatric Pulmonology
OP	Pediatric Orthopedics	PDR	Pediatric Radiology
OPH	Ophthalmology	PDS	Pediatric Surgery (Surgery)
ORS	Orthopedic Surgery	PE	Pediatric Emergency Medicine (Emergency Medicine)
OS	Other (i.e., a specialty other than those appearing above)	PEM	Pediatric Emergency Medicine (Pediatrics)
OSM	Sports Medicine (Orthopedic Surgery)	PFP	Forensic Psychiatry
OSS	Orthopedic Surgery of the Spine	PG	Pediatric Gastroenterology
OTO	Otolaryngology	PHL	Phlebology
OTR	Orthopedic Trauma	PHM	Pharmaceutical Medicine
P	Psychiatry	PHO	Pediatric Hematology/Oncology

Table 5.6

DOs by Self-Designated Specialty and Activity (166 Specialties), 2006, continued

Specialty	Total Physicians	Patient Care		Hospital Based		Other Professional Activity			
		Total Patient Care	Office Based	Resid./ Fellows	Phys. Staff	Admin.	Med. Teach.	Research	Other
PHP	37	20	14		6	14		2	1
PLM	6	4	4			1	1		
PM	1,050	1,037	708	271	58	6	5	1	1
PMD	29	29	25		4				
PMM	4	4	3	1					
PMP	9	9		9					
PN	5	5	3	1	1				
PO	3	3	3						
PP	4	4	3	1					
PPM	2	2		2					
PPR	2	2		2					
PRO	7	7	7						
PS	66	63	60	2	1	1		2	
PSM	3	3	2	1					
PTH	364	347	171	118	58	5	6	2	4
PTX	3	3	1	1	1				
PUD	218	209	192	3	14	1	5	3	
PYA	1	1	1						
PYG	17	16	10	4	2		1		
PYN	1	1		1					
R	262	247	197		50	5	7		3
REN	13	13	11		2				
RHU	185	177	129	33	15	3	2	2	1
RNR	72	72	58	12	2				
RO	76	74	65	5	4	1	1		
SCI	3	3	2	1					
SME	9	9	8	1					
SO	4	4	3		1				
SP	7	7	3	4					
TRS	13	13	10	1	2				
TS	68	66	54	5	7	1		1	
U	191	186	159	12	15	1	1	1	2
UCM	23	23	20		3				
UM	7	7	5		2				
UP	2	2	2						
US	5,935	5,907	4,547	1,123	237	5	7	1	15
VIR	35	35	26	3	6				
VM	6	6	6						
VN	1	1		1					
VS	72	70	61	8	1		1		1
Inactive	3,556								
Not Class	3,129								

PHP	Public Health and General Preventive Medicine		R	Radiology
PLM	Palliative Medicine		REN	Reproductive Endocrinology
PM	Physical Medicine & Rehabilitation		RHU	Rheumatology
PMD	Pain Medicine		RNR	Neuroradiology
PMM	Sports Medicine (Physical Medicine & Rehabilitation)		RO	Radiation Oncology
PMP	Pain Management (Physical Medicine & Rehabilitation)		SCI	Spinal Cord Injury Medicine
PN	Pediatric Nephrology		SME	Sleep Medicine
PO	Pediatric Ophthalmology		SO	Surgical Oncology
PP	Pediatric Pathology		SP	Selective Pathology
PPM	Pediatrics/Physical Medicine & Rehabilitation		TRS	Trauma Surgery
PPR	Pediatric Rheumatology		TS	Thoracic Surgery
PRO	Proctology		U	Urology
PS	Plastic Surgery		UCM	Urgent Care Medicine
PSM	Sports Medicine (Pediatrics)		UM	Underseas Medicine (Preventive Medicine)
PTH	Anatomic/Clinical Pathology		UP	Pediatric Urology
PTX	Medical Toxicology (Preventive Medicine)		US	Unspecified
PUD	Pulmonary Disease		VIR	Vascular and Interventional Radiology
PYA	Psychoanalysis		VM	Vascular Medicine
PYG	Geriatric Psychiatry		VN	Vascular Neurology
PYN	Psychiatry/Neurology		VS	Vascular Surgery

Table 5.7

DOs by Self-Designated Specialty and Activity, 2006

Specialty	Total Physicians	Patient Care				Other Professional Activity			
		Total Patient Care	Office Based	Hospital Based		Admin.	Med. Teach.	Research	Other
				Resid./ Fellows	Phys. Staff				
Total Physicians	59,560	51,765	39,515	7,783	4,467	447	406	132	125
GP/FM Prac	17,730	17,395	14,583	1,379	1,433	138	149	15	33
FM	14,553	14,264	11,734	1,379	1,151	106	139	14	30
GP	3,177	3,131	2,849		282	32	10	1	3
Med. Spec.	11,504	11,262	7,996	2,487	779	72	90	64	16
AI	113	109	91	10	8	2	2		
CD	701	676	552	90	34	4	8	11	2
D	423	418	351	42	25	1	2	1	1
GE	386	379	303	52	24	2	2	3	
IM	6,813	6,688	4,729	1,475	484	44	42	31	8
PD	2,636	2,572	1,657	739	176	17	28	14	5
PDC	17	17	9	5	3				
PUD	415	403	304	74	25	2	6	4	
Sur. Spec.	5,588	5,498	4,326	680	492	26	45	8	11
CRS	23	23	18	3	2				
GS	1,114	1,096	763	225	108	5	12		1
NS	75	74	61	5	8		1		
OBG	2,133	2,107	1,576	348	183	10	10	2	4
OPH	383	380	340	15	25		2	1	
ORS	1,163	1,137	964	47	126	7	15	1	3
OTO	357	351	316	18	17	1	4		1
PS	79	76	73	2	1	1		2	
TS	68	66	54	5	7	1		1	
U	193	188	161	12	15	1	1	1	2
Oth. Spec.	18,053	17,610	12,610	3,237	1,763	211	122	45	65
AM	98	83	53	2	28	10	1	3	1
AN	2,560	2,532	1,783	527	222	10	13	4	1
CHP	263	254	190	43	21	4	3	2	
DR	746	727	486	149	92	2	7		10
EM	3,416	3,329	2,260	413	656	49	25	9	4
FOP	20	15	11	2	2	1			4
GPM	211	194	145	17	32	11	2	2	2
MG	6	6	4	2					
N	632	616	473	110	33	1	8	5	2
NM	49	44	29	5	10	1	2	1	1
OM	241	200	157	2	41	29	4	2	6
P	1,473	1,428	918	341	169	26	14	4	1
PHP	37	20	14		6	14		2	1
PM	1,057	1,044	713	273	58	6	5	1	1
PTH	437	416	218	133	65	5	8	2	6
R	407	390	307	21	62	5	7		5
RO	76	74	65	5	4	1	1		
OTH	315	257	231	1	25	31	15	7	5
UNSP	6,003	5,975	4,547	1,191	237	5	7	1	15
VM	6	6	6						
Inactive	3,129								
Not Class	3,556								

Subspecialties in this table are condensed into major specialties. See Appendix A.

Table 5.8

Male DOs by Self-Designated Specialty and Activity, 2006

Specialty	Total Physicians	Total Patient Care	Office Based	Resid./ Fellows	Phys. Staff	Admin.	Med. Teach.	Research	Other
		Patient Care		Hospital Based		Other Professional Activity			
Total Physicians	43,452	37,504	29,519	4,537	3,448	378	306	104	96
GP/FM Prac	12,898	12,645	10,829	705	1,111	121	101	7	24
FM	10,202	9,990	8,404	705	881	92	93	6	21
GP	2,696	2,655	2,425		230	29	8	1	3
Med. Spec.	7,726	7,538	5,607	1,407	524	61	66	50	11
AI	87	83	69	10	4	2	2		
CD	614	590	488	73	29	4	8	10	2
D	313	309	262	30	17	1	1	1	1
GE	350	343	277	44	22	2	2	3	
IM	4,815	4,717	3,468	911	338	37	32	24	5
PD	1,185	1,143	772	278	93	15	16	8	3
PDC	13	13	8	4	1				
PUD	349	340	263	57	20		5	4	
Sur. Spec.	4,305	4,230	3,451	375	404	21	40	6	8
CRS	21	21	17	2	2				
GS	954	936	667	179	90	5	12		1
NS	70	69	57	5	7		1		
OBG	1,213	1,196	965	105	126	7	7	1	2
OPH	329	328	293	10	25		1		
ORS	1,080	1,057	897	42	118	6	14	1	2
OTO	325	320	290	15	15		4		1
PS	71	68	65	2	1	1		2	
TS	65	63	51	5	7	1		1	
U	177	172	149	10	13	1	1	1	2
Oth. Spec.	13,459	13,091	9,632	2,050	1,409	175	99	41	53
AM	91	78	49	1	28	8	1	3	1
AN	2,091	2,064	1,480	397	187	9	13	4	1
CHP	155	147	110	24	13	4	2	2	
DR	590	573	386	111	76	2	6		9
EM	2,708	2,633	1,830	268	535	44	20	8	3
FOP	15	10	7	1	2	1			4
GPM	153	139	105	11	23	9	1	2	2
MG	3	3	2	1					
N	449	435	344	69	22	1	7	5	1
NM	42	37	24	4	9	1	2	1	1
OM	193	162	128	1	33	23	4	1	3
P	951	917	620	179	118	18	12	4	
PHP	23	10	9		1	11		1	1
PM	776	768	544	184	40	4	2	1	1
PTH	314	295	164	76	55	5	8	1	5
R	360	344	273	12	59	4	7		5
RO	63	61	52	5	4	1	1		
OTH	255	209	184	1	24	25	9	7	5
UNSP	4,221	4,200	3,315	705	180	5	4	1	11
VM	6	6	6						
Inactive	2,819								
Not Class	2,245								

Subspecialties in this table are condensed into major specialties. See Appendix A.

Table 5.9

Female DOs by Self-Designated Specialty and Activity, 2006

Specialty	Total Physicians	Patient Care				Other Professional Activity			
		Total Patient Care	Office Based	Hospital Based		Admin.	Med. Teach.	Research	Other
				Resid./ Fellows	Phys. Staff				
Total Physicians	16,108	14,261	9,996	3,246	1,019	69	100	28	29
GP/FM Prac	4,832	4,750	3,754	674	322	17	48	8	9
FM	4,351	4,274	3,330	674	270	14	46	8	9
GP	481	476	424		52	3	2		
Med. Spec.	3,778	3,724	2,389	1,080	255	11	24	14	5
AI	26	26	22		4				
CD	87	86	64	17	5			1	
D	110	109	89	12	8		1		
GE	36	36	26	8	2				
IM	1,998	1,971	1,261	564	146	7	10	7	3
PD	1,451	1,429	885	461	83	2	12	6	2
PDC	4	4	1	1	2				
PUD	66	63	41	17	5	2	1		
Sur. Spec.	1,283	1,268	875	305	88	5	5	2	3
CRS	2	2	1	1					
GS	160	160	96	46	18				
NS	5	5	4		1				
OBG	920	911	611	243	57	3	3	1	2
OPH	54	52	47	5			1	1	
ORS	83	80	67	5	8	1	1		1
OTO	32	31	26	3	2	1			
PS	8	8	8						
TS	3	3	3						
U	16	16	12	2	2				
Oth. Spec.	4,594	4,519	2,978	1,187	354	36	23	4	12
AM	7	5	4	1		2			
AN	469	468	303	130	35	1			
CHP	108	107	80	19	8		1		
DR	156	154	100	38	16		1		1
EM	708	696	430	145	121	5	5	1	1
FOP	5	5	4	1					
GPM	58	55	40	6	9	2	1		
MG	3	3	2	1					
N	183	181	129	41	11		1		1
NM	7	7	5	1	1				
OM	48	38	29	1	8	6		1	3
P	522	511	298	162	51	8	2		1
PHP	14	10	5		5	3		1	
PM	281	276	169	89	18	2	3		
PTH	123	121	54	57	10			1	1
R	47	46	34	9	3	1			
RO	13	13	13						
OTH	60	48	47		1	6	6		
UNSP	1,782	1,775	1,232	486	57		3		4
Inactive	310								
Not Class	1,311								

Subspecialties in this table are condensed into major specialties. See Appendix A.

Table 5.10

DOs by Race/Ethnicity, 2006

Specialty	Total	White	Black	Hispanic	Asian	Other	American Indian/ Alaskan Native	Unknown
Total Physicians	59,560	20,377	423	696	1,675	188	45	36,156
Aerospace Medicine	98	35			1	1		61
Allergy/Immunology	113	71		1	8			33
Anesthesiology	2,560	1,149	17	27	108	15		1,244
Cardiovascular Disease	701	420	6	1	32	3		239
Child Psychiatry	263	166	5	8	23		2	59
Colon/Rectal Surgery	23	16						7
Dermatology	423	152	2	2	8	2		257
Diagnostic Radiology	746	333	8	8	24	2		371
Emergency Medicine	3,416	1,312	14	35	63	14	3	1,975
Family Medicine	14,553	5,432	91	181	385	57	15	8,392
Forensic Pathology	20	17	1					2
Gastroenterology	386	222	2	3	28	3		128
General Practice	3,177	687	7	11	11	5	2	2,454
General Preventive Medicine	211	108	3		7		1	92
General Surgery	1,114	361	7	14	18			714
Internal Medicine	6,813	2,756	77	116	392	42	6	3,424
Medical Genetics	6	3						3
Neurological Surgery	75	28		1	1			45
Neurology	632	360	7	8	40	2	1	214
Nuclear Medicine	49	20			2			27
Obstetrics/Gynecology	2,133	930	31	31	51	8		1,082
Occupational Medicine	241	120	2		7	3		109
Ophthalmology	383	172		4	8	3		196
Orthopedic Surgery	1,163	348	1	2	8	1	1	802
Otolaryngology	357	148		1	2	1		205
Pathology-Anatomic/Clinical	437	224	1	1	10	1		200
Pediatric Cardiology	17	12			2			3
Pediatrics	2,636	1,141	36	90	94	8	3	1,264
Physical Medicine & Rehabilitation	1,057	495	14	12	56	1	3	476
Plastic Surgery	79	38		2	2			37
Psychiatry	1,473	737	24	24	51	5	1	631
Public Health & General Preventive Medicine	37	21	1		1			14
Pulmonary Diseases	415	243	1	6	26			139
Radiation Oncology	76	42			5	1	1	27
Radiology	407	170	2	4	20	2	1	208
Thoracic Surgery	68	35		2	1			30
Urological Surgery	193	77	1	2	4			109
Vascular Medicine	6	4						2
Other Specialty	315	135	2		2	2	1	173
Unspecified	6,003	96	7	7	6		1	5,886
Inactive	3,129	988	13	10	10	3		2,105
Not Classified	3,556	553	40	82	158	3	3	2,717

Table 5.11

Male DOs by Race/Ethnicity, 2006

Specialty	Total	White	Black	Hispanic	Asian	Other	American Indian/ Alaskan Native	Unknown
Total Physicians	43,452	15,166	229	430	1,112	139	31	26,345
Aerospace Medicine	91	33				1		57
Allergy/Immunology	87	52			7			28
Anesthesiology	2,091	926	11	21	86	10		1,037
Cardiovascular Disease	614	366	3	1	27	1		216
Child Psychiatry	155	103	1	3	9		1	38
Colon/Rectal Surgery	21	14						7
Dermatology	313	132	2	1	4	2		172
Diagnostic Radiology	590	271	5	6	14	2		292
Emergency Medicine	2,708	1,080	12	31	45	12	3	1,525
Family Medicine	10,202	3,904	37	117	251	39	11	5,843
Forensic Pathology	15	12	1					2
Gastroenterology	350	202	2	3	24	2		117
General Practice	2,696	577	6	10	8	4	2	2,089
General Preventive Medicine	153	72	2		7		1	71
General Surgery	954	314	4	13	14			609
Internal Medicine	4,815	1,983	50	75	263	30	6	2,408
Medical Genetics	3	1						2
Neurological Surgery	70	26		1	1			42
Neurology	449	260	3	7	27	2		150
Nuclear Medicine	42	17			2			23
Obstetrics/Gynecology	1,213	588	17	13	27	6		562
Occupational Medicine	193	96	1		6	3		87
Ophthalmology	329	153		2	7	2		165
Orthopedic Surgery	1,080	325	1	2	8	1	1	742
Otolaryngology	325	138		1	2	1		183
Pathology-Anatomic/Clinical	314	168	1		6			139
Pediatric Cardiology	13	8			2			3
Pediatrics	1,185	536	13	37	32	5	1	561
Physical Medicine & Rehabilitation	776	377	10	7	40	1	2	339
Plastic Surgery	71	34		2	2			33
Psychiatry	951	497	10	10	35	5		394
Public Health & General Preventive Medicine	23	15						8
Pulmonary Diseases	349	206		5	19			119
Radiation Oncology	63	34			4	1	1	23
Radiology	360	152	1	4	16	2		185
Thoracic Surgery	65	32		2	1			30
Urological Surgery	177	73	1	2	3			98
Vascular Medicine	6	4						2
Other Specialty	255	109	1		1	1		143
Unspecified	4,221	79	6	6	4			4,126
Inactive	2,819	877	12	8	7	3		1,912
Not Classified	2,245	320	16	40	101	3	2	1,763

Table 5.12

Female DOs by Race/Ethnicity, 2006

Specialty	Total	White	Black	Hispanic	Asian	Other	American Indian/ Alaskan Native	Unknown
Total Physicians	16,108	5,211	194	266	563	49	14	9,811
Aerospace Medicine	7	2			1			4
Allergy/Immunology	26	19		1	1			5
Anesthesiology	469	223	6	6	22	5		207
Cardiovascular Disease	87	54	3		5	2		23
Child Psychiatry	108	63	4	5	14		1	21
Colon/Rectal Surgery	2	2						
Dermatology	110	20		1	4			85
Diagnostic Radiology	156	62	3	2	10			79
Emergency Medicine	708	232	2	4	18	2		450
Family Medicine	4,351	1,528	54	64	134	18	4	2,549
Forensic Pathology	5	5						
Gastroenterology	36	20			4	1		11
General Practice	481	110	1	1	3	1		365
General Preventive Medicine	58	36	1					21
General Surgery	160	47	3	1	4			105
Internal Medicine	1,998	773	27	41	129	12		1,016
Medical Genetics	3	2						1
Neurological Surgery	5	2						3
Neurology	183	100	4	1	13		1	64
Nuclear Medicine	7	3						4
Obstetrics/Gynecology	920	342	14	18	24	2		520
Occupational Medicine	48	24	1		1			22
Ophthalmology	54	19		2	1	1		31
Orthopedic Surgery	83	23						60
Otolaryngology	32	10						22
Pathology-Anatomic/Clinical	123	56		1	4	1		61
Pediatric Cardiology	4	4						
Pediatrics	1,451	605	23	53	62	3	2	703
Physical Medicine & Rehabilitation	281	118	4	5	16		1	137
Plastic Surgery	8	4						4
Psychiatry	522	240	14	14	16		1	237
Public Health & General Preventive Medicine	14	6	1		1			6
Pulmonary Diseases	66	37	1	1	7			20
Radiation Oncology	13	8			1			4
Radiology	47	18	1		4		1	23
Thoracic Surgery	3	3						
Urological Surgery	16	4			1			11
Other Specialty	60	26	1		1	1	1	30
Unspecified	1,782	17	1	1	2		1	1,760
Inactive	310	111	1	2	3			193
Not Classified	1,311	233	24	42	57		1	954

Table 5.13

DOs by Age and State of Location, 2006

State	Total Physicians	< 35	35-44	45-54	55-64	≥ 65
Total Physicians	59,560	12,060	16,736	15,436	7,975	7,353
Alabama	385	51	135	121	64	14
Alaska	134	15	44	45	25	5
Arizona	1,789	257	495	443	300	294
Arkansas	267	35	76	82	50	24
California	3,604	872	1,184	875	391	282
Colorado	1,028	142	274	308	170	134
Connecticut	443	144	154	107	13	25
Delaware	270	50	77	80	32	31
District Of Columbia	108	57	26	14	6	5
Florida	4,288	556	1,197	1,113	558	864
Georgia	825	137	239	245	127	77
Hawaii	213	71	55	51	21	15
Idaho	229	31	83	68	36	11
Illinois	2,469	721	755	572	224	197
Indiana	859	127	234	272	138	88
Iowa	1,177	194	273	347	231	132
Kansas	680	125	165	208	122	60
Kentucky	409	101	132	90	52	34
Louisiana	114	25	25	35	17	12
Maine	655	119	168	216	93	59
Maryland	665	180	249	158	41	37
Massachusetts	672	205	196	166	64	41
Michigan	5,740	921	1,356	1,400	796	1,267
Minnesota	452	100	137	151	43	21
Mississippi	326	79	96	101	33	17
Missouri	2,098	347	426	590	415	320
Montana	128	8	41	45	27	7
Nebraska	169	54	47	36	22	10
Nevada	490	69	153	150	69	49
New Hampshire	221	43	86	70	13	9
New Jersey	2,961	528	930	764	364	375
New Mexico	268	32	49	89	54	44
New York	3,431	980	1,202	723	215	311
North Carolina	713	178	300	154	49	32
North Dakota	65	10	15	27	10	3
Ohio	4,273	1,079	1,099	1,080	566	449
Oklahoma	1,625	273	427	463	271	191
Oregon	603	64	174	173	120	72
Pennsylvania	6,177	1,370	1,597	1,512	829	869
Rhode Island	221	36	60	83	20	22
South Carolina	389	89	132	93	50	25
South Dakota	108	16	32	37	11	12
Tennessee	548	106	148	162	80	52
Texas	3,625	711	951	876	645	442
Utah	257	47	115	54	27	14
Vermont	66	8	15	25	6	12
Virginia	836	194	247	238	83	74
Washington	814	149	196	226	151	92
West Virginia	688	151	187	213	97	40
Wisconsin	758	149	199	226	115	69
Wyoming	81	12	22	28	12	7
Possessions	15	1	7	4	1	2
APO's and FPO's	131	41	54	27	6	3

Table 5.14

Male DOs by Age and State of Location, 2006

State	Total Physicians	< 35	35-44	45-54	55-64	≥ 65
Total Physicians	43,452	7,048	11,380	11,613	6,963	6,448
Alabama	312	36	104	100	61	11
Alaska	83	7	22	28	22	4
Arizona	1,356	156	341	329	268	262
Arkansas	206	24	57	63	43	19
California	2,468	499	787	620	334	228
Colorado	765	79	182	226	153	125
Connecticut	277	70	106	72	12	17
Delaware	193	26	49	62	30	26
District Of Columbia	65	26	20	11	5	3
Florida	3,310	338	824	871	495	782
Georgia	621	84	166	185	116	70
Hawaii	159	53	41	38	16	11
Idaho	189	20	72	57	31	9
Illinois	1,670	398	511	410	192	159
Indiana	654	80	156	205	130	83
Iowa	876	110	191	259	205	111
Kansas	508	70	122	163	105	48
Kentucky	297	60	98	72	41	26
Louisiana	83	16	17	26	14	10
Maine	439	64	99	147	75	54
Maryland	417	99	156	102	31	29
Massachusetts	449	112	126	121	53	37
Michigan	4,294	555	915	1,034	678	1,112
Minnesota	296	50	90	108	30	18
Mississippi	257	54	74	83	32	14
Missouri	1,648	211	309	473	373	282
Montana	101	3	34	36	24	4
Nebraska	121	38	33	25	18	7
Nevada	397	47	122	117	64	47
New Hampshire	142	23	53	49	11	6
New Jersey	2,136	304	596	555	334	347
New Mexico	207	22	31	71	45	38
New York	2,188	554	729	480	178	247
North Carolina	511	104	219	117	43	28
North Dakota	54	6	12	25	9	2
Ohio	3,230	651	773	877	505	424
Oklahoma	1,212	180	284	349	228	171
Oregon	430	38	108	123	103	58
Pennsylvania	4,502	772	1,071	1,162	737	760
Rhode Island	167	20	37	71	18	21
South Carolina	271	43	99	66	42	21
South Dakota	74	10	18	29	9	8
Tennessee	418	69	111	130	64	44
Texas	2,709	427	653	671	565	393
Utah	213	33	99	47	22	12
Vermont	48	3	10	19	5	11
Virginia	580	112	168	178	69	53
Washington	615	92	144	166	124	89
West Virginia	496	72	140	166	85	33
Wisconsin	558	84	137	175	98	64
Wyoming	66	9	17	22	11	7
Possessions	11	1	4	3	1	2
APO's and FPO's	103	34	43	19	6	1

Table 5.15

Female DOs by Age and State of Location, 2006

State	Total Physicians	< 35	35-44	45-54	55-64	≥ 65
Total Physicians	16,108	5,012	5,356	3,823	1,012	905
Alabama	73	15	31	21	3	3
Alaska	51	8	22	17	3	1
Arizona	433	101	154	114	32	32
Arkansas	61	11	19	19	7	5
California	1,136	373	397	255	57	54
Colorado	263	63	92	82	17	9
Connecticut	166	74	48	35	1	8
Delaware	77	24	28	18	2	5
District Of Columbia	43	31	6	3	1	2
Florida	978	218	373	242	63	82
Georgia	204	53	73	60	11	7
Hawaii	54	18	14	13	5	4
Idaho	40	11	11	11	5	2
Illinois	799	323	244	162	32	38
Indiana	205	47	78	67	8	5
Iowa	301	84	82	88	26	21
Kansas	172	55	43	45	17	12
Kentucky	112	41	34	18	11	8
Louisiana	31	9	8	9	3	2
Maine	216	55	69	69	18	5
Maryland	248	81	93	56	10	8
Massachusetts	223	93	70	45	11	4
Michigan	1,446	366	441	366	118	155
Minnesota	156	50	47	43	13	3
Mississippi	69	25	22	18	1	3
Missouri	450	136	117	117	42	38
Montana	27	5	7	9	3	3
Nebraska	48	16	14	11	4	3
Nevada	93	22	31	33	5	2
New Hampshire	79	20	33	21	2	3
New Jersey	825	224	334	209	30	28
New Mexico	61	10	18	18	9	6
New York	1,243	426	473	243	37	64
North Carolina	202	74	81	37	6	4
North Dakota	11	4	3	2	1	1
Ohio	1,043	428	326	203	61	25
Oklahoma	413	93	143	114	43	20
Oregon	173	26	66	50	17	14
Pennsylvania	1,675	598	526	350	92	109
Rhode Island	54	16	23	12	2	1
South Carolina	118	46	33	27	8	4
South Dakota	34	6	14	8	2	4
Tennessee	130	37	37	32	16	8
Texas	916	284	298	205	80	49
Utah	44	14	16	7	5	2
Vermont	18	5	5	6	1	1
Virginia	256	82	79	60	14	21
Washington	199	57	52	60	27	3
West Virginia	192	79	47	47	12	7
Wisconsin	200	65	62	51	17	5
Wyoming	15	3	5	6	1	
Possessions	4		3	1		
APO's and FPO's	28	7	11	8		2

Table 5.16

DOs by State of Location and Major Professional Activity, 2006

State	Total Physicians	Patient Care				Other Professional Activity			
		Total Patient Care	Office Based	Hospital Based		Admin.	Med. Teach.	Research	Other*
				Resid./ Fellows	Phys. Staff				
Total Physicians	59,560	51,765	39,515	7,783	4,467	447	406	132	6,810
Alabama	385	355	284	37	34	2	6	1	21
Alaska	134	126	106	2	18	1	1		6
Arizona	1,789	1,512	1,201	187	124	15	7	3	252
Arkansas	267	245	196	27	22	1			21
California	3,604	3,183	2,400	566	217	24	18	4	375
Colorado	1,028	912	761	75	76	12	2	1	101
Connecticut	443	397	239	128	30	2	4		40
Delaware	270	238	175	49	14	4		1	27
District Of Columbia	108	94	27	54	13	3	3		8
Florida	4,288	3,627	3,059	274	294	31	32	9	589
Georgia	825	708	542	85	81	9	11	4	93
Hawaii	213	186	106	50	30	1			26
Idaho	229	213	186	9	18				16
Illinois	2,469	2,187	1,501	522	164	21	13	10	238
Indiana	859	778	620	82	76	5	5	2	69
Iowa	1,177	1,056	825	133	98	10	5	1	105
Kansas	680	605	471	84	50	4	1	2	68
Kentucky	409	347	263	45	39	3	2		57
Louisiana	114	99	60	23	16	1	1		13
Maine	655	572	423	82	67	4	4		75
Maryland	665	572	395	102	75	11	4	6	72
Massachusetts	672	583	364	181	38	5	1	2	81
Michigan	5,740	4,849	3,797	561	491	42	43	8	798
Minnesota	452	420	297	82	41	4	1		27
Mississippi	326	294	210	45	39	2	4		26
Missouri	2,098	1,836	1,377	247	212	20	17	1	224
Montana	128	118	104	1	13				10
Nebraska	169	151	91	46	14	1	2		15
Nevada	490	440	375	30	35	3	3		44
New Hampshire	221	199	154	24	21	2	1		19
New Jersey	2,961	2,565	2,128	283	154	21	20	12	343
New Mexico	268	229	189	15	25	1	3		35
New York	3,431	2,996	2,011	779	206	23	17	5	390
North Carolina	713	643	449	103	91	4	1	3	62
North Dakota	65	58	40	7	11				7
Ohio	4,273	3,637	2,788	619	230	22	46	11	557
Oklahoma	1,625	1,381	1,149	89	143	12	14	2	216
Oregon	603	521	439	40	42	3	5		74
Pennsylvania	6,177	5,282	3,975	890	417	48	47	23	777
Rhode Island	221	195	144	30	21	2		3	21
South Carolina	389	353	261	57	35		2	1	33
South Dakota	108	91	70	17	4	1			16
Tennessee	548	491	357	72	62	4	1		52
Texas	3,625	3,166	2,464	476	226	38	31	13	377
Utah	257	234	178	36	20				23
Vermont	66	56	43	6	7			1	9
Virginia	836	725	486	145	94	10	9		92
Washington	814	723	566	95	62	5	4		82
West Virginia	688	630	485	85	60	2	9		47
Wisconsin	758	694	552	95	47	5	4	3	52
Wyoming	81	64	48	7	9	3	2		12
Possessions	15	11	8		3				4
APO's and FPO's	131	118	76	4	38				13

* Includes Other, Inactive and Not Classified Physicians

Table 5.17

Male DOs by State of Location and Major Professional Activity, 2006

State	Total Physicians	Patient Care		Hospital Based		Other Professional Activity			
		Total Patient Care	Office Based	Resid./Fellows	Phys. Staff	Admin.	Med. Teach.	Research	Other*
Total Physicians	43,452	37,504	29,519	4,537	3,448	378	306	104	5,160
Alabama	312	289	230	27	32	2	5		16
Alaska	83	79	66	1	12				4
Arizona	1,356	1,129	928	102	99	14	6	2	205
Arkansas	206	192	155	18	19	1			13
California	2,468	2,186	1,691	329	166	20	13	3	246
Colorado	765	665	562	41	62	9	2	1	88
Connecticut	277	250	166	64	20		3		24
Delaware	193	168	130	26	12	4		1	20
District Of Columbia	65	55	20	25	10	2	3		5
Florida	3,310	2,742	2,353	161	228	27	28	9	504
Georgia	621	531	418	52	61	8	10	2	70
Hawaii	159	136	78	35	23	1			22
Idaho	189	174	153	5	16				15
Illinois	1,670	1,482	1,066	294	122	16	12	8	152
Indiana	654	593	479	56	58	4	3	2	52
Iowa	876	782	634	74	74	7	3	1	83
Kansas	508	449	359	51	39	4		1	54
Kentucky	297	252	195	27	30	3	1		41
Louisiana	83	74	47	16	11	1	1		7
Maine	439	383	288	48	47	3	2		51
Maryland	417	357	250	59	48	8	3	6	43
Massachusetts	449	390	261	98	31	4	1	1	53
Michigan	4,294	3,584	2,869	341	374	39	34	6	631
Minnesota	296	275	202	46	27	4	1		16
Mississippi	257	231	171	30	30	2	4		20
Missouri	1,648	1,435	1,114	144	177	16	10	1	186
Montana	101	93	83	1	9				8
Nebraska	121	107	64	31	12	1	1		12
Nevada	397	357	308	20	29	3	2		35
New Hampshire	142	129	99	14	16	1			12
New Jersey	2,136	1,827	1,552	161	114	19	14	9	267
New Mexico	207	176	148	11	17	1	2		28
New York	2,188	1,904	1,319	448	137	17	9	5	253
North Carolina	511	465	333	68	64	4	1	2	39
North Dakota	54	48	36	2	10				6
Ohio	3,230	2,724	2,156	381	187	18	39	11	438
Oklahoma	1,212	1,026	867	47	112	11	10	2	163
Oregon	430	375	325	18	32	2	3		50
Pennsylvania	4,502	3,837	3,004	507	326	41	35	15	574
Rhode Island	167	146	113	16	17	2		3	16
South Carolina	271	241	185	28	28		1	1	28
South Dakota	74	63	50	9	4	1			10
Tennessee	418	374	275	48	51	3			41
Texas	2,709	2,355	1,899	275	181	31	21	11	291
Utah	213	194	152	25	17				19
Vermont	48	39	31	3	5			1	8
Virginia	580	493	342	78	73	10	7		70
Washington	615	541	423	64	54	4	3		67
West Virginia	496	448	359	40	49	2	9		37
Wisconsin	558	506	407	63	36	5	2		45
Wyoming	66	53	40	5	8	3	2		8
Possessions	11	7	5		2				4
APO's and FPO's	103	93	59	4	30				10

* Includes Other, Inactive and Not Classified Physicians

Table 5.18

Female DOs by State of Location and Major Professional Activity, 2006

State	Total Physicians	Patient Care				Other Professional Activity			
		Total Patient Care	Office Based	Hospital Based		Admin.	Med. Teach.	Research	Other*
				Resid./ Fellows	Phys. Staff				
Total Physicians	16,108	14,261	9,996	3,246	1,019	69	100	28	1,650
Alabama	73	66	54	10	2		1	1	5
Alaska	51	47	40	1	6	1	1		2
Arizona	433	383	273	85	25	1	1	1	47
Arkansas	61	53	41	9	3				8
California	1,136	997	709	237	51	4	5	1	129
Colorado	263	247	199	34	14	3			13
Connecticut	166	147	73	64	10	2	1		16
Delaware	77	70	45	23	2				7
District Of Columbia	43	39	7	29	3	1			3
Florida	978	885	706	113	66	4	4		85
Georgia	204	177	124	33	20	1	1	2	23
Hawaii	54	50	28	15	7				4
Idaho	40	39	33	4	2				1
Illinois	799	705	435	228	42	5	1	2	86
Indiana	205	185	141	26	18	1	2		17
Iowa	301	274	191	59	24	3	2		22
Kansas	172	156	112	33	11		1	1	14
Kentucky	112	95	68	18	9		1		16
Louisiana	31	25	13	7	5				6
Maine	216	189	135	34	20	1	2		24
Maryland	248	215	145	43	27	3	1		29
Massachusetts	223	193	103	83	7	1		1	28
Michigan	1,446	1,265	928	220	117	3	9	2	167
Minnesota	156	145	95	36	14				11
Mississippi	69	63	39	15	9				6
Missouri	450	401	263	103	35	4	7		38
Montana	27	25	21		4				2
Nebraska	48	44	27	15	2		1		3
Nevada	93	83	67	10	6		1		9
New Hampshire	79	70	55	10	5	1	1		7
New Jersey	825	738	576	122	40	2	6	3	76
New Mexico	61	53	41	4	8		1		7
New York	1,243	1,092	692	331	69	6	8		137
North Carolina	202	178	116	35	27			1	23
North Dakota	11	10	4	5	1				1
Ohio	1,043	913	632	238	43	4	7		119
Oklahoma	413	355	282	42	31	1	4		53
Oregon	173	146	114	22	10	1	2		24
Pennsylvania	1,675	1,445	971	383	91	7	12	8	203
Rhode Island	54	49	31	14	4				5
South Carolina	118	112	76	29	7		1		5
South Dakota	34	28	20	8					6
Tennessee	130	117	82	24	11	1	1		11
Texas	916	811	565	201	45	7	10	2	86
Utah	44	40	26	11	3				4
Vermont	18	17	12	3	2				1
Virginia	256	232	144	67	21		2		22
Washington	199	182	143	31	8	1	1		15
West Virginia	192	182	126	45	11				10
Wisconsin	200	188	145	32	11		2	3	7
Wyoming	15	11	8	2	1				4
Possessions	4	4	3		1				
APO's and FPO's	28	25	17		8				3

* Includes Other, Inactive and Not Classified Physicians

Table 5.19

DOs by State, Self-Designated Specialty, and Activity, 2006
Alabama

Specialty	Total Physicians	Patient Care		Hospital Based		Other Professional Activity			
		Total Patient Care	Office Based	Resid./ Fellows	Phys. Staff	Admin.	Med. Teach.	Research	Other
Total Physicians	385	355	284	37	34	2	6	1	
GP/FM Prac.	143	140	124	4	12		3		
FM	127	124	110	4	10		3		
GP	16	16	14		2				
Med. Prac.	78	75	51	19	5	1	1	1	
AI	2	2	2						
CD	5	5	4		1				
D	1	1	1						
GE	4	4	2	1	1				
IM	52	49	36	10	3	1	1	1	
PD	14	14	6	8					
Sur. Spec.	36	36	26	5	5				
GS	13	13	9	3	1				
OBG	8	8	8						
OPH	5	5	3		2				
ORS	6	6	3	2	1				
OTO	3	3	2		1				
U	1	1	1						
Oth. Spec.	107	104	83	9	12	1	2		
AM	1	1			1				
AN	23	23	18	3	2				
CHP	2	1	1			1			
DR	3	3	3						
EM	17	17	13		4				
GPM	3	3	2		1				
N	8	7	6	1				1	
NM	1							1	
P	6	6	5		1				
PM	10	10	9	1					
PTH	3	3	2	1					
R	2	2	2						
UNSP	28	28	22	3	3				
Not Class	8								
Inactive	13								

Note: Excludes Address Unknown.

Subspecialties in this table are condensed into major specialties. See Appendix A.

Table 5.19

DOs by State, Self-Designated Specialty, and Activity, 2006, continued
Alaska

| Specialty | Total Physicians | Patient Care | | | | Other Professional Activity | | | |
| | | Total Patient Care | Office Based | Hospital Based | | Admin. | Med. Teach. | Research | Other |
				Resid./ Fellows	Phys. Staff				
Total Physicians	134	126	106	2	18	1	1		1
GP/FM Prac.	61	59	46	2	11	1	1		
FM	51	49	36	2	11	1	1		
GP	10	10	10						
Med. Prac.	27	27	25		2				
CD	2	2	2						
D	1	1	1						
GE	1	1	1						
IM	13	13	13						
PD	8	8	6		2				
PDC	2	2	2						
Sur. Spec.	9	9	8		1				
GS	2	2	2						
OBG	2	2	2						
ORS	4	4	3		1				
OTO	1	1	1						
Oth. Spec.	32	31	27		4				1
AM	1	1	1						
AN	3	3	3						
CHP	1	1	1						
DR	3	2	2						1
EM	4	4	2		2				
GPM	1	1	1						
OM	1	1	1						
P	8	8	6		2				
PM	1	1	1						
UNSP	9	9	9						
Not Class	3								
Inactive	2								

Note: Excludes Address Unknown.

Subspecialties in this table are condensed into major specialties. See Appendix A.

Table 5.19

DOs by State, Self-Designated Specialty, and Activity, 2006, continued
Arizona

| Specialty | Total Physicians | Patient Care | | Hospital Based | | Other Professional Activity | | | |
		Total Patient Care	Office Based	Resid./Fellows	Phys. Staff	Admin.	Med. Teach.	Research	Other
Total Physicians	1,789	1,512	1,201	187	124	15	7	3	8
GP/FM Prac.	530	520	431	38	51	3	2	2	3
FM	431	421	348	38	35	3	2	2	3
GP	99	99	83		16				
Med. Prac.	350	344	256	74	14	2	2		2
AI	1	1	1						
CD	29	29	22	6	1				
D	22	22	22						
GE	9	9	7	2					
IM	197	194	144	42	8	2			1
PD	78	77	48	24	5				1
PUD	14	12	12				2		
Sur. Spec.	165	161	137	14	10	2	2		
CRS	1	1	1						
GS	37	34	24	6	4	2	1		
NS	1	1	1						
OBG	58	58	46	8	4				
OPH	8	8	7		1				
ORS	35	34	33		1		1		
OTO	9	9	9						
PS	6	6	6						
TS	2	2	2						
U	8	8	8						
Oth. Spec.	500	487	377	61	49	8	1	1	3
AM	6	6	2		4				
AN	64	63	55	5	3				1
CHP	10	10	6	2	2				
DR	19	19	16	2	1				
EM	87	86	60	9	17		1		
FOP	2	1	1						1
GPM	4	3	3			1			
N	24	24	20	3	1				
NM	3	3	2		1				
OM	4	3	1		2	1			
P	43	41	26	14	1	1			1
PM	15	14	13		1			1	
PTH	13	13	6	4	3				
R	14	14	11		3				
RO	2	2	2						
OTH	8	4	4			4			
UNSP	182	181	149	22	10	1			
Not Class	95								
Inactive	149								

Note: Excludes Address Unknown.

Subspecialties in this table are condensed into major specialties. See Appendix A.

Table 5.19

DOs by State, Self-Designated Specialty, and Activity, 2006, continued
Arkansas

| Specialty | Total Physicians | Patient Care | | | | Other Professional Activity | | | |
		Total Patient Care	Office Based	Resid./ Fellows	Phys. Staff	Admin.	Med. Teach.	Research	Other
				Hospital Based					
Total Physicians	267	245	196	27	22	1			
GP/FM Prac.	119	119	107	7	5				
FM	97	97	86	7	4				
GP	22	22	21		1				
Med. Prac.	51	50	32	9	9	1			
CD	6	6	6						
D	1	1	1						
GE	1	1	1						
IM	27	26	18	1	7	1			
PD	16	16	6	8	2				
Sur. Spec.	19	19	17	2					
GS	4	4	2	2					
NS	3	3	3						
OBG	5	5	5						
OPH	4	4	4						
ORS	3	3	3						
Oth. Spec.	57	57	40	9	8				
AM	1	1			1				
AN	10	10	6	2	2				
CHP	1	1	1						
DR	2	2	1	1					
EM	13	13	8	3	2				
N	3	3	2		1				
NM	1	1	1						
OM	1	1	1						
P	2	2			2				
PM	9	9	7	2					
PTH	1	1		1					
R	1	1	1						
RO	1	1	1						
OTH	2	2	2						
UNSP	9	9	9						
Not Class	11								
Inactive	267	245	196	27	22	1			

Note: Excludes Address Unknown.

Subspecialties in this table are condensed into major specialties. See Appendix A.

Table 5.19

DOs by State, Self-Designated Specialty, and Activity, 2006, continued
California

| Specialty | Total Physicians | Patient Care | | Hospital Based | | Other Professional Activity | | | |
		Total Patient Care	Office Based	Resid./ Fellows	Phys. Staff	Admin.	Med. Teach.	Research	Other
Total Physicians	3,604	3,183	2,400	566	217	24	18	4	6
GP/FM Prac.	1,250	1,233	980	182	71	9	6		2
FM	1,117	1,101	860	182	59	8	6		2
GP	133	132	120		12	1			
Med. Prac.	711	701	495	167	39	5	3	2	
AI	3	3	2		1				
CD	22	22	20	1	1				
D	29	29	24	2	3				
GE	12	12	11		1				
IM	472	464	328	113	23	5	2	1	
PD	153	151	96	46	9		1	1	
PUD	20	20	14	5	1				
Sur. Spec.	275	267	199	41	27	2	4		2
CRS	1	1	1						
GS	54	53	24	22	7				1
NS	6	6	4	1	1				
OBG	110	109	81	16	12				1
OPH	16	16	14		2				
ORS	57	53	47	1	5	1	3		
OTO	17	15	14	1		1	1		
PS	5	5	5						
TS	2	2	2						
U	7	7	7						
Oth. Spec.	999	982	726	176	80	8	5	2	2
AM	4	3	2		1	1			
AN	134	133	104	22	7		1		
CHP	26	25	19	5	1			1	
DR	34	34	22	8	4				
EM	180	178	134	22	22	1	1		
FOP	2	1		1					1
GPM	20	20	14	5	1				
N	41	40	31	6	3			1	
NM	7	7	5	2					
OM	19	16	13	1	2	2			1
P	118	116	68	29	19	2			
PHP	7	6	3		3	1			
PM	62	62	45	16	1				
PTH	35	35	19	11	5				
R	13	12	11		1		1		
RO	3	3	1	1	1				
OTH	16	14	13		1	1	1		
UNSP	278	277	222	47	8		1		
Not Class	278								
Inactive	91								

Note: Excludes Address Unknown.

Subspecialties in this table are condensed into major specialties. See Appendix A.

Table 5.19

DOs by State, Self-Designated Specialty, and Activity, 2006, continued
Colorado

Specialty	Total Physicians	Patient Care				Other Professional Activity			
		Total Patient Care	Office Based	Hospital Based		Admin.	Med. Teach.	Research	Other
				Resid./ Fellows	Phys. Staff				
Total Physicians	1,028	912	761	75	76	12	2	1	
GP/FM Prac.	403	399	322	44	33	3	1		
FM	334	331	260	44	27	2	1		
GP	69	68	62		6	1			
Med. Prac.	132	130	112	11	7	1		1	
AI	1	1	1						
CD	5	5	3	2					
D	8	8	7		1				
GE	5	5	3		2				
IM	85	83	72	8	3	1		1	
PD	21	21	19	1	1				
PUD	7	7	7						
Sur. Spec.	92	92	77	3	12				
GS	17	17	10	2	5				
OBG	33	33	27	1	5				
OPH	7	7	7						
ORS	23	23	21		2				
OTO	6	6	6						
PS	2	2	2						
TS	2	2	2						
U	2	2	2						
Oth. Spec.	300	291	250	17	24	8	1		
AM	4	4	4						
AN	47	46	40	2	4	1			
CHP	8	7	6	1		1			
DR	14	13	7	2	4		1		
EM	59	58	54	2	2	1			
GPM	7	5	2	1	2	2			
N	7	6	5	1		1			
OM	6	6	6						
P	21	21	12	4	5				
PHP	3	1	1			2			
PM	19	19	17	1	1				
PTH	8	8	7	1					
R	4	4	3		1				
RO	2	2	2						
OTH	4	4	3		1				
UNSP	87	87	81	2	4				
Not Class	30								
Inactive	71								

Note: Excludes Address Unknown.

Subspecialties in this table are condensed into major specialties. See Appendix A.

Table 5.19

DOs by State, Self-Designated Specialty, and Activity, 2006, continued
Connecticut

Specialty	Total Physicians	Patient Care				Other Professional Activity			
		Total Patient Care	Office Based	Hospital Based		Admin.	Med. Teach.	Research	Other
				Resid./ Fellows	Phys. Staff				
Total Physicians	443	397	239	128	30	2	4		
GP/FM Prac.	55	54	40	8	6	1			
FM	53	52	39	8	5	1			
GP	2	2	1		1				
Med. Prac.	163	161	94	61	6		2		
AI	1	1	1						
CD	5	5	3	2					
D	3	3	3						
GE	2	2	2						
IM	103	103	55	43	5				
PD	39	37	25	12			2		
PUD	10	10	5	4	1				
Sur. Spec.	50	49	24	23	2		1		
GS	4	3	2	1			1		
OBG	38	38	15	21	2				
OPH	1	1	1						
ORS	7	7	6	1					
Oth. Spec.	135	133	81	36	16	1	1		
AN	27	27	15	12					
CHP	2	2	1	1					
DR	8	8	5	3					
EM	44	43	17	12	14		1		
N	4	4	3	1					
OM	3	2	2			1			
P	10	10	5	3	2				
PM	6	6	6						
PTH	5	5	3	2					
R	3	3	3						
OTH	5	5	5						
UNSP	18	18	16	2					
Not Class	33								
Inactive	7								

Note: Excludes Address Unknown.

Subspecialties in this table are condensed into major specialties. See Appendix A.

Table 5.19

DOs by State, Self-Designated Specialty, and Activity, 2006, continued
Delaware

Specialty	Total Physicians	Patient Care				Other Professional Activity			
		Total Patient Care	Office Based	Hospital Based		Admin.	Med. Teach.	Research	Other
				Resid./ Fellows	Phys. Staff				
Total Physicians	270	238	175	49	14	4		1	
GP/FM Prac.	75	74	62	6	6	1			
FM	68	68	57	6	5				
GP	7	6	5		1	1			
Med. Prac.	68	66	42	21	3	1		1	
AI	1	1	1						
CD	10	10	10						
D	1	1	1						
GE	1	1	1						
IM	31	30	16	12	2			1	
PD	21	20	11	9		1			
PDC	1	1			1				
PUD	2	2	2						
Sur. Spec.	39	39	29	9	1				
GS	4	4	1	3					
OBG	19	19	13	6					
OPH	1	1	1						
ORS	9	9	8		1				
OTO	5	5	5						
TS	1	1	1						
Oth. Spec.	61	59	42	13	4	2			
AN	9	9	7	1	1				
DR	6	6	1	5					
EM	10	10	7	2	1				
N	3	3	3						
OM	1						1		
P	3	3	2		1				
PHP	1						1		
PM	4	4	4						
R	3	3	2		1				
RO	1	1	1						
UNSP	20	20	15	5					
Not Class	14								
Inactive	13								

Note: Excludes Address Unknown.

Subspecialties in this table are condensed into major specialties. See Appendix A.

Table 5.19

DOs by State, Self-Designated Specialty, and Activity, 2006, continued
District of Columbia

| Specialty | Total Physicians | Patient Care | | Hospital Based | | Other Professional Activity | | | |
		Total Patient Care	Office Based	Resid./ Fellows	Phys. Staff	Admin.	Med. Teach.	Research	Other
Total Physicians	108	94	27	54	13	3	3		
GP/FM Prac.	16	16	5	7	4				
FM	16	16	5	7	4				
Med. Prac.	39	37	10	22	5		2		
AI	3	2		1	1		1		
D	1	1			1				
GE	1	1	1						
IM	26	25	7	15	3		1		
PD	6	6	2	4					
PUD	2	2		2					
Sur. Spec.	5	5	1	4					
GS	1	1	1						
OBG	4	4		4					
Oth. Spec.	40	36	11	21	4	3	1		
AN	5	5	3	2					
CHP	1	1		1					
DR	2	2		2					
GPM	2	2			2				
N	4	4		4					
P	6	4	2	2		1	1		
PM	10	10	2	6	2				
PTH	4	3	2	1		1			
OTH	1					1			
UNSP	5	5	2	3					
Not Class	5								
Inactive	3								

Note: Excludes Address Unknown.

Subspecialties in this table are condensed into major specialties. See Appendix A.

Table 5.19

DOs by State, Self-Designated Specialty, and Activity, 2006, continued
Florida

Specialty	Total Physicians	Patient Care				Other Professional Activity			
		Total Patient Care	Office Based	Hospital Based		Admin.	Med. Teach.	Research	Other
				Resid./ Fellows	Phys. Staff				
Total Physicians	4,288	3,627	3,059	274	294	31	32	9	6
GP/FM Prac.	1,237	1,210	1,073	42	95	13	13		1
FM	992	971	853	42	76	9	11		1
GP	245	239	220		19	4	2		
Med. Prac.	717	701	576	71	54	2	8	5	1
AI	8	8	5	3					
CD	42	39	35	3	1		2	1	
D	66	65	60	2	3			1	
GE	31	31	26	3	2				
IM	411	405	337	36	32	1	2	3	
PD	133	127	89	23	15	1	4		1
PUD	26	26	24	1	1				
Sur. Spec.	377	370	326	16	28	2	5		
CRS	3	3	3						
GS	71	70	58	5	7		1		
NS	8	7	7				1		
OBG	109	108	89	8	11		1		
OPH	38	38	37		1				
ORS	89	85	77	3	5	2	2		
OTO	31	31	30		1				
PS	6	6	6						
TS	3	3	3						
U	19	19	16		3				
Oth. Spec.	1,374	1,346	1,084	145	117	14	6	4	4
AM	12	11	7	1	3	1			
AN	166	166	136	21	9				
CHP	9	9	8	1					
DR	40	40	33	3	4				
EM	253	244	187	10	47	4	1	3	1
GPM	23	23	17	2	4				
N	48	46	40	3	3		2		
NM	4	4	4						
OM	15	13	11		2	2			
P	68	65	54	2	9	1	1	1	
PHP	3	1	1			2			
PM	56	56	50	4	2				
PTH	24	23	18		5				1
R	44	42	34		8	2			
RO	4	4	4						
OTH	33	28	25		3	2	2		1
UNSP	570	569	453	98	18				1
VM	2	2	2						
Not Class	191								
Inactive	392								

Note: Excludes Address Unknown.

Subspecialties in this table are condensed into major specialties. See Appendix A.

Table 5.19

DOs by State, Self-Designated Specialty, and Activity, 2006, continued
Georgia

Specialty	Total Physicians	Patient Care				Other Professional Activity			
		Total Patient Care	Office Based	Hospital Based		Admin.	Med. Teach.	Research	Other
				Resid./ Fellows	Phys. Staff				
Total Physicians	825	708	542	85	81	9	11	4	2
GP/FM Prac.	290	281	232	22	27	3	4	1	1
FM	244	237	193	22	22	2	4	1	
GP	46	44	39		5	1			1
Med. Prac.	117	114	84	15	15		3		
CD	6	6	5		1				
D	3	3	3						
GE	7	7	5	1	1				
IM	78	76	54	11	11		2		
PD	18	17	13	3	1		1		
PDC	1	1			1				
PUD	4	4	4						
Sur. Spec.	97	95	73	10	12		2		
CRS	1	1	1						
GS	17	16	9	5	2		1		
OBG	34	33	28	2	3		1		
OPH	3	3	2		1				
ORS	32	32	23	3	6				
OTO	5	5	5						
U	5	5	5						
Oth. Spec.	230	218	153	38	27	6	2	3	1
AM	2	1	1					1	
AN	35	35	22	7	6				
CHP	5	5	4		1				
DR	12	12	7	3	2				
EM	50	48	32	12	4		1	1	
GPM	11	10	7	1	2	1			
N	4	4	4						
NM	2	2			2				
OM	5	3	2		1	2			
P	24	23	17	3	3	1			
PHP	2							1	1
PM	14	13	9	4		1			
PTH	8	7	5	1	1		1		
R	1	1			1				
RO	2	2	2						
OTH	2	1	1			1			
UNSP	51	51	40	7	4				
Not Class	44								
Inactive	47								

Note: Excludes Address Unknown.

Subspecialties in this table are condensed into major specialties. See Appendix A.

Table 5.19

DOs by State, Self-Designated Specialty, and Activity, 2006, continued
Hawaii

Specialty	Total Physicians	Patient Care				Other Professional Activity			
		Total Patient Care	Office Based	Hospital Based		Admin.	Med. Teach.	Research	Other
				Resid./ Fellows	Phys. Staff				
Total Physicians	213	186	106	50	30	1			
GP/FM Prac.	62	62	40	8	14				
FM	51	51	31	8	12				
GP	11	11	9		2				
Med. Prac.	33	33	15	11	7				
CD	1	1	1						
D	1	1			1				
IM	20	20	9	7	4				
PD	10	10	4	4	2				
PUD	1	1	1						
Sur. Spec.	22	22	10	12					
GS	6	6	1	5					
OBG	10	10	4	6					
OPH	3	3	2	1					
OTO	2	2	2						
PS	1	1	1						
Oth. Spec.	70	69	41	19	9	1			
AN	4	4	3	1					
CHP	7	7	3	3	1				
DR	6	6		5	1				
EM	11	11	9		2				
N	3	3	1		2				
OM	2	2	2						
P	12	11	6	5		1			
PHP	1	1			1				
PM	4	4	3	1					
PTH	1	1	1						
RO	1	1			1				
OTH	1	1	1						
UNSP	17	17	12	4	1				
Not Class	17								
Inactive	9								

Note: Excludes Address Unknown.

Subspecialties in this table are condensed into major specialties. See Appendix A.

Table 5.19

DOs by State, Self-Designated Specialty, and Activity, 2006, continued
Idaho

Specialty	Total Physicians	Patient Care		Hospital Based		Other Professional Activity			
		Total Patient Care	Office Based	Resid./ Fellows	Phys. Staff	Admin.	Med. Teach.	Research	Other
Total Physicians	229	213	186	9	18				
GP/FM Prac.	102	102	85	9	8				
FM	97	97	80	9	8				
GP	5	5	5						
Med. Prac.	23	23	20		3				
CD	5	5	4		1				
D	1	1	1						
GE	2	2	2						
IM	8	8	6		2				
PD	7	7	7						
Sur. Spec.	14	14	13		1				
GS	2	2	1		1				
OBG	8	8	8						
ORS	3	3	3						
OTO	1	1	1						
Oth. Spec.	74	74	68		6				
AM	1	1	1						
AN	6	6	5		1				
CHP	5	5	3		2				
DR	5	5	5						
EM	13	13	11		2				
GPM	2	2	2						
N	3	3	3						
P	4	4	4						
PM	3	3	3						
PTH	1	1	1						
R	2	2	2						
OTH	4	4	4						
UNSP	25	25	24		1				
Not Class	10								
Inactive	6								

Note: *Excludes Address Unknown.*

Subspecialties in this table are condensed into major specialties. See Appendix A.

Table 5.19

DOs by State, Self-Designated Specialty, and Activity, 2006, continued
Illinois

Specialty	Total Physicians	Patient Care				Other Professional Activity			
		Total Patient Care	Office Based	Hospital Based		Admin.	Med. Teach.	Research	Other
				Resid./ Fellows	Phys. Staff				
Total Physicians	2,469	2,187	1,501	522	164	21	13	10	5
GP/FM Prac.	658	649	512	96	41	4	4	1	
FM	590	581	452	96	33	4	4	1	
GP	68	68	60		8				
Med. Prac.	537	520	325	169	26	6	2	7	2
AI	5	5	5						
CD	35	34	23	9	2	1			
D	7	7	6	1					
GE	16	16	12	4					
IM	319	306	187	100	19	4	2	5	2
PD	139	136	81	50	5	1		2	
PUD	16	16	11	5					
Sur. Spec.	236	233	170	41	22		1	1	1
GS	45	44	30	8	6		1		
NS	1	1	1						
OBG	122	120	79	31	10			1	1
OPH	18	18	16		2				
ORS	27	27	25		2				
OTO	11	11	11						
PS	3	3	3						
TS	1	1	1						
U	8	8	4	2	2				
Oth. Spec.	805	785	494	216	75	11	6	1	2
AN	124	123	71	45	7	1			
CHP	12	12	8	4					
DR	40	39	20	16	3	1			
EM	209	201	136	30	35	5	2		1
GPM	3	2	2			1			
N	26	26	19	5	2				
NM	2	1			1		1		
OM	17	17	13		4				
P	41	38	22	9	7	1	1	1	
PM	50	49	23	21	5	1			
PTH	17	16	5	5	6		1		
R	19	17	13	3	1	1			1
RO	5	5	5						
OTH	9	8	7		1		1		
UNSP	231	231	150	78	3				
Not Class	187								
Inactive	46								

Note: Excludes Address Unknown.

Subspecialties in this table are condensed into major specialties. See Appendix A.

Table 5.19

DOs by State, Self-Designated Specialty, and Activity, 2006, continued
Indiana

Specialty	Total Physicians	Patient Care		Hospital Based		Other Professional Activity			
		Total Patient Care	Office Based	Resid./ Fellows	Phys. Staff	Admin.	Med. Teach.	Research	Other
Total Physicians	859	778	620	82	76	5	5	2	
GP/FM Prac.	295	291	234	27	30	2	2		
FM	231	230	180	27	23		1		
GP	64	61	54		7	2	1		
Med. Prac.	139	138	103	29	6	1			
AI	4	4	4						
CD	23	23	22	1					
D	1	1	1						
GE	6	6	6						
IM	75	74	52	20	2	1			
PD	26	26	16	6	4				
PDC	1	1		1					
PUD	3	3	2	1					
Sur. Spec.	98	97	89	1	7			1	
CRS	2	2	2						
GS	12	12	9		3				
OBG	42	42	39		3				
OPH	5	5	5						
ORS	32	31	29	1	1			1	
OTO	4	4	4						
U	1	1	1						
Oth. Spec.	258	252	194	25	33	2	3	1	
AM	3	3	2		1				
AN	53	51	36	10	5		2		
CHP	2	2		1	1				
DR	11	10	6		4		1		
EM	57	55	43	2	10	2			
GPM	3	3	3						
N	5	5	5						
NM	1	1	1						
OM	4	4	4						
P	14	14	9	4	1				
PM	15	15	10	3	2				
PTH	3	3		2	1				
R	8	8	6		2				
RO	1	1	1						
OTH	8	7	7					1	
UNSP	70	70	61	3	6				
Not Class	25								
Inactive	44								

Note: Excludes Address Unknown.

Subspecialties in this table are condensed into major specialties. See Appendix A.

Table 5.19

DOs by State, Self-Designated Specialty, and Activity, 2006, continued

Iowa

		Patient Care				Other Professional Activity			
				Hospital Based					
Specialty	Total Physicians	Total Patient Care	Office Based	Resid./ Fellows	Phys. Staff	Admin.	Med. Teach.	Research	Other
Total Physicians	1,177	1,056	825	133	98	10	5	1	1
GP/FM Prac.	511	504	410	57	37	3	4		
FM	442	435	352	57	26	3	4		
GP	69	69	58		11				
Med. Prac.	211	209	148	41	20	1	1		
AI	2	2	2						
CD	14	14	13		1				
D	4	4	3		1				
GE	7	7	6		1				
IM	124	123	85	24	14		1		
PD	56	55	35	17	3	1			
PUD	4	4	4						
Sur. Spec.	92	90	78	1	11	2			
GS	19	19	15		4				
OBG	29	28	25	1	2	1			
OPH	6	6	5		1				
ORS	24	24	21		3				
OTO	5	5	5						
PS	3	3	3						
TS	2	1	1			1			
U	4	4	3		1				
Oth. Spec.	259	253	189	34	30	4		1	1
AN	52	50	33	12	5	1		1	
CHP	3	3	3						
DR	11	11	8		3				
EM	47	46	37	2	7	1			
GPM	4	4	3		1				
N	7	7	6	1					
OM	5	4	3	1		1			
P	32	32	21	3	8				
PM	8	8	7		1				
PTH	9	8	7		1				1
R	4	4	4						
RO	1	1	1						
OTH	3	2	2			1			
UNSP	73	73	54	15	4				
Not Class	33								
Inactive	71								

Note: Excludes Address Unknown.

Subspecialties in this table are condensed into major specialties. See Appendix A.

Table 5.19

DOs by State, Self-Designated Specialty, and Activity, 2006, continued
Kansas

Specialty	Total Physicians	Patient Care		Hospital Based		Other Professional Activity			
		Total Patient Care	Office Based	Resid./ Fellows	Phys. Staff	Admin.	Med. Teach.	Research	Other
Total Physicians	680	605	471	84	50	4	1	2	
GP/FM Prac.	276	275	237	17	21	1			
FM	209	208	174	17	17	1			
GP	67	67	63		4				
Med. Prac.	98	96	68	23	5	1		1	
AI	4	3	2		1	1			
CD	6	6	6						
D	2	2	2						
GE	3	3	2		1				
IM	55	55	35	18	2				
PD	25	24	18	5	1			1	
PUD	3	3	3						
Sur. Spec.	63	63	50	9	4				
GS	19	19	15	4					
NS	1	1		1					
OBG	27	27	21	3	3				
OPH	4	4	4						
ORS	4	4	3		1				
OTO	5	5	5						
U	3	3	2	1					
Oth. Spec.	175	171	116	35	20	2	1	1	
AN	18	17	8	9		1			
CHP	9	8	6		2		1		
DR	13	13	8	4	1				
EM	22	22	15		7				
FOP	1	1	1						
GPM	4	4	4						
N	6	6	4	2					
OM	3	3	2		1				
P	23	23	13	7	3				
PM	10	10	7	2	1				
PTH	8	7	4	3				1	
R	4	3	1		2	1			
OTH	1	1	1						
UNSP	53	53	42	8	3				
Not Class	40								
Inactive	28								

Note: *Excludes Address Unknown.*

Subspecialties in this table are condensed into major specialties. See Appendix A.

Table 5.19

DOs by State, Self-Designated Specialty, and Activity, 2006, continued
Kentucky

Specialty	Total Physicians	Patient Care				Other Professional Activity			
		Total Patient Care	Office Based	Hospital Based		Admin.	Med. Teach.	Research	Other
				Resid./ Fellows	Phys. Staff				
Total Physicians	409	347	263	45	39	3	2		
GP/FM Prac.	123	121	98	9	14	2			
FM	103	101	80	9	12	2			
GP	20	20	18		2				
Med. Prac.	72	72	50	15	7				
CD	2	2	2						
D	2	2	1	1					
GE	3	3	3						
IM	42	42	31	7	4				
PD	20	20	11	6	3				
PUD	3	3	2	1					
Sur. Spec.	43	43	37	2	4				
GS	9	9	8	1					
NS	1	1	1						
OBG	20	20	17	1	2				
ORS	5	5	4		1				
OTO	4	4	3		1				
U	4	4	4						
Oth. Spec.	114	111	78	19	14	1	2		
AM	1	1			1				
AN	27	27	17	6	5				
CHP	2	1	1			1			
DR	5	5	2	2	1				
EM	10	9	8		1		1		
N	3	2	1	1			1		
OM	3	3	2		1				
P	12	12	10	2					
PM	3	3	2	1					
PTH	4	4	1	3					
R	1	1	1						
RO	1	1	1						
OTH	2	2	2						
UNSP	40	40	30	5	5				
Not Class	42								
Inactive	15								

Note: Excludes Address Unknown.

Subspecialties in this table are condensed into major specialties. See Appendix A.

Table 5.19

DOs by State, Self-Designated Specialty, and Activity, 2006, continued
Louisiana

Specialty	Total Physicians	Patient Care				Other Professional Activity			
		Total Patient Care	Office Based	Hospital Based		Admin.	Med. Teach.	Research	Other
				Resid./ Fellows	Phys. Staff				
Total Physicians	114	99	60	23	16	1	1		
GP/FM Prac.	25	24	16	3	5		1		
FM	24	23	15	3	5		1		
GP	1	1	1						
Med. Prac.	35	35	22	11	2				
CD	1	1	1						
GE	1	1	1						
IM	22	22	12	8	2				
PD	9	9	6	3					
PUD	2	2	2						
Sur. Spec.	8	8	5	2	1				
CRS	1	1	1						
OBG	4	4	3	1					
ORS	1	1		1					
OTO	1	1	1						
U	1	1			1				
Oth. Spec.	33	32	17	7	8	1			
AN	4	4	3		1				
CHP	1	1	1						
DR	1	1			1				
EM	8	8	3	4	1				
N	1	1	1						
P	4	4	3	1					
PM	4	4	2		2				
PTH	3	3	1	1	1				
OTH	1					1			
UNSP	6	6	3	1	2				
Not Class	8								
Inactive	5								

Note: Excludes Address Unknown.

Subspecialties in this table are condensed into major specialties. See Appendix A.

Table 5.19

DOs by State, Self-Designated Specialty, and Activity, 2006, continued
Maine

Specialty	Total Physicians	Patient Care				Other Professional Activity			
		Total Patient Care	Office Based	Hospital Based		Admin.	Med. Teach.	Research	Other
				Resid./ Fellows	Phys. Staff				
Total Physicians	655	572	423	82	67	4	4		
GP/FM Prac.	265	260	216	23	21	2	3		
FM	225	221	180	23	18	1	3		
GP	40	39	36		3	1			
Med. Prac.	105	105	70	27	8				
AI	1	1	1						
CD	6	6	5	1					
D	1	1	1						
GE	3	3	3						
IM	61	61	38	18	5				
PD	27	27	18	6	3				
PUD	6	6	4	2					
Sur. Spec.	53	51	38	3	10	1	1		
GS	12	12	8		4				
OBG	19	19	13	3	3				
OPH	1	1			1				
ORS	17	15	14		1	1	1		
OTO	3	3	3						
U	1	1			1				
Oth. Spec.	157	156	99	29	28	1			
AM	2	2	2						
AN	17	17	11	2	4				
CHP	5	5	4		1				
DR	4	4	1	2	1				
EM	32	32	17	3	12				
GPM	1	1			1				
N	3	3	3						
OM	4	4	2		2				
P	22	22	14	3	5				
PM	10	9	9			1			
PTH	2	2	1		1				
R	4	4	3		1				
OTH	3	3	3						
UNSP	48	48	29	19					
Not Class	39								
Inactive	36								

Note: Excludes Address Unknown.

Subspecialties in this table are condensed into major specialties. See Appendix A.

Table 5.19

DOs by State, Self-Designated Specialty, and Activity, 2006, continued
Maryland

Specialty	Total Physicians	Patient Care		Hospital Based		Other Professional Activity			
		Total Patient Care	Office Based	Resid./ Fellows	Phys. Staff	Admin.	Med. Teach.	Research	Other
Total Physicians	665	572	395	102	75	11	4	6	3
GP/FM Prac.	114	112	93	4	15	1	1		
FM	102	100	83	4	13	1	1		
GP	12	12	10		2				
Med. Prac.	166	162	113	26	23	2	1	1	
AI	4	4	3		1				
CD	10	9	6	1	2	1			
D	5	5	1	1	3				
GE	3	3	3						
IM	101	99	71	13	15	1		1	
PD	37	36	24	10	2		1		
PDC	1	1	1						
PUD	5	5	4	1					
Sur. Spec.	72	71	42	19	10	1			
GS	20	20	10	8	2				
OBG	22	21	13	5	3	1			
OPH	7	7	5	1	1				
ORS	15	15	11	2	2				
OTO	6	6	1	3	2				
U	2	2	2						
Oth. Spec.	244	227	147	53	27	7	2	5	3
AM	3	3	2		1				
AN	39	38	21	15	2		1		
CHP	6	6	3	2	1				
DR	4	4	4						
EM	35	35	28	2	5				
FOP	1	1	1						
GPM	12	9	6		3		1	1	1
MG	2	2	1	1					
N	11	11	6	4	1				
OM	9	5	4		1	3		1	
P	29	25	12	10	3	3		1	
PHP	2					1		1	
PM	30	30	21	6	3				
PTH	3	3	1	1	1				
R	3	3	2		1				
OTH	6	4	2		2			1	1
UNSP	49	48	33	12	3				1
Not Class	60								
Inactive	9								

Note: Excludes Address Unknown.

Subspecialties in this table are condensed into major specialties. See Appendix A.

Table 5.19

DOs by State, Self-Designated Specialty, and Activity, 2006, continued
Massachusetts

Specialty	Total Physicians	Patient Care				Other Professional Activity			
		Total Patient Care	Office Based	Hospital Based		Admin.	Med. Teach.	Research	Other
				Resid./ Fellows	Phys. Staff				
Total Physicians	672	583	364	181	38	5	1	2	3
GP/FM Prac.	111	109	93	10	6				2
FM	96	94	81	10	3				2
GP	15	15	12		3				
Med. Prac.	219	214	127	73	14	3	1		1
AI	1	1	1						
CD	9	8	4	3	1		1		
D	3	3	3						
GE	4	4	4						
IM	160	156	91	54	11	3			1
PD	38	38	23	13	2				
PUD	4	4	1	3					
Sur. Spec.	54	54	32	19	3				
GS	14	14	3	10	1				
OBG	27	27	18	8	1				
OPH	2	2	2						
ORS	10	10	8	1	1				
OTO	1	1	1						
Oth. Spec.	210	206	112	79	15	2		2	
AN	53	53	25	27	1				
CHP	2	2	2						
DR	7	7	3	3	1				
EM	37	35	23	5	7			2	
FOP	1	1	1						
GPM	3	3	1	2					
N	10	10	5	5					
OM	4	4	3		1				
P	20	19	9	8	2	1			
PM	28	28	11	15	2				
PTH	5	5	1	4					
R	5	5	4	1					
RO	1	1	1						
OTH	6	5	5			1			
UNSP	27	27	17	9	1				
VM	1	1	1						
Not Class	61								
Inactive	17								

Note: Excludes Address Unknown.

Subspecialties in this table are condensed into major specialties. See Appendix A.

Table 5.19

DOs by State, Self-Designated Specialty, and Activity, 2006, continued
Michigan

Specialty	Total Physicians	Patient Care		Hospital Based		Other Professional Activity			
		Total Patient Care	Office Based	Resid./ Fellows	Phys. Staff	Admin.	Med. Teach.	Research	Other
Total Physicians	5,740	4,849	3,797	561	491	42	43	8	19
GP/FM Prac.	1,466	1,440	1,251	48	141	12	8	2	4
FM	1,126	1,107	944	48	115	6	8	2	3
GP	340	333	307		26	6			1
Med. Prac.	827	799	629	92	78	9	14	3	2
AI	8	8	6	1	1				
CD	59	55	51	1	3		1	2	1
D	52	50	40	10			1		1
GE	23	22	18	2	2		1		
IM	489	477	386	39	52	5	6	1	
PD	160	152	99	37	16	4	4		
PDC	2	2	1	1					
PUD	34	33	28	1	4		1		
Sur. Spec.	604	594	484	37	73	1	7	1	1
CRS	1	1	1						
GS	115	115	98	12	5				
NS	8	8	4		4				
OBG	191	188	147	12	29	1	2		
OPH	50	49	42	3	4		1		
ORS	153	149	114	7	28		3		1
OTO	42	42	39	2	1				
PS	4	4	3	1					
TS	11	10	9		1			1	
U	29	28	27		1		1		
Oth. Spec.	2,064	2,016	1,433	384	199	20	14	2	12
AM	1	1	1						
AN	210	206	142	32	32	2	2		
CHP	16	15	15				1		
DR	85	83	62	10	11				2
EM	320	316	223	30	63	4			
GPM	12	12	11		1				
N	63	61	50	7	4		1	1	
NM	3	3	3						
OM	26	23	18		5	2			1
P	129	125	89	24	12	3	1		
PHP	4	2	1		1	2			
PM	74	70	48	20	2	1	3		
PTH	30	28	21	4	3	1			1
R	59	55	39	5	11		2		2
RO	9	9	9						
OTH	32	26	22	1	3	4	1		1
UNSP	991	981	679	251	51	1	3	1	5
Not Class	390								
Inactive	389								

Note: Excludes Address Unknown.

Subspecialties in this table are condensed into major specialties. See Appendix A.

Table 5.19

DOs by State, Self-Designated Specialty, and Activity, 2006, continued
Minnesota

| Specialty | Total Physicians | Patient Care | | | | Other Professional Activity | | | |
| | | Total Patient Care | Office Based | Hospital Based | | Admin. | Med. Teach. | Research | Other |
				Resid./ Fellows	Phys. Staff				
Total Physicians	452	420	297	82	41	4	1		
GP/FM Prac.	153	150	115	23	12	3			
FM	135	133	102	23	8	2			
GP	18	17	13		4	1			
Med. Prac.	92	92	53	28	11				
AI	1	1		1					
CD	2	2	1	1					
D	2	2	1		1				
GE	1	1	1						
IM	54	54	29	18	7				
PD	24	24	17	4	3				
PUD	8	8	4	4					
Sur. Spec.	51	51	37	8	6				
GS	14	14	9	2	3				
OBG	19	19	12	4	3				
OPH	2	2	2						
ORS	13	13	12	1					
U	3	3	2	1					
Oth. Spec.	129	127	92	23	12	1	1		
AN	17	17	15	1	1				
CHP	10	10	7	2	1				
DR	6	6	5	1					
EM	15	14	7	1	6		1		
GPM	1	1	1						
N	9	9	7	2					
OM	2	2	1		1				
P	18	18	10	7	1				
PM	20	20	13	7					
PTH	2	1		1		1			
R	4	4	4						
RO	2	2	2						
OTH	1	1	1						
UNSP	22	22	19	1	2				
Not Class	15								
Inactive	12								

Note: Excludes Address Unknown.

Subspecialties in this table are condensed into major specialties. See Appendix A.

Table 5.19

DOs by State, Self-Designated Specialty, and Activity, 2006, continued
Mississippi

| Specialty | Total Physicians | Patient Care | | | | Other Professional Activity | | | |
| | | Total Patient Care | Office Based | Hospital Based | | Admin. | Med. Teach. | Research | Other |
				Resid./ Fellows	Phys. Staff				
Total Physicians	326	294	210	45	39	2	4		
GP/FM Prac.	128	123	96	8	19	1	4		
FM	111	106	84	8	14	1	4		
GP	17	17	12		5				
Med. Prac.	66	66	47	14	5				
CD	2	2	1	1					
D	1	1	1						
GE	4	4	2	1	1				
IM	37	37	28	8	1				
PD	18	18	12	3	3				
PUD	4	4	3	1					
Sur. Spec.	33	33	20	10	3				
GS	9	9	2	6	1				
OBG	16	16	11	3	2				
OPH	4	4	3	1					
OTO	2	2	2						
TS	2	2	2						
Oth. Spec.	73	72	47	13	12	1			
AM	1	1			1				
AN	13	13	6	6	1				
CHP	1	1			1				
DR	2	2	2						
EM	27	27	19	3	5				
N	3	3	1		2				
OM	1	1	1						
P	3	3	1	1	1				
PM	3	3	3						
PTH	3	3	2	1					
OTH	5	4	3		1	1			
UNSP	11	11	9	2					
Not Class	15								
Inactive	11								

Note: Excludes Address Unknown.

Subspecialties in this table are condensed into major specialties. See Appendix A.

Table 5.19

DOs by State, Self-Designated Specialty, and Activity, 2006, continued
Missouri

Specialty	Total Physicians	Patient Care				Other Professional Activity			
		Total Patient Care	Office Based	Hospital Based		Admin.	Med. Teach.	Research	Other
				Resid./ Fellows	Phys. Staff				
Total Physicians	2,098	1,836	1,377	247	212	20	17	1	6
GP/FM Prac.	700	693	576	35	82	2	4	1	
FM	484	478	385	35	58	1	4	1	
GP	216	215	191		24	1			
Med. Prac.	333	324	208	89	27	5	3		1
AI	3	2	2			1			
CD	12	12	10		2				
D	9	9	6	3					
GE	10	10	9	1					
IM	197	192	132	43	17	2	2		1
PD	95	94	45	41	8	1			
PUD	7	5	4	1		1	1		
Sur. Spec.	216	207	167	25	15	2	6		1
GS	45	43	37	1	5	1	1		
NS	3	3	2		1				
OBG	79	77	52	20	5		2		
OPH	11	11	11						
ORS	53	50	46		4	1	2		
OTO	14	13	10	3			1		
PS	2	2	2						
TS	4	4	3	1					
U	5	4	4						1
Oth. Spec.	631	612	426	98	88	11	4		4
AM	3	3	2		1				
AN	100	98	70	20	8	1	1		
CHP	8	8	6	1	1				
DR	29	29	14	9	6				
EM	101	98	49	4	45	3			
GPM	8	6	6			2			
N	16	16	14	1	1				
NM	3	2	2						1
OM	9	7	4		3	1			1
P	46	43	26	12	5	2	1		
PHP	1	1	1						
PM	26	25	13	11	1		1		
PTH	21	20	12	7	1				1
R	11	11	10		1				
OTH	11	11	9		2				
UNSP	238	234	188	33	13	2	1		1
Not Class	83								
Inactive	135								

Note: Excludes Address Unknown.

Subspecialties in this table are condensed into major specialties. See Appendix A.

Table 5.19

DOs by State, Self-Designated Specialty, and Activity, 2006, continued
Montana

Specialty	Total Physicians	Patient Care		Hospital Based		Other Professional Activity			
		Total Patient Care	Office Based	Resid./ Fellows	Phys. Staff	Admin.	Med. Teach.	Research	Other
Total Physicians	128	118	104	1	13				1
GP/FM Prac.	51	50	43	1	6				1
FM	42	41	36	1	4				1
GP	9	9	7		2				
Med. Prac.	19	19	17		2				
AI	1	1			1				
CD	3	3	2		1				
GE	1	1	1						
IM	11	11	11						
PD	2	2	2						
PDC	1	1	1						
Sur. Spec.	11	11	10		1				
GS	4	4	3		1				
OBG	4	4	4						
ORS	1	1	1						
OTO	1	1	1						
TS	1	1	1						
Oth. Spec.	38	38	34		4				
AN	7	7	6		1				
CHP	1	1	1						
EM	5	5	4		1				
GPM	1	1	1						
N	4	4	4						
P	6	6	4		2				
PM	3	3	3						
RO	1	1	1						
UNSP	10	10	10						
Not Class	3								
Inactive	6								

Note: Excludes Address Unknown.

Subspecialties in this table are condensed into major specialties. See Appendix A.

Table 5.19

DOs by State, Self-Designated Specialty, and Activity, 2006, continued
Nebraska

Specialty	Total Physicians	Patient Care				Other Professional Activity			
		Total Patient Care	Office Based	Hospital Based		Admin.	Med. Teach.	Research	Other
				Resid./ Fellows	Phys. Staff				
Total Physicians	169	151	91	46	14	1	2		
GP/FM Prac.	55	52	28	20	4	1	2		
FM	50	47	23	20	4	1	2		
GP	5	5	5						
Med. Prac.	32	32	15	14	3				
AI	1	1	1						
GE	1	1	1						
IM	14	14	8	5	1				
PD	13	13	5	7	1				
PUD	3	3		2	1				
Sur. Spec.	20	20	13	5	2				
GS	4	4	3		1				
OBG	13	13	7	5	1				
OPH	1	1	1						
ORS	1	1	1						
TS	1	1	1						
Oth. Spec.	47	47	35	7	5				
AN	10	10	6	3	1				
DR	2	2	2						
EM	8	8	6	1	1				
N	1	1	1						
P	4	4	2	2					
PM	5	5	3		2				
PTH	4	4	3	1					
R	1	1	1						
RO	1	1	1						
OTH	1	1	1						
UNSP	10	10	9		1				
Not Class	9								
Inactive	6								

Note: *Excludes Address Unknown.*

Subspecialties in this table are condensed into major specialties. See Appendix A.

Table 5.19

DOs by State, Self-Designated Specialty, and Activity, 2006, continued
Nevada

Specialty	Total Physicians	Patient Care		Hospital Based		Other Professional Activity			
		Total Patient Care	Office Based	Resid./ Fellows	Phys. Staff	Admin.	Med. Teach.	Research	Other
Total Physicians	490	440	375	30	35	3	3		
GP/FM Prac.	143	141	121	3	17	2			
FM	106	105	92	3	10	1			
GP	37	36	29		7	1			
Med. Prac.	94	93	76	14	3		1		
CD	3	3	2		1				
D	5	5	5						
GE	1	1	1						
IM	61	60	54	5	1		1		
PD	24	24	14	9	1				
Sur. Spec.	39	38	34		4		1		
GS	5	5	3		2				
NS	1	1	1						
OBG	11	10	10				1		
OPH	5	5	4		1				
ORS	10	10	9		1				
OTO	5	5	5						
PS	2	2	2						
Oth. Spec.	170	168	144	13	11	1	1		
AM	1	1	1						
AN	27	26	25		1		1		
CHP	2	2	2						
DR	4	4	4						
EM	42	42	32	3	7				
FOP	2	2	2						
GPM	1					1			
N	4	4	4						
OM	3	3	3						
P	11	11	8	1	2				
PM	3	3	3						
PTH	2	2	1	1					
R	4	4	4						
RO	1	1	1						
OTH	3	3	3						
UNSP	60	60	51	8	1				
Not Class	24								
Inactive	20								

Note: Excludes Address Unknown.

Subspecialties in this table are condensed into major specialties. See Appendix A.

Table 5.19

DOs by State, Self-Designated Specialty, and Activity, 2006, continued
New Hampshire

| Specialty | Total Physicians | Patient Care | | Hospital Based | | Other Professional Activity | | | |
		Total Patient Care	Office Based	Resid./ Fellows	Phys. Staff	Admin.	Med. Teach.	Research	Other
Total Physicians	221	199	154	24	21	2	1		
GP/FM Prac.	76	75	63	6	6		1		
FM	73	72	60	6	6		1		
GP	3	3	3						
Med. Prac.	52	52	34	11	7				
AI	1	1	1						
CD	2	2	2						
GE	1	1	1						
IM	39	39	23	10	6				
PD	8	8	7		1				
PUD	1	1		1					
Sur. Spec.	18	17	14	2	1	1			
GS	3	3	2	1					
OBG	3	3	2	1					
OPH	1	1	1						
ORS	9	8	7		1	1			
OTO	2	2	2						
Oth. Spec.	56	55	43	5	7	1			
AN	14	14	11	1	2				
DR	2	2	2						
EM	8	8	7		1				
GPM	1	1		1					
N	7	7	4	2	1				
OM	1	1	1						
P	3	2	2			1			
PM	6	6	5		1				
PTH	4	4	3	1					
UNSP	10	10	8		2				
Not Class	13								
Inactive	6								

Note: Excludes Address Unknown.

Subspecialties in this table are condensed into major specialties. See Appendix A.

Table 5.19

DOs by State, Self-Designated Specialty, and Activity, 2006, continued
New Jersey

Specialty	Total Physicians	Patient Care		Hospital Based		Other Professional Activity			
		Total Patient Care	Office Based	Resid./ Fellows	Phys. Staff	Admin.	Med. Teach.	Research	Other
Total Physicians	2,961	2,565	2,128	283	154	21	20	12	10
GP/FM Prac.	667	649	599	24	26	3	10		5
FM	556	539	492	24	23	2	10		5
GP	111	110	107		3	1			
Med. Prac.	811	796	616	134	46	4	2	9	
AI	7	7	7						
CD	67	63	53	7	3	1		3	
D	24	24	23		1				
GE	36	35	33	2			1		
IM	440	434	336	72	26	1	1	4	
PD	193	190	128	50	12	2		1	
PDC	1	1	1						
PUD	43	42	35	3	4			1	
Sur. Spec.	300	296	249	26	21	3			1
CRS	1	1	1						
GS	40	40	27	7	6				
OBG	138	136	112	17	7	2			
OPH	18	18	18						
ORS	58	57	49	2	6	1			
OTO	19	19	19						
PS	10	10	9		1				
TS	6	6	5		1				
U	10	9	9						1
Oth. Spec.	850	824	664	99	61	11	8	3	4
AM	3	3	3						
AN	132	131	103	16	12			1	
CHP	15	14	14			1			
DR	34	33	23	7	3				1
EM	171	163	123	17	23	6	2		
FOP	2	1	1			1			
MG	1	1	1						
N	38	36	30	6				2	
NM	3	2	1		1	1			
OM	3	3	3						
P	71	69	50	16	3	1	1		
PM	69	69	55	11	3				
PTH	17	16	9	2	5		1		
R	28	25	20	2	3		3		
RO	5	4	3	1		1			
OTH	18	17	16		1		1		
UNSP	240	237	209	21	7				3
Not Class	168								
Inactive	165								

Note: Excludes Address Unknown.

Subspecialties in this table are condensed into major specialties. See Appendix A.

Table 5.19

DOs by State, Self-Designated Specialty, and Activity, 2006, continued
New Mexico

| Specialty | Total Physicians | Patient Care | | | | Other Professional Activity | | | |
| | | Total Patient Care | Office Based | Hospital Based | | Admin. | Med. Teach. | Research | Other |
				Resid./ Fellows	Phys. Staff				
Total Physicians	268	229	189	15	25	1	3		
GP/FM Prac.	101	100	89	5	6	1			
FM	79	78	68	5	5	1			
GP	22	22	21		1				
Med. Prac.	30	28	22	4	2		2		
AI	1	1	1						
CD	1	1	1						
D	4	3	2	1			1		
IM	14	14	11	1	2				
PD	9	8	6	2			1		
PUD	1	1	1						
Sur. Spec.	24	24	21		3				
GS	3	3	2		1				
OBG	7	7	6		1				
OPH	3	3	3						
ORS	9	9	8		1				
OTO	2	2	2						
Oth. Spec.	78	77	57	6	14		1		
AN	12	12	9		3				
CHP	5	5	3	2					
DR	4	4	4						
EM	13	13	7		6				
GPM	3	3	3						
N	2	2	1	1					
OM	3	3	3						
P	6	5	3	1	1		1		
PM	4	4	4						
PTH	1	1		1					
R	1	1			1				
RO	1	1	1						
OTH	1	1	1						
UNSP	22	22	18	1	3				
Not Class	13								
Inactive	22								

Note: Excludes Address Unknown.

Subspecialties in this table are condensed into major specialties. See Appendix A.

Table 5.19

DOs by State, Self-Designated Specialty, and Activity, 2006, continued
New York

Specialty	Total Physicians	Patient Care		Hospital Based		Other Professional Activity			
		Total Patient Care	Office Based	Resid./ Fellows	Phys. Staff	Admin.	Med. Teach.	Research	Other
Total Physicians	3,431	2,996	2,011	779	206	23	17	5	9
GP/FM Prac.	731	716	602	51	63	6	8		1
FM	646	634	529	51	54	5	6		1
GP	85	82	73		9	1	2		
Med. Prac.	1,029	1,014	623	351	40	5	3	3	4
AI	11	11	10	1					
CD	41	41	28	12	1				
D	29	29	24	4	1				
GE	31	31	22	9					
IM	593	581	346	210	25	4	2	3	3
PD	281	278	164	103	11	1	1		1
PDC	1	1			1				
PUD	42	42	29	12	1				
Sur. Spec.	283	282	201	69	12	1			
CRS	1	1	1						
GS	62	61	36	21	4	1			
NS	5	5	4	1					
OBG	146	146	100	41	5				
OPH	12	12	10	1	1				
ORS	39	39	34	3	2				
OTO	6	6	5	1					
PS	5	5	5						
TS	1	1	1						
U	6	6	5	1					
Oth. Spec.	1,007	984	585	308	91	11	6	2	4
AN	151	151	81	64	6				
CHP	18	17	10	5	2			1	
DR	38	38	21	13	4				
EM	184	176	86	54	36	5	2		1
GPM	9	9	8	1					
MG	2	2	1	1					
N	59	59	41	17	1				
NM	4	4	1	2	1				
OM	3	3	3						
P	130	127	58	53	16	1	2		
PHP	4	2	2			2			
PM	144	144	79	57	8				
PTH	24	23	7	13	3			1	
R	16	15	7	4	4				1
RO	4	4	3		1				
OTH	12	7	7			3	2		
UNSP	205	203	170	24	9				2
Not Class	282								
Inactive	99								

Note: Excludes Address Unknown.

Subspecialties in this table are condensed into major specialties. See Appendix A.

Table 5.19

DOs by State, Self-Designated Specialty, and Activity, 2006, continued
North Carolina

Specialty	Total Physicians	Patient Care				Other Professional Activity			
		Total Patient Care	Office Based	Hospital Based		Admin.	Med. Teach.	Research	Other
				Resid./ Fellows	Phys. Staff				
Total Physicians	713	643	449	103	91	4	1	3	
GP/FM Prac.	225	223	137	49	37		1	1	
FM	214	212	131	49	32		1	1	
GP	11	11	6		5				
Med. Prac.	148	145	108	21	16	2		1	
CD	13	13	11	2					
D	11	10	7	1	2	1			
GE	4	4	3	1					
IM	81	81	62	9	10				
PD	37	35	25	6	4	1		1	
PDC	1	1		1					
PUD	1	1		1					
Sur. Spec.	64	64	42	9	13				
GS	13	13	7	2	4				
OBG	30	30	19	7	4				
OPH	5	5	5						
ORS	9	9	5		4				
OTO	5	5	4		1				
U	2	2	2						
Oth. Spec.	214	211	162	24	25	2		1	
AM	1					1			
AN	28	28	18	5	5				
CHP	6	6	6						
DR	14	14	11	2	1				
EM	62	62	50	4	8				
GPM	5	5	4		1				
N	9	9	7	2					
OM	1	1	1						
P	21	20	14	4	2	1			
PHP	1	1			1				
PM	13	13	8	3	2				
PTH	4	4	2	1	1				
R	5	5	5						
OTH	3	2	1		1			1	
UNSP	41	41	35	3	3				
Not Class	41								
Inactive	21								

Note: Excludes Address Unknown.

Subspecialties in this table are condensed into major specialties. See Appendix A.

Table 5.19

DOs by State, Self-Designated Specialty, and Activity, 2006, continued
North Dakota

| Specialty | Total Physicians | Patient Care | | | | Other Professional Activity | | | |
| | | Total Patient Care | Office Based | Hospital Based | | Admin. | Med. Teach. | Research | Other |
				Resid./ Fellows	Phys. Staff				
Total Physicians	65	58	40	7	11				
GP/FM Prac.	15	15	10		5				
FM	13	13	8		5				
GP	2	2	2						
Med. Prac.	15	15	14		1				
CD	1	1	1						
IM	9	9	8		1				
PD	5	5	5						
Sur. Spec.	10	10	6	1	3				
GS	4	4	2	1	1				
NS	1	1			1				
OBG	1	1			1				
ORS	2	2	2						
OTO	1	1	1						
U	1	1	1						
Oth. Spec.	18	18	10	6	2				
AN	1	1	1						
CHP	1	1	1						
EM	3	3	2		1				
OM	1	1	1						
P	6	6	2	3	1				
PM	2	2	1	1					
R	1	1	1						
UNSP	3	3	1	2					
Not Class	5								
Inactive	2								

Note: Excludes Address Unknown.

Subspecialties in this table are condensed into major specialties. See Appendix A.

Table 5.19

DOs by State, Self-Designated Specialty, and Activity, 2006, continued
Ohio

Specialty	Total Physicians	Patient Care				Other Professional Activity			
		Total Patient Care	Office Based	Hospital Based		Admin.	Med. Teach.	Research	Other
				Resid./ Fellows	Phys. Staff				
Total Physicians	4,273	3,637	2,788	619	230	22	46	11	6
GP/FM Prac.	1,034	996	902	33	61	9	24	3	2
FM	796	763	683	33	47	8	21	2	2
GP	238	233	219		14	1	3	1	
Med. Prac.	721	706	512	156	38	1	7	6	1
AI	5	5	4		1				
CD	53	50	44	6			1	1	1
D	29	29	20	6	3				
GE	23	22	19	2	1			1	
IM	442	435	320	91	24	1	5	1	
PD	142	139	87	45	7		1	2	
PDC	1	1		1					
PUD	26	25	18	5	2			1	
Sur. Spec.	458	450	368	53	29	1	6	1	
CRS	3	3	2	1					
GS	101	99	74	18	7	1	1		
NS	14	14	13	1					
OBG	146	145	113	24	8		1		
OPH	38	37	31	3	3		1		
ORS	99	96	84	4	8		3		
OTO	28	28	27		1				
PS	8	7	7					1	
TS	8	8	6		2				
U	13	13	11	2					
Oth. Spec.	1,509	1,485	1,006	377	102	11	9	1	3
AM	2	2	1	1					
AN	194	192	135	39	18	1	1		
CHP	16	15	13	2			1		
DR	61	59	44	6	9		2		
EM	290	286	199	50	37	1	3		
FOP	2	1			1				1
GPM	8	8	5		3				
N	32	31	24	4	3			1	
NM	5	5	5						
OM	17	13	8		5	4			
P	91	88	52	30	6	2	1		
PHP	1					1			
PM	42	42	29	11	2				
PTH	42	40	20	14	6	1	1		
R	35	35	27	2	6				
RO	2	2	2						
OTH	15	12	11		1	1			2
UNSP	652	652	429	218	5				
VM	2	2	2						
Not Class	288								
Inactive	263								

Note: Excludes Address Unknown.

Subspecialties in this table are condensed into major specialties. See Appendix A.

Table 5.19

DOs by State, Self-Designated Specialty, and Activity, 2006, continued
Oklahoma

Specialty	Total Physicians	Patient Care				Other Professional Activity			
		Total Patient Care	Office Based	Hospital Based		Admin.	Med. Teach.	Research	Other
				Resid./ Fellows	Phys. Staff				
Total Physicians	1,625	1,381	1,149	89	143	12	14	2	4
GP/FM Prac.	576	565	496	25	44	4	6		1
FM	456	446	392	25	29	3	6		1
GP	120	119	104		15	1			
Med. Prac.	194	183	153	18	12	3	6	1	1
CD	10	10	9		1				
D	4	4	4						
GE	7	7	7						
IM	99	93	78	9	6	3	2	1	
PD	66	62	50	8	4		3		1
PUD	8	7	5	1	1		1		
Sur. Spec.	160	157	130	7	20	2	1		
GS	35	35	32		3				
NS	5	5	5						
OBG	49	46	30	5	11	2	1		
OPH	18	18	16		2				
ORS	35	35	31	1	3				
OTO	10	10	9		1				
PS	3	3	3						
TS	1	1	1						
U	4	4	3	1					
Oth. Spec.	483	476	370	39	67	3	1	1	2
AM	4	3	3			1			
AN	67	67	52	9	6				
CHP	2	2	2						
DR	22	22	12	3	7				
EM	92	91	55	1	35		1		
FOP	1								1
GPM	1	1	1						
N	7	7	6		1				
NM	1	1	1						
OM	8	8	7		1				
P	38	38	27	8	3				
PHP	1	1	1						
PM	8	7	6	1		1			
PTH	8	8	7	1					
R	7	7	5		2				
RO	1	1	1						
OTH	6	4	3		1	1		1	
UNSP	209	208	181	16	11				1
Not Class	122								
Inactive	90								

Note: Excludes Address Unknown.

Subspecialties in this table are condensed into major specialties. See Appendix A.

Table 5.19

DOs by State, Self-Designated Specialty, and Activity, 2006, continued
Oregon

Specialty	Total Physicians	Patient Care		Hospital Based		Other Professional Activity			
		Total Patient Care	Office Based	Resid./ Fellows	Phys. Staff	Admin.	Med. Teach.	Research	Other
Total Physicians	603	521	439	40	42	3	5		1
GP/FM Prac.	211	208	184	9	15		3		
FM	174	171	151	9	11		3		
GP	37	37	33		4				
Med. Prac.	113	112	81	25	6	1			
CD	2	2	2						
D	3	3	3						
GE	4	4	4						
IM	81	81	53	22	6				
PD	21	20	18	2		1			
PUD	2	2	1	1					
Sur. Spec.	46	45	38	2	5				1
GS	8	8	5	2	1				
OBG	14	13	13						1
OPH	4	4	4						
ORS	15	15	12		3				
OTO	3	3	2		1				
U	2	2	2						
Oth. Spec.	160	156	136	4	16	2	2		
AM	1	1			1				
AN	19	19	18	1					
CHP	4	4	3		1				
DR	8	8	8						
EM	29	28	21		7		1		
GPM	2	2	2						
MG	1	1	1						
N	8	8	8						
P	14	14	11	1	2				
PM	6	6	5		1				
PTH	5	5	3	1	1				
R	4	4	4						
OTH	7	4	4			2	1		
UNSP	52	52	48	1	3				
Not Class	29								
Inactive	44								

Note: Excludes Address Unknown.

Subspecialties in this table are condensed into major specialties. See Appendix A.

Table 5.19

DOs by State, Self-Designated Specialty, and Activity, 2006, continued
Pennsylvania

Specialty	Total Physicians	Patient Care				Other Professional Activity			
		Total Patient Care	Office Based	Resid./ Fellows	Phys. Staff	Admin.	Med. Teach.	Research	Other
Total Physicians	6,177	5,282	3,975	890	417	48	47	23	15
GP/FM Prac.	1,717	1,680	1,436	120	124	20	11	2	4
FM	1,423	1,389	1,159	120	110	17	11	2	4
GP	294	291	277		14	3			
Med. Prac.	1,326	1,290	920	296	74	8	16	11	1
AI	10	10	8	2					
CD	106	100	78	17	5		3	3	
D	31	31	27	3	1				
GE	69	67	51	15	1	1		1	
IM	796	781	551	183	47	3	10	2	
PD	259	249	163	68	18	3	2	4	1
PUD	55	52	42	8	2	1	1	1	
Sur. Spec.	566	555	419	87	49	1	6	2	2
CRS	5	5	2	2	1				
GS	119	115	75	33	7		4		
NS	5	5	4		1				
OBG	213	211	152	39	20			1	1
OPH	41	41	40	1					
ORS	92	91	74	3	14				1
OTO	43	41	34	5	2		2		
PS	10	9	8	1				1	
TS	10	10	7	1	2				
U	28	27	23	2	2	1			
Oth. Spec.	1,806	1,757	1,200	387	170	19	14	8	8
AM	4	4	2		2				
AN	258	253	170	67	16	1	2	2	
CHP	12	12	9	2	1				
DR	82	78	47	23	8		1		3
EM	330	324	181	64	79	3	1	1	1
FOP	2	2	2						
GPM	12	11	10	1			1		
N	60	57	41	13	3		1		2
NM	4	3	1		2			1	
OM	23	15	12		3	5	1	1	1
P	133	127	95	16	16	3	2	1	
PHP	3	2	2			1			
PM	104	103	72	27	4	1			
PTH	35	34	15	11	8		1		
R	45	44	36	1	7		1		
RO	14	13	10	3			1		
OTH	31	23	21		2	4	2	2	
UNSP	654	652	474	159	19	1			1
Not Class	397								
Inactive	365								

Note: Excludes Address Unknown.

Subspecialties in this table are condensed into major specialties. See Appendix A.

Table 5.19

DOs by State, Self-Designated Specialty, and Activity, 2006, continued
Puerto Rico

Specialty	Total Physicians	Patient Care		Hospital Based		Other Professional Activity			
		Total Patient Care	Office Based	Resid./ Fellows	Phys. Staff	Admin.	Med. Teach.	Research	Other
Total Physicians	2	1	1						
GP/FM Prac.	1	1	1						
FM	1	1	1						
Inactive	1								

Note: Excludes Address Unknown.

Subspecialties in this table are condensed into major specialties. See Appendix A.

Table 5.19

**DOs by State, Self-Designated Specialty, and Activity, 2006, continued
Rhode Island**

Specialty	Total Physicians	Patient Care		Hospital Based		Other Professional Activity			
		Total Patient Care	Office Based	Resid./ Fellows	Phys. Staff	Admin.	Med. Teach.	Research	Other
Total Physicians	221	195	144	30	21	2		3	
GP/FM Prac.	76	76	65	8	3				
FM	60	60	49	8	3				
GP	16	16	16						
Med. Prac.	63	60	45	8	7			3	
CD	3	3	3						
D	1	1	1						
GE	5	5	4		1				
IM	45	42	31	6	5			3	
PD	5	5	3	1	1				
PUD	4	4	3	1					
Sur. Spec.	12	12	10	1	1				
OBG	5	5	5						
OPH	1	1	1						
ORS	1	1	1						
OTO	3	3	2		1				
PS	1	1	1						
U	1	1		1					
Oth. Spec.	49	47	24	13	10	2			
AN	9	9	7		2				
CHP	1	1			1				
DR	1						1		
EM	11	10	3	4	3	1			
N	2	2	1	1					
OM	1	1	1						
P	12	12	5	4	3				
PM	1	1		1					
PTH	2	2	1	1					
UNSP	9	9	6	2	1				
Not Class	9								
Inactive	12								

Note: Excludes Address Unknown.

Subspecialties in this table are condensed into major specialties. See Appendix A.

Table 5.19

DOs by State, Self-Designated Specialty, and Activity, 2006, continued
South Carolina

| Specialty | Total Physicians | Patient Care | | | | Other Professional Activity | | | |
| | | Total Patient Care | Office Based | Hospital Based | | Admin. | Med. Teach. | Research | Other |
				Resid./ Fellows	Phys. Staff				
Total Physicians	389	353	261	57	35		2	1	
GP/FM Prac.	106	106	81	13	12				
FM	91	91	70	13	8				
GP	15	15	11		4				
Med. Prac.	105	104	71	25	8		1		
AI	3	3	3						
CD	4	4	4						
D	1	1	1						
GE	4	4	4						
IM	67	67	44	18	5				
PD	20	19	11	6	2		1		
PUD	6	6	4	1	1				
Sur. Spec.	37	37	26	9	2				
CRS	1	1	1						
GS	10	10	4	5	1				
NS	1	1		1					
OBG	13	13	10	3					
OPH	1	1	1						
ORS	5	5	4		1				
OTO	1	1	1						
PS	1	1	1						
U	4	4	4						
Oth. Spec.	108	106	83	10	13		1	1	
AM	1	1			1				
AN	13	13	12		1				
CHP	4	4	3	1					
DR	5	4	4				1		
EM	32	32	24	1	7				
GPM	1	1		1					
N	8	8	6	2					
P	10	10	6	3	1				
PM	3	3	3						
PTH	1	1	1						
R	1	1	1						
OTH	3	2	1		1			1	
UNSP	25	25	21	2	2				
VM	1	1	1						
Not Class	17								
Inactive	16								

Note: Excludes Address Unknown.

Subspecialties in this table are condensed into major specialties. See Appendix A.

Table 5.19

DOs by State, Self-Designated Specialty, and Activity, 2006, continued
South Dakota

| Specialty | Total Physicians | Patient Care | | Hospital Based | | Other Professional Activity | | | |
		Total Patient Care	Office Based	Resid./ Fellows	Phys. Staff	Admin.	Med. Teach.	Research	Other
Total Physicians	108	91	70	17	4	1			
GP/FM Prac.	36	35	24	10	1	1			
FM	32	31	20	10	1	1			
GP	4	4	4						
Med. Prac.	20	20	17	2	1				
CD	1	1	1						
D	1	1	1						
IM	14	14	11	2	1				
PD	3	3	3						
PUD	1	1	1						
Sur. Spec.	12	12	11		1				
GS	2	2	2						
OBG	4	4	4						
ORS	3	3	2		1				
OTO	3	3	3						
Oth. Spec.	24	24	18	5	1				
AN	1	1	1						
DR	2	2	2						
EM	4	4	3		1				
N	2	2	2						
P	7	7	5	2					
PM	1	1	1						
PTH	2	2		2					
R	1	1	1						
UNSP	4	4	3	1					
Not Class	8								
Inactive	8								

Note: Excludes Address Unknown.

Subspecialties in this table are condensed into major specialties. See Appendix A.

Table 5.19

DOs by State, Self-Designated Specialty, and Activity, 2006, continued
Tennessee

| Specialty | Total Physicians | Patient Care | | | | Other Professional Activity | | | |
| | | Total Patient Care | Office Based | Hospital Based | | Admin. | Med. Teach. | Research | Other |
				Resid./ Fellows	Phys. Staff				
Total Physicians	548	491	357	72	62	4	1		
GP/FM Prac.	200	197	154	24	19	2	1		
FM	158	155	114	24	17	2	1		
GP	42	42	40		2				
Med. Prac.	106	106	76	21	9				
AI	1	1	1						
CD	3	3	3						
D	2	2	2						
GE	2	2	1		1				
IM	75	75	55	13	7				
PD	22	22	13	8	1				
PDC	1	1	1						
Sur. Spec.	53	53	35	10	8				
GS	9	9	7	2					
OBG	28	28	19	7	2				
ORS	11	11	7		4				
OTO	3	3	2		1				
TS	1	1		1					
U	1	1			1				
Oth. Spec.	137	135	92	17	26	2			
AM	2	2	1		1				
AN	25	25	18	2	5				
CHP	1	1		1					
DR	5	5	5						
EM	34	33	23		10	1			
GPM	2	2	2						
N	5	5	3	1	1				
NM	6	5	3		2	1			
P	12	12	7	3	2				
PM	6	6	6						
PTH	7	7	1	5	1				
R	2	2		1	1				
RO	1	1	1						
OTH	1	1	1						
UNSP	28	28	21	4	3				
Not Class	30								
Inactive	22								

Note: Excludes Address Unknown.

Subspecialties in this table are condensed into major specialties. See Appendix A.

Table 5.19

DOs by State, Self-Designated Specialty, and Activity, 2006, continued
Texas

| Specialty | Total Physicians | Patient Care | | Hospital Based | | Other Professional Activity | | | |
		Total Patient Care	Office Based	Resid./ Fellows	Phys. Staff	Admin.	Med. Teach.	Research	Other
Total Physicians	3,625	3,166	2,464	476	226	38	31	13	6
GP/FM Prac.	1,194	1,168	1,002	89	77	13	10	1	2
FM	908	884	738	89	57	12	9	1	2
GP	286	284	264		20	1	1		
Med. Prac.	644	630	416	157	57	4	4	6	
AI	11	10	9	1			1		
CD	38	36	27	7	2	1		1	
D	23	23	18	5					
GE	24	22	9	7	6	1		1	
IM	349	344	229	84	31	2	1	2	
PD	177	174	110	51	13		2	1	
PDC	2	2	2						
PUD	20	19	12	2	5			1	
Sur. Spec.	327	321	254	50	17	3	1	1	1
GS	66	66	47	16	3				
NS	9	9	9						
OBG	124	120	91	20	9	3	1		
OPH	18	18	15	2	1				
ORS	67	66	57	8	1				1
OTO	23	23	20	2	1				
PS	5	5	5						
TS	5	5	3	2					
U	10	9	7		2			1	
Oth. Spec.	1,089	1,047	792	180	75	18	16	5	3
AM	20	15	11		4	3		2	
AN	173	172	127	28	17		1		
CHP	13	13	10	3					
DR	34	32	27	3	2		1		1
EM	218	205	143	38	24	7	4	2	
FOP	2	2	2						
GPM	17	15	12	1	2	1		1	
N	25	24	22	2			1		
NM	2	2		1	1				
OM	12	7	5		2	2	2		1
P	87	85	52	26	7		2		
PHP	2	2	2						
PM	67	65	41	22	2		1		1
PTH	42	39	17	18	4	1	2		
R	28	27	25	2		1			
RO	3	3	3						
OTH	23	19	18		1	3	1		
UNSP	321	320	275	36	9		1		
Not Class	176								
Inactive	195								

Note: Excludes Address Unknown.

Subspecialties in this table are condensed into major specialties. See Appendix A.

Table 5.19

DOs by State, Self-Designated Specialty, and Activity, 2006, continued
Utah

Specialty	Total Physicians	Patient Care				Other Professional Activity			
		Total Patient Care	Office Based	Hospital Based		Admin.	Med. Teach.	Research	Other
				Resid./ Fellows	Phys. Staff				
Total Physicians	257	234	178	36	20				1
GP/FM Prac.	106	105	76	22	7				1
FM	100	99	70	22	7				1
GP	6	6	6						
Med. Prac.	27	27	18	6	3				
AI	1	1	1						
CD	1	1			1				
D	1	1	1						
IM	13	13	8	3	2				
PD	9	9	7	2					
PDC	1	1		1					
PUD	1	1	1						
Sur. Spec.	25	25	23		2				
GS	5	5	5						
OBG	14	14	13		1				
OPH	1	1			1				
ORS	5	5	5						
Oth. Spec.	77	77	61	8	8				
AM	1	1	1						
AN	16	16	15	1					
CHP	1	1	1						
DR	1	1	1						
EM	11	11	10		1				
GPM	1	1		1					
N	1	1		1					
P	14	14	10	3	1				
PM	9	9	7	1	1				
R	3	3	1		2				
OTH	2	2	2						
UNSP	17	17	13	1	3				
Not Class	15								
Inactive	7								

Note: Excludes Address Unknown.

Subspecialties in this table are condensed into major specialties. See Appendix A.

Table 5.19

DOs by State, Self-Designated Specialty, and Activity, 2006, continued
Vermont

Specialty	Total Physicians	Patient Care				Other Professional Activity			
		Total Patient Care	Office Based	Hospital Based		Admin.	Med. Teach.	Research	Other
				Resid./ Fellows	Phys. Staff				
Total Physicians	66	56	43	6	7			1	
GP/FM Prac.	19	19	14		5				
FM	14	14	11		3				
GP	5	5	3		2				
Med. Prac.	12	11	7	3	1			1	
CD	1	1	1						
IM	7	6	3	2	1			1	
PD	3	3	3						
PUD	1	1		1					
Sur. Spec.	7	7	7						
GS	1	1	1						
OBG	2	2	2						
OPH	1	1	1						
ORS	3	3	3						
Oth. Spec.	19	19	15	3	1				
AN	1	1	1						
DR	1	1	1						
EM	3	3	2		1				
N	2	2	2						
PM	1	1	1						
PTH	1	1		1					
R	1	1	1						
OTH	1	1	1						
UNSP	8	8	6	2					
Not Class	2								
Inactive	7								

Note: Excludes Address Unknown.

Subspecialties in this table are condensed into major specialties. See Appendix A.

Table 5.19

DOs by State, Self-Designated Specialty, and Activity, 2006, continued
Virginia

Specialty	Total Physicians	Patient Care				Other Professional Activity			
		Total Patient Care	Office Based	Hospital Based		Admin.	Med. Teach.	Research	Other
				Resid./ Fellows	Phys. Staff				
Total Physicians	836	725	486	145	94	10	9		5
GP/FM Prac.	224	217	161	33	23	2	4		1
FM	199	193	138	33	22	2	3		1
GP	25	24	23		1		1		
Med. Prac.	161	158	110	34	14	1	2		
AI	1	1			1				
CD	8	8	6	1	1				
D	12	12	10		2				
GE	2	2	2						
IM	87	85	61	18	6	1	1		
PD	44	43	26	13	4		1		
PUD	7	7	5	2					
Sur. Spec.	68	67	47	10	10				1
CRS	1	1			1				
GS	16	16	12	2	2				
NS	1	1	1						
OBG	25	25	16	5	4				
OPH	3	3	3						
ORS	16	16	12	1	3				
OTO	5	4	3	1					1
U	1	1		1					
Oth. Spec.	296	283	168	68	47	7	3		3
AM	6	1			1	3	1		1
AN	48	48	26	11	11				
CHP	3	3	2	1					
DR	10	10	6	1	3				
EM	52	49	32	8	9	2	1		
FOP	1	1		1					
GPM	11	10	3		7	1			
N	11	11	7	4					
NM	1	1	1						
OM	6	4	2		2	1			1
P	21	21	13	5	3				
PM	27	27	15	8	4				
PTH	8	7	1	2	4				1
R	3	3	3						
RO	1	1	1						
OTH	6	6	5		1				
UNSP	81	80	51	27	2		1		
Not Class	67								
Inactive	20								

Note: Excludes Address Unknown.

Subspecialties in this table are condensed into major specialties. See Appendix A.

Table 5.19

DOs by State, Self-Designated Specialty, and Activity, 2006, continued
Virgin Islands

| Specialty | Total Physicians | Patient Care | | Hospital Based | | Other Professional Activity | | | |
		Total Patient Care	Office Based	Resid./ Fellows	Phys. Staff	Admin.	Med. Teach.	Research	Other
Total Physicians	2	2	2						
Med. Prac.	1	1	1						
IM	1	1	1						
Sur. Spec.	1	1	1						
OBG	1	1	1						

Note: Excludes Address Unknown.

Subspecialties in this table are condensed into major specialties. See Appendix A.

Table 5.19

DOs by State, Self-Designated Specialty, and Activity, 2006, continued
Washington

| Specialty | Total Physicians | Patient Care | | | | Other Professional Activity | | | |
		Total Patient Care	Office Based	Resid./ Fellows	Phys. Staff	Admin.	Med. Teach.	Research	Other
Total Physicians	814	723	566	95	62	5	4		
GP/FM Prac.	329	325	262	38	25	2	2		
FM	264	261	204	38	19	1	2		
GP	65	64	58		6	1			
Med. Prac.	94	94	68	17	9				
AI	2	2	2						
CD	4	4	3		1				
D	4	4	4						
GE	2	2	2						
IM	58	58	37	15	6				
PD	22	22	18	2	2				
PUD	2	2	2						
Sur. Spec.	84	84	68	9	7				
GS	13	13	9	3	1				
OBG	30	30	26	3	1				
OPH	5	5	4	1					
ORS	28	28	23	2	3				
OTO	6	6	5		1				
U	2	2	1		1				
Oth. Spec.	225	220	168	31	21	3	2		
AM	3	3	2		1				
AN	29	29	21	5	3				
CHP	3	3	1	2					
DR	15	15	8	6	1				
EM	46	45	34	3	8	1			
FOP	1	1			1				
GPM	6	5	4		1	1			
N	10	9	6	3			1		
NM	1	1			1				
OM	3	3	3						
P	18	18	16	1	1				
PHP	1					1			
PM	16	16	14	2					
PTH	3	3	1	2					
R	3	3	3						
RO	1	1	1						
OTH	9	8	6		2		1		
UNSP	57	57	48	7	2				
Not Class	39								
Inactive	43								

Note: *Excludes Address Unknown.*

Subspecialties in this table are condensed into major specialties. See Appendix A.

Table 5.19

DOs by State, Self-Designated Specialty, and Activity, 2006, continued
West Virginia

| Specialty | Total Physicians | Patient Care | | | | Other Professional Activity | | | |
| | | Total Patient Care | Office Based | Hospital Based | | Admin. | Med. Teach. | Research | Other |
				Resid./ Fellows	Phys. Staff				
Total Physicians	688	630	485	85	60	2	9		1
GP/FM Prac.	295	291	246	19	26	1	3		
FM	219	216	175	19	22		3		
GP	76	75	71		4	1			
Med. Prac.	119	119	85	28	6				
CD	6	6	4	2					
D	8	8	7	1					
GE	2	2	1		1				
IM	68	68	50	15	3				
PD	31	31	21	9	1				
PUD	4	4	2	1	1				
Sur. Spec.	50	49	37	8	4		1		
CRS	1	1	1						
GS	11	10	7	3			1		
OBG	20	20	15	4	1				
OPH	3	3	2	1					
ORS	11	11	8		3				
OTO	2	2	2						
U	2	2	2						
Oth. Spec.	178	171	117	30	24	1	5		1
AN	27	25	17	5	3	1	1		
DR	5	4	2		2				1
EM	51	51	35	4	12				
GPM	1	1	1						
N	1	1		1					
OM	1						1		
P	12	12	10	1	1				
PM	3	3	3						
PTH	3	2	1		1		1		
R	1	1	1						
RO	3	3	2		1				
OTH	5	3	3				2		
UNSP	65	65	42	19	4				
Not Class	29								
Inactive	17								

Note: Excludes Address Unknown.

Subspecialties in this table are condensed into major specialties. See Appendix A.

Table 5.19

DOs by State, Self-Designated Specialty, and Activity, 2006, continued
Wisconsin

Specialty	Total Physicians	Patient Care				Other Professional Activity			
		Total Patient Care	Office Based	Hospital Based		Admin.	Med. Teach.	Research	Other
				Resid./ Fellows	Phys. Staff				
Total Physicians	758	694	552	95	47	5	4	3	4
GP/FM Prac.	294	288	243	32	13	3		1	2
FM	248	245	203	32	10	1		1	1
GP	46	43	40		3	2			1
Med. Prac.	135	130	102	23	5	1	3	1	
AI	3	3	3						
CD	9	9	6	3					
D	2	2		1	1				
GE	6	6	5	1					
IM	74	73	56	14	3	1			
PD	39	35	30	4	1		3	1	
PUD	2	2	2						
Sur. Spec.	73	71	59	6	6	1		1	
CRS	13	13	8	3	2				
NS	1	1	1						
OBG	33	33	26	3	4				
OPH	6	5	5					1	
ORS	10	10	10						
OTO	4	4	4						
PS	1					1			
TS	3	3	3						
U	2	2	2						
Oth. Spec.	208	205	148	34	23		1		2
AN	28	28	19	8	1				
CHP	1	1			1				
DR	14	14	8	3	3				
EM	40	39	28	3	8		1		
GPM	1	1	1						
N	15	15	11	3	1				
NM	1	1	1						
OM	4	4	4						
P	19	19	13	5	1				
PM	19	19	10	7	2				
PTH	7	6	4	1	1				1
R	7	6	5		1				1
RO	1	1	1						
OTH	4	4	4						
UNSP	47	47	39	4	4				
Not Class	14								
Inactive	34								

Note: Excludes Address Unknown.

Subspecialties in this table are condensed into major specialties. See Appendix A.

Table 5.19

DOs by State, Self-Designated Specialty, and Activity, 2006, continued
Wyoming

Specialty	Total Physicians	Patient Care		Hospital Based		Other Professional Activity			
		Total Patient Care	Office Based	Resid./ Fellows	Phys. Staff	Admin.	Med. Teach.	Research	Other
Total Physicians	81	64	48	7	9	3	2		1
GP/FM Prac.	30	27	19	5	3	1	2		
FM	28	25	18	5	2	1	2		
GP	2	2	1		1				
Med. Prac.	6	5	5			1			
CD	1	1	1						
IM	4	3	3			1			
PD	1	1	1						
Sur. Spec.	6	6	5		1				
OBG	1	1	1						
OPH	1	1	1						
ORS	1	1	1						
PS	1	1	1						
TS	1	1			1				
U	1	1	1						
Oth. Spec.	28	26	19	2	5	1			1
AN	6	6	5		1				
DR	4	3	3						1
EM	7	6	3		3	1			
P	3	3	2		1				
PM	1	1	1						
UNSP	7	7	5	2					
Not Class	5								
Inactive	6								

Note: Excludes Address Unknown.

Subspecialties in this table are condensed into major specialties. See Appendix A.

Table 5.19

DOs by State, Self-Designated Specialty, and Activity, 2006, continued
Pacific Islands

| Specialty | Total Physicians | Patient Care | | | | Other Professional Activity | | | |
| | | Total Patient Care | Office Based | Hospital Based | | Admin. | Med. Teach. | Research | Other |
				Resid./ Fellows	Phys. Staff				
Total Physicians	11	8	5		3				
GP/FM Prac.	4	4	3		1				
FM	3	3	2		1				
GP	1	1	1						
Med. Prac.	1	1			1				
PD	1	1			1				
Oth. Spec.	3	3	2		1				
EM	1	1	1						
P	1	1	1						
UNSP	1	1			1				
Not Class	2								
Inactive	1								

Note: Excludes Address Unknown.

Subspecialties in this table are condensed into major specialties. See Appendix A.

Table 5.20

DOs in Metropolitan Areas by Self-Designated Specialty and Activity, 2006

Specialty	Total Physicians	Major Professional Activity								
		Patient Care					Other Professional Activity			
		Total Patient Care	Office Based	Locum Tenens	Hospital Based		Admin.	Med. Teach.	Research	Other
					Resid./ Fellows	Phys. Staff				
Total Physicians	42,097	36,515	27,408	53	6,075	2,979	333	297	105	95
GP/FM Prac	11,828	11,592	9,599	27	1,090	876	98	105	12	21
FM	9,779	9,575	7,748	25	1,090	712	75	98	11	20
GP	2,049	2,017	1,851	2		164	23	7	1	1
Med. Spec.	8,639	8,447	5,884	6	2,001	556	61	72	46	13
AI	91	87	73		8	6	2	2		
CD	528	505	411		68	26	4	7	10	2
D	303	300	258	1	24	17		2		1
GE	272	268	220	1	37	10	1	1	2	
IM	5,135	5,035	3,462	2	1,224	347	37	35	21	7
PD	1,980	1,929	1,222	2	575	130	15	22	11	3
PDC	11	11	8		1	2				
PUD	319	312	230		64	18	2	3	2	
Sur. Spec.	3,851	3,795	2,921	4	556	314	17	25	6	8
CRS	16	16	12		2	2				
GS	765	753	494	2	188	69	2	9		1
NS	62	62	52		3	7				
OBG	1,497	1,480	1,079		290	111	8	5	1	3
OPH	261	259	229	1	8	21		2		
ORS	781	767	648		38	81	5	6	1	2
OTO	235	232	209	1	12	10		2		1
PS	57	54	51		2	1	1		2	
TS	50	49	42		5	2			1	
U	127	123	105		8	10	1	1	1	1
Oth. Spec.	13,027	12,681	9,004	16	2,428	1,233	157	95	41	53
AM	63	52	33		1	18	7	1	2	1
AN	1,891	1,870	1,298	1	414	157	6	10	4	1
CHP	202	195	147		32	16	4	1	2	
DR	531	515	337	3	112	63	1	6		9
EM	2,457	2,387	1,590	5	339	453	36	22	9	3
FOP	17	14	10		2	2	1			2
GPM	142	130	99		12	19	8	1	2	1
MG	5	5	3		2					
N	475	462	350	1	87	24		7	4	2
NM	35	33	21		4	8		1	1	
OM	188	154	124		1	29	24	3	2	5
P	1,073	1,036	661		248	127	21	11	4	1
PHP	26	14	10			4	9		2	1
PM	865	853	585		220	48	5	5	1	1
PTH	317	301	151		100	50	4	6	1	5
R	316	303	235	2	15	51	4	4		5
RO	57	55	46	1	5	3	1	1		
OTH	218	175	157		1	17	24	10	6	3
UNSP	4,145	4,123	3,143	3	833	144	2	6	1	13
VM	4	4	4							
Not Class	2,172									
Inactive	2,580									

Note: Does not include 18 physicians whose counties could not be determined as rural or metropolitan.

Subspecialties in this table are condensed into major specialties. See Appendix A.

Table 5.21

DOs in Rural Areas by Self-Designated Specialty and Activity, 2006

Specialty	Total Physicians	Total Patient Care	Office Based	Locum Tenens	Resid./ Fellows	Phys. Staff	Admin.	Med. Teach.	Research	Other
Total Physicians	17,445	15,234	12,039	1,707	1,488	114	109	27	30	
GP/FM Prac	5,895	5,796	4,951	288	557	40	44	3	12	
FM	4,767	4,682	3,955	288	439	31	41	3	10	
GP	1,128	1,114	996		118	9	3		2	
Med. Spec.	2,865	2,815	2,106	486	223	11	18	18	3	
AI	22	22	18	2	2					
CD	173	171	141	22	8		1	1		
D	120	118	92	18	8	1		1		
GE	114	111	82	15	14	1	1	1		
IM	1,678	1,653	1,265	251	137	7	7	10	1	
PD	656	643	433	164	46	2	6	3	2	
PDC	6	6	1	4	1					
PUD	96	91	74	10	7		3	2		
Sur. Spec.	1,736	1,702	1,400	124	178	9	20	2	3	
CRS	7	7	6	1						
GS	359	353	277	37	39	3	3			
NS	13	12	9	2	1		1			
OBG	636	627	497	58	72	2	5	1	1	
OPH	122	121	110	7	4			1		
ORS	382	370	316	9	45	2	9		1	
OTO	122	119	106	6	7	1	2			
PS	12	12	12							
TS	18	17	12		5	1				
U	65	64	55	4	5				1	
Oth. Spec.	5,018	4,921	3,582	809	530	54	27	4	12	
AM	35	31	20	1	10	3		1		
AN	669	662	484	113	65	4	3			
CHP	61	59	43	11	5		2			
DR	213	210	144	37	29	1	1		1	
EM	957	940	663	74	203	13	3		1	
FOP	3	1	1						2	
GPM	69	64	46	5	13	3	1		1	
MG	1	1	1							
N	157	154	122	23	9	1	1	1		
NM	14	11	8	1	2	1	1		1	
OM	53	46	33	1	12	5	1		1	
P	400	392	257	93	42	5	3			
PHP	11	6	4		2	5				
PM	191	190	127	53	10	1				
PTH	120	115	67	33	15	1	2	1	1	
R	91	87	70	6	11	1	3			
RO	19	19	18		1					
OTH	97	82	74		8	7	5	1	2	
UNSP	1,855	1,849	1,398	358	93	3	1		2	
VM	2	2	2							
Not Class	956									
Inactive	975									

Note: Does not include 18 physicians whose counties could not be determined as rural or metropolitan.

Subspecialties in this table are condensed into major specialties. See Appendix A.

Table 5.22

DOs by Metropolitan Areas, 2006

Metropolitan Areas	Total Physicians	Total Patient Care	FM/GP Practice	Medical Specialties	Surgical Specialties	Other Specialties	Hospital Based Practice	Other Professional Activity	Inactive	Not Classified
Total Metros	42,083	36,508	9,623	5,889	2,924	9,020	9,052	827	2,168	2,580
Abilene TX	30	28	11	2	6	8	1			2
Albany GA	5	5		3		1	1			
Albany NY*	144	125	42	22	4	26	31	1	3	15
Albuquerque NM	96	78	29	5	4	26	14	3	12	3
Alexandria LA	1	1					1			
Allentown PA*	467	393	96	82	35	79	101	8	23	43
Altoona PA	61	59	18	10	5	12	14			2
Amarillo TX	31	24	10	5	1	3	5	2	4	1
Anchorage AK	65	59	19	13	3	13	11	2	2	2
Anniston AL	8	8	3	1	1		3			
Appleton WI*	48	44	13	9	2	10	10	1	2	1
Asheville NC	16	13	4	1	1	2	5		2	1
Athens GA	10	8	2	1		5			2	
Atlanta GA	286	244	85	36	27	59	37	13	15	14
Auburn AL*	4	4	2	1		1				
Augusta GA*	125	112	14	14	7	12	65	2	1	10
Austin TX*	166	152	51	36	7	35	23	3	5	6
Bakersfield CA	65	57	9	7	6	19	16	2	3	3
Bangor ME	71	61	26	4	2	7	22		2	8
Barnstable MA*	29	22	5	8	1	6	2	2	2	3
Baton Rouge LA*	15	12	1	2	2	2	5		1	2
Beaumont TX*	49	44	25	3	2	14		1	2	2
Bellingham WA	12	10	3	3	2	2			1	1
Benton Harbor MI	33	29	14	7	3	4	1		4	
Billings MT	23	23	4	5		10	4			
Biloxi MS*	73	53	10	13	6	8	16	5	4	11
Binghamton NY	51	47	16	9	2	5	15	1		3
Birmingham AL	49	44	16	7	2	4	15	3		2
Bismarck ND	13	12	1	6	1	3	1			1
Bloomington IL*	37	31	7	5	1	9	9		2	4
Bloomington IN	9	9	2	4	1	1	1			
Boise City ID	66	62	21	7	3	23	8		1	3
Boston MA*	787	689	159	120	36	138	236	12	20	66
Brownsville TX*	25	23	9	2	2	5	5		2	
Bryan TX*	10	9	1			2	6			1
Buffalo NY*	138	120	29	27	11	27	26	5	7	6
Burlington VT	13	10	5	2		1	2		1	2
Canton OH*	143	119	33	13	9	28	36	4	10	10
Casper WY	13	9	4	1		1	3	3		1
Cedar Rapids IA	30	26	9	3	1	7	6		3	1
Champaign IL*	25	24	7	5	2	6	4	1		
Charleston SC*	79	73	14	11	2	17	29	2	1	3
Charleston WV	102	94	29	18	4	14	29	1	2	5
Charlotte NC*	118	112	29	31	2	31	19		2	4
Charlottesville VA	7	6		2	2	2		1		
Chattanooga TN	63	60	15	9	6	10	20	1	1	1
Cheyenne WY	8	6	1	1		3	1	1		1
Chicago IL*	1,733	1,547	326	254	119	361	487	36	34	116
Chico CA*	26	25	12	6	1	4	2			1
Cincinnati OH*	203	176	49	23	11	48	45	2	13	12
Clarksville TN*	29	28	6	5	2	3	12			1
Cleveland OH*	711	619	150	93	44	181	151	15	43	34
Colorado Springs CO	66	57	20	7	4	19	7	2	3	4
Columbia MO	48	43	5	3	3	13	19		3	2

Table 5.22

DOs by Metropolitan Areas, 2006, continued

Metropolitan Areas	Total Physicians	Total Patient Care	Office-Based Practice				Hospital Based Practice	Other Professional Activity	Inactive	Not Classified
			FM/GP Practice	Medical Specialties	Surgical Specialties	Other Specialties				
Columbia SC	35	31	3	8		4	16		1	3
Columbus GA	53	45	15	3	2	9	16	2	1	5
Columbus OH	681	561	147	77	61	170	106	19	44	57
Corpus Christi TX	21	18	8	4	1	3	2		3	
Corvalis OR	15	14	5	2	2	3	2			1
Cumberland MD	7	7	2	2	2	1				
Dallas TX*	1,396	1,224	385	193	98	338	210	41	72	59
Danville VA	9	9	3	1	2	3				
Davenport IA*	94	85	24	11	7	26	17		7	2
Daytona Beach FL	85	64	25	9	4	16	10	3	16	2
Dayton OH	430	358	70	46	42	110	90	10	31	31
Decatur AL	11	11	2	5		3	1			
Decatur IL	9	7	2	2	2	1			1	1
Denver CO*	465	413	151	52	35	106	69	7	32	13
Des Moines IA	367	326	92	53	22	63	96	11	21	9
Detroit MI*	2,951	2,470	581	342	233	741	573	50	205	226
Dothan AL	10	9	1	2	1	4	1		1	
Dover DE	27	26	11	7	2	6			1	
Dubuque IA	9	9	5	1	1	1	1			
Duluth MN*	26	25	3	5	5	6	6			1
Eau Claire WI	23	19	7	1	1	5	5	1	2	1
Elkhart IN*	32	31	9	1	6	11	4		1	
Elmira NY	13	13	3	4	1	2	3			
El Paso TX	106	97	16	8	8	23	42	1	2	6
Enid OK	25	23	7	3	4	8	1		2	
Erie PA	262	212	76	28	15	50	43	8	18	24
Eugene OR*	27	25	8	2	1	9	5		2	
Evansville IN*	28	24	8	1	3	9	3		3	1
Fargo ND*	8	8	1	1	1	2	3			
Fayetteville AR*	40	37	11	3	6	5	12		3	
Fayetteville NC	49	46	5	6	2	13	20	1		2
Flagstaff AZ	18	16	6	1	1	3	5		2	
Florence AL	18	18	7	2	3	6				
Florence SC	7	7	3	1			3			
Fort Collins CO*	46	44	13	4	5	16	6		1	1
Fort Myers FL*	173	148	55	30	23	26	14	3	20	2
Fort Pierce FL*	73	62	19	9	4	19	11		8	3
Fort Smith AR	55	53	19	12	7	12	3		1	1
Fort Wayne IN	64	63	21	10	2	15	15	1		
Fresno CA	78	69	16	11	1	12	29		5	4
Ft Walton Beach FL	24	18	4	2	4	5	3	1	2	3
Gadsden AL	11	11	5	1	1	4				
Gainsesville FL	61	51	7	2	1	16	25		2	8
Glens Falls NY	12	12	6	3		2	1			
Goldsboro NC	14	14	2	1	5	4	2			
Grand Forks ND	12	11	1	3	1	2	4			1
Grand Junction CO	56	46	14	8	10	8	6		8	2
Grand Rapids MI*	342	306	94	37	27	100	48	4	25	7
Great Falls MT	21	20	7	3	4	4	2			1
Green Bay WI	37	36	7	11	4	11	3		1	
Greensboro NC*	66	58	11	14	3	12	18		2	6
Greenville NC	31	30	3	8	1	9	9		1	
Greenville SC*	74	68	15	9	4	18	22	1	3	2
Harrisburg PA*	309	254	58	45	20	49	82	9	20	26
Hartford CT	172	157	17	40	4	34	62	1	3	11
Hattiesburg MS	21	20	7	6	1	5	1			1

Table 5.22

DOs by Metropolitan Areas, 2006, continued

Metropolitan Areas	Total Physicians	Total Patient Care	Office-Based Practice				Hospital Based Practice	Other Professional Activity	Inactive	Not Classified
			FM/GP Practice	Medical Specialties	Surgical Specialties	Other Specialties				
Hickory NC*	15	13	2	1	1	6	3			2
Honolulu HI	128	113	20	9	5	21	58		7	8
Houma LA	4	3	1	1		1			1	
Houston TX*	427	352	114	35	22	85	96	15	25	35
Huntington WV*	46	44	18	5	4	8	9		2	
Huntsville AL	40	36	12	3	1	14	6	1	2	1
Indianapolis IN	202	179	40	21	18	35	65	3	10	10
Iowa City IA	61	48	3	4		9	32		2	11
Jackson MI	40	35	15	6	3	8	3	1	3	1
Jackson MS	64	63	9	3	6	11	34			1
Jackson TN	18	18	4	3	1	2	8			
Jacksonville FL	228	202	58	27	11	42	64	7	5	14
Jacksonville NC	28	24	3	3		4	14	1	1	2
Jamestown NY	17	12	3	4		2	3		5	
Janesville WI*	10	10	5		1	2	2			
Johnson City TN*	56	52	14	11	1	6	20	1		3
Johnstown PA	56	48	17	4	5	11	11		4	4
Jonesboro AR	14	14	5	3	1	2	3			
Joplin MO	76	69	17	3	8	19	22		4	3
Kalamazoo MI*	134	120	36	18	9	33	24	4	5	5
Kansas City MO	488	424	101	62	34	91	136	11	27	26
Kileen-Temple TX	62	60	8	3	1	9	39			2
Knoxville TN	45	38	8	7	1	10	12		3	4
Kokomo IN	5	5	3		1	1				
La Crosse WI	17	17	7	4	1	1	4			
Lafayette IN	16	16	4	1	2	6	3			
Lafayette LA	3	3		2			1			
Lake Charles LA	4	3				1	2		1	
Lakeland FL*	46	37	10	4	5	16	2		6	3
Lancaster PA	210	173	52	31	29	35	26	1	23	13
Lansing MI*	594	495	107	55	50	164	119	26	28	45
Laredo TX	7	7	3		3	1				
Las Cruces NM	25	24	12	2	2	7	1			1
Las Vegas NV	389	347	93	52	33	116	53	5	16	21
Lawrence KS	18	17	7		1	3	6	1		
Lawton OK	36	32	13	1	4	6	8		2	2
Lewiston ME*	35	31	11	4	3	4	9	1	1	2
Lexington KY	47	40	6	5	3	14	12		2	5
Lima OH	25	24	2	5	6	10	1		1	
Lincoln NE	22	20	3	4		7	6		1	1
Little Rock AR*	45	43	9	7		7	20			2
Longview TX*	19	19	2	7		9	1			
Los Angeles CA*	1,555	1,361	442	212	82	308	317	13	36	145
Louisville KY	42	35	3	9	1	15	7	2	1	4
Lubbock TX	44	39	10	6	7	9	7	1	4	
Lynchburg VA	13	12	7	3			2		1	
Macon GA	35	26	11	1	5	5	4	1	3	5
Madison WI	61	59	12	10	2	13	22			2
Mansfield OH	29	26	4	4	3	9	6		3	
McAllen TX	19	17	5	1	4	6	1			2
Medford OR	56	50	24	3	2	18	3		5	1
Melbourne FL*	63	55	12	8	5	27	3	1	6	1
Memphis TN	41	38	10	6	1	5	16		1	2
Merced CA	12	11	4		1	3	3			1
Miami FL*	468	384	105	60	24	108	87	12	30	42
Milwaukee WI*	251	228	84	27	17	48	52	8	11	4

Table 5.22

DOs by Metropolitan Areas, 2006, continued

Metropolitan Areas	Total Physicians	Total Patient Care	Major Professional Activity				Hospital Based Practice	Other Professional Activity	Inactive	Not Classified
			Patient Care							
			Office-Based Practice							
			FM/GP Practice	Medical Specialties	Surgical Specialties	Other Specialties				
Minneapolis MN*	174	160	34	20	10	41	55	2	5	7
Missoula MT	14	13	8	1		3	1			1
Mobile AL	52	48	8	6	7	6	21	1	2	1
Modesto CA	39	37	10	3	2	11	11	1		1
Monroe LA	6	5	3		1	1		1		
Montgomery AL	38	33	9	9		10	5	1	2	2
Muncie IN	10	10	5			1	4			
Mytle Beach SC	34	30	7	8	2	9	4		1	3
Naples FL	75	53	13	10	5	19	6	1	20	1
Nashville TN	67	56	19	4	4	17	12	1	4	6
New London CT*	23	21	8	4		4	5		1	1
New Orleans LA	42	38	4	11	1	8	14			4
New York NY*	3,822	3,355	634	753	267	714	987	64	121	282
Norfolk VA*	164	139	20	23	13	17	66	4	4	17
Ocala FL	42	33	13	3	3	11	3	2	6	1
Odessa TX*	17	13	3	1	3	5	1		2	2
Oklahoma City OK	358	313	89	31	25	99	69	4	16	25
Omaha NE	91	81	11	9	7	19	35	1	2	7
Orlando FL	346	297	82	38	34	96	47	8	23	18
Owensboro KY	10	7	5			1	1	1	2	
Panama City FL	20	18	6		4	7	1		2	
Parkersburg WV*	63	54	23	5	7	15	4	1	3	5
Pensacola FL	92	81	21	2	12	22	24	1	2	8
Peoria IL*	81	73	15	7	3	9	39	3	1	4
Philadelphia PA*	3,450	2,916	796	551	209	750	610	98	238	198
Phoenix AZ*	1,236	1,048	286	189	96	254	223	19	93	76
Pine Bluff AR	16	12	6		2	1	3			4
Pittsburgh PA	558	494	104	106	36	88	160	14	13	37
Pittsfield MA	32	27	1	5	2	5	14		1	4
Pocatello ID	15	14	5	2		6	1			1
Portland ME	183	159	51	23	14	38	33	3	13	8
Portland OR*	346	286	98	46	20	70	52	7	27	26
Providence RI*	139	119	43	28	9	12	27	4	9	7
Provo UT*	44	42	15	3	4	8	12		1	1
Pueblo CO	26	25	10	3	3	3	6	1		
Punta Gorda FL	30	28	10	5	3	9	1		2	
Raleigh NC*	81	66	15	4	3	19	25	4	3	8
Rapid City SD	14	14	3		1	3	7			
Reading PA	108	91	30	12	5	19	25	2	7	8
Redding CA	43	41	18	5	2	7	9		1	1
Reno NV	57	51	16	12		15	8		4	2
Richland WA*	29	28	10	4	3	8	3		1	
Richmond VA*	103	86	9	11	5	14	47	1	2	14
Roanoke VA	53	45	7	5	1	15	17	2	2	4
Rochester MN	37	34	5	4	2	4	19	2	1	
Rochester NY	79	70	13	13	4	23	17		4	5
Rockford IL	35	32	8	3	6	7	8	1	1	1
Rocky Mount NC	4	4	1		1	1	1			
Sacramento CA*	178	151	48	22	4	35	42	4	7	16
Saginaw MI*	155	136	42	13	9	40	32	1	11	7
Saint Cloud MN	18	18	4	6	1	3	4			
Saint Joseph MO	7	7	3	2		1	1			
Saint Louis MO	407	349	95	42	28	74	110	11	18	29
Salinas CA	28	27	13	7		2	5	1		
Salt Lake City UT*	76	70	16	8	9	20	17		1	5
San Angelo TX	12	10	3	3	1	2	1		2	

Table 5.22

DOs by Metropolitan Areas, 2006, continued

Metropolitan Areas	Total Physicians	Major Professional Activity								
		Patient Care						Hospital Based Practice	Other Professional Activity	Inactive	Not Classified
		Total Patient Care	Office-Based Practice							
			FM/GP Practice	Medical Specialties	Surgical Specialties	Other Specialties				
San Antonio TX	252	219	41	30	11	48	89	7	10	16
San Diego CA	425	380	103	38	26	79	134	6	14	25
San Francisco CA*	494	434	104	100	34	104	92	12	9	39
San Luis Obispo CA*	21	18	8	4		4	2		3	
Santa Barbara CA*	31	27	8	7	2	4	6		1	3
Santa Fe NM	16	13	4	1	2	4	2		1	2
Sarasota FL*	151	125	36	21	9	46	13	2	20	4
Savannah GA	27	23	8	3	3	6	3		2	2
Scranton PA*	184	167	47	36	19	30	35	4	9	4
Seattle WA*	450	401	135	32	41	101	92	5	19	25
Sharon PA	94	77	25	12	11	15	14		12	5
Sheboygan WI	9	7	2	1		2	2	1	1	
Sherman TX*	13	10	5		1	4			1	2
Shreveport LA*	15	13		1		3	9		1	1
Sioux City IA	33	30	12	2	1	8	7		2	1
Sioux Falls SD	42	37	6	5	4	10	12	1		4
South Bend IN	82	65	25	6	7	15	12	3	12	2
Spokane WA	64	59	19	8	3	13	16		2	3
Springfield IL	13	12	4			2	6			1
Springfield MA	17	14	1	4		3	6			3
Springfield MO	108	94	29	16	6	21	22	1	10	3
State College PA	36	36	6	4	4	18	4			
Steubenville OH*	11	9	3	2		3	1	1	1	
Stockton CA*	50	46	15	10	2	11	8		2	2
Sumter SC	12	11	2	2	2	3	2			1
Syracuse NY	90	77	17	11	5	8	36		4	9
Tallahassee FL	27	21	4	5	2	10		1	5	
Tampa FL*	677	586	171	113	50	161	91	7	64	20
Terre Haute IN	23	20	3	3	4	3	7		1	2
Texarkana TX-AR	7	6	3		1	2			1	
Toledo OH	170	138	23	14	20	42	39	3	9	20
Topeka KS	33	30	13	6		9	2	1	1	1
Tucson AZ	201	172	53	34	14	43	28	6	20	3
Tulsa OK	646	542	181	81	57	134	89	18	42	44
Tuscaloosa AL	6	6	3	1		2				
Tyler TX	40	34	8	2	6	12	6	1	5	
Utica NY*	43	37	14	4	3	5	11	2	2	2
Victoria TX	14	14	5	2	3	3	1			
Visalia CA*	22	21	5	4	3	6	3	1		
Waco TX	33	29	11	4	1	7	6	1	2	1
Washington DC*	737	635	100	114	34	160	227	32	15	55
Waterloo IA*	41	40	14	6	4	10	6		1	
Wausau WI	28	27	7	5	7	6	2		1	
West Palm Beach FL*	270	230	70	52	32	61	15	2	31	7
Wheeling WV	7	5	1			4			1	1
Wichita Falls TX	22	20	5	3		8	4		1	1
Wichita KS	174	157	65	14	11	26	41	1	6	10
Williamsport PA	33	30	7	5	5	7	6	1	1	1
Wilmington NC	34	31	8	4	1	5	13		3	
Yakima WA	43	33	18	3	2	8	2	2	7	1
York PA	215	188	46	23	23	52	44		13	14
Youngstown OH*	316	283	105	47	19	66	46	7	18	8
Yuba City CA	23	21	9	3	2	6	1	1		1
Yuma AZ	24	22	8	3		10	1			2

Note: Does not include 16 physicians whose MSA could not be determined.

* MSA name is abbreviated.

Table 5.23

DOs by Self-Designated Primary Care Specialty, Activity, and Sex, 2006

Specialty	Total Physicians	Patient Care					Other Professional Activity			
		Total Patient Care	Office Based	Locum Tenens	Resid./ Fellows	Phys. Staff	Admin.	Med. Teach.	Research	Other
Both Sexes										
Total Physicians	59,560	51,765	39,432	83	7,783	4,467	447	406	132	125
Active Physicians	56,431	51,765	39,432	83	7,783	4,467	447	406	132	125
Primary Care	27,215	26,743	21,125	47	3,451	2,120	183	210	34	45
Family Medicine	14,373	14,090	11,563	34	1,350	1,143	102	137	14	30
General Practice	3,177	3,131	2,843	6		282	32	10	1	3
Internal Medicine	5,524	5,448	3,837	4	1,211	396	28	32	10	6
Obstetrics/Gynecology	2,025	2,006	1,491	1	348	166	7	9	1	2
Pediatrics	2,116	2,068	1,391	2	542	133	14	22	8	4
Prim. Care Subspec.	2,190	2,110	1,440	5	503	162	27	19	29	5
FM Subspecialties	170	164	135	2	19	8	4	2		
IM Subspecialties	1,422	1,370	968	1	307	94	17	11	22	2
OBG Subspecialties	108	101	84			17	3	1	1	2
PD Subspecialties	490	475	253	2	177	43	3	5	6	1
All Other Specialties	23,470	22,912	16,867	31	3,829	2,185	237	177	69	75
Inactive	3,129									
Not Classified	3,556									
Male										
Total Physicians	43,452	37,504	29,464	55	4,537	3,448	378	306	104	96
Active Physicians	40,633	37,504	29,464	55	4,537	3,448	378	306	104	96
Primary Care	18,681	18,327	15,024	30	1,714	1,559	159	142	22	31
Family Medicine	10,064	9,857	8,275	21	686	875	88	92	6	21
General Practice	2,696	2,655	2,420	5		230	29	8	1	3
Internal Medicine	3,901	3,841	2,810	3	748	280	24	23	9	4
Obstetrics/Gynecology	1,135	1,122	905	1	105	111	5	7		1
Pediatrics	885	852	614		175	63	13	12	6	2
Prim. Care Subspec.	1,501	1,445	1,027	3	305	110	21	13	19	3
FM Subspecialties	133	128	106	2	14	6	4	1		
IM Subspecialties	1,009	970	709	1	199	61	13	9	16	1
OBG Subspecialties	78	74	59			15	2		1	1
PD Subspecialties	281	273	153		92	28	2	3	2	1
All Other Specialties	18,206	17,732	13,413	22	2,518	1,779	198	151	63	62
Inactive	2,819									
Not Classified	2,245									
Female										
Total Physicians	16,108	14,261	9,968	28	3,246	1,019	69	100	28	29
Active Physicians	15,798	14,261	9,968	28	3,246	1,019	69	100	28	29
Primary Care	8,534	8,416	6,101	17	1,737	561	24	68	12	14
Family Medicine	4,309	4,233	3,288	13	664	268	14	45	8	9
General Practice	481	476	423	1		52	3	2		
Internal Medicine	1,623	1,607	1,027	1	463	116	4	9	1	2
Obstetrics/Gynecology	890	884	586		243	55	2	2	1	1
Pediatrics	1,231	1,216	777	2	367	70	1	10	2	2
Prim. Care Subspec.	689	665	413	2	198	52	6	6	10	2
FM Subspecialties	37	36	29		5	2		1		
IM Subspecialties	413	400	259		108	33	4	2	6	1
OBG Subspecialties	30	27	25			2	1	1		1
PD Subspecialties	209	202	100	2	85	15	1	2	4	
All Other Specialties	5,264	5,180	3,454	9	1,311	406	39	26	6	13
Inactive	310									
Not Classified	1,311									

Table 5.24

DOs by Self-Designated Primary Care Specialty, Age, and Sex, 2006

Specialty	Total Physicians	< 35	35-44	45-54	55-64	≥ 65
			Both Sexes			
Total Physicians	59,560	12,060	16,736	15,436	7,975	7,353
Active Physicians	56,431	12,057	16,653	15,127	7,578	5,016
Primary Care	27,215	4,858	7,982	7,926	4,033	2,416
Family Medicine	14,373	2,276	4,539	4,408	1,991	1,159
General Practice	3,177	8	260	1,140	1,063	706
Internal Medicine	5,524	1,394	1,827	1,446	519	338
Obstetrics/Gynecology	2,025	437	705	531	258	94
Pediatrics	2,116	743	651	401	202	119
Prim. Care Subspec.	2,190	564	762	542	245	77
FM Subspecialties	170	39	57	33	23	18
IM Subspecialties	1,422	352	516	370	157	27
OBG Subspecialties	108		9	46	36	17
PD Subspecialties	490	173	180	93	29	15
All Other Specialties	23,470	4,781	6,945	6,451	3,242	2,051
Inactive	3,129	3	83	309	397	2,337
Not Classified	3,556	1,854	964	208	58	472
			Male			
Total Physicians	43,452	7,048	11,380	11,613	6,963	6,448
Active Physicians	40,633	7,046	11,334	11,391	6,618	4,244
Primary Care	18,681	2,426	4,950	5,730	3,497	2,078
Family Medicine	10,064	1,167	2,935	3,235	1,707	1,020
General Practice	2,696	2	194	884	945	671
Internal Medicine	3,901	884	1,224	1,076	456	261
Obstetrics/Gynecology	1,135	130	359	356	226	64
Pediatrics	885	243	238	179	163	62
Prim. Care Subspec.	1,501	332	503	390	206	70
FM Subspecialties	133	27	45	27	17	17
IM Subspecialties	1,009	224	353	270	137	25
OBG Subspecialties	78		5	29	28	16
PD Subspecialties	281	81	100	64	24	12
All Other Specialties	18,206	3,171	5,257	5,152	2,872	1,754
Inactive	2,819	2	46	222	345	2,204
Not Classified	2,245	1,117	624	119	43	342
			Female			
Total Physicians	16,108	5,012	5,356	3,823	1,012	905
Active Physicians	15,798	5,011	5,319	3,736	960	772
Primary Care	8,534	2,432	3,032	2,196	536	338
Family Medicine	4,309	1,109	1,604	1,173	284	139
General Practice	481	6	66	256	118	35
Internal Medicine	1,623	510	603	370	63	77
Obstetrics/Gynecology	890	307	346	175	32	30
Pediatrics	1,231	500	413	222	39	57
Prim. Care Subspec.	689	232	259	152	39	7
FM Subspecialties	37	12	12	6	6	1
IM Subspecialties	413	128	163	100	20	2
OBG Subspecialties	30		4	17	8	1
PD Subspecialties	209	92	80	29	5	3
All Other Specialties	5,264	1,610	1,688	1,299	370	297
Inactive	310	1	37	87	52	133
Not Classified	1,311	737	340	89	15	130

Table 5.25

DOs by Self-Designated Primary Care Specialty and State of Location, 2006

State	Total Physicians	Total Primary Care	Family Medicine	General Practice	Internal Medicine	OB/Gyn	Pediatrics	Subspec- ialties	All Other Special- ties	Not Class- ified	Inactive/ Address Un- known
Totals	59,560	27,215	14,373	3,177	5,524	2,025	2,116	2,190	23,470	3,556	3,129
AL	385	199	127	16	37	8	11	18	147	8	13
AK	134	79	50	10	11	2	6	7	43	3	2
AZ	1,789	797	424	99	157	57	60	67	681	95	149
AR	267	158	97	22	21	5	13	9	79	11	10
CA	3,604	1,886	1,103	133	418	106	126	105	1,244	278	91
CO	1,028	522	330	69	73	31	19	23	382	30	71
CT	443	202	52	2	82	37	29	35	166	33	7
DE	270	123	65	7	23	18	10	18	102	14	13
DC	108	44	16		19	4	5	10	46	5	3
FL	4,288	1,767	977	245	329	106	110	131	1,807	191	392
GA	825	392	243	46	61	30	12	28	314	44	47
HI	213	95	50	11	16	10	8	6	86	17	9
ID	229	125	97	5	8	8	7		88	10	6
IL	2,469	1,132	585	68	264	111	104	105	999	187	46
IN	859	400	229	64	51	40	16	39	351	25	44
IA	1,177	694	441	69	106	27	51	26	353	33	71
KS	680	365	205	67	49	25	19	19	228	40	28
KY	409	192	103	20	36	20	13	15	145	42	15
LA	114	49	24	1	16	3	5	11	41	8	5
ME	655	354	224	40	49	18	23	21	205	39	36
MD	665	242	100	12	81	21	28	32	322	60	9
MA	672	300	92	15	138	25	30	36	258	61	17
MI	5,740	2,165	1,114	340	394	183	134	148	2,648	390	389
MN	452	225	132	18	41	16	18	32	168	15	12
MS	326	180	111	17	25	16	11	21	99	15	11
MO	2,098	1,005	476	216	163	76	74	68	807	83	135
MT	128	67	42	9	10	4	2	2	50	3	6
NE	169	94	50	5	13	13	13	4	56	9	6
NV	490	224	104	37	54	9	20	15	207	24	20
NH	221	120	73	3	33	3	8	7	75	13	6
NJ	2,961	1,284	546	111	337	125	165	165	1,179	168	165
NM	268	129	79	22	13	7	8	2	102	13	22
NY	3,431	1,575	640	85	465	143	242	199	1,276	282	99
NC	713	336	206	11	63	29	27	36	279	41	21
ND	65	23	13	2	5	1	2	6	29	5	2
OH	4,273	1,645	782	238	375	141	109	126	1,951	288	263
OK	1,625	749	451	120	78	47	53	42	622	122	90
OR	603	308	173	37	68	12	18	21	201	29	44
PA	6,177	2,748	1,396	294	637	201	220	245	2,422	397	365
RI	221	121	60	16	37	5	3	11	68	9	12
SC	389	186	91	15	51	12	17	20	150	17	16
SD	108	54	32	4	12	4	2	4	34	8	8
TN	548	306	157	42	67	27	13	20	170	30	22
TX	3,625	1,717	904	286	266	118	143	130	1,407	176	195
UT	257	135	100	6	11	12	6	8	92	15	7
VT	66	28	14	5	6	2	1	3	26	2	7
VA	836	343	193	25	70	23	32	30	376	67	20
WA	814	424	262	65	52	26	19	15	293	39	43
WV	688	397	218	76	61	20	22	16	229	29	17
WI	758	408	245	46	58	33	26	29	273	14	34
WY	81	36	28	2	4	1	1		34	5	6
POSS.	146	66	47	3	10	4	2	4	60	14	2

Notes:

Total Physicians include Active, Inactive, and Address Unknown.

FM subspecialties include FPG and FSM.

IM subspecialties include AMI, CCM, DIA, END, HEM, HEP, HO, ICE, ID, ILI, IMG, ISM, NEP, NTR, ON, PCC, and RHU.

OBG subspecialties include GO, GYN, MFM, OBS, OCC, and REN.

PD subspecialties include ADL, CCP, MPD, NPM, PDA, PDC, PDE, PDI, PDP, PDT, PEM, PG, PHO, PLI, PN, PPR, and PSM.

Chapter 6
Physician Trends

Increased demand for health services in the last two decades, along with forecasts of health care resources and the number of physicians per capita through the year 2000, resulted in concern throughout the medical community that the physician workforce would prove inadequate to meet the emerging health needs of the nation. To ensure the supply of physicians, a variety of measures were implemented. Complicated immigration regulations were modified to more readily allow the entry of foreign physicians into US medicine. Earlier exchange programs were extended to allow aliens to waive the two-year foreign residence requirement in the home or third country after studying in the US if their admission was in the public interest,[1] and medical schools received additional funding to expand capacities and accommodate larger enrollments. Government at the state and federal levels authorized financing procedures and programs to achieve new health care objectives, and private foundations and medical associations undertook measures to parallel these efforts.

The 1970s and, in some cases, the early 1980s witnessed additional environmental developments that promised to have important effects on organized medicine. Some of these included a change in the demographic characteristics and growth rate of the US population, a shift in migration patterns, and an overall change in the composition of the physician supply.[2]

An examination of the historical physician profile reflects some of these general trends. Although these historical data should be useful to workforce planners and health policy analysts, readers should not interpret these data as indicative of misdistribution, oversupply, or undersupply.

Collection and Classification Systems

The *Re-Classification of Physicians' Professional Activities* project was initiated in 1967.[3] The purpose of the project was to increase the validity and reliability of physicians' records and to facilitate the classification of the physician workforce in functional categories.

Traditionally, the physician population was distributed between the two categories of Private Practice and Not in Private Practice, a classification scheme affected more by the type of employer and fee-for-service vs salary forms of remuneration than by the actual activity of individual physicians. The new system introduced the functional categories Patient Care and Other Professional Activity. This classification concept is based on the extent to which a physician is engaged in direct care of patients and is, therefore, more meaningful than a concept based on the financial characteristics of a practice.

A good example of how the earlier system was based on employment rather than activity was the category Medical School Faculty. Most physicians who were employed by medical schools were placed in this category, even though many of them spent more time in Research, Administration, or even in Patient Care than in actual teaching. In the new system, Medical Teaching replaced Medical School Faculty to emphasize that only physicians who are actively teaching are included in this category.

Under the new system, the Not Classified category was introduced as a contingency category for physicians for whom no information is available. Physicians are temporarily assigned to this category until additional follow-up information can be obtained that can ensure proper classification. Also in 1968, as part of the reclassification effort, Fellows were classified in Research rather than in Residency programs to reflect the assessment that a majority of Fellows were engaged in medical research at that time. In 1986, a separate category was added for Clinical Fellows, which previously had been included in Research. (See the "Definitions" section in the Introduction for more information on physician classifications.) In 1994, the separate category of Fellows was discontinued; Fellows were tabulated as Residents/Fellows.

Total US Physicians

Major Categories

Table 11 demonstrates the total population of physicians in the US, with a numeric distribution of physicians in such major categories as Patient Care, the primary care specialties, school of graduation,

and sex from 1970 to 2006. An analysis of the table reveals that the vast majority of US physicians have remained in Patient Care: 83.4% (1970), 80.5% (1980), and 78.4% (2006). The proportion of female physicians to total physicians more than tripled between 1970 and 2006, from 7.6% to 27.8%.

Although physicians in the primary care specialties showed a fairly steady decline as a percentage of the total physician population in the 36-year period—40.2% (1970), 36.5% (1980), 34.7% (1990), 32.6% (2006) —they demonstrated a percentage growth of 124.0% from 134,354 physicians in 1970 to 300,907 physicians in 2006.

Table 11 also suggests some striking distribution patterns for international and US medical graduates. International Medical Graduates (IMGs), for example, comprised 17.1% of total physicians in 1970, but in 2006, they constituted 25.7%. US medical graduates accounted for 81.0% of all physicians in 1970 and 73.0% three decades later.

Activity

The major professional activity classification of physicians indicates whether a physician is engaged

---

Mini-Table 11

Total US Physicians by Major Categories, 1970–2006

Category	1970	1980	1990	2006
Total Physicians*	**334,028**	**467,679**	**615,421**	**921,904**
Patient Care	278,535	376,512	503,870	723,118
Non-patient Care	32,310	38,404	43,440	43,718
Primary Care†	134,354	170,705	213,514	300,907
Primary Care Subspecialties‡	25,401	16,642	30,911	67,519
Male	308,627	413,395	511,227	665,647
Female	25,401	54,284	104,194	256,257
US Graduates§	270,637	362,307	475,394	673,081
IMGs	57,217	97,726	131,764	236,669
Canadian Graduates	6,174	7,646	8,263	12,154

*Address Unknown is excluded from all Federal/Nonfederal categories, and Not-Classified, Inactive, and Address Unknown are excluded from Patient Care/Non-patient Care categories.

† Includes General Specialties of Family Medicine, General Practice, Internal Medicine, Obstetrics/Gynecology, and Pediatrics.

‡ Includes primary care subspecialties as listed in footnote for Family Medicine, General Practice, Internal Medicine, Obstetrics/Gynecology, and Pediatrics on Table 4.7,

§ Includes graduates from Inactive Schools.

Source: Tables 1.1, 1.17, and Table 4.1

in direct care of patients or in Other Professional Activity. Patient Care is further subcategorized into Office-Based and Hospital-Based practice, which includes Residents/Fellows and full-time Hospital Staff. Other Professional Activity includes Medical Teaching, Administration, Research, and the category of Other. Other was introduced in 1968 for physicians engaged in such activities as journalism, law, or sales or employed by pharmaceutical companies, medical societies, and so on. (The "Definitions" section of the Introduction explains the categories in Major Professional Activity.)

During the 10-year period from 1975 to 1985 (Table 6.1), the number of physicians in Patient Care increased by 136,883 for a gain of 43.9%. Between 1980 and 2006, 346,606 physicians were added to the Patient Care physician population for an increase of 92.1%. Within the Patient Care category between 1975 and 1985 there were increases of 53.3% in Office-Based practice and 22.9% in Hospital-Based practice. Since 1980, the complement of Office-Based physicians grew by 106.0%, and that in Hospital-Based practice did so by 55.7%.

Proportionate percentages of physicians in residency/fellowship training since 1975 showed little fluctuation until recently: 14.7% (1975), 13.3% (1980), 13.6% (1985), 15.0% (1990), and 10.5% (2006). However, the total number of Residents/Fellows since 1975 grew by 39,300, or 68.0%. Figure 8 displays the distribution of the total physician population between 1975 and 2006 and the distribution of physicians in Patient Care, Office-Based, and Hospital-Based practice.

Table 12 displays a profile of country and year of graduation for physicians as of 2006. Of the 236,669 IMGs included in the US physician workforce in 2006, nearly three in ten (24.7%), or 58,367, received their MD degrees before 1970, whereas one fifth (20.2%) of the graduates from US active schools, or 135,721 physicians, did so in the same time period. Table 12 shows that fewer than one quarter of physicians graduated from medical schools before 1970 (21.5%). This percentage is greater for graduates of Canadian medical schools. For Canadian graduates, nearly one third (31.2%) graduated before 1970.

Specialty

Tables 6.2 through 6.4 demonstrate the relationship between specialization and physician supply between 1975 and 2006. The number of physicians in General Practice greatly diminished in the 31-year period, decreasing by 31,881. The decline may be explained in part by the establishment in 1975 of the discipline of Family Medicine. Between 1975 and 2006, Family Medicine showed an increase of 70,683 physicians.

Between 1975 and 1985, the total physician population increased by 40.4% (Table 6.4). However, the number of physicians in General Practice decreased by 36.2% in this same interval. By contrast, in absolute numbers, Internal Medicine demonstrated a dramatic increase of 63.6% from 1975 (54,331) to 1985 (88,862). Between 1980 and 2006, Internal Medicine increased by 117.7% for a gain of 84,174 physicians. In 1975, Diagnostic Radiology accounted for only 3,544

Mini-Table 12

Physicians by Year and Country of Graduation, 2006

Country of Graduation	Number				Percentage			
	Total	Prior to 1970	1970-1988	1990 & Later	Total	Prior to 1970	1970-1989	1990 & Later
Total Physicians	**921,904**	**198,266**	**381,019**	**342,619**	**100.0**	**21.5**	**41.3**	**37.2**
US Medical Schools								
Active Schools	671,554	135,721	269,645	266,188	100.0	20.2	40.2	39.6
Inactive Schools	1,527	381	610	536	100.0	25.0	39.9	35.1
Canadian Schools	12,154	3,797	5,215	3,142	100.0	31.2	42.9	25.9
International Schools	236,669	58,367	105,549	72,753	100.0	24.7	44.6	30.7

Source: Table 1.17

Figure 8

Physicians by Major Professional Activity, 1975–2006

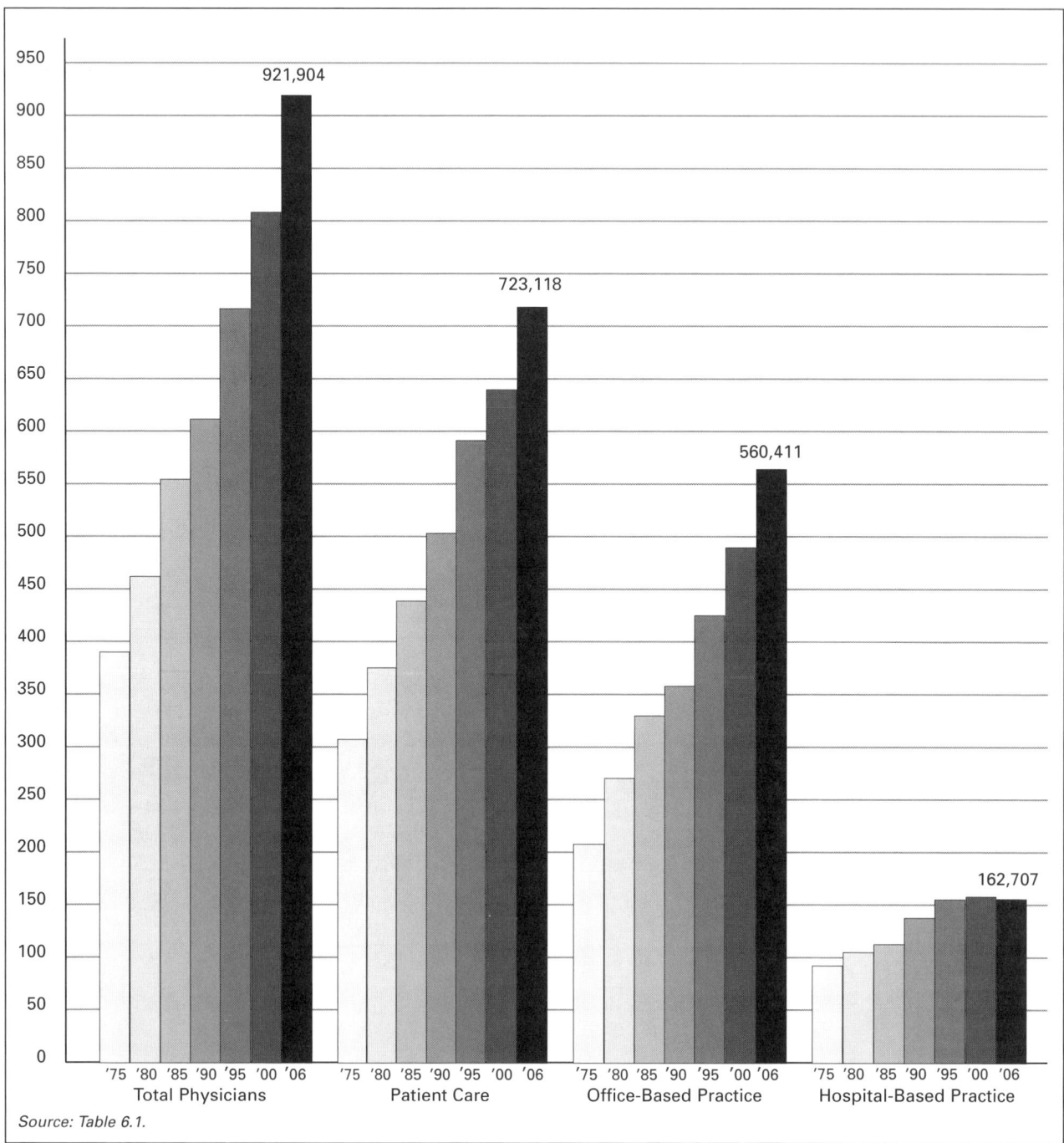

Source: Table 6.1.

physicians of a total physician workforce of 393,742, or 0.9%. In 2006, however, Diagnostic Radiologists numbered 24,231, representing 2.7% of all physicians for the year. Figure 9 demonstrates trends in the five largest specialties in 2006 for selected years 1975 to 2006.

Age and Sex

An age and sex profile of all physicians in the US (Table 6.5) indicated that a little more than half were younger than 45 years in each of the selected years 1975 to 1990. In 2006, this proportion was 38.5%. This trend was also true of the male physician population, but the female physician popula-

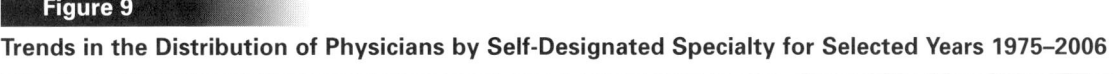

Figure 9

Trends in the Distribution of Physicians by Self-Designated Specialty for Selected Years 1975–2006

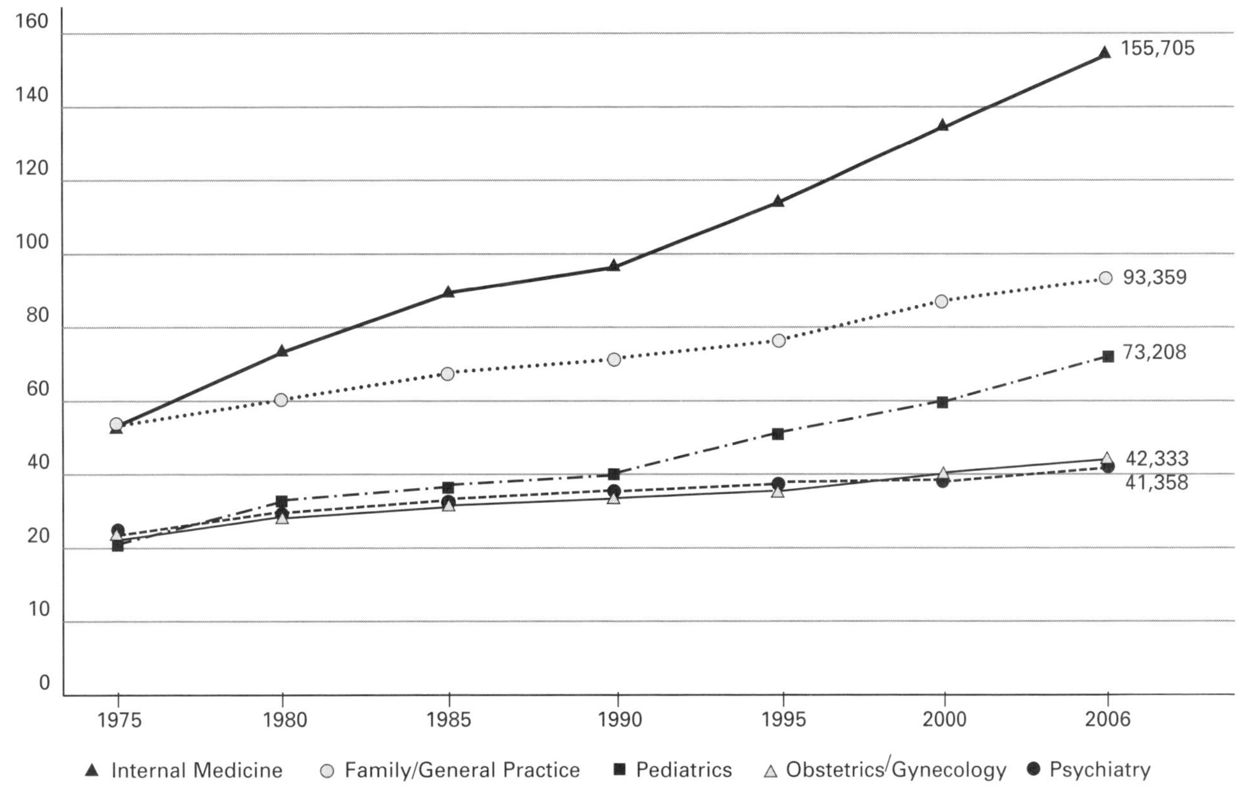

[Line graph showing trends from 1975 to 2006. Y-axis ranges from 0 to 160 (thousands). End-of-line values for 2006: Internal Medicine 155,705; Family/General Practice 93,359; Pediatrics 73,208; Obstetrics/Gynecology 42,333; Psychiatry 41,358.]

▲ Internal Medicine   ○ Family/General Practice   ■ Pediatrics   △ Obstetrics/Gynecology   ● Psychiatry

Source: Table 6.2

tion consistently showed higher percentages in the young age groups compared with the male population. In 1975, 62.3% of female physicians were younger than 45 years compared with 72.9% in 1985 and 56.2% in 2006. Between 1975 and 2006, the number of female physicians younger than 45 years showed a more than sixfold increase.

Nearly one in four total physicians were female in 2006 (27.8%) with to approximately 1 in 11 in 1975 (9.1%).

The total number of physicians 65 years and older more than tripled from 50,993 in 1975 to 177,232 in 2006, and the percentage of total physicians increased from 13.0% to 19.2%. The male/female distribution in this group has shown little change during the period, with physicians 65 years or older being 92.8% male and 7.2% female in 1975 and 89.7% male and 10.3% female in 2006.

International Medical Graduates (IMGs)

Activity

A trend analysis of Tables 6.6 through 6.8 compared with Table 6.1 reveals that the total number of physicians increased by 528,162 between 1975 and 2006, or 134.1%; IMGs accounted for more than one fourth (29.5%) of this increase by gaining 155,821 physicians. In the 31-year period, the number of non-IMGs grew by 119.0%, whereas the number of IMGs increased by 192.7%. Table 13 further reveals that in 1980, IMGs accounted for 20.9% of the total physician count of 467,679. The percentage climbed to 25.7% of the total count of 921,904 physicians in 2006.

As a study of Table 13 and Table 6.9 indicates, however, the percentage of IMGs in full-time staff positions decreased from 16.1% in 1980 to 8.6% 26

Mini-Table 13

Total Physicians and International Medical Graduates by Activity, 1980 and 2006

Activity	1980		2006	
	Total	IMGs	Total	IMGs
Total Physicians	**467,679**	**97,726**	**921,904**	**236,669**
Patient Care	376,512	72,935	723,118	185,045
Office-Based Practice	272,000	45,764	560,411	137,115
Hospital-Based Practice	104,512	27,171	162,707	47,930
Residents/Fellows	62,042	11,424	97,102	27,579
Full-Time Staff	42,470	15,747	65,605	20,351
Other Prof. Activity	38,404	8,656	43,718	7,446
Medical Teaching	7,942	1,569	14,575	1,958
Administration	12,209	1,533	10,273	1,714
Research	15,377	4,918	14,475	2,829
Other	2,876	636	4,395	945
Not Classified	20,629	10,235	46,252	21,255
Inactive	25,744	2,731	108,344	22,838
Address Unknown	6,390	3,169	472	85

Source: Tables 6.1 and 6.9.

years later. This decrease may be attributed in large part to the variety of questions raised in the 1970s regarding the escalating number of alien physicians in the US and the enactment of federal legislation in 1976 that placed limitations on the immigration of foreign nationals.* Figure 10 depicts the percentage change of IMGs and total physicians by major professional activity categories from 1980 to 2006.

Specialty

All specialties listed in Table 6.6 except Aerospace Medicine, General Practice, Public Health, and Radiology had a larger number of IMGs in 2006 than in 1975. The following specialties increased more than 100% from 1975 to 2006: Allergy and Immunology, Anesthesiology, Cardiovascular Diseases, Child Psychiatry, Colon and Rectal Surgery, Diagnostic Radiology, Family Medicine, Forensic Pathology, Gastroenterology, General Preventive Medicine, Internal Medicine, Neurology, Occupational Medicine, Pediatrics, Pediatric Cardiology, Physical Medicine and

Rehabilitation, Plastic Surgery, Psychiatry, Pulmonary Diseases, Radiation Oncology, and Thoracic Surgery. Table 14 displays the percentage of total IMGs among the largest IMG specialties, ranked by size, in 2006. The table also provides percentages and ranks for 1980.

Table 6.9 shows changes in major professional activity for IMGs from 1975 to 2006. Although most IMGs were in Patient Care for the years surveyed, the percentage in Patient Care has remained about the same. However, Office-Based practice increased from 1975 to 2006 (40.6% and 57.9%).

Female Physicians

Activity

Between 1980 and 2006, the total number of physicians in the US grew by 97.1% (Table 15), whereas the total number of female physicians increased 372.1%. Female physicians in Patient Care increased by 434.5%, which was largely accounted for by the high increase in the number of female physicians in Office-Based practice (640.0%). The next largest increase was in female Full-Time Staff (216.6%).

Table 15 also indicates increased representation of women in residency programs, growing from

---

* Health Professions Educational Assistance Act of 1976 (P.L. 94484). Title VI of P.L. 94484 "Limitation of Foreign Medical Graduates" as amended by the Health Services Extension Act of 1977 further required IMGs emigrating to the US for Graduate Medical Education to take and pass the VISA Qualifying Examination (VQE).

Figure 10

Percentage Change in Total Physicians and International Medical Graduates by Major Professional Activity, 1980–2006

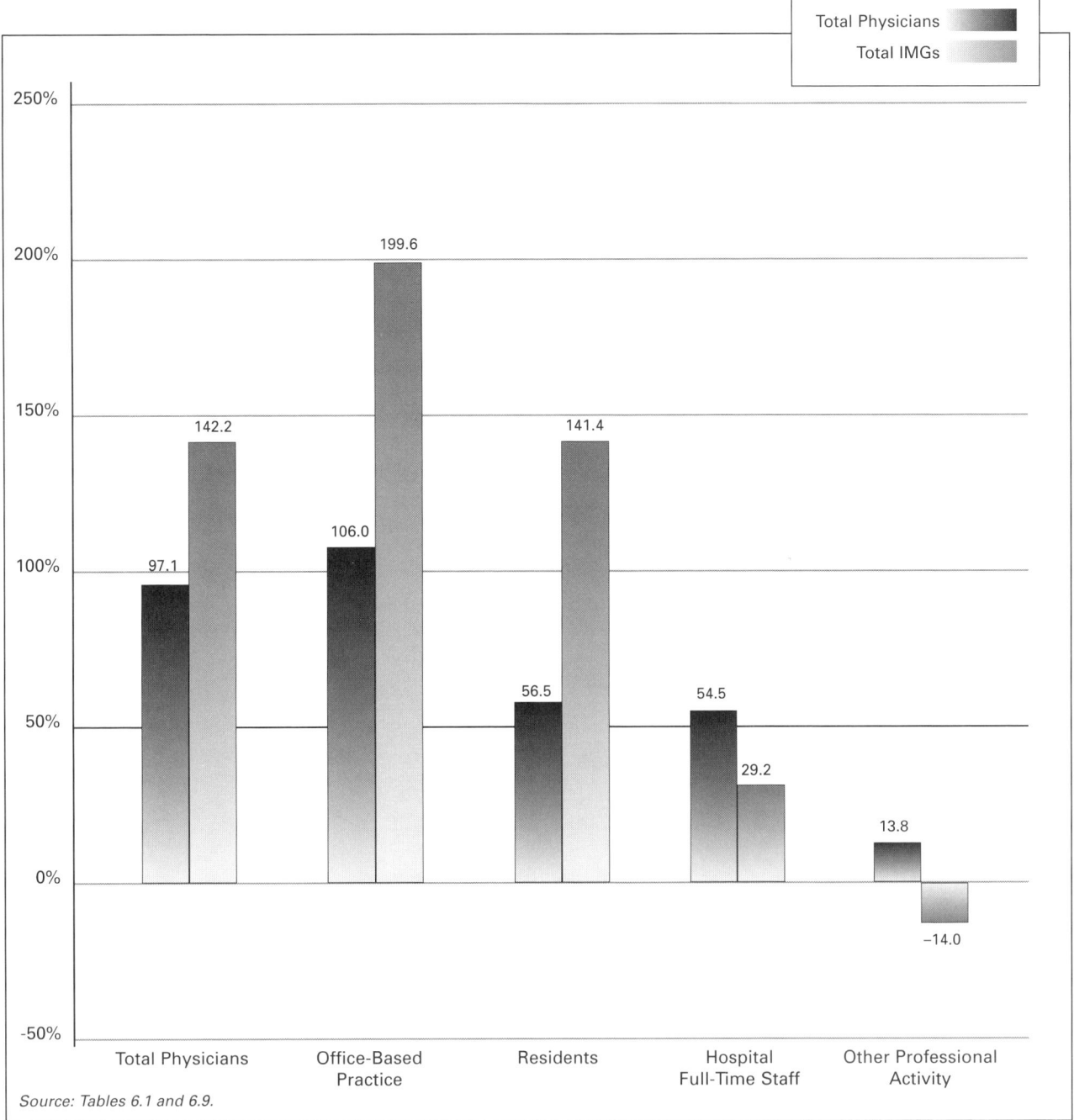

Source: Tables 6.1 and 6.9.

21.5% of total Resident physicians in 1980 to 43.3% in 2006. Women also demonstrated considerable percentage increases in Patient Care, from 10.6% of all physicians in the category in 1980 to 29.5% in 2006 (see also Table 6.13).

Specialty

The total number of female physicians increased more than six-fold between 1975 and 2006 from 35,626 to 256,257 physicians (Table 6.10). In 1975, only seven specialties had more than 1,000 female physicians: Pediatrics (5,135), Internal Medicine (4,006), Psychiatry (3,144),

Percentage of IMGs in Highest IMG Self-Designated Specialties Ranked by Size, 2006

	Total IMGs (%)		Rank	
Specialty	1980	2006	1980	2006
Internal Medicine	13.4%	24.1%	1	1
General/Family Practice	9.4%	9.4%	2	2
Pediatrics	6.8%	8.6%	5	3
Psychiatry	7.0%	5.5%	3	4
Anesthesiology	6.0%	4.9%	6	5
General Surgery	6.9%	3.2%	4	6
Obstetrics/Gynecology	5.4%	3.1%	7	7
Cardiovascular Disease	2.3%	2.9%	9	8
Pathology	4.0%	2.7%	8	9

Source: Table 6.7.

General/Family Medicine (2,866), Anesthesiology (1,819), Obstetrics/Gynecology (1,777), and Pathology (1,674). By 2006, there were 10 specialties with more than 5,000 female physicians:

- Internal Medicine (49,541)

- Pediatrics (39,468)

- General/Family Medicine (30,471)

- Obstetrics/Gynecology (18,520)

- Psychiatry (14,066)

- Anesthesiology (9,369)

- Emergency Medicine (6,830)

- Pathology (6,620)

- General Surgery (5,718)

- Diagnostic Radiology (5,524)

Although rankings changed over time, all seven of the specialties with the most female physicians in 1975 remained among the top ranking in 2006. In 1975, these seven represented more than half of the total female physician population (57.3%), and in 2006, 65.6%. Pediatrics had the highest count of female physicians in 1975 and 1980, but Internal Medicine had the most female physicians in 1985, 1990, 1995, 2000, and 2006.

The total number of female physicians more than doubled between 1975 and 1985 (Table 6.12). In that decade, 10 specialties grew four times or more in the numbers of female physicians: Family Medicine, Diagnostic Radiology, Thoracic Surgery, Urological Surgery, Forensic Pathology, Gastro-enterology, Neurological Surgery, Orthopedic Surgery, Aerospace Medicine, and Otolaryngology.

As Table 6.12 indicates, from 1990 to 2006, the total number of female physicians increased by 145.9%. During these 16 years, eight specialties exhibited growth of 200% or more in numbers of female physicians: Thoracic Surgery (648.0%), Colon & Rectal Surgery (496.8%), Urological Surgery (335.1%), Family Medicine (244.5%),

Total Physicians and Female Physicians by Activity, 1980 and 2006

	1980		2006	
Activity	Total	Women	Total	Women
Total Physicians	**467,679**	**54,284**	**921,904**	**256,257**
Patient Care	376,512	39,969	723,118	213,644
Office-Based Practice	272,000	20,609	560,411	152,504
Hospital-Based Practice	104,512	19,360	162,707	61,140
Residents/Fellows	62,042	13,322	97,102	42,024
Full-Time Staff	42,470	6,038	65,605	19,116
Other Prof. Activity	38,404	4,737	43,718	9,701
Medical Teaching	7,942	1,090	14,575	2,758
Administration	12,209	1,178	10,273	2,655
Research	15,377	2,077	14,475	3,081
Other	2,876	392	4,395	1,207
Not Classified	20,629	4,030	46,252	18,894
Inactive	25,744	3,773	108,344	13,875
Address Unknown	6,390	1,775	472	143

Source: Table 6.1 and Table 6.13.

Emergency Medicine (231.9), General Preventive Medicine (228.1%), Gastroenterology (214.7), and Pulmonary Diseases (211.6%).

Table 6.13 shows that although the number of women in each of the activities increased from 1975 to 2006, the percentage distributions decreased for most of the activities. Prominent among the few activities seeing distributional increases, Patient Care accounted for 68.3% of female physicians' activity in 1975 and 83.4% in 2006. Office-Based practice represented 35.1% of female physicians' activity in 1975 and more than half (59.5%) in 2006.

Physician-Population Ratios

The physician-population ratios and rank by state in Chapter 6 should not be interpreted as indicative of oversupply, misdistribution, or undersupply. Although some have used aggregate physician-population ratios to suggest availability or shortage, the ratios alone should not be construed as constituting an adequate measure of the quantity or quality of health care received by the American public. An analysis of health care requirements, ancillary medical resources, demographic and socioeconomic factors, and geographic location, among other factors, is required to assess equitable or optimal access to services. The ratios are provided, therefore, as general guidelines to allow comparisons of the distribution of physicians over time and among the states, as well as of selected specialties.

National Ratios

An analysis of Table 6.16 indicates that the number of physicians increased by 215.6% between 1965 and 2006, whereas the US population did so by only 51.9%. The ratios of Patient Care physicians per 100,000 civilians between 1965 and 2006 showed similar patterns. Physicians in Patient Care totaled 259,418 in 1965 and 723,118 in 2006, a 178.7% gain. As a result, in 1965 there were 132 Patient Care physicians per 100,000 people, but by 2006 there were 242, an increase of 83.3%. The number of people per physician in Patient Care

steadily declined between 1965 and 2006 from 760 (1965) to 414 (2006).

State Ratios

Although the number of physicians per 100,000 population averaged 303 in 2006 (Table 6.17), one state in 2006 had a ratio less than 200: Oklahoma (199). However, no state, the District of Columbia, or Possessions have seen a decrease in this ratio since 1975.

In 2006, 17 states (including the District of Columbia) demonstrated physician-population ratios in Patient Care at or above the national average of 242 physicians per 100,000 people (Table 6.19). In this group, the District of Columbia (638), Massachusetts (383), Maryland (342), New York (338), and Vermont (317) had the highest Patient Care ratios. Mississippi (164), Idaho (162), and Oklahoma (158) had the lowest. Thirty-four states exceeded the 2006 national average of 414 patients per one physician in Patient Care. The lowest ratios were indicated for the District of Columbia (157), Massachusetts (261), Maryland (292), New York (296), and Vermont (315). The five states in this group with the most patients per physician were Oklahoma (632), Idaho (618), Mississippi (609), Iowa (602), and Nevada (579).

Specialty Ratios

As Table 6.21 indicates, ratios between 1980 and 2006 showed increases of 55.2% for Office-Based physicians, from 120.6 per 100,000 (1980) to 187.2 per 100,000 (2006), and more than 48.5% for total physicians: 207.3 (1980) to 307.9 (2006). As General Practice ratios in Office-Based practice declined in the 1980s, Family Medicine ratios demonstrated continuous increases: 8.1 (1980), 15.2 (1990), and 22.1 (2006).

The ratio spread was small between total physicians and Office-Based physicians in General Practice in 1980 (14.4 per 100,000 vs 13.1 per 100,000) and 2006 (3.5 vs 3.0). Pathology, conversely, illustrates that physicians in this discipline are not Office Based in as large numbers as are General Practitioners: 6.0 vs 2.7 (1980) and 6.6 vs 4.0 (2006).

References

1. *Foreign Medical Graduates in the US 1970.* Center for Health Services Research and Development, American Medical Association; 1971.

2. *The Environment of Medicine: Report of the Council on Long Range Planning and Development.* American Medical Association; December 1983.

3. *Reclassification of Physicians, 1968.* Center for Health Services Research and Development, American Medical Association; 1971.

Table 6.1

Physicians by Activity, 1975–2006

	1975	1980	1985	1990	1995	2000	2006
				Number			
Total Physicians	393,742	467,679	552,716	615,421	720,325	813,770	921,904
Patient Care	311,937	376,512	448,820	503,870	582,131	647,430	723,118
Office-Based Practice	215,429	272,000	330,197	360,995	427,275	490,398	560,411
Hospital-Based Practice	96,508	104,512	118,623	142,875	154,856	157,032	162,707
Residents/Fellows*	57,802	62,042	75,411	92,080	96,352	95,725	97,102
Full-Time Staff	38,706	42,470	43,212	50,795	58,504	61,307	65,605
Other Prof. Activity	28,343	38,404	48,320	43,440	43,312	44,938	43,718
Administration	11,161	12,209	13,810	14,819	16,345	16,210	14,575
Medical Teaching	6,445	7,942	7,832	8,090	9,469	10,214	10,273
Research**	7,944	15,377	23,268	16,930	14,340	14,598	14,475
Other	2,793	2,876	3,410	3,601	3,158	3,916	4,395
Inactive	21,449	25,744	38,646	52,653	72,326	75,168	108,344
Not Classified	26,145	20,629	13,950	12,678	20,579	45,136	46,252
Address Unknown	5,868	6,390	2,980	2,780	1,977	1,098	472
				Percent Distribution			
Total Physicians	100.0	100.0	100.0	100.0	100.0	100.0	100.0
Patient Care	79.2	80.5	81.2	81.9	80.8	79.6	78.4
Office-Based Practice	54.7	58.2	59.7	58.7	59.3	60.3	60.8
Hospital-Based Practice	24.5	22.3	21.5	23.2	21.5	19.3	17.6
Residents/Fellows*	14.7	13.3	13.6	15.0	13.4	11.8	10.5
Full-Time Staff	9.8	9.1	7.8	8.3	8.1	7.5	7.1
Other Prof. Activity	7.2	8.2	8.7	7.1	6.0	5.5	4.7
Administration	2.8	2.6	2.5	2.4	2.3	2.0	1.6
Medical Teaching	1.6	1.7	1.4	1.3	1.3	1.3	1.1
Research**	2.0	3.3	4.2	2.8	2.0	1.8	1.6
Other	0.7	0.6	0.6	0.6	0.4	0.5	0.5
Inactive	5.4	5.5	7.0	8.6	10.0	9.2	11.8
Not Classified	6.6	4.4	2.5	2.1	2.9	5.5	5.0
Address Unknown	1.5	1.4	0.5	0.5	0.3	0.1	0.1

				Percent Change			
	1975-2006	1975-1985	1985-1995	1975-1980	1980-1985	1985-1990	1990-2006
Total Physicians	134.1	40.4	30.3	18.8	18.2	11.3	49.8
Patient Care	131.8	43.9	29.7	20.7	19.2	12.3	43.5
Office-Based Practice	160.1	53.3	29.4	26.3	21.4	9.3	55.2
Hospital-Based Practice	68.6	22.9	30.5	8.3	13.5	20.4	13.9
Residents/Fellows*	68.0	30.5	27.8	7.3	21.5	22.1	5.5
Full-Time Staff	69.5	11.6	35.4	9.7	1.7	17.5	29.2
Other Prof. Activity	54.2	70.5	-10.4	35.5	25.8	-10.1	0.6
Administration	126.1	23.7	18.4	9.4	13.1	7.3	80.2
Medical Teaching	-8.0	21.5	20.9	23.2	-1.4	3.3	-30.7
Research**	82.2	192.9	-38.4	93.6	51.3	-27.2	-14.5
Other	57.4	22.1	-7.4	3.0	18.6	5.6	22.0
Inactive	405.1	80.2	87.2	20.0	50.1	36.2	105.8
Not Classified	76.9	-46.6	47.5	-21.1	-32.4	-9.1	264.8
Address Unknown	-92.0	-49.2	-33.7	8.9	-53.4	-6.7	-83.0

Note: Data for 1990 through 1994 are as of January 1; data prior to 1990 and for 1995-2006 are as of December 31.

*Includes all years of residency.

**Includes physicians in research activities and Research Fellows.

Table 6.2

Physicians by Self-Designated Specialty, 1975–2006

Specialty	1975	1980	1985	1990	1995	2000	2006
Total Physicians	393,742	467,679	552,716	615,421	720,325	813,770	921,904
Aerospace Medicine	684	587	674	687	575	473	473
Allergy/Immunology	1,716	1,518	3,060	3,388	3,775	3,998	4,196
Anesthesiology	12,861	15,958	22,021	25,981	32,853	35,715	41,193
Cardiovascular Dis.	6,933	9,823	13,224	15,862	18,998	21,025	22,426
Child Psychiatry	2,581	3,271	3,783	4,343	5,542	6,158	7,260
Colon/Rectal Surgery	661	719	817	882	990	1,127	1,340
Dermatology	4,661	5,660	6,582	7,557	8,563	9,675	10,744
Diagnostic Radiology	3,544	7,048	12,887	15,412	19,808	21,104	24,624
Emergency Medicine*	0	5,699	11,283	14,243	19,112	23,064	29,987
Family Medicine	12,183	27,530	40,021	47,639	59,345	71,635	82,866
Forensic Pathology	190	240	311	414	496	577	657
Gastroenterology	2,381	4,046	5,917	7,493	9,551	10,627	12,268
General Practice	42,374	32,519	27,030	22,841	16,867	15,213	10,493
Gen. Preventive Med.	789	810	933	1,036	1,269	1,718	2,161
General Surgery	31,562	34,034	38,169	38,376	37,569	36,716	37,707
Internal Medicine	54,331	71,531	88,862	98,349	115,168	134,539	155,705
Medical Genetics**	0	0	0	0	179	361	533
Neurological Surgery	2,926	3,341	4,019	4,358	4,888	4,997	5,425
Neurology	4,131	5,685	7,776	9,237	11,397	12,333	14,554
Nuclear Medicine*	0	0	1,352	1,340	1,435	1,448	1,477
Obstetrics/Gynecology	21,731	26,305	30,867	33,697	37,652	40,241	42,333
Occupational Medicine	2,355	2,358	2,640	2,744	3,031	2,990	2,641
Ophthalmology	11,129	12,974	14,881	16,073	17,464	18,126	18,058
Orthopedic Surgery	11,379	13,996	17,166	19,138	22,037	22,287	24,296
Otolaryngology	5,745	6,553	7,267	8,138	9,086	9,417	9,974
Path.-Anatomic/Clin.	11,720	13,402	15,456	16,170	17,824	18,220	19,171
Pediatric Cardiology	538	659	813	1,006	1,336	1,536	1,877
Pediatrics	22,192	28,803	36,026	40,893	50,620	62,386	73,208
Physical Med./Rehab.	1,664	2,146	3,258	4,105	5,565	6,512	7,736
Plastic Surgery	2,236	2,980	3,951	4,590	5,493	6,200	7,063
Psychiatry	23,922	27,481	32,255	35,163	38,098	39,457	41,385
Public Health	2,665	2,316	2,060	2,015	1,760	1,830	1,434
Pulmonary Diseases	2,335	3,715	5,083	6,080	7,453	8,706	10,232
Radiation Oncology	1,169	1,581	2,272	2,821	3,630	3,904	4,424
Radiology	11,527	11,653	8,757	8,492	8,038	8,661	8,886
Thoracic Surgery	1,979	2,133	2,183	2,063	2,310	4,953	4,807
Urological Surgery	6,667	7,743	8,836	9,372	9,886	10,302	10,518
Other Specialty	7,277	5,810	6,398	7,254	7,307	5,810	5,192
Unspecified	7,542	12,289	8,250	8,058	8,473	8,327	7,512
Inactive	21,449	25,744	38,646	52,653	72,326	75,168	108,344
Not Classified	26,145	20,629	13,950	12,678	20,579	45,136	46,252
Address Unknown	5,868	6,390	2,980	2,780	1,977	1,098	472

Note: Data for 1990 are as of January 1; data for all other years, December 31.

*Data were not available for Emergency Medicine prior to 1980 and Nuclear Medicine prior to 1985.

**Data on Medical Genetics were not available prior to 1994.

Table 6.3

Percent Distribution of Physicians by Self-Designated Specialty, 1975–2006

Specialty	1975	1980	1985	1990	1995	2000	2006
Total Physicians	100.0	100.0	100.0	100.0	100.0	100.0	100.0
Aerospace Medicine	0.2	0.1	0.1	0.1	0.1	0.1	0.1
Allergy/Immunology	0.4	0.3	0.6	0.6	0.5	0.5	0.5
Anesthesiology	3.3	3.4	4.0	4.2	4.6	4.4	4.5
Cardiovascular Dis.	1.8	2.1	2.4	2.6	2.6	2.6	2.4
Child Psychiatry	0.7	0.7	0.7	0.7	0.8	0.8	0.8
Colon/Rectal Surgery	0.2	0.2	0.1	0.1	0.1	0.1	0.1
Dermatology	1.2	1.2	1.2	1.2	1.2	1.2	1.2
Diagnostic Radiology	0.9	1.5	2.3	2.5	2.7	2.6	2.7
Emergency Medicine*	*	1.2	2.0	2.3	2.7	2.8	3.3
Family Medicine	3.1	5.9	7.2	7.7	8.2	8.8	9.0
Forensic Pathology	0.0	0.1	0.1	0.1	0.1	0.1	0.1
Gastroenterology	0.6	0.9	1.1	1.2	1.3	1.3	1.3
General Practice	10.8	7.0	4.9	3.7	2.3	1.9	1.1
Gen. Preventive Med.	0.2	0.2	0.2	0.2	0.2	0.2	0.2
General Surgery	8.0	7.3	6.9	6.2	5.2	4.5	4.1
Internal Medicine	13.8	15.3	16.1	16.0	16.0	16.5	16.9
Medical Genetics**	**	**	**	**	0.0	0.0	0.1
Neurological Surgery	0.7	0.7	0.7	0.7	0.7	0.6	0.6
Neurology	1.0	1.2	1.4	1.5	1.6	1.5	1.6
Nuclear Medicine*	*	*	0.2	0.2	0.2	0.2	0.2
Obstetrics/Gynecology	5.5	5.6	5.6	5.5	5.2	4.9	4.6
Occupational Medicine	0.6	0.5	0.5	0.4	0.4	0.4	0.3
Ophthalmology	2.8	2.8	2.7	2.6	2.4	2.2	2.0
Orthopedic Surgery	2.9	3.0	3.1	3.1	3.1	2.7	2.6
Otolaryngology	1.5	1.4	1.3	1.3	1.3	1.2	1.1
Path.-Anatomic/Clin.	3.0	2.9	2.8	2.6	2.5	2.2	2.1
Pediatric Cardiology	0.1	0.1	0.1	0.2	0.2	0.2	0.2
Pediatrics	5.6	6.2	6.5	6.6	7.0	7.7	7.9
Physical Med./Rehab.	0.4	0.5	0.6	0.7	0.8	0.8	0.8
Plastic Surgery	0.6	0.6	0.7	0.7	0.8	0.8	0.8
Psychiatry	6.1	5.9	5.8	5.7	5.3	4.8	4.5
Public Health	0.7	0.5	0.4	0.3	0.2	0.2	0.2
Pulmonary Diseases	0.6	0.8	0.9	1.0	1.0	1.1	1.1
Radiation Oncology	0.3	0.3	0.4	0.5	0.5	0.5	0.5
Radiology	2.9	2.5	1.6	1.4	1.1	1.1	1.0
Thoracic Surgery	0.5	0.5	0.4	0.3	0.3	0.6	0.5
Urological Surgery	1.7	1.7	1.6	1.5	1.4	1.3	1.1
Other Specialty	1.8	1.2	1.2	1.2	1.0	0.7	0.6
Unspecified	1.9	2.6	1.5	1.3	1.2	1.0	0.8
Inactive	5.4	5.5	7.0	8.6	10.0	9.2	11.8
Not Classified	6.6	4.4	2.5	2.1	2.9	5.5	5.0
Address Unknown	1.5	1.4	0.5	0.5	0.3	0.1	0.1

Note: Data for 1990 are as of January 1; data for all other years, December 31.

Data were not available for Emergency Medicine prior to 1980 and Nuclear Medicine prior to 1985.

**Data on Medical Genetics were not available prior to 1994.*

Table 6.4

Percent Change of Physicians by Self-Designated Specialty, 1975–2006

Specialty	1975-2006	1975-1985	1985-1995	1975-1980	1980-1985	1985-1990	1990-2006
Total Physicians	134.1	40.4	30.3	18.8	18.2	11.3	49.8
Aerospace Medicine	-30.8	-1.5	-14.7	-14.2	14.8	1.9	-31.1
Allergy/Immunology	144.5	78.3	23.4	-11.5	101.6	10.7	23.8
Anesthesiology	220.3	71.2	49.2	24.1	38.0	18.0	58.6
Cardiovascular Dis.	223.5	90.7	43.7	41.7	34.6	19.9	41.4
Child Psychiatry	181.3	46.6	46.5	26.7	15.7	14.8	67.2
Colon/Rectal Surgery	102.7	23.6	21.2	8.8	13.6	8.0	51.9
Dermatology	130.5	41.2	30.1	21.4	16.3	14.8	42.2
Diagnostic Radiology	594.8	263.6	53.7	98.9	82.8	19.6	59.8
Emergency Medicine*	*	*	69.4	*	98.0	26.2	110.5
Family Medicine	580.2	228.5	48.3	126.0	45.4	19.0	73.9
Forensic Pathology	245.8	63.7	59.5	26.3	29.6	33.1	58.7
Gastroenterology	415.2	148.5	61.4	69.9	46.2	26.6	63.7
General Practice	-75.2	-36.2	-37.6	-23.3	-16.9	-15.5	-54.1
Gen. Preventive Med.	173.9	18.3	36.0	2.7	15.2	11.0	108.6
General Surgery	19.5	20.9	-1.6	7.8	12.1	0.5	-1.7
Internal Medicine	186.6	63.6	29.6	31.7	24.2	10.7	58.3
Medical Genetics**	**	**	**	**	**	**	**
Neurological Surgery	85.4	37.4	21.6	14.2	20.3	8.4	24.5
Neurology	252.3	88.2	46.6	37.6	36.8	18.8	57.6
Nuclear Medicine*	*	*	6.1	*	*	-0.9	10.2
Obstetrics/Gynecology	94.8	42.0	22.0	21.0	17.3	9.2	25.6
Occupational Medicine	12.1	12.1	14.8	0.1	12.0	3.9	-3.8
Ophthalmology	62.3	33.7	17.4	16.6	14.7	8.0	12.3
Orthopedic Surgery	113.5	50.9	28.4	23.0	22.6	11.5	27.0
Otolaryngology	73.6	26.5	25.0	14.1	10.9	12.0	22.6
Path.-Anatomic/Clin.	63.6	31.9	15.3	14.4	15.3	4.6	18.6
Pediatric Cardiology	248.9	51.1	64.3	22.5	23.4	23.7	86.6
Pediatrics	229.9	62.3	40.5	29.8	25.1	13.5	79.0
Physical Med./Rehab.	364.9	95.8	70.8	29.0	51.8	26.0	88.5
Plastic Surgery	215.9	76.7	39.0	33.3	32.6	16.2	53.9
Psychiatry	73.0	34.8	18.1	14.9	17.4	9.0	17.7
Public Health	-46.2	-22.7	-14.6	-13.1	-11.1	-2.2	-28.8
Pulmonary Diseases	338.2	117.7	46.6	59.1	36.8	19.6	68.3
Radiation Oncology	278.4	94.4	59.8	35.2	43.7	24.2	56.8
Radiology	-22.9	-24.0	-8.2	1.1	-24.9	-3.0	4.6
Thoracic Surgery	142.9	10.3	5.8	7.8	2.3	-5.5	133.0
Urological Surgery	57.8	32.5	11.9	16.1	14.1	6.1	12.2
Other Specialty	-28.7	-12.1	14.2	-20.2	10.1	13.4	-28.4
Unspecified	-0.4	9.4	2.7	62.9	-32.9	-2.3	-6.8
Inactive	405.1	80.2	87.2	20.0	50.1	36.2	105.8
Not Classified	76.9	-46.6	47.5	-21.1	-32.4	-9.1	264.8
Address Unknown	-92.0	-49.2	-33.7	8.9	-53.4	-6.7	-83.0

Note: Data for 1990 are as of January 1; data for all other years, December 31.

*Data were not available for Emergency Medicine prior to 1980 and Nuclear Medicine prior to 1985.

**Data on Medical Genetics were not available prior to 1994.

Table 6.5

Physicians by Age and Sex, 1975–2006

Year and Sex	Total Physicians	< 35	35-44	45-54	55-64	≥ 65
	Number					
1975						
Total Physicians	393,742	108,393	96,368	82,166	55,822	50,993
Male	358,106	94,863	87,687	76,027	52,190	47,339
Female	35,636	13,530	8,681	6,139	3,632	3,654
1980						
Total Physicians	467,679	128,506	118,840	88,063	68,239	64,031
Male	413,395	105,507	104,160	81,106	63,278	59,344
Female	54,284	22,999	14,680	6,957	4,961	4,687
1985						
Total Physicians	552,716	141,622	154,752	99,692	78,987	77,663
Male	471,991	107,357	130,148	89,786	72,859	71,841
Female	80,725	34,265	24,604	9,906	6,128	5,822
1990						
Total Physicians	615,421	134,872	184,743	116,803	83,614	95,389
Male	511,227	96,856	147,545	102,052	76,833	87,941
Female	104,194	38,016	37,198	14,751	6,781	7,448
2000						
Total Physicians	813,770	136,704	211,873	201,646	118,608	144,939
Male	618,233	81,473	145,043	156,782	102,522	132,413
Female	195,537	55,231	66,830	44,864	16,086	12,526
2006						
Total Physicians	921,904	141,492	213,311	223,864	166,005	177,232
Male	665,647	77,168	133,515	160,253	135,790	158,921
Female	256,257	64,324	79,796	63,611	30,215	18,311
	Percentage					
1975						
Total Physicians	100.0%	100.0%	100.0%	100.0%	100.0%	100.0%
Male	90.9%	87.5%	91.0%	92.5%	93.5%	92.8%
Female	9.1%	12.5%	9.0%	7.5%	6.5%	7.2%
1980						
Total Physicians	100.0%	100.0%	100.0%	100.0%	100.0%	100.0%
Male	88.4%	82.1%	87.6%	92.1%	92.7%	92.7%
Female	11.6%	17.9%	12.4%	7.9%	7.3%	7.3%
1985						
Total Physicians	100.0%	100.0%	100.0%	100.0%	100.0%	100.0%
Male	85.4%	75.8%	84.1%	90.1%	92.2%	92.5%
Female	14.6%	24.2%	15.9%	9.9%	7.8%	7.5%
1990						
Total Physicians	100.0%	100.0%	100.0%	100.0%	100.0%	100.0%
Male	83.1%	71.8%	79.9%	87.4%	91.9%	92.2%
Female	16.9%	28.2%	20.1%	12.6%	8.1%	7.8%
2000						
Total Physicians	100.0%	100.0%	100.0%	100.0%	100.0%	100.0%
Male	76.0%	59.6%	68.5%	77.8%	86.4%	91.4%
Female	24.0%	40.4%	31.5%	22.2%	13.6%	8.6%
2006						
Total Physicians	100.0%	100.0%	100.0%	100.0%	100.0%	100.0%
Male	72.2%	54.5%	62.6%	71.6%	81.8%	89.7%
Female	27.8%	45.5%	37.4%	28.4%	18.2%	10.3%

Note: Data for 1990 are as of January 1; data for all other years, December 31.

Table 6.6

International Medical Graduates by Self-Designated Specialty, 1975–2006

Specialty	1975	1980	1985	1990	1995	2000	2006
Total Physicians	80,848	97,726	118,875	131,764	165,498	196,961	236,669
Aerospace Medicine	40	40	41	52	47	43	37
Allergy/Immunology	205	189	218	682	855	999	1,033
Anesthesiology	4,585	5,886	7,558	7,863	9,182	10,844	11,712
Cardiovascular Dis.	1,383	2,248	3,343	4,085	5,249	6,178	6,822
Child Psychiatry	580	749	973	1,107	1,318	1,630	2,139
Colon/Rectal Surgery	89	128	194	212	225	247	263
Dermatology	414	468	541	560	587	638	645
Diagnostic Radiology	626	1,299	2,090	2,185	2,378	2,873	2,858
Emergency Medicine*	*	*	1,768	1,997	2,225	2,296	2,664
Family Medicine	1,007	3,192	5,443	6,743	9,662	11,920	17,268
Forensic Pathology	53	65	85	114	128	136	152
Gastroenterology	437	796	1,298	1,630	2,192	2,735	3,298
General Practice	6,748	5,970	6,510	6,569	6,215	6,108	4,982
Gen. Preventive Med.	99	96	137	148	171	252	309
General Surgery	6,786	6,729	7,831	7,692	7,783	7,354	7,457
Internal Medicine	10,538	13,065	18,713	21,423	34,730	42,762	57,029
Medical Genetics**	**	**	**	**	23	76	131
Neurological Surgery	477	552	658	682	720	722	752
Neurology	933	1,180	1,784	2,153	3,077	3,606	4,644
Nuclear Medicine*	*	*	*	400	479	480	536
Obstetrics/Gynecology	4,209	5,268	6,504	6,844	7,048	7,159	7,446
Occupational Medicine	182	228	310	332	404	407	384
Ophthalmology	950	1,173	1,350	1,382	1,432	1,493	1,423
Orthopedic Surgery	1,095	1,500	1,734	1,759	1,842	1,709	1,610
Otolaryngology	777	955	1,121	1,120	1,061	1,007	932
Path.-Anatomic/Clin.	3,848	3,933	4,659	4,806	5,468	6,003	6,361
Pediatric Cardiology	164	180	213	238	337	382	466
Pediatrics	5,137	6,597	9,419	10,849	15,123	17,115	20,318
Physical Med./Rehab.	675	950	1,473	1,559	1,740	2,154	2,374
Plastic Surgery	319	469	680	755	794	816	851
Psychiatry	6,122	6,793	8,763	9,344	11,255	12,009	12,999
Public Health	287	271	274	249	203	220	168
Pulmonary Diseases	563	858	1,143	1,390	1,945	2,527	3,376
Radiation Oncology	354	481	695	727	775	833	791
Radiology	1,991	2,095	1,996	1,539	1,461	1,505	1,670
Thoracic Surgery	442	496	536	522	507	1,065	1,052
Urological Surgery	1,050	1,447	1,781	1,805	1,782	1,731	1,588
Other Specialty	1,420	2,201	1,280	1,465	1,515	1,100	982
Unspecified	2,112	3,044	2,009	1,444	2,368	3,303	2,969
Inactive	2,131	2,731	4,827	7,651	11,127	13,244	22,838
Not Classified	10,087	10,235	7,527	8,397	9,486	18,913	21,255
Address Unknown	1,933	3,169	1,388	1,290	579	367	85

Note: Data for 1990 are as of January 1; data for all other years, December 31.

*Data were not available for Emergency Medicine prior to 1980 and Nuclear Medicine prior to 1985.

**Data on Medical Genetics were not available prior to 1994.

Table 6.7

Percent Distribution of International Medical Graduates by Self-Designated Specialty, 1975–2006

Specialty	1975	1980	1985	1990	1995	2000	2006
Total Physicians	100.0	100.0	100.0	100.0	100.0	100.0	100.0
Aerospace Medicine	0.0	0.0	0.0	0.0	0.0	0.0	0.0
Allergy/Immunology	0.3	0.2	0.2	0.5	0.5	0.5	0.4
Anesthesiology	5.7	6.0	6.4	6.0	5.5	5.5	4.9
Cardiovascular Dis.	1.7	2.3	2.8	3.1	3.2	3.1	2.9
Child Psychiatry	0.7	0.8	0.8	0.8	0.8	0.8	0.9
Colon/Rectal Surgery	0.1	0.1	0.2	0.2	0.1	0.1	0.1
Dermatology	0.5	0.5	0.5	0.4	0.4	0.3	0.3
Diagnostic Radiology	0.8	1.3	1.8	1.7	1.4	1.5	1.2
Emergency Medicine*	*	*	1.5	1.5	1.3	1.2	1.1
Family Medicine	1.2	3.3	4.6	5.1	5.8	6.1	7.3
Forensic Pathology	0.1	0.1	0.1	0.1	0.1	0.1	0.1
Gastroenterology	0.5	0.8	1.1	1.2	1.3	1.4	1.4
General Practice	8.3	6.1	5.5	5.0	3.8	3.1	2.1
Gen. Preventive Med.	0.1	0.1	0.1	0.1	0.1	0.1	0.1
General Surgery	8.4	6.9	6.6	5.8	4.7	3.7	3.2
Internal Medicine	13.0	13.4	15.7	16.3	21.0	21.7	24.1
Medical Genetics**	**	**	**	**	0.0	0.0	0.1
Neurological Surgery	0.6	0.6	0.6	0.5	0.4	0.4	0.3
Neurology	1.2	1.2	1.5	1.6	1.9	1.8	2.0
Nuclear Medicine*	*	*	*	0.3	0.3	0.2	0.2
Obstetrics/Gynecology	5.2	5.4	5.5	5.2	4.3	3.6	3.1
Occupational Medicine	0.2	0.2	0.3	0.3	0.2	0.2	0.2
Ophthalmology	1.2	1.2	1.1	1.0	0.9	0.8	0.6
Orthopedic Surgery	1.4	1.5	1.5	1.3	1.1	0.9	0.7
Otolaryngology	1.0	1.0	0.9	0.9	0.6	0.5	0.4
Path.-Anatomic/Clin.	4.8	4.0	3.9	3.6	3.3	3.0	2.7
Pediatric Cardiology	0.2	0.2	0.2	0.2	0.2	0.2	0.2
Pediatrics	6.4	6.8	7.9	8.2	9.1	8.7	8.6
Physical Med./Rehab.	0.8	1.0	1.2	1.2	1.1	1.1	1.0
Plastic Surgery	0.4	0.5	0.6	0.6	0.5	0.4	0.4
Psychiatry	7.6	7.0	7.4	7.1	6.8	6.1	5.5
Public Health	0.4	0.3	0.2	0.2	0.1	0.1	0.1
Pulmonary Diseases	0.7	0.9	1.0	1.1	1.2	1.3	1.4
Radiation Oncology	0.4	0.5	0.6	0.6	0.5	0.4	0.3
Radiology	2.5	2.1	1.7	1.2	0.9	0.8	0.7
Thoracic Surgery	0.5	0.5	0.5	0.4	0.3	0.5	0.4
Urological Surgery	1.3	1.5	1.5	1.4	1.1	0.9	0.7
Other Specialty	1.8	2.3	1.1	1.1	0.9	0.6	0.4
Unspecified	2.6	3.1	1.7	1.1	1.4	1.7	1.3
Inactive	2.6	2.8	4.1	5.8	6.7	6.7	9.6
Not Classified	12.5	10.5	6.3	6.4	5.7	9.6	9.0
Address Unknown	2.4	3.2	1.2	1.0	0.3	0.2	0.0

Note: Data for 1990 are as of January 1; data for all other years, December 31.

*Data were not available for Emergency Medicine prior to 1980 and Nuclear Medicine prior to 1985.

**Data on Medical Genetics were not available prior to 1994.

Table 6.8

Percent Change of International Medical Graduates by Self-Designated Specialty, 1975–2006

Specialty	1975-2006	1975-1985	1985-1995	1975-1980	1980-1995	1985-1990	1990-2006
Total Physicians	192.7	47.0	39.2	20.9	21.6	10.8	79.6
Aerospace Medicine	-7.5	2.5	14.6	0.0	2.5	26.8	-28.8
Allergy/Immunology	403.9	6.3	292.2	-7.8	15.3	212.8	51.5
Anesthesiology	155.4	64.8	21.5	28.4	28.4	4.0	49.0
Cardiovascular Dis.	393.3	141.7	57.0	62.5	48.7	22.2	67.0
Child Psychiatry	268.8	67.8	35.5	29.1	29.9	13.8	93.2
Colon/Rectal Surgery	195.5	118.0	16.0	43.8	51.6	9.3	24.1
Dermatology	55.8	30.7	8.5	13.0	15.6	3.5	15.2
Diagnostic Radiology	356.5	233.9	13.8	107.5	60.9	4.5	30.8
Emergency Medicine*	*	*	25.8	*	*	13.0	33.4
Family Medicine	1614.8	440.5	77.5	217.0	70.5	23.9	156.1
Forensic Pathology	186.8	60.4	50.6	22.6	30.8	34.1	33.3
Gastroenterology	654.7	197.0	68.9	82.2	63.1	25.6	102.3
General Practice	-26.2	-3.5	-4.5	-11.5	9.0	0.9	-24.2
Gen. Preventive Med.	212.1	38.4	24.8	-3.0	42.7	8.0	108.8
General Surgery	9.9	15.4	-0.6	-0.8	16.4	-1.8	-3.1
Internal Medicine	441.2	77.6	85.6	24.0	43.2	14.5	166.2
Medical Genetics**	**	**	**	**	**	**	**
Neurological Surgery	57.7	37.9	9.4	15.7	19.2	3.6	10.3
Neurology	397.7	91.2	72.5	26.5	51.2	20.7	115.7
Nuclear Medicine*	*	*	*	*	*	*	34.0
Obstetrics/Gynecology	76.9	54.5	8.4	25.2	23.5	5.2	8.8
Occupational Medicine	111.0	70.3	30.3	25.3	36.0	7.1	15.7
Ophthalmology	49.8	42.9	5.4	23.5	16.8	1.8	3.0
Orthopedic Surgery	47.0	58.4	6.2	37.0	15.6	1.4	-8.5
Otolaryngology	19.9	44.3	-5.4	22.9	17.4	-0.1	-16.8
Path.-Anatomic/Clin.	65.3	21.1	17.4	2.2	18.5	3.2	32.4
Pediatric Cardiology	184.1	29.9	58.2	9.8	18.3	11.7	95.8
Pediatrics	295.5	83.4	60.6	28.4	42.8	15.2	87.3
Physical Med./Rehab.	251.7	118.2	18.1	40.7	55.1	5.8	52.3
Plastic Surgery	166.8	113.2	16.8	47.0	45.0	11.0	12.7
Psychiatry	112.3	43.1	28.4	11.0	29.0	6.6	39.1
Public Health	-41.5	-4.5	-25.9	-5.6	1.1	-9.1	-32.5
Pulmonary Diseases	499.6	103.0	70.2	52.4	33.2	21.6	142.9
Radiation Oncology	123.4	96.3	11.5	35.9	44.5	4.6	8.8
Radiology	-16.1	0.3	-26.8	5.2	-4.7	-22.9	8.5
Thoracic Surgery	138.0	21.3	-5.4	12.2	8.1	-2.6	101.5
Urological Surgery	51.2	69.6	0.1	37.8	23.1	1.3	-12.0
Other Specialty	-30.8	-9.9	18.4	55.0	-41.8	14.5	-33.0
Unspecified	40.6	-4.9	17.9	44.1	-34.0	-28.1	105.6
Inactive	971.7	126.5	130.5	28.2	76.7	58.5	198.5
Not Classified	110.7	-25.4	26.0	1.5	-26.5	11.6	153.1
Address Unknown	-95.6	-28.2	-58.3	63.9	-56.2	-7.1	-93.4

Note: Data for 1990 are as of January 1; data for all other years, December 31.

*Data were not available for Emergency Medicine prior to 1980 and Nuclear Medicine prior to 1985.

**Data on Medical Genetics were not available prior to 1994.

Table 6.9

International Medical Graduates by Activity, 1975–2006

Activity	1975	1980	1985	1990	1995	2000	2006
				Number			
Total Physicians	80,848	97,726	118,875	131,764	165,498	196,961	236,669
Patient Care	61,416	72,935	95,362	106,515	136,812	156,810	185,045
Office-Based Practice	32,796	45,764	66,076	74,824	94,920	113,936	137,115
Hospital-Based Practice	28,620	27,171	29,286	31,691	41,892	42,874	47,930
Residents/Fellows*	16,447	11,424	12,837	13,496	22,552	22,419	27,579
Full-Time Staff	12,173	15,747	16,449	18,195	19,340	20,455	20,351
Other Prof. Activity	5,248	8,656	9,771	7,911	7,494	7,627	7,446
Administration	1,319	1,533	1,743	1,936	2,217	1,718	1,958
Medical Teaching	1,317	1,569	1,443	1,438	1,672	2,164	1,714
Research**	2,071	4,918	5,768	3,683	2,835	2,901	2,829
Other	541	636	817	854	770	844	945
Inactive	2,131	2,731	4,827	7,651	11,127	18,913	22,838
Not Classified	10,120	10,235	7,527	8,397	9,486	13,244	21,255
Address Unknown	1,933	3,169	1,388	1,290	579	367	85
				Percent Distribution			
Total Physicians	100.0	100.0	100.0	100.0	100.0	100.0	100.0
Patient Care	76.0	74.6	80.2	80.8	82.7	79.6	78.2
Office-Based Practice	40.6	46.8	55.6	56.8	57.4	57.8	57.9
Hospital-Based Practice	35.4	27.8	24.6	24.1	25.3	21.8	20.3
Residents/Fellows*	20.3	11.7	10.8	10.2	13.6	11.4	11.7
Full-Time Staff	15.1	16.1	13.8	13.8	11.7	10.4	8.6
Other Prof. Activity	6.5	8.9	8.2	6.0	4.5	3.9	3.1
Administration	1.6	1.6	1.5	1.5	1.3	0.9	0.8
Medical Teaching	1.6	1.6	1.2	1.1	1.0	1.1	0.7
Research**	2.6	5.0	4.9	2.8	1.7	1.5	1.2
Other	0.7	0.7	0.7	0.6	0.5	0.4	0.4
Inactive	2.6	2.8	4.1	5.8	6.7	9.6	9.6
Not Classified	12.5	10.5	6.3	6.4	5.7	6.7	9.0
Address Unknown	2.4	3.2	1.2	1.0	0.3	0.2	0.0

	Percent Change						
	1975-2006	1975-1985	1985-1995	1975-1980	1980-1985	1985-1990	1990-2006
Total Physicians	192.7	47.0	39.2	20.9	21.6	10.8	79.6
Patient Care	201.3	55.3	43.5	18.8	30.7	11.7	73.7
Office-Based Practice	318.1	101.5	43.7	39.5	44.4	13.2	83.3
Hospital-Based Practice	67.5	2.3	43.0	-5.1	7.8	8.2	51.2
Residents/Fellows*	67.7	-21.9	75.7	-30.5	12.4	5.1	104.3
Full-Time Staff	67.2	35.1	17.6	29.4	4.5	10.6	11.8
Other Prof. Activity	41.9	86.2	-23.3	64.9	12.9	-19.0	-5.9
Administration	48.7	32.1	27.2	16.2	13.7	11.1	36.2
Medical Teaching	29.9	9.6	15.9	19.1	-8.0	-0.3	-11.5
Research**	36.6	178.5	-50.8	137.5	17.3	-36.1	-23.2
Other	74.7	51.0	-5.8	17.6	28.5	4.5	10.7
Inactive	971.7	126.5	130.5	28.2	76.7	58.5	198.5
Not Classified	110.0	-25.6	26.0	1.1	-26.5	11.6	153.1
Address Unknown	-95.6	-28.2	-58.3	63.9	-56.2	-7.1	-93.4

Note: Data for 1990 are as of January 1; all other years, December 31.

*Includes all years of Residency and Clinical Fellows.

**Includes physicians in research activities and Research Fellows.

e Physicians by Self-Designated Specialty, 1975–2006

Specialty	1975	1980	1985	1990	1995	2000	2006
Total Physicians	35,626	54,284	80,725	104,194	149,404	195,537	256,257
Aerospace Medicine	7	13	32	35	32	31	38
Allergy/Immunology	124	116	138	506	736	883	1,154
Anesthesiology	1,819	2,388	3,710	4,608	6,422	7,343	9,369
Cardiovascular Dis.	185	327	598	839	1,293	1,623	2,192
Child Psychiatry	659	896	1,193	1,489	2,146	2,504	3,326
Colon/Rectal Surgery	5	5	15	31	52	91	185
Dermatology	375	628	1,082	1,641	2,453	3,189	4,262
Diagnostic Radiology	228	656	1,781	2,418	3,757	4,129	5,524
Emergency Medicine*	0	0	1,348	2,058	3,297	4,351	6,830
Family Medicine	590	2,638	5,657	8,248	13,971	20,401	28,416
Forensic Pathology	10	26	53	92	130	168	220
Gastroenterology	52	118	269	456	729	927	1,435
General Practice	2,276	2,039	2,339	2,354	2,361	2,338	2,055
Gen. Preventive Med.	98	109	199	249	399	586	817
General Surgery	567	1,150	1,987	2,406	3,302	4,024	5,718
Internal Medicine	4,006	8,130	14,716	19,171	27,609	37,073	49,541
Medical Genetics**	0	0	0	0	75	162	253
Neurological Surgery	18	48	91	139	213	233	331
Neurology	341	580	1,059	1,462	2,166	2,609	3,698
Nuclear Medicine*	0	0	168	184	254	248	298
Obstetrics/Gynecology	1,777	3,243	5,597	7,551	11,231	14,124	18,520
Occupational Medicine	79	118	210	291	482	490	542
Ophthalmology	395	657	1,120	1,550	2,227	2,628	3,380
Orthopedic Surgery	60	144	293	421	677	774	1,163
Otolaryngology	69	141	287	426	693	838	1,216
Path.-Anatomic/Clin.	1,674	2,215	3,217	3,716	4,891	5,408	6,620
Pediatric Cardiology	99	125	146	199	324	390	541
Pediatrics	5,135	8,189	12,440	15,675	22,646	30,322	39,468
Physical Med./Rehab.	322	515	920	1,193	1,767	2,143	2,675
Plastic Surgery	62	120	219	309	478	610	872
Psychiatry	3,144	4,361	6,539	8,170	10,392	11,648	14,066
Public Health	533	470	440	471	458	516	430
Pulmonary Diseases	166	239	352	501	826	1,097	1,561
Radiation Oncology	103	191	360	498	786	857	1,068
Radiology	675	895	680	842	953	1,136	1,386
Thoracic Surgery	4	14	26	25	50	132	187
Urological Surgery	16	39	98	134	244	334	583
Other Specialty	615	1,027	734	961	1,111	902	953
Unspecified	930	2,136	1,767	1,968	2,571	2,937	2,452
Inactive	3,440	3,773	5,267	7,438	8,755	9,406	13,875
Not Classified	4,173	4,030	2,894	2,844	5,924	15,621	18,894
Address Unknown	795	1,775	684	625	521	311	143

Note: Data for 1990 are as of January 1; data for all other years, December 31.

*Data were not available for Emergency Medicine prior to 1980 and Nuclear Medicine prior to 1985.

**Data on Medical Genetics were not available prior to 1994.

Table 6.11

Percent Distribution of Female Physicians by Self-Designated Specialty, 1975–2006

Specialty	1975	1980	1985	1990	1995	2000	2006
Total Physicians	100.0	100.0	100.0	100.0	100.0	100.0	100.0
Aerospace Medicine	0.0	0.0	0.0	0.0	0.0	0.0	0.0
Allergy/Immunology	0.3	0.2	0.2	0.5	0.5	0.5	0.5
Anesthesiology	5.1	4.4	4.6	4.4	4.3	3.8	3.7
Cardiovascular Dis.	0.5	0.6	0.7	0.8	0.9	0.8	0.9
Child Psychiatry	1.8	1.7	1.5	1.4	1.4	1.3	1.3
Colon/Rectal Surgery	0.0	0.0	0.0	0.0	0.0	0.0	0.1
Dermatology	1.1	1.2	1.3	1.6	1.6	1.6	1.7
Diagnostic Radiology	0.6	1.2	2.2	2.3	2.5	2.1	2.2
Emergency Medicine*	*	*	1.7	2.0	2.2	2.2	2.7
Family Medicine	1.7	4.9	7.0	7.9	9.4	10.4	11.1
Forensic Pathology	0.0	0.0	0.1	0.1	0.1	0.1	0.1
Gastroenterology	0.1	0.2	0.3	0.4	0.5	0.5	0.6
General Practice	6.4	3.8	2.9	2.3	1.6	1.2	0.8
Gen. Preventive Med.	0.3	0.2	0.2	0.2	0.3	0.3	0.3
General Surgery	1.6	2.1	2.5	2.3	2.2	2.1	2.2
Internal Medicine	11.2	15.0	18.2	18.4	18.5	19.0	19.3
Medical Genetics**	**	**	**	**	0.1	0.1	0.1
Neurological Surgery	0.1	0.1	0.1	0.1	0.1	0.1	0.1
Neurology	1.0	1.1	1.3	1.4	1.4	1.3	1.4
Nuclear Medicine*	*	*	*	0.2	0.2	0.1	0.1
Obstetrics/Gynecology	5.0	6.0	6.9	7.2	7.5	7.2	7.2
Occupational Medicine	0.2	0.2	0.3	0.3	0.3	0.3	0.2
Ophthalmology	1.1	1.2	1.4	1.5	1.5	1.3	1.3
Orthopedic Surgery	0.2	0.3	0.4	0.4	0.5	0.4	0.5
Otolaryngology	0.2	0.3	0.4	0.4	0.5	0.4	0.5
Path.-Anatomic/Clin.	4.7	4.1	4.0	3.6	3.3	2.8	2.6
Pediatric Cardiology	0.3	0.2	0.2	0.2	0.2	0.2	0.2
Pediatrics	14.4	15.1	15.4	15.0	15.2	15.5	15.4
Physical Med./Rehab.	0.9	0.9	1.1	1.1	1.2	1.1	1.0
Plastic Surgery	0.2	0.2	0.3	0.3	0.3	0.3	0.3
Psychiatry	8.8	8.0	8.1	7.8	7.0	6.0	5.5
Public Health	1.5	0.9	0.5	0.5	0.3	0.3	0.2
Pulmonary Diseases	0.5	0.4	0.4	0.5	0.6	0.6	0.6
Radiation Oncology	0.3	0.4	0.4	0.5	0.5	0.4	0.4
Radiology	1.9	1.6	0.8	0.8	0.6	0.6	0.5
Thoracic Surgery	0.0	0.0	0.0	0.0	0.0	0.1	0.1
Urological Surgery	0.0	0.1	0.1	0.1	0.2	0.2	0.2
Other Specialty	1.7	1.9	0.9	0.9	0.7	0.5	0.4
Unspecified	2.6	3.9	2.2	1.9	1.7	1.5	1.0
Inactive	9.7	7.0	6.5	7.1	5.9	4.8	5.4
Not Classified	11.7	7.4	3.6	2.7	4.0	8.0	7.4
Address Unknown	2.2	3.3	0.8	0.6	0.3	0.2	0.1

Note: Data for 1990 are as of January 1; data for all other years, December 31.

*Data were not available for Emergency Medicine prior to 1980 and Nuclear Medicine prior to 1985.

**Data on Medical Genetics were not available prior to 1994.

Table 6.12

Percent Change of Female Physicians by Self-Designated Specialty, 1975–2006

Specialty	1975-2006	1975-1985	1985-1995	1975-1980	1980-1985	1985-1990	1990-2006
Total Physicians	619.3	126.6	85.1	52.4	48.7	29.1	145.9
Aerospace Medicine	442.9	357.1	0.0	85.7	146.2	9.4	8.6
Allergy/Immunology	830.6	11.3	433.3	-6.5	19.0	266.7	128.1
Anesthesiology	415.1	104.0	73.1	31.3	55.4	24.2	103.3
Cardiovascular Dis.	1084.9	223.2	116.2	76.8	82.9	40.3	161.3
Child Psychiatry	404.7	81.0	79.9	36.0	33.1	24.8	123.4
Colon/Rectal Surgery	3600.0	200.0	246.7	0.0	200.0	106.7	496.8
Dermatology	1036.5	188.5	126.7	67.5	72.3	51.7	159.7
Diagnostic Radiology	2322.8	681.1	110.9	187.7	171.5	35.8	128.5
Emergency Medicine*	*	*	144.6	*	*	52.7	231.9
Family Medicine	4716.3	858.8	147.0	347.1	114.4	45.8	244.5
Forensic Pathology	2100.0	430.0	145.3	160.0	103.8	73.6	139.1
Gastroenterology	2659.6	417.3	171.0	126.9	128.0	69.5	214.7
General Practice	-9.7	2.8	0.9	-10.4	14.7	0.6	-12.7
Gen. Preventive Med.	733.7	103.1	100.5	11.2	82.6	25.1	228.1
General Surgery	908.5	250.4	66.2	102.8	72.8	21.1	137.7
Internal Medicine	1136.7	267.3	87.6	102.9	81.0	30.3	158.4
Medical Genetics**	**	**	**	**	**	**	**
Neurological Surgery	1738.9	405.6	134.1	166.7	89.6	52.7	138.1
Neurology	984.5	210.6	104.5	70.1	82.6	38.1	152.9
Nuclear Medicine*	*	*	51.2	*	*	9.5	62.0
Obstetrics/Gynecology	942.2	215.0	100.7	82.5	72.6	34.9	145.3
Occupational Medicine	586.1	165.8	129.5	49.4	78.0	38.6	86.3
Ophthalmology	755.7	183.5	98.8	66.3	70.6	38.4	118.1
Orthopedic Surgery	1838.3	388.3	131.1	140.0	103.5	43.7	176.2
Otolaryngology	1662.3	315.9	141.5	104.3	103.5	48.4	185.4
Path.-Anatomic/Clin.	295.5	92.2	52.0	32.3	45.2	15.5	78.1
Pediatric Cardiology	446.5	47.5	121.9	26.3	16.8	36.3	171.9
Pediatrics	668.6	142.3	82.0	59.5	51.9	26.0	151.8
Physical Med./Rehab.	730.7	185.7	92.1	59.9	78.6	29.7	124.2
Plastic Surgery	1306.5	253.2	118.3	93.5	82.5	41.1	182.2
Psychiatry	347.4	108.0	58.9	38.7	49.9	24.9	72.2
Public Health	-19.3	-17.4	4.1	-11.8	-6.4	7.0	-8.7
Pulmonary Diseases	840.4	112.0	134.7	44.0	47.3	42.3	211.6
Radiation Oncology	936.9	249.5	118.3	85.4	88.5	38.3	114.5
Radiology	105.3	0.7	40.1	32.6	-24.0	23.8	64.6
Thoracic Surgery	4575.0	550.0	92.3	250.0	85.7	-3.8	648.0
Urological Surgery	3543.8	512.5	149.0	143.8	151.3	36.7	335.1
Other Specialty	55.0	19.3	51.4	67.0	-28.5	30.9	-0.8
Unspecified	163.7	90.0	45.5	129.7	-17.3	11.4	24.6
Inactive	303.3	53.1	66.2	9.7	39.6	41.2	86.5
Not Classified	352.8	-30.6	104.7	-3.4	-28.2	-1.7	564.3
Address Unknown	-82.0	-14.0	-23.8	123.3	-61.5	-8.6	-77.1

Note: Data for 1990 are as of January 1; data for all other years, December 31.

*Data were not available for Emergency Medicine prior to 1980 and Nuclear Medicine prior to 1985.

**Data on Medical Genetics were not available prior to 1994.

Table 6.13

Female Physicians by Activity, 1975–2006

Activity	1975	1980	1985	1990	1995	2000	2006
				Number			
Total Physicians	35,626	54,284	80,725	104,194	149,404	195,537	256,257
Patient Care	24,345	39,969	64,424	86,376	126,583	161,837	213,644
Office-Based Practice	12,497	20,609	36,526	49,249	79,843	108,120	152,504
Hospital-Based Practice	11,848	19,360	27,898	37,127	46,740	53,717	61,140
Residents/Fellows*	7,512	13,322	19,778	26,838	32,797	37,363	42,024
Full-Time Staff	4,336	6,038	8,120	10,289	13,943	16,354	19,116
Other Prof. Activity	2,873	4,737	7,456	6,911	7,621	8,362	9,701
Administration	1,020	1,178	1,484	1,816	2,399	2,310	2,758
Medical Teaching	795	1,090	1,319	1,584	2,142	2,580	2,655
Research**	743	2,077	4,062	2,856	2,442	2,700	3,081
Other	315	392	591	655	638	772	1,207
Inactive	3,440	3,773	5,267	7,438	8,755	9,406	13,875
Not Classified	4,173	4,030	2,894	2,844	5,924	15,621	18,894
Address Unknown	795	1,775	684	625	521	311	143
				Percent Distribution			
Total Physicians	100.0	100.0	100.0	100.0	100.0	100.0	100.0
Patient Care	68.3	73.6	79.8	82.9	84.7	82.8	83.4
Office-Based Practice	35.1	38.0	45.2	47.3	53.4	55.3	59.5
Hospital-Based Practice	33.3	35.7	34.6	35.6	31.3	27.5	23.9
Residents/Fellows*	21.1	24.5	24.5	25.8	22.0	19.1	16.4
Full-Time Staff	12.2	11.1	10.1	9.9	9.3	8.4	7.5
Other Prof. Activity	8.1	8.7	9.2	6.6	5.1	4.3	3.8
Administration	2.9	2.2	1.8	1.7	1.6	1.2	1.1
Medical Teaching	2.2	2.0	1.6	1.5	1.4	1.3	1.0
Research**	2.1	3.8	5.0	2.7	1.6	1.4	1.2
Other	0.9	0.7	0.7	0.6	0.4	0.4	0.5
Inactive	9.7	7.0	6.5	7.1	5.9	4.8	5.4
Not Classified	11.7	7.4	3.6	2.7	4.0	8.0	7.4
Address Unknown	2.2	3.3	0.8	0.6	0.3	0.2	0.1

	Percent Change						
	1975-2006	1975-1985	1985-1995	1975-1980	1980-1985	1985-1990	1990-2006
Total Physicians	619.3	126.6	85.1	52.4	48.7	29.1	145.9
Patient Care	777.6	164.6	96.5	64.2	61.2	34.1	147.3
Office-Based Practice	1120.3	192.3	118.6	64.9	77.2	34.8	209.7
Hospital-Based Practice	416.0	135.5	67.5	63.4	44.1	33.1	64.7
Residents/Fellows*	459.4	163.3	65.8	77.3	48.5	35.7	56.6
Full-Time Staff	340.9	87.3	71.7	39.3	34.5	26.7	85.8
Other Prof. Activity	237.7	159.5	2.2	64.9	57.4	-7.3	40.4
Administration	246.9	45.5	61.7	15.5	26.0	22.4	74.1
Medical Teaching	160.3	65.9	62.4	37.1	21.0	20.1	46.2
Research**	314.7	446.7	-39.9	179.5	95.6	-29.7	7.9
Other	283.2	87.6	8.0	24.4	50.8	10.8	84.3
Inactive	303.3	53.1	66.2	9.7	39.6	41.2	86.5
Not Classified	352.8	-30.6	104.7	-3.4	-28.2	-1.7	564.3
Address Unknown	-82.0	-14.0	-23.8	123.3	-61.5	-8.6	-77.1

Note: Data for 1990 are as of January 1; all other years, December 31.
*Includes all years of Residency and Clinical Fellows.
**Includes physicians in research activities and Research Fellows.

Table 6.14

Trends in the Distribution of Physicians by Metropolitan/Nonmetropolitan Status, 1980–2006

Totals Activity Specialty Group	Total (100.0%)	1980 Metropolitan Number	%	Nonmetropolitan Number	%
Total Physicians*	443,502	385,365	86.9	58,137	13.1
Total Patient Care	361,915	312,687	86.4	49,228	13.6
Office-Based Practice	271,268	228,922	84.4	42,346	15.6
General/Family Practice	47,772	32,876	68.8	14,896	31.2
Medical Specialty	75,883	67,697	89.2	8,186	10.8
Surgical Specialty	81,877	70,042	85.5	11,835	14.5
Other Specialty	65,736	58,307	88.7	7,429	11.3
Hospital-Based Practice	90,647	83,765	92.4	6,882	7.6
Other Professional Activity	35,214	33,221	94.3	1,993	5.7
Not Classified	20,629	18,553	89.9	2,076	10.1
Inactive	25,744	20,904	81.2	4,840	18.8

Totals Activity Specialty Group	Total (100.0%)	1990 Metropolitan Number	%	Nonmetropolitan Number	%
Total Physicians*	592,166	521,668	88.1	70,498	11.9
Total Patient Care	487,796	429,396	88.0	58,400	12.0
Office-Based Practice	359,932	309,381	86.0	50,551	14.0
General/Family Practice	57,571	41,120	71.4	16,451	28.6
Medical Specialty	112,773	101,106	89.7	11,667	10.3
Surgical Specialty	100,277	86,955	86.7	13,322	13.3
Other Specialty	89,311	80,200	89.8	9,111	10.2
Hospital-Based Practice	127,864	120,015	93.9	7,849	6.1
Other Professional Activity	39,039	37,193	95.3	1,846	4.7
Not Classified	12,678	11,379	89.8	1,299	10.2
Inactive	52,653	43,700	83.0	8,953	17.0

Totals Activity Specialty Group	Total (100.0%)	2006 Metropolitan Number	%	Nonmetropolitan Number	%
Total Physicians*	921,229	709,321	77.0	211,908	23.0
Total Patient Care	722,981	558,108	77.2	164,873	22.8
Office-Based Practice	560,299	428,015	76.4	132,284	23.6
General/Family Medicine	93,331	62,968	67.5	30,363	32.5
Medical Specialty	290,606	230,614	79.4	59,992	20.6
Surgical Specialty	161,347	124,670	77.3	36,677	22.7
Other Specialty	221,405	174,369	78.8	47,036	21.2
Hospital-Based Practice	162,682	130,093	80.0	32,589	20.0
Other Professional Activity	43,708	34,513	79.0	9,195	21.0
Not Classified	46,248	36,629	79.2	9,619	20.8
Inactive	108,292	80,071	73.9	28,221	26.1

Note: Data for 1990 are as of January 1. Data for 1980 and 2006 are as of December 31.

Note: 1980 and 1990 figures are for nonfederal physicians only. 2005 figures include both federal and nonfederal physicians. Federal status is defined as fulltime employment by the federal government, including the Army, Navy, Air Force, Veterans' Administration, Public Health Service, and other federally funded agencies.

*Excludes address unknown. Metropolitan and Nonmetropolitan totals additionally exclude 195 physicians whose counties could not be determined.

Table 6.15

Percent Distribution and Percent Change for Physicians by Metropolitan/Nonmetropolitan Status, 1980–2006

Totals Activity Specialty Group	% Distribution 1980			% Change 1980-1990		
	Total	Metro	Nonmetro	Total	Metro	Nonmetro
Total Physicians*	100.0	100.0	100.0	33.5	35.4	21.3
Total Patient Care	81.6	81.1	84.7	34.8	37.3	18.6
Office-Based Practice	61.2	59.4	72.8	32.7	35.1	19.4
General/Family Practice	10.8	8.5	25.6	20.5	25.1	10.4
Medical Specialty	17.1	17.6	14.1	48.6	49.4	42.5
Surgical Specialty	18.5	18.2	20.4	22.5	24.1	12.6
Other Specialty	14.8	15.1	12.8	35.9	37.5	22.6
Hospital-Based Practice	20.4	21.7	11.8	41.1	43.3	14.1
Other Professional Activity	7.9	8.6	3.4	10.9	12.0	-7.4
Not Classified	4.7	4.8	3.6	-38.5	-38.7	-37.4
Inactive	5.8	5.4	8.3	104.5	109.1	85.0

Totals Activity Specialty Group	% Distribution 1990			% Change 1990-2006		
	Total	Metro	Nonmetro	Total	Metro	Nonmetro
Total Physicians*	100.0	100.0	100.0	55.6	36.0	200.6
Total Patient Care	82.4	82.3	82.8	48.2	30.0	182.3
Office-Based Practice	60.8	59.3	71.7	55.7	38.3	161.7
General/Family Medicine	9.7	7.9	23.3	62.1	53.1	84.6
Medical Specialty	19.0	19.4	16.5	157.7	128.1	414.2
Surgical Specialty	16.9	16.7	18.9	60.9	43.4	175.3
Other Specialty	15.1	15.4	12.9	147.9	117.4	416.3
Hospital-Based Practice	21.6	23.0	11.1	27.2	8.4	315.2
Other Professional Activity	6.6	7.1	2.6	12.0	-7.2	398.1
Not Classified	2.1	2.2	1.8	264.8	221.9	640.5
Inactive	8.9	8.4	12.7	105.7	83.2	215.2

Totals Activity Specialty Group	% Distribution 2006			% Change 1980-2006		
	Total	Metro	Nonmetro	Total	Metro	Nonmetro
Total Physicians*	100.0	100.0	100.0	107.7	84.1	264.5
Total Patient Care	78.5	78.7	77.8	99.8	78.5	234.9
Office-Based Practice	60.8	60.3	62.4	106.5	87.0	212.4
General/Family Medicine	10.1	8.9	14.3	95.4	91.5	103.8
Medical Specialty	31.5	32.5	28.3	283.0	240.7	632.9
Surgical Specialty	17.5	17.6	17.3	97.1	78.0	209.9
Other Specialty	24.0	24.6	22.2	236.8	199.1	533.1
Hospital-Based Practice	17.7	18.3	15.4	79.5	55.3	373.5
Other Professional Activity	4.7	4.9	4.3	24.1	3.9	361.4
Not Classified***	5.0	5.2	4.5	124.2	97.4	363.3
Inactive	11.8	11.3	13.3	320.6	283.0	483.1

Note: Data for 1990 are as of January 1. Data for 1980 and 2006 are as of December 31.

Note: 1980 and 1990 figures are for nonfederal physicians only. 2006 figures include both federal and nonfederal physicians. Federal status is defined as fulltime employment by the federal government, including the Army, Navy, Air Force, Veterans' Administration, Public Health Service, and other federally funded agencies.

*Excludes address unknown.

Physicians, Population, and Physician/Population Ratios, 1965–2006

Year	Total Physicians*	Total Population (in thousands)	Physicians/ 100,00 Population	Pop./One Physician	Patient Care Physicians**	Patient Care Phy/100,000 Population	Pop./One Patient Care Physician
1965	292,088	197,147	148	675	259,418	132	760
1970	334,028	208,066	161	623	278,535	134	747
1975	393,742	219,272	180	557	311,937	142	703
1980	467,679	231,266	202	494	376,512	163	614
1981	485,123	233,459	208	481	389,369	167	600
1982	501,958	235,691	213	470	408,663	173	577
1983	519,546	238,139	218	458	423,361	178	562
1984	536,986	240,543	223	448	437,089	182	550
1985	552,716	242,946	228	440	448,820	185	541
1986	569,160	245,163	232	431	462,126	188	531
1987	585,597	247,488	237	423	478,511	193	517
1989	600,789	249,876	240	416	493,159	197	507
1990	615,421	252,164	244	410	503,870	200	500
1992	653,062	256,570	255	393	535,220	209	479
1993	670,336	259,250	259	387	550,448	212	471
1994	684,414	260,341	263	380	562,456	216	463
1995	720,325	262,755	274	365	582,131	222	451
2000	813,770	282,217	288	347	647,430	229	436
2006	921,904	299,398	308	325	723,118	242	414

Note: Data for 1989-1994 are as of January 1. Data for 1995, 2000, 2002, and prior to 1989 are as of December 31.

*Includes Active and Inactive Physicians in the US. Excludes physicians located in the Possessions (Pacific Islands, Puerto Rico, Virgin Islands, and Canal Zone prior to 1980).

**Includes Office-Based Practice, Residents, and Hospital Staff physicians.

Sources: US Bureau of the Census, Current Population Reports, Series P-25, No. St-99-2, 1044, 1045, 1106, and 1127. US Government Printing Office, Washington, DC, March 1990 and 1992, November 1993, and March 1994 and 1995. Also prior nos. 460, 876, 911. Also, US Census Bureau, Population Division, Annual Population Estimates and Estimated Components of Change for the United States and States: April 1, 2000 to July 1, 2006; Source: Population Division, US Census Bureau. Physician Characteristics and Distribution in the US, Dept. of Physician Practice and Communications Information, Division of Survey and Data Resources, American Medical Association, 2004 and prior editions.

Table 6.17

Physicians, Population, and Physician/Population Ratios, 1980–2006

State	1980			1985		
	Total Nonfederal	Population (in thousands)	Physician/ Population Ratio	Total Nonfederal	Population (in thousands)	Physician/ Population Ratio
Total*	439,301	225,552	195	542,343	237,924	228
Alabama	5,039	3,871	130	6,335	3,973	159
Alaska	509	380	134	845	532	159
Arizona	5,535	2,706	205	7,323	3,184	230
Arkansas	2,939	2,289	128	3,698	2,327	159
California	58,368	23,499	248	72,089	26,441	273
Colorado	5,999	2,863	210	7,347	3,209	229
Connecticut	8,177	3,100	264	9,725	3,201	304
Delaware	1,001	591	169	1,299	618	210
Dist. Of Col.	3,626	629	576	4,157	635	655
Florida	20,374	9,786	208	27,534	11,351	243
Georgia	8,060	5,414	149	10,851	5,963	182
Hawaii	2,020	911	222	2,743	1,040	264
Idaho	1,089	942	116	1,382	994	139
Illinois	21,740	11,392	191	25,503	11,400	224
Indiana	7,415	5,483	135	8,667	5,459	159
Iowa	3,847	2,912	132	4,420	2,830	156
Kansas	3,893	2,342	166	4,546	2,427	187
Kentucky	5,059	3,628	139	6,134	3,695	166
Louisiana	6,752	4,190	161	8,541	4,408	194
Maine	1,865	1,117	167	2,302	1,163	198
Maryland	11,745	4,183	281	16,053	4,413	364
Massachusetts	16,342	5,730	285	19,693	5,881	335
Michigan	15,347	9,244	166	17,456	9,076	192
Minnesota	8,150	4,080	200	9,517	4,184	227
Mississippi	2,797	2,500	112	3,551	2,588	137
Missouri	8,331	4,903	170	10,011	5,000	200
Montana	1,100	784	140	1,337	822	163
Nebraska	2,442	1,560	157	2,815	1,585	178
Nevada	1,171	797	147	1,679	951	177
New Hampshire	1,655	920	180	2,117	997	212
New Jersey	14,799	7,353	201	18,617	7,566	246
New Mexico	2,143	1,290	166	2,822	1,438	196
New York	49,105	17,549	280	57,492	17,792	323
North Carolina	9,354	5,791	162	11,810	6,254	189
North Dakota	919	643	143	1,190	677	176
Ohio	18,342	10,790	170	21,838	10,735	203
Oklahoma	4,031	3,008	134	5,107	3,271	156
Oregon	5,119	2,635	194	5,923	2,673	222
Pennsylvania	23,347	11,868	197	28,185	11,771	239
Rhode Island	2,102	943	223	2,478	969	256
South Carolina	4,362	3,061	143	5,637	3,303	171
South Dakota	809	684	118	1,089	698	156
Tennessee	7,460	4,574	163	9,252	4,715	196
Texas	22,571	14,182	159	30,238	16,273	186
Utah	2,492	1,466	170	3,130	1,643	191
Vermont	1,185	512	231	1,471	530	278
Virginia	9,682	5,216	186	12,756	5,715	223
Washington	7,921	4,098	193	10,319	4,400	235
West Virginia	2,745	1,950	141	3,417	1,907	179
Wisconsin	7,859	4,727	166	9,151	4,748	193
Wyoming	567	471	120	751	500	150

* Excludes physicians located in the Possessions (Pacific Islands, Puerto Rico, Virgin Islands, and Canal Zone prior to 1980), and physicians whose address is unknown.

Note: 1980 figures are for nonfederal physicians only. All other figures include both federal and nonfederal physicians. Federal status is defined as full-time employment by the federal government, including the Army, Navy, Air Force, Veterans' Administration, Public Health Service, and other federally funded agencies.

Table 6.17

Physicians, Population, and Physician/Population Ratios, 1980–2006, continued

State	1990 Total	1990 Population (in thousands)	1990 Physician/ Population Ratio	1995 Total	1995 Population (in thousands)	1995 Physician/ Population Ratio
Total*	604,089	249,464	242	708,951	262,803	270
Alabama	7,246	4,049	179	8,793	4,263	206
Alaska	915	553	165	1,092	601	182
Arizona	8,560	3,679	233	10,383	4,307	241
Arkansas	4,120	2,354	175	4,921	2,480	198
California	80,874	29,950	270	88,553	31,494	281
Colorado	8,037	3,304	243	9,999	3,738	267
Connecticut	10,892	3,289	331	12,278	3,265	376
Delaware	1,500	669	224	1,804	718	251
Dist. Of Col.	4,318	604	715	4,296	551	779
Florida	32,425	13,018	249	38,918	14,185	274
Georgia	12,689	6,507	195	16,120	7,189	224
Hawaii	3,097	1,113	278	3,562	1,180	302
Idaho	1,495	1,012	148	1,936	1,165	166
Illinois	27,140	11,447	237	31,845	11,885	268
Indiana	9,693	5,555	174	11,743	5,792	203
Iowa	4,831	2,780	174	5,463	2,841	192
Kansas	5,037	2,481	203	5,865	2,587	227
Kentucky	6,878	3,693	186	8,259	3,855	214
Louisiana	8,929	4,219	212	10,616	4,328	245
Maine	2,604	1,231	211	2,956	1,237	239
Maryland	18,291	4,797	381	21,345	5,024	425
Massachusetts	21,904	6,019	364	25,831	6,062	426
Michigan	18,872	9,310	203	22,404	9,660	232
Minnesota	10,661	4,387	243	12,512	4,605	272
Mississippi	3,956	2,577	153	4,482	2,691	167
Missouri	11,057	5,126	216	12,781	5,325	240
Montana	1,513	800	189	1,896	869	218
Nebraska	3,063	1,581	194	3,679	1,635	225
Nevada	2,006	1,219	165	2,806	1,526	184
New Hampshire	2,582	1,112	232	2,908	1,146	254
New Jersey	20,882	7,757	269	24,236	7,966	304
New Mexico	3,289	1,520	216	4,030	1,682	240
New York	61,628	18,003	342	71,637	18,151	395
North Carolina	13,990	6,657	210	17,527	7,185	244
North Dakota	1,246	637	195	1,475	642	230
Ohio	23,729	10,862	218	27,435	11,155	246
Oklahoma	5,310	3,147	169	5,929	3,266	182
Oregon	6,756	2,859	236	8,000	3,141	255
Pennsylvania	31,369	11,896	264	36,780	12,045	305
Rhode Island	2,822	1,005	281	3,302	989	334
South Carolina	6,415	3,499	183	7,999	3,700	216
South Dakota	1,159	697	166	1,437	728	197
Tennessee	10,643	4,891	218	13,301	5,241	254
Texas	33,357	17,045	196	40,243	18,680	215
Utah	3,511	1,730	203	4,320	1,977	219
Vermont	1,673	565	296	1,878	583	322
Virginia	14,656	6,214	236	17,423	6,601	264
Washington	11,955	4,901	244	14,609	5,431	269
West Virginia	3,490	1,792	195	4,066	1,821	223
Wisconsin	10,258	4,902	209	12,399	5,137	241
Wyoming	766	453	169	879	478	184

Excludes physicians located in the Possessions (Pacific Islands, Puerto Rico, Virgin Islands, and Canal Zone prior to 1980), and physicians whose address is unknown.

Table 6.17

Physicians, Population, and Physician/Population Ratios, 1980–2006, continued

State	2000 Total	2000 Population (in thousands)	2000 Physician/ Population Ratio	2006 Total	2006 Population (in thousands)	2006 Physician/ Population Ratio
Total*	802,156	282,217	284	908,065	299,398	303
Alabama	9,887	4,452	222	10,994	4,599	239
Alaska	1,362	628	217	1,697	670	253
Arizona	12,250	5,167	237	15,127	6,166	245
Arkansas	5,711	2,679	213	6,464	2,811	230
California	97,213	34,008	286	110,406	36,458	303
Colorado	11,692	4,327	270	14,175	4,753	298
Connecticut	13,279	3,413	389	14,488	3,505	413
Delaware	2,099	787	267	2,414	853	283
Dist. Of Col.	4,488	571	786	5,023	582	864
Florida	46,013	16,050	287	53,566	18,090	296
Georgia	19,324	8,231	235	22,805	9,364	244
Hawaii	3,887	1,212	321	4,599	1,285	358
Idaho	2,370	1,300	182	2,934	1,466	200
Illinois	35,943	12,441	289	39,240	12,832	306
Indiana	13,461	6,092	221	15,229	6,314	241
Iowa	5,927	2,929	202	6,428	2,982	216
Kansas	6,486	2,693	241	7,079	2,764	256
Kentucky	9,468	4,049	234	10,828	4,206	257
Louisiana	12,207	4,470	273	12,643	4,288	295
Maine	3,598	1,277	282	4,197	1,322	318
Maryland	23,449	5,312	441	25,969	5,616	462
Massachusetts	28,886	6,363	454	32,575	6,437	506
Michigan	25,209	9,957	253	27,877	10,096	276
Minnesota	14,257	4,934	289	16,756	5,167	324
Mississippi	5,399	2,849	190	5,890	2,911	202
Missouri	14,061	5,607	251	15,586	5,843	267
Montana	2,188	904	242	2,548	945	270
Nebraska	4,300	1,713	251	4,852	1,768	274
Nevada	4,025	2,018	199	5,384	2,496	216
New Hampshire	3,438	1,241	277	4,079	1,315	310
New Jersey	27,462	8,434	326	30,183	8,725	346
New Mexico	4,565	1,822	251	5,424	1,955	277
New York	78,524	19,000	413	83,826	19,306	434
North Carolina	21,118	8,079	261	25,385	8,857	287
North Dakota	1,603	641	250	1,745	636	274
Ohio	30,229	11,364	266	34,091	11,478	297
Oklahoma	6,565	3,455	190	7,111	3,579	199
Oregon	9,312	3,432	271	11,741	3,701	317
Pennsylvania	39,603	12,287	322	42,204	12,441	339
Rhode Island	3,814	1,051	363	4,368	1,068	409
South Carolina	9,689	4,024	241	11,241	4,321	260
South Dakota	1,708	756	226	1,975	782	253
Tennessee	15,360	5,703	269	17,791	6,039	295
Texas	46,904	20,952	224	54,971	23,508	234
Utah	5,041	2,243	225	6,093	2,550	239
Vermont	2,318	610	380	2,659	624	426
Virginia	20,362	7,105	287	23,545	7,643	308
Washington	16,693	5,912	282	19,864	6,396	311
West Virginia	4,442	1,808	246	4,710	1,818	259
Wisconsin	13,954	5,375	260	16,154	5,557	291
Wyoming	1,013	494	205	1,132	515	220

* Excludes physicians located in the Possessions (Pacific Islands, Puerto Rico, Virgin Islands, and Canal Zone prior to 1980), and physicians whose address is unknown.

Sources: US Bureau of the Census, Current Population Reports, Series P-25, No. St-99-2, 1044, 1045, 1106, and 1127. US Government Printing Office, Washington, DC, March 1990 and 1992, November 1993, and March 1994 and 1995. Also prior nos. 460, 876, 911. Also, Historical Annual Time Series of State Population Estimates and Demographic Components of Change 1900 to 1990 Total Population Estimates; Source: US Census Bureau, Population Division, Annual Population Estimates and Estimated Components of Change for the United States and States: April 1, 2000 to July 1, 2005; Physician Characteristics and Distribution in the US, Dept. of Physician Practice and Communications Information, Division of Survey and Data Resources, American Medical Association, 2006 and prior editions.

Table 6.18

Population Ratios per One Physician by State, 1980–2006

State	Individuals per One Physican					
	1980	1985	1990	1995	2000	2006
Total*	513	439	413	371	352	330
Alabama	768	627	559	485	450	418
Alaska	747	630	605	551	461	395
Arizona	489	435	430	415	422	408
Arkansas	779	629	571	504	469	435
California	403	367	370	356	350	330
Colorado	477	437	411	374	370	335
Connecticut	379	329	302	266	257	242
Delaware	590	476	446	398	375	354
Dist. Of Col.	173	153	140	128	127	116
Florida	480	412	401	364	349	338
Georgia	672	550	513	446	426	411
Hawaii	451	379	359	331	312	280
Idaho	865	719	677	602	548	500
Illinois	524	447	422	373	346	327
Indiana	739	630	573	493	453	415
Iowa	757	640	575	520	494	464
Kansas	602	534	492	441	415	390
Kentucky	717	602	537	467	428	388
Louisiana	621	516	473	408	366	339
Maine	599	505	473	419	355	315
Maryland	356	275	262	235	227	216
Massachusetts	351	299	275	235	220	198
Michigan	602	520	493	431	395	362
Minnesota	501	440	412	368	346	308
Mississippi	894	729	652	600	528	494
Missouri	589	499	464	417	399	375
Montana	713	615	529	458	413	371
Nebraska	639	563	516	444	398	364
Nevada	681	566	607	544	501	464
New Hampshire	556	471	431	394	361	322
New Jersey	497	406	371	329	307	289
New Mexico	602	510	462	417	399	360
New York	357	309	292	253	242	230
North Carolina	619	530	476	410	383	349
North Dakota	700	569	512	435	400	364
Ohio	588	492	458	407	376	337
Oklahoma	746	641	593	551	526	503
Oregon	515	451	423	393	369	315
Pennsylvania	508	418	379	327	310	295
Rhode Island	449	391	356	300	276	244
South Carolina	702	586	545	463	415	384
South Dakota	845	641	601	507	443	396
Tennessee	613	510	460	394	371	339
Texas	628	538	511	464	447	428
Utah	588	525	493	458	445	419
Vermont	432	360	337	310	263	235
Virginia	539	448	424	379	349	325
Washington	517	426	410	372	354	322
West Virginia	710	558	514	448	407	386
Wisconsin	601	519	478	414	385	344
Wyoming	831	665	591	544	488	455

* Excludes physicians located in the Possessions (Pacific Islands, Puerto Rico, Virgin Islands, and Canal Zone prior to 1980), and physicians whose address is unknown.

Note: 1980 and 1990 figures are for nonfederal physicians only. 2005 figures include both federal and nonfederal physicians. Federal status is defined as fulltime employment by the federal government, including the Army, Navy, Air Force, Veterans' Administration, Public Health Service, and other federally funded agencies.

Sources: US Bureau of the Census, Current Population Reports, Series P-25, No. St-99-2, 1044, 1045, 1106, and 1127. US Government Printing Office, Washington, DC, March 1990 and 1992, November 1993, and March 1994 and 1995. Also prior nos. 460, 876, 911. Also, US Census Bureau, Population Division, Annual Population Estimates and Estimated Components of Change for the United States and States: April 1, 2000 to July 1, 2005; Physician Characteristics and Distribution in the US, Dept. of Physician Practice and Communications Information, Division of Survey and Data Resources, American Medical Association, 2006 and prior editions.

Table 6.19

Physician-Population Ratios and Rank by State, 2006

State	Physicians per 100,000 Population		Rank by Physician/ Population Ratio		Individuals per One Physician	
	Total	Patient Care	Total	Patient Care	Total	Patient Care
Total*	303	242			330	414
Alabama	239	198	42	40	418	506
Alaska	253	214	37	31	395	466
Arizona	245	188	39	45	408	531
Arkansas	230	189	45	44	435	529
California	303	233	18	23	330	429
Colorado	298	235	19	21	335	425
Connecticut	413	320	6	6	242	312
Delaware	283	226	26	26	354	443
Dist. Of Col.	864	638	1	1	116	157
Florida	296	222	21	27	338	450
Georgia	244	197	40	41	411	508
Hawaii	358	282	8	8	280	354
Idaho	200	162	50	50	500	618
Illinois	306	244	17	13	327	409
Indiana	241	199	41	39	415	503
Iowa	216	166	48	48	464	602
Kansas	256	203	36	38	390	493
Kentucky	257	210	35	35	388	477
Louisiana	295	242	22	16	339	413
Maine	318	246	12	12	315	407
Maryland	462	342	3	3	216	292
Massachusetts	506	383	2	2	198	261
Michigan	276	218	28	29	362	459
Minnesota	324	258	11	11	308	388
Mississippi	202	164	49	49	494	609
Missouri	267	215	32	30	375	464
Montana	270	211	31	34	371	474
Nebraska	274	219	30	28	364	456
Nevada	216	173	47	47	464	579
New Hampshire	310	242	15	17	322	414
New Jersey	346	277	9	9	289	362
New Mexico	277	213	27	32	360	470
New York	434	338	4	4	230	296
North Carolina	287	226	25	24	349	442
North Dakota	274	226	29	25	364	442
Ohio	297	234	20	22	337	428
Oklahoma	199	158	51	51	503	632
Oregon	317	244	13	14	315	410
Pennsylvania	339	260	10	10	295	385
Rhode Island	409	324	7	5	244	309
South Carolina	260	212	33	33	384	472
South Dakota	253	208	38	36	396	481
Tennessee	295	241	23	18	339	415
Texas	234	191	44	43	428	525
Utah	239	191	43	42	419	524
Vermont	426	317	5	7	235	315
Virginia	308	243	16	15	325	412
Washington	311	237	14	19	322	422
West Virginia	259	207	34	37	386	483
Wisconsin	291	236	24	20	344	423
Wyoming	220	175	46	46	455	

* Excludes physicians located in the Possessions (Pacific Islands, Puerto Rico, Virgin Islands, and Canal Zone prior to 1980), and physicians whose address is unknown.

Source: US Census Bureau, Population Division, Annual Population Estimates and Estimated Components of Change for the United States and States: April 1, 2000 to July 1, 2005; Physician Characteristics and Distribution in the US, Dept. of Physician Practice and Communications Information, Division of Survey and Data Resources, American Medical Association, 2006 and prior editions.

Table 6.20

Total and Office-Based Physicians by Self-Designated Specialty, 1980–2006

Specialty	1980 Fed & Nonfed Physicians		1990 Fed & Nonfed Physicians		2006 Fed & Nonfed Physicians	
	Total	Office-Based	Total	Office-Based	Total	Office-Based
Total Physicians	467,679	272,000	615,421	360,995	921,904	560,411
Allergy/Immunology	1,518	1,371	3,388	2,453	4,196	3,310
Anesthesiology	15,958	11,338	25,981	17,803	41,193	31,746
Cardiovascular Dis.	9,823	6,729	15,862	10,680	22,426	17,480
Child Psychiatry	3,271	1,961	4,343	2,615	7,260	5,345
Dermatology	5,660	4,378	7,557	6,006	10,744	8,920
Diagnostic Radiology	7,048	4,191	15,412	9,815	24,624	17,577
Emergency Medicine	5,699	3,362	14,243	8,420	29,987	20,055
Family Practice	27,530	18,378	47,639	37,476	82,866	66,028
Gastroenterology	4,046	2,737	7,493	5,200	12,268	9,881
General Practice	32,519	29,642	22,841	20,517	10,493	8,872
General Surgery	34,034	22,426	38,376	24,520	37,707	25,706
Internal Medicine	71,531	40,616	98,349	57,950	155,705	107,284
Neurological Surgery	3,341	2,468	4,358	3,092	5,425	4,103
Neurology	5,685	3,253	9,237	5,595	14,554	10,423
Obstetrics/Gynecology	26,305	19,513	33,697	25,485	42,333	34,225
Ophthalmology	12,974	10,603	16,073	13,068	18,058	15,765
Orthopedic Surgery	13,996	10,728	19,138	14,199	24,296	19,220
Otolaryngology	6,553	5,266	8,138	6,367	9,974	8,199
Pathology-1	13,642	6,081	16,584	7,494	19,828	11,874
Pediatrics-2	29,462	18,209	41,899	27,073	75,085	53,058
Physical Med./Rehab.	2,146	1,014	4,105	2,183	7,736	5,634
Plastic Surgery	2,980	2,438	4,590	3,835	7,063	6,016
Psychiatry	27,481	16,004	35,163	20,146	41,385	27,387
Pulmonary Diseases	3,715	2,048	6,080	3,662	10,232	7,377
Radiation Oncology	1,581	1,027	2,821	1,968	4,424	3,419
Radiology	11,653	7,802	8,492	6,060	8,886	6,954
Urological Surgery	7,743	6,228	9,372	7,398	10,518	8,850
Other Specialty	5,810	2,418	7,254	2,656	5192	2,257
Other Surgical Spec.-3	2,852	2,261	2,945	2,389	6,147	5,148
Other Remaining Spec.-4	6,071	2,549	7,822	3,316	8,719	4,343
Unspecified	12,289	4,959	8,058	1,554	7,512	3,955
Not Classified	20,629		12,678		46,252	
Other Categories-5	32,134		55,433		108,816	

Note: Data for 1990 are as of January 1. Data for 1980 and 2006 are as of December 31.

1 - Includes Pathology and Forensic Pathology

2 - Includes Pediatrics and Pediatric Cardiology. Also includes Pediatric Allergy for 1980.

3 - Includes Colon and Rectal Surgery and Thoracic Surgery.

4 - Includes Aerospace Medicine, General Preventive Medicine, Nuclear Medicine, Occupational Medicine, Medical Genetics, and Public Health.

5 - Includes Inactive and Address Unknown. These categories are included in Total Physicians only, not in Office-Based Practice.

Table 6.21

Physician-Population Ratios for Total and Office-Based Physicians by Self-Designated Specialty, 1980–2006

Specialty	1980 Physicians per 100,000 Population		1990 Physicians per 100,000 Population		2006 Physicians per 100,000 Population	
	Total	Office-Based	Total	Office-Based	Total	Office-Based
Total Physicians	207.3	120.6	249.6	146.4	307.9	187.2
Allergy/Immunology	0.7	0.6	1.4	1.0	1.4	1.1
Anesthesiology	7.1	5.0	10.5	7.2	13.8	10.6
Cardiovascular Dis.	4.4	3.0	6.4	4.3	7.5	5.8
Child Psychiatry	1.5	0.9	1.8	1.1	2.4	1.8
Dermatology	2.5	1.9	3.1	2.4	3.6	3.0
Diagnostic Radiology	3.1	1.9	6.3	4.0	8.2	5.9
Emergency Medicine	2.5	1.5	5.8	3.4	10.0	6.7
Family Practice	12.2	8.1	19.3	15.2	27.7	22.1
Gastroenterology	1.8	1.2	3.0	2.1	4.1	3.3
General Practice	14.4	13.1	9.3	8.3	3.5	3.0
General Surgery	15.1	9.9	15.6	9.9	12.6	8.6
Internal Medicine	31.7	18.0	39.9	23.5	52.0	35.8
Neurological Surgery	1.5	1.1	1.8	1.3	1.8	1.4
Neurology	2.5	1.4	3.7	2.3	4.9	3.5
Obstetrics/Gynecology	11.7	8.7	13.7	10.3	14.1	11.4
Ophthalmology	5.8	4.7	6.5	5.3	6.0	5.3
Orthopedic Surgery	6.2	4.8	7.8	5.8	8.1	6.4
Otolaryngology	2.9	2.3	3.3	2.6	3.3	2.7
Pathology-1	6.0	2.7	6.7	3.0	6.6	4.0
Pediatrics-2	13.1	8.1	17.0	11.0	25.1	17.7
Physical Med./Rehab.	1.0	0.4	1.7	0.9	2.6	1.9
Plastic Surgery	1.3	1.1	1.9	1.6	2.4	2.0
Psychiatry	12.2	7.1	14.3	8.2	13.8	9.1
Pulmonary Diseases	1.6	0.9	2.5	1.5	3.4	2.5
Radiation Oncology	0.7	0.5	1.1	0.8	1.5	1.1
Radiology	5.2	3.5	3.4	2.5	3.0	2.3
Urological Surgery	3.4	2.8	3.8	3.0	3.5	3.0
Other Specialty	2.6	1.1	2.9	1.1	1.7	0.8
Other Surgical Spec.-3	1.3	1.0	1.2	1.0	2.1	1.7
Other Remaining Spec.-4	2.7	1.1	3.2	1.3	2.9	1.5
Unspecified	5.4	2.2	3.3	0.6	2.5	1.3
Not Classified	9.1		5.1		15.4	
Other Categories-5	14.2		22.5		36.3	

Note: Data for 1990 are as of January 1. Data for 1980 and 2006 are as of December 31.

1 - Includes Pathology and Forensic Pathology

2 - Includes Pediatrics and Pediatric Cardiology. Also includes Pediatric Allergy for 1980.

3 - Includes Colon and Rectal Surgery and Thoracic Surgery.

4 - Includes Aerospace Medicine, General Preventive Medicine, Nuclear Medicine, Occupational Medicine, Medical Genetics, and Public Health.

5 - Includes Inactive and Address Unknown. These categories are included in Total Physicians only, not in Office-Based Practice.

Source: US Census Bureau, Population Division, Annual Population Estimates and Estimated Components of Change for the United States and States: April 1, 2000 to July 1, 2006; Physician Characteristics and Distribution in the US, Dept. of Physician Practice and Communications Information, Division of Survey and Data Resources, American Medical Association, 2006 and prior editions.

Appendix A

Self-Designated Practice Specialties

Allergy & Immunology (AI)

Allergy (A)

Allergy & Immunology/Clinical & Laboratory
  Immunology (ALI)

Immunology (IG)

Aerospace Medicine (AM)

Anesthesiology (AN)

Pain Management (APM)

Critical Care (Anesthesiology) (CCA)

Cardiovascular Disease (CD)

Child & Adolescent Psychiatry (CHP)

Colon & Rectal Surgery (CRS)

Proctology (PRO)

Dermatology (D)

Clinical & Laboratory Dermatological Immunology (DDL)

Procedural Dermatology (PRD)

Diagnostic Radiology (DR)

Cardiothoracic Radiology (CTR)

Emergency Medicine (EM)

Sports Medicine (Emergency Medicine) (ESM)

Medical Toxicology (Emergency Medicine) (ETX)

Pediatric Emergency Medicine (Emergency Medicine) (PE)

Urgent Care Medicine (UCM)

Underseas Medicine (Emergency Medicine) (UME)

Forensic Pathology (FOP)

Family Medicine (FM)

Geriatric Medicine (Family Medicine) (FPG)

Family Medicine/Psychiatry (FPP)

Sports Medicine (Family Medicine) (FSM)

Internal Medicine/Family Medicine (IFP)

Gastroenterology (GE)

General Practice (GP)

General Preventive Medicine (GPM)

Medical Toxicology (Preventive Medicine) (PTX)

Underseas Medicine (UM)

General Surgery (GS)

Abdominal Surgery (AS)

Surgical Critical Care (Surgery) (CCS)

Craniofacial Surgery (CFS)

Dermatologic Surgery (DS)

Head & Neck Surgery (HNS)

Hand Surgery (HS)

Hand Surgery (Surgery) (HSS)

Oral & Maxillofacial Surgery (OMF)

Pediatric Cardiothoracic Surgery (PCS)

Pediatric Surgery (Surgery) (PDS)

Surgical Oncology (SO)

Trauma Surgery (TRS)

Vascular Surgery (VS)

Internal Medicine (IM)

Adolescent Medicine (AMI)

Critical Care Medicine (Internal Medicine) (CCM)

Diabetes (DIA)

Endocrinology, Diabetes & Metabolism (END)

Hematology (Internal Medicine) (HEM)

Hepatology (HEP)

Hematology/Oncology (HO)

Hospitalist (HOS)

Interventional Cardiology (IC)

Cardiac Electrophysiology (ICE)

Infectious Diseases (ID)

Clinical & Laboratory Immunology (Internal Medicine) (ILI)

Internal Medicine/Dermatology (IMD)

Geriatric Medicine (IMG)

Internal Medicine (Preventive Medicine) (IPM)

Sports Medicine (Internal Medicine) (ISM)

Internal Medicine (Emergency Medicine) (MEM)

Internal Medicine & Neurology (MN)

Internal Medicine/Psychiatry (MP)

Nuclear Cardiology (NC)

Nephrology (NEP)

Nutrition (NTR)

Medical Oncology (ON)

Rheumatology (RHU)

Medical Genetics (MG)

Clinical Biochemical Genetics (CBG)

Clinical Cytogenetics (CCG)

Clinical Genetics (CG)

Clinical Molecular Genetics (CMG)

Neurology (N)

Child Neurology (CHN)

Clinical Neurophysiology (CN)

Vascular Neurology (VN)

Nuclear Medicine (NM)

Neurological Surgery (NS)

Endovascular Surgical Neuroradiology (ESN)

Neurology/Diagnostic Radiology/Neuroradiology (NRN)

Pediatric Surgery (Neurology) (NSP)

Obstetrics & Gynecology (OBG)

Gynecological Oncology (GO)

Gynecology (GYN)

Maternal & Fetal Medicine (MFM)

Obstetrics (OBS)

Critical Care Medicine (Obstetrics & Gynecology) (OCC)

Reproductive Endocrinology (REN)

Occupational Medicine (OM)

Ophthalmology (OPH)

Pediatric Ophthalmology (PO)

Orthopedic Surgery (ORS)

Hand Surgery (Orthopedic Surgery) (HSO)

Adult Reconstructive Orthopedics (OAR)

Orthopedics, Foot & Ankle (OFA)

Osteopathic Manipulative Medicine (OMM)

Musculoskeletal Oncology (OMO)

Pediatric Orthopedics (OP)

Sports Medicine (Orthopedic Surgery) (OSM)

Orthopedic Surgery of the Spine (OSS)

Orthopedic Trauma (OTR)

Other Specialty (OS)

Addiction Medicine (ADM)

Epidemiology (EP)

Legal Medicine (LM)

Medical Management (MDM)

Clinical Pharmacology (PA)

Phlebology (PHL)

Pharmaceutical Medicine (PHM)

Palliative Medicine (PLM)

Pain Medicine (PMD)

Sleep Medicine (SME)

Otolaryngology (OTO)

Otology/Neurotology (NO)

Pediatric Otolaryngology (PDO)

Psychiatry (P)

Addiction Psychiatry (ADP)

Pediatric Psychiatry/Child Psychiatry (CPP)

Neurodevelopmental Disabilities (Psychiatry & Neurology) (NDN)

Neuropsychiatry (NUP)

Forensic Psychiatry (PFP)

Psychoanalysis (PYA)

Geriatric Psychiatry (PYG)

Psychosomatic Medicine (PYM)

Psychiatry/Neurology (PYN)

Pediatrics (PD)

Adolescent Medicine (ADL)

Pediatric Critical Care Medicine (CCP)

Developmental/Behavioral Pediatrics (DBP)

Pediatrics/Emergency Medicine (EMP)

Internal Medicine/Pediatrics (MPD)

Neurodevelopmental Disabilities (Pediatrics) (NDP)

Neonatal-Perinatal Medicine (NPM)

Pediatric Anesthesiology (PAN)

Pediatric Allergy (PDA)

Pediatric Endocrinology (PDE)

Pediatric Infectious Disease (PDI)

Pediatrics/Dermatology (PDM)

Pediatric Pulmonology (PDP)

Medical Toxicology (Pediatrics) (PDT)

Pediatric Emergency Medicine (Pediatrics) (PEM)

Pediatric Gastroenterology (PG)

Pediatric Hematology/Oncology (PHO)

Clinical & Laboratory Immunology (Pediatrics) (PLI)

Pediatrics/Medical Genetics (PMG)

Pain Management (Physical Medicine & Rehabilitation) (PMP)

Pediatric Nephrology (PN)

Pediatrics/Physical Medicine & Rehabilitation (PPM)

Pediatric Rheumatology (PPR)

Sports Medicine (Pediatrics) (PSM)

Pediatric Rehabilitation Medicine (RPM)

Pediatric Cardiology (PDC)

Public Health & General Preventive Medicine (PHP)

Physical Medicine & Rehabilitation (PM)

Neuromuscular Medicine (NMN)

Sports Medicine (Physical Medicine & Rehabilitation) (PMM)

Spinal Cord Injury (SCI)

Plastic Surgery (PS)

Cosmetic Surgery (CS)

Facial Plastic Surgery (FPS)

Surgery of the Hand (Plastic Surgery) (HSP)

Plastic Surgery Within the Head & Neck (PSH)

Anatomic/Clinical Pathology (PTH)

Anatomic Pathology (ATP)

Blood Banking/Transfusion Medicine (BBK)

Clinical Pathology (CLP)

Dermatopathology (DMP)

Hematology (HMP)

Molecular Genetic Pathology (MGP)

Medical Microbiology (MM)

Neuropathology (NP)

Chemical Pathology (PCH)

Cytopathology (PCP)

Pediatric Pathology (PP)

Selective Pathology (SP)

Pulmonary Disease (PUD)

Pulmonary Critical Care Medicine (PCC)

Radiology (R)

Abdominal Radiology (AR)

Musculoskeletal Radiology (MSR)

Nuclear Radiology (NR)

Pediatric Radiology (PDR)

Neuroradiology (RNR)

Radiological Physics (RP)

Vascular & Interventional Radiology (VIR)

Radiation Oncology (RO)

Thoracic Surgery (TS)

Transplant Surgery (TTS)

Urology (U)

Pediatric Urology (UP)

Vascular Medicine (VM)

Unspecified (US)

Appendix B

American Specialty Boards

American Board of	Certifies in Specialties of
Allergy and Immunology	Allergy and Immunology*
Anesthesiology	Anesthesiology,* Critical Care Medicine,** Pain Medicine**
Colon and Rectal Surgery	Colon & Rectal Surgery*
Dermatology	Dermatology,* Clinical & Laboratory Dermatological Immunology,** Dermatopathology,** Pediatric Dermatology**
Emergency Medicine	Emergency Medicine,* Medical Toxicology,** Pediatric Emergency Medicine,** Sports Medicine,** Undersea & Hyperbaric Medicine**
Family Medicine	Family Medicine,* Adolescent Medicine,** Geriatric Medicine,** Sports Medicine**
Internal Medicine	Internal Medicine,* Adolescent Medicine,** Cardiovascular Disease,** Cardiac Electrophysiology,** Critical Care Medicine,** Endocrinology, Diabetes & Metabolism,** Gastroenterology,** Geriatric Medicine,** Hematology,** Infectious Diseases,** Interventional Cardiology,** Medical Oncology,** Nephrology,** Pulmonary Disease,** Rheumatology,** Sleep Medicine,** Sports Medicine,** Transplant Hepatology**
Medical Genetics	Clinical Biochemical Genetics,* Clinical Cytogenetics,* Clinical Genetics—MD,* Clinical Molecular Genetics,* Ph.D. Medical Genetics,* Molecular Genetic Pathology**
Neurological Surgery	Neurological Surgery*
Nuclear Medicine	Nuclear Medicine*
Obstetrics and Gynecology	Obstetrics & Gynecology,* Critical Care Medicine,** Gynecologic Oncology,** Maternal & Fetal Medicine,** Reproductive Endocrinology**
Ophthalmology	Ophthalmology*
Orthopaedic Surgery	Orthopaedic Surgery,* Hand Surgery,** Sports Medicine**
Otolaryngology	Otolaryngology,* Neurotology,** Pediatric Otolaryngology,** Plastic Surgery Within the Head & Neck,** Sleep Medicine**
Pathology	Anatomic & Clinical Pathology,* Anatomic Pathology,* Clinical Pathology,* Blood Banking,** Chemical Pathology,** Cytopathology,** Dermatopathology,** Forensic Pathology,** Hematology,** Medical Microbiology,** Molecular Genetic Pathology,** Neuropathology,** Pediatric Pathology**
Pediatrics	Pediatrics,* Adolescent Medicine,** Blood Banking,** Developmental-Behavioral Pediatrics,** Medical Toxicology,** Neonatal-Perinatal Medicine,** Neurodevelopmental Disabilities,** Pediatric Cardiology,** Pediatric Critical Care Medicine,** Pediatric Emergency Medicine,** Pediatric Endocrinology,** Pediatric Gastroenterology,** Pediatric Hematology-Oncology,** Pediatric Infectious Disease,** Pediatric Nephrology,** Pediatric Pulmonology,** Pediatric Rheumatology,** Pediatric Transplant Hepatology,** Sleep Medicine,** Sports Medicine**

American Board of	Certifies in Specialties of
Physical Medicine and Rehabilitation	Physical Medicine & Rehabilitation,* Pain Medicine,** Neuromuscular Medicine, Pediatric Rehabilitation Medicine,** Spinal Cord Injury Medicine,** Sports Medicine**
Plastic Surgery	Plastic Surgery,* Plastic Surgery Within the Head and Neck,** Surgery of the Hand**
Preventive Medicine	Aerospace Medicine,* Occupational Medicine,* Public Health & General Preventive Medicine,* Medical Toxicology,** Undersea & Hyperbaric Medicine**
Psychiatry and Neurology	Neurology,* Neurology With Special Qualifications in Child Neurology,* Psychiatry,* Addiction Psychiatry,** Child & Adolescent Psychiatry,** Clinical Neurophysiology,** Forensic Psychiatry,** Geriatric Psychiatry,** Neurodevelopmental Disabilities,** Pain Medicine,** Psychosomatic Medicine,** Sleep Medicine,** Vascular Neurology**
Radiology	Diagnostic Radiology,* Radiation Oncology,* Radiological Physics,* Neuroradiology,** Nuclear Radiology,** Pediatric Radiology,** Vascular & Interventional Radiology**
Surgery	Surgery,* Vascular Surgery,* Pediatric Surgery,** Surgery of the Hand,** Surgical Critical Care**
Thoracic Surgery	Thoracic Surgery*
Urology	Urology*

Note: includes current name of certificate. Excludes certificates that were issued during selected years prior to 1990.

Source: Annual Report and Reference Handbook—1994. The American Board of Medical Specialties Research & Education Foundation.

* General Certification

** Subspecialty Certification

Appendix C
List of Metropolitan Statistical Areas (MSAs)

The 280 Metropolitan Statistical Areas (MSAs) in this publication are comprised of the following counties:

Abilene, TX—Taylor

Aguadilla, PR—Aguada, Aguadilla, Moca

Albany, GA—Dougherty, Lee

Albany-Schenectady-Troy, NY—Albany, Montgomery, Rensselaer, Saratoga, Schenectady, Schoharie

Albuquerque, NM—Bernalillo, Sandoval, Valencia

Alexandria, LA—Rapides

Allentown-Bethlehem-Easton, PA—Carbon, Lehigh, Northampton

Altoona, PA—Blair

Amarillo, TX—Potter, Randall

Anchorage, AK—Anchorage

Anniston, AL—Calhoun

Appleton-Oshkosh-Neenah, WI—Calumet, Outagamie, Winnebago

Asheville, NC—Buncombe, Madison

Athens, GA—Clarke, Jackson, Madison, Oconee

Atlanta, GA—Barrow, Barton, Carroll, Cherokee, Clayton, Cobb, Coweta, De Kalb, Douglas, Fayette, Forsyth, Fulton, Gwinnett, Henry, Newton, Paulding, Pickens, Rockdale, Spalding, Walton

Auburn-Opelika, AL—Lee

Augusta-Aiken, GA-SC—
    Georgia Portion—Columbia, McDuffie, Richmond
    South Carolina Portion—Aiken, Edgefield

Austin-San Marcos, TX—Bastrop, Calhoun, Hays, Travis, Williamson

Bakersfield, CA—Kern

Bangor, ME—Penobscot, Waldo

Barnstable-Yarmouth, MA—Barnstable

Baton Rouge, LA—Ascension, East Baton Rouge, Livingston, West Baton Rouge

Beaumont-Port Arthur, TX—Hardin, Jefferson, Orange

Bellingham, WA—Whatcom

Benton Harbor, MI—Berrien

Billings, MT—Yellowstone

Biloxi-Gulfport, MS—Hancock, Harrison, Jackson

Binghamton, NY—Broome, Tioga

Birmingham, AL—Blount, Jefferson, St. Clair, Shelby

Bismarck, ND—Burleigh, Morton

Bloomington, IN—Monroe

Bloomington-Normal, IL—McLean

Boise, ID—Ada, Canyon

Boston-Worcester-Lawrence, CT-MA-ME-NH—
    Connecticut Portion—Windham
    Maine Portion—York
    Massachusetts Portion—Bristol, Essex, Hampden, Middlesex, Norfolk, Plymouth, Suffolk, Worcester
    New Hampshire Portion—Rockingham, Hillsborough, Merrimack, Strafford

Brownsville-Harlingen, TX—Cameron

Bryan-College Station, TX—Brazos

Buffalo-Niagara Falls, NY—Erie, Niagara

Burlington, VT—Chittenden, Franklin, Grand Isle

Canton-Massillon, OH—Carroll, Stark

Casper, WY—Natrona

Cedar Rapids, IA—Linn

Champaign-Urbana-Rantoul, IL—Champaign

Charleston-North Charleston, SC—Berkeley, Charleston, Dorchester

Charleston, WV—Kanawha, Putnam

Charlotte-Gastonia Rock Hill, NC—
    North Carolina Portion—Cabarrus, Gaston, Lincoln, Mecklenburg, Rowan, Union
    South Carolina Portion—York

Charlottesville, VA—Albermarle, Charlottesville, Fluvanna, Greene

Chattanooga, TN—
    Georgia Portion—Catoosa, Dade, Walker
    Tennessee Portion—Hamilton, Marion

Cheyenne, WY—Laramie

Chicago-Gary-Kenosha, IL-IN-WI—
    Illinois Portion—Cook, DeKalb, DuPage, Grundy, Kane, Kankakee, Kendall, Lake, McHenry, Will
    Indiana Portion—Gary
    Wisconsin Portion—Kenosha

Chico-Paradise, CA—Butte

Cincinnati-Hamilton, OH-KY-IN—
    Indiana Portion—Dearborn, Ohio
    Kentucky Portion—Boone, Campbell, Gallatin, Grant, Kenton, Pendleton
    Ohio Portion—Brown, Butler, Clermont, Hamilton, Warren

Clarksville-Hopkinsville, TN-KY—
  Kentucky Portion—Christian
  Tennessee Portion—Montgomery
Cleveland-Akron, OH—Ashtabula, Cuyahoga, Geauga,
  Lake, Lorain, Medina, Portage, Summit
Colorado Springs CO—El Paso
Columbia, MO—Boone
Columbia, SC—Lexington, Richland
Columbus, GA-AL—
  Alabama Portion—Russell
  Georgia Portion—Chattahoochee, Harris, Muscogee
Columbus, OH—Delaware, Fairfield, Franklin, Licking,
  Madison, Pickaway
Corpus Christi, TX—Nueces, San Patricio
Corvallis, OR—Benton
Cumberland, MD-WV—
  Maryland Portion—Allegany
  West Virginia Portion—Mineral
Dallas-Fort Worth, TX—Collin, Dallas, Denton, Ellis,
  Henderson, Hood, Hunt, Johnson,
  Kaufman, Parker, Rockwall, Tarrant
Danville, VA—Danville, Pittsylvania
Davenport-Moline-Rock Island, IL-IA—
  Illinois Portion—Henry, Rock Island
  Iowa Portion—Scott
Dayton-Springfield, OH—Clark, Greene, Miami,
  Montgomery
Daytona Beach, FL—Flagler, Volusia
Decatur, AL—Lawrence, Morgan
Decatur, IL—Macon
Denver-Boulder-Greeley, CO—Adams, Arapahoe, Boulder,
  Denver, Douglas, Jefferson, Weld
Des Moines, IA—Dallas, Polk, Warren
Detroit-Ann Arbor-Flint, MI—Genesee, Lapeer, Lenawee,
  Livingston, Macomb, Monroe,
  Oakland, St. Clair, Washtenaw, Wayne
Dothan, AL—Dale, Houston
Dover, DE—Kent
Dubuque, IA—Dubuque
Duluth-Superior, MN-WI—
  Minnesota Portion—St. Louis
  Wisconsin Portion—Douglas
Eau Claire, WI—Chippewa, Eau Claire
El Paso, TX—El Paso
Elkhart-Goshen, IN—Elkhart
Elmira, NY—Chemung
Enid, OK—Garfield
Erie, PA—Erie
Eugene-Springfield, OR—Lane
Evansville-Henderson, IN—
  Indiana Portion—Posey, Vanderburgh, Warrick
  Kentucky Portion—Henderson
Fargo-Moorhead, NDMN—
  Minnesota Portion—Clay
  North Dakota Portion—Cass
Fayetteville, NC—Cumberland

Fayetteville-Springdale-Rogers, AR—Benton, Washington
Flagstaff, AZ-UT—
  Arizona Portion—Coconino
  Utah Portion—Kane
Florence, AL—Colbert, Lauderdale
Florence, SC—Florence
Fort Collins-Loveland, CO—Larimer
Fort Myers-Cape Coral, FL—Lee
Fort Pierce-Port St. Lucie, FL—Martin, St. Lucie
Fort Smith, AR-OK—
  Arkansas Portion—Crawford, Sebastian
  Oklahoma Portion—Sequoyah
Fort Walton Beach, FL—Okaloosa
Fort Wayne, IN—Adams, Allen, DeKalb, Huntington,
  Wells, Whitley
Fresno, CA—Fresno, Madera
Gadsden, AL—Etowah
Gainesville, FL—Alachua
Glens Falls, NY—Warren, Washington
Goldsboro, NC—Wayne
Grand Forks, ND-MN—
  North Dakota Portion—Grand Forks
  Minnesota Portion—Polk
Grand Junction, CO—Mesa
Grand Rapids-Muskegon-Holland, MI—Allegan, Kent,
  Muskegon, Ottawa
Great Falls, MT—Cascade
Green Bay, WI—Brown
Greensboro-Winston-Salem-High Point, NC—Alamance,
  Davidson, Davie, Forsyth, Guilford, Randolph, Stokes,
  Yadkin
Greenville, NC—Pitt
Greenville-Spartanburg-Anderson, SC—Anderson,
  Cherokee, Greenville, Pickens, Spartanburg
Harrisburg-Lebanon-Carlisle, PA—Cumberland, Dauphin,
  Lebanon, Perry
Hartford, CT—Hartford, Litchfield, Middlesex, New
  London, Tolland, Windham
Hattiesburg, MS—Forrest, Lamar
Hickory-Morganton-Lenoir, NC—Alexander, Burke,
  Caldwell, Catawba
Honolulu, HI—Honolulu
Houma, LA—Lafourche, Terrebonne
Houston-Galveston-Brazoria, TX—Brazoria, Chambers,
  Fort Bend, Galveston, Harris, Liberty,
  Montgomery, Waller
Huntington-Ashland, WV-KY-OH—
  Kentucky Portion—Boyd, Carter, Greenup
  Ohio Portion—Lawrence
  West Virginia Portion—Cabell, Wayne
Huntsville, AL—Limestone, Madison
Indianapolis, IN—Boone, Hamilton, Hancock, Hendricks,
  Johnson, Madison, Marion, Morgan, Shelby
Iowa City, IA—Johnson
Jackson, MI—Jackson
Jackson, MS—Hinds, Madison, Rankin
Jackson, TN—Chester, Madison

Jacksonville, FL—Clay, Duval, Nassau, St. Johns

Jacksonville, NC—Onslow

Jamestown, NY—Chautauqua

Janesville-Beloit, WI—Rock

Johnson City-Kingsport-Bristol, TN-VA—
  Tennessee Portion—Carter, Hawkins, Sullivan, Unicoi, Washington
  Virginia Portion—Bristol, Scott, Washington

Johnstown, PA—Cambria, Somerset

Jonesboro, AR—Craighead

Joplin, MO—Jasper, Newton

Kalamazoo-Battle Creek, MI—Calhoun, Kalamazoo, Van Buren

Kansas City, MO-KS—
  Kansas Portion—Johnson, Leavenworth, Miami, Wyandotte
  Missouri Portion—Cass, Clay, Clinton, Jackson, Lafayette, Platte, Ray

Killeen-Temple, TX—Bell, Coryell

Knoxville, TN—Anderson, Blount, Knox, Loudon, Sevier, Union

Kokomo, IN—Howard, Tipton

La Crosse, WI-MN—
  Minnesota Portion—Houston
  Wisconsin Portion—La Crosse

Lafayette, IN—Clinton, Tippecanoe

Lafayette, LA—Arcadia, Lafayette, St. Landry, St. Martin

Lake Charles, LA—Calcasieu

Lakeland-Winter Haven, FL—Polk

Lancaster, PA—Lancaster

Lansing-East Lansing, MI—Clinton, Eaton, Ingham

Laredo, TX—Webb

Las Cruces, NM—Dona Ana

Las Vegas, NV-AZ—
  Arizona Portion—Mohave
  Nevada Portion—Clark, Nye

Lawrence, KS—Douglas

Lawton, OK—Comanche

Lewiston-Auburn, ME—Androscoggin

Lexington, KY—Bourbon, Clark, Fayette, Jessamine, Madison, Scott, Woodford

Lima, OH—Allen, Augiaize

Lincoln, NE—Lancaster

Little Rock-North Little Rock, AR—Faulkner, Lonoke, Pulaski, Saline

Longview-Marshall, TX—Gregg, Harrison, Upshur

Los Angeles-Riverside-Orange County, CA—Los Angeles, Orange, Riverside, San Bernardino, Ventura

Louisville, KY-IN—
  Indiana Portion—Clark, Floyd, Harrison, Scott
  Kentucky Portion—Bullitt, Jefferson, Oldham

Lubbock, TX—Lubbock

Lynchburg, VA—Amherst, Bedford, Bedford City, Campbell, Lynchburg

Macon, GA—Bibb, Houston, Jones, Peach, Twiggs

Madison, WI—Dane

Mansfield, OH—Crawford, Richland

Mayaguez, PR—Anasco, Cabo Rojo, Hormigueros, Mayaquez, Sabana Grande, San German

McAllen-Edinburg-Mission, TX—Hidalgo

Medford-Ashland, OR—Jackson

Melbourne-Titusville-Palm Bay, FL—Brevard

Memphis, TN-AR-MS—
  Arkansas Portion—Crittenden
  Mississippi Portion—DeSoto
  Tennessee Portion—Fayette, Shelby, Tipton

Merced, CA—Merced

Miami-Fort Lauderdale, FL—Broward, Miami-Dade

Milwaukee-Racine, WI—Milwaukee, Ozaukee, Racine, Washington, Waukesha

Minneapolis-St. Paul, MN-WI—
  Minnesota Portion—Anoka, Carver, Chisago, Dakota, Hennepin, Isanti, Ramsey, Scott, Sherburne, Washington, Wright
  Wisconsin Portion—Pierce, St. Croix

Missoula, MT—Missoula

Mobile, AL—Baldwin, Mobile

Modesto, CA—Stanislaus

Monroe, LA—Ouachita

Montgomery, AL—Autauqa, Elmore, Montgomery

Muncie, IN—Delaware

Myrtle Beach, SC—Horry

Naples, FL—Collier

Nashville, TN—Cheatham, Davidson, Dickson, Robertson, Rutherford, Sumner, Williamson, Wilson

New London-Norwich, CT—Middlesex, New London, Windham, Washington

New Orleans, LA—Jefferson, Orleans, Plaquemines, St. Bernard, St. Charles, St. James, St. John the Baptist, St. Tammany

New York-Northern New Jersey-Long Island, NY-NJ-CT-PA—
  Connecticut Portion—Fairfield, Litchfield, New Haven
  New Jersey Portion—Bergen, Essex, Hudson, Hunterdon, Mercer, Middlesex, Monmouth, Morris, Nassau, Ocean, Passaic, Somerset, Suffolk, Sussex, Union, Warren
  New York Portion—Bronx, Dutchess, Kings, New York, Orange, Putnam, Queens, Richmond, Rockland, Westchester
  Pennsylvania Portion—Pike

Norfolk-Virginia Beach-Newport News, VA-NC—
  North Carolina Portion—Currituck
  Virginia Portion—Chesapeake, Gloucester, Isle of Wight, Hampton, James, Mathews, Newport News, Norfolk, Poquoson, Portsmouth, Suffolk, Virginia Beach, Williamsburg, York

Ocala, FL—Marion

Odessa-Midland, TX—Ector, Midland

Oklahoma City, OK—Canadian, Cleveland, Logan, McClain, Oklahoma, Pottawatomie

Omaha, NE-IA—
  Iowa Portion—Pottawatamie
  Nebraska Portion—Cass, Douglas, Sarpy, Washington

Orlando, FL—Lake, Orange, Osceola, Seminole

Owensboro, KY—Daviess

Panama City, FL—Bay

Parkersburg-Marietta, WV-OH—
Ohio Portion—Washington
West Virginia Portion—Wood

Pensacola, FL—Escambia, Santa Rosa

Peoria-Pekin, IL—Peoria, Tazewell, Woodford

Philadelphia-Wilmington-Atlantic City, PA-NJ-DE-MD—
Delaware Portion—New Castle
Maryland Portion—Cecil
New Jersey Portion—Burlington, Camden, Cumberland,
Gloucester, Salem
Pennsylvania Portion—Bucks, Chester, Delaware,
Montgomery, Philadelphia

Phoenix-Mesa, AZ—Maricopa, Pinal

Pine Bluff, AR—Jefferson

Pittsburgh, PA—Allegheny, Beaver, Butler, Fayette,
Washington, Westmoreland

Pittsfield, MA—Berkshire

Pocatello, ID—Banrock

Ponce, PR—Guayanilla, Juana Diaz, Penuelas, Ponce,
Villalba, Yauco

Portland, ME—Cumberland, York

Portland-Salem, OR-WA—
Oregon Portion—Clackamas, Columbia, Marion,
Multnomah, Polk, Washington, Yamhill
Washington Portion—Clark

Providence-Fall River-Warwick, RI-MA—
Massachusetts Portion—Bristol
Rhode Island Portion—Bristol, Kent, Newport,
Providence, Washington

Provo-Orem, UT—Utah

Pueblo, CO—Pueblo

Punta Gorda, FL—Charlotte

Raleigh-Durham-Chapel Hill, NC—Chatham, Durham,
Franklin, Johnston, Orange, Wake

Rapid City, SD—Pennington

Reading, PA—Berks

Redding, CA—Shasta

Reno, NV—Washoe

Richland-Kennewick-Pasco, WA—Benton, Franklin

Richmond-Petersburg, VA—Charles City, Chesterfield,
Colonial Heights City, Dinwiddie, Goochland, Hanover,
Henrico, Hopewell City, New Kent, Petersburg City,
Powhatan, Prince George, Richmond City

Roanoke, VA—Botetourt, Roanoke, Roanoke City, Salem
City

Rochester, MN—Olmsted

Rochester, NY—Genessee, Livingston, Monroe, Ontario,
Orleans, Wayne

Rockford, IL—Boone, Ogle, Winnebago

Rocky Mount, NC—Edgecombe, Nash

Sacramento-Yolo, CA—El Dorado, Placer, Sacramento,
Yolo

Saginaw-Bay City-Midland, MI—Bay, Midland, Saginaw

St. Cloud, MN—Benton, Stearns

St. Joseph, MO—Andrew, Buchanan

St. Louis, MO-IL—
Illinois Portion—Clinton, Jersey, Madison, Monroe,
St. Clair
Missouri Portion—Crawford, Franklin, Jefferson,
Lincoln, St. Charles, St. Louis, St. Louis City, Warren

Salinas, CA—Monterey

Salt Lake City-Ogden, UT—Davis, Salt Lake, Weber

San Angelo, TX—Tom Green

San Antonio, TX—Bexar, Comal, Guadalupe, Wilson

San Diego, CA—San Diego

San Francisco-Oakland-San Jose, CA—Alamdea, Contra
Costa, Marin, Napa, San Francisco, San Mateo, Santa
Clara, Santa Cruz, Solano, Sonoma

San Juan-Caguas-Arecibo, PR—Aguas Buenas, Arecibo,
Barceloneta, Bayamon, Caguas, Camuy, Canovanas,
Carolina, Catano, Ceiba, Cayey, Ceiba, Cidra, Comerio,
Corozal, Dorado, Fajardo, Florida, Guaynabo, Gurabo,
Hatillo, Humacao, Juncos, Las Piedras, Loiza, Luquillo,
Manati, Morovis, Naguabo, Naranjito, Rio Grande, San
Juan, San Lorenzo, Toa Alta, Toa Baja, Trujillo Alto,
Vega Alta, Vega Baja, Yabucoa

San Luis Obisbo-Atascadero-Paso, CA—San Luis Obisbo

Santa Barbara-Santa Maria-Lompoc, CA—Santa Barbara

Santa Fe, NM—Los Alamos, Santa Fe

Sarasota-Bradenton, FL—Manatee, Sarasota

Savannah, GA—Bryan, Chatham, Effingham

Scranton-Wilkes-Barre-Hazleton, PA—Columbia,
Lackawanna, Luzerne, Wyoming

Seattle-Tacoma-Bremerton, WA—Island, King, Kitsap,
Pierce, Snohomish, Thurston

Sharon, PA—Mercer

Sheboygan, WI—Sheboygan

Sherman-Denison, TX—Grayson

Shreveport-Bossier City, LA—Bossier, Caddo, Webster

Sioux City, IA-NE—
Iowa Portion—Woodbury
Nebraska Portion—Dakota

Sioux Falls, SD—Lincoln, Minnehaha

South Bend, IN—St. Joseph

Spokane, WA—Spokane

Springfield, IL—Menard, Sangamon

Springfield, MA—Franklin, Hampden, Hampshire

Springfield, MO—Christian, Greene, Webster

State College, PA—Centre

Steubenville-Weirton, OH-WV—
Ohio Portion—Jefferson
West Virginia Portion—Brooke, Hancock

Stockton-Lodi, CA—San Joaquin

Sumter, SC—Sumter

Syracuse, NY—Cayuga, Madison, Onondaga, Oswego

Tallahassee, FL—Gadsden, Leon

Tampa-St Petersburg-Clearwater, FL—Hernando,
Hillsborough, Pasco, Pinellas

Terre Haute, IN—Clay, Vermillion, Vigo

Texarkana, TX-AR
   Arkansas Portion—Miller
   Texas Portion—Bowie
Toledo, OH—Fulton, Lucas, Wood
Topeka, KS—Shawnee
Tucson, AZ—Pima
Tulsa, OK—Creek, Osage, Rogers, Tulsa, Wagoner
Tuscaloosa, AL—Tuscaloosa
Tyler, TX—Smith
Utica-Rome, NY—Herkimer, Oneida
Victoria, TX—Victoria
Visalia-Tulare-Porterville, CA—Tulare
Waco, TX—McLennan
Washington, DC-MD-VA-WV—
   District of Columbia Portion—District of Columbia
   Maryland Portion—Anne Arundel, Baltimore, Baltimore City, Calvert, Carroll, Charles, Frederick, Harford, Howard, Montgomery, Prince George's, Queen Anne's, Washington
   Virginia Portion—Alexandria City, Arlington, Clarke, Culpeper, Fairfax, Fairfax City, Falls Church City, Fauquier, Fredericksburg City, King George, Loudoun, Manassas City, Manassas Park City, Prince William, Spotsylvania, Stafford, Warren
   West Virginia Portion—Berkeley, Jefferson
Waterloo-Cedar Falls, IA—Black Hawk
Wausau, WI—Marathon
West Palm Beach-Boca Raton, FL—Palm Beach

Wheeling, WV-OH—
   Ohio Portion—Belmont
   West Virginia Portion—Marshall, Ohio
Wichita, KS—Butler, Harvey, Sedgwick
Wichita Falls, TX—Archer, Wichita
Williamsport, PA—Lycoming
Wilmington, NC—Brunswick, New Hanover
Yakima, WA—Yakima
York, PA—York
Youngstown-Warren, OH—Columbiana, Mahoning, Trumbull
Yuba City, CA—Sutter, Yuba
Yuma, AZ—Yuma

Appendix D

Regions, Divisions, and States

Census Region
Census Division
State

Northeast

Middle Atlantic
New Jersey
New York
Pennsylvania

New England
Connecticut
Maine
Massachusetts
New Hampshire
Rhode Island
Vermont

North Central

East North Central
Illinois
Indiana
Michigan
Ohio
Wisconsin

West North Central
Iowa
Kansas
Minnesota
Missouri
Nebraska
North Dakota
South Dakota

South

East South Central
Alabama
Kentucky
Mississippi
Tennessee

South Atlantic
Delaware
District of Columbia
Florida
Georgia
Maryland
North Carolina
South Carolina
Virginia
West Virginia

West South Central
Arkansas
Louisiana
Oklahoma
Texas

West

Mountain
Arizona
Colorado
Idaho
Montana
Nevada
New Mexico
Utah
Wyoming

Pacific
Alaska
California
Hawaii
Oregon
Washington

Possessions
Puerto Rico
Virgin Islands
Pacific Islands

Appendix E
Demographic County Classifications

9 = Counties in MSAs with 5,000,000 or more inhabitants

8 = Counties in MSAs with 1,000,000 to 4,999,999 inhabitants

7 = Counties in MSAs with 500,000 to 999,999 inhabitants

6 = Counties in MSAs with 50,000 to 499,999 inhabitants

4 = Nonmetropolitan counties with over 50,000 inhabitants

3 = Nonmetropolitan counties with 25,000 to 49,999 inhabitants

2 = Nonmetropolitan counties with 10,000 to 24,999 inhabitants

1 = Nonmetropolitan counties with under 9,999 inhabitants

0 = Not Available

Index

Abdominal radiology, number of physicians, by activity, 20

Abdominal surgery, number of physicians, by activity, 20

Activity. *See* Major professional activity

Activity, other. *See* Other activity

Addiction medicine, number of physicians, by activity, 20

Addiction psychiatry, number of physicians, by activity, 20

Administration
 definition, explanation of term, xvii
 trends data, 398, 400, 403, 411, 415
 See also Major professional activity

Adolescent medicine, number of physicians, by activity, 20

Adult reconstructive orthopedics, number of physicians, by activity, 22

Aerospace medicine
 number of physicians, by activity, 20
 See also Specialties

African-American physicians. *See* Ethnicity

Age
 data presentation, xx
 international medical graduates, primary care, 290
 major professional activity, sex distribution and, 1, 2, 8, 42, 43
 mean age, specialty and activity, 15-24, 309-312
 primary care specialties, 275, 281
 specialty and, 9-14, 305-308
 state and, 47-52, 323-325
 trends data, 396-397, 407

Alabama
 by activity and county, 213-214
 by activity and county group, 209
 female, by specialty and activity, 149
 by specialty and activity, 95
 See also State data

Alabama, University of, physician graduates, by year of graduation, 32
 female, 38
 male, 35
 primary care, 283

Alaska
 by activity and county, 214
 by activity and county group, 211
 boroughs, census areas, xxi
 female physicians, by specialty and activity, 150
 by specialty and activity, 96
 See also State data

Alaskan Native physicians. *See* Ethnicity

Albany Medical College, physician graduates, by year of graduation, 33
 female, 39
 male, 36
 primary care, 284

Albert Einstein College of Medicine, physician graduates, by year of graduation, 33
 female, 39
 male, 36
 primary care, 284

Allergy, number of physicians, by activity, 20

Allergy and immunology
 number of physicians, by activity, 20
 See also Specialties

American Indian physicians. *See* Ethnicity

Anatomic/clinical pathology, number of physicians, by activity, 24

Anatomic pathology, number of physicians, by activity, 20

Anesthesiology
 number of physicians, by activity, 20
 See also Specialties

Arizona
 by activity and county, 214
 by activity and county group, 210
 female, by specialty and activity, 151
 by specialty and activity, 97
 See also State data

Arizona, University of, physician graduates, by year of graduation, 32
 female, 38
 male, 35
 primary care, 283

Arkansas
  by activity and county, 214-216
  by activity and county group, 210
  female, by specialty and activity, 152
  by specialty and activity, 98
  See also State data
Arkansas, University of, physician graduates, by year of
    graduation, 32
  female, 38
  male, 35
  primary care, 283
Asian-American physicians. *See* Ethnicity

Baylor College of Medicine, physician graduates, by year of
    graduation, 33
  female, 39
  male, 36
  primary care, 285
Black physicians. *See* Ethnicity
Blood banking transfusion medicine, number of physicians,
    by activity, 20
Board certification
  definition, explanation, xix
primary care specialties, 276, 282
  specialty data, 5-6, 29-31
Boston University, physician graduates, by year of
    graduation, 32
  female, 38
  male, 36
  primary carc, 283
Bowman Gray, physician graduates, by year of graduation,
    33
  female, 39
  male, 36
  primary care, 284
Brown University, physician graduates, by year of
    graduation, 33
  female, 39
  male, 36
  primary care, 284

California
  by activity and county, 216-217
  by activity and county group, 212
  female, by specialty and activity, 153
  by specialty and activity, 99
  See also State data
California, University of (Davis), physician graduates, by
    year of graduation, 32
  female, 38
  male, 35
  primary care, 283
California, University of (Irvine), physician graduates, by
    year of graduation, 32
  female, 38
  male, 35
  primary care, 283

California, University of (Los Angeles), physician graduates,
    by year of graduation, 32
  female, 38
  male, 35
  primary care, 283
California, University of (San Diego), physician graduates,
    by year of graduation, 32
  female, 38
  male, 35
  primary care, 283
California, University of (San Francisco), physician
    graduates, by year of graduation, 32
  female, 38
  male, 35
  primary care, 283
Canada
  graduates, primary care, by state, 293
  graduates, trends data, 394-395
Cardiac electrophysiology, number of physicians, by activity,
    21
Cardiothoracic radiology, number of physicians, by activity,
    20
Cardiovascular disease
  number of physicians, by activity, 20
  See also Specialties
Case Western Reserve, physician graduates, by year of
    graduation, 33
  female, 39
  male, 36
  primary care, 244
Census divisions
  by activity and county group, 203-204
  physician/population ratios, 61
  by specialty and activity, 70-79
Census regions
  by specialty and activity, 65-69
Central del Caribe, Universidad, physician graduates, by
    year of graduation, 33
  female, 39
  male, 36
  primary care, 284
Certification. *See* Board certification
Chemical pathology, number of physicians, by activity, 23
Characteristics of physicians. *See* Age; Ethnicity; Female
    physicians; International medical graduates; Major
    professional activity; Male physicians; Medical
    schools; Specialties
Characteristics of physicians, geographic. *See* Census
    divisions; Census regions; County data; County
    groups; Metropolitan statistical areas; State data
Chicago Medical School, physician graduates, by year of
    graduation, 32
  female, 38
  male, 35
  primary care, 283

Chicago, University of/Pritzker, physician graduates, by year of graduation, 32
  female, 38
  male, 35
  primary care, 283
Child and adolescent psychiatry
  number of physicians, by activity, 20
  See also Specialties
Child neurology, number of physicians, by activity, 20
Cincinnati, University of, physician graduates, by year of graduation, 33
  female, 39
  male, 36
  primary care, 284
Cities. *See* Metropolitan statistical areas
Clinical and laboratory dermatological immunology, number of physicians, by activity, 20
Clinical and laboratory immunology
  number of physicians, by activity, 20, 21, 23
Clinical biochemical genetics, number of physicians, by activity, 20
Clinical cardiac electrophysiology, number of physicians, by activity, 21
Clinical cytogenetics, number of physicians, by activity, 20
Clinical genetics, number of physicians, by activity, 20
Clinical molecular genetics, number of physicians, by activity, 20
Clinical neurophysiology, number of physicians, by activity, 20
Clinical pathology, number of physicians, by activity, 20
Clinical pharmacology, number of physicians, by activity, 23
Collection and classification systems, physician trends, 393-394
Colon/rectal surgery
  number of physicians, by activity, 20
  See also Specialties
Colorado
  by activity and county, 217-218
  by activity and county group, 210
  female, by specialty and activity, 154
  by specialty and activity, 100
  See also State data
Colorado, University of, physician graduates, by year of graduation, 32
  female, 38
  male, 35
  primary care, 283
Columbia University, physician graduates, by year of graduation, 33
  female, 39
  male, 36
  primary care, 284
Connecticut
  by activity and county, 218
  by activity and county group, 205
  female, by specialty and activity, 155
  by specialty and activity, 101
  See also State data

Connecticut, University of, physician graduates, by year of graduation, 32
  female, 38
  male, 30
  primary care, 283
Cornell University, physician graduates, by year of graduation, 33
  female, 39
  male, 36
  primary care, 284
Cosmetic surgery, number of physicians, by activity, 20
County data
  definition, explanation, xx-xxi
  physicians, by activity, 213-266
County groups
  by activity and census division, 203-212
  definition, explanation, xx
Craniofacial surgery, number of physicians, by activity, 20
Creighton University, physician graduates, by year of graduation, 32
  female, 39
  male, 36
  primary care, 284
Critical care medicine, number of physicians, by activity, 20, 22
Cytopathology, number of physicians, by activity, 23

Dartmouth Medical School, physician graduates, by year of graduation, 33
  female, 39
  male, 36
  primary care, 284
Definitions, xvii-xxi
Delaware
  by activity and county, 218
  by activity and county group, 208
  female, by specialty and activity, 156
  by specialty and activity, 102
  See also State data
Demographic County Classification, xx. *See also* County groups
Dermatologic surgery, number of physicians, by activity, 20
Dermatology
  number of physicians, by activity, 20
  See also Specialties
Dermatopathology, number of physicians, by activity, 20
Developmental behavioral pediatrics, number of physicians, by activity, 20
Diabetes, number of physicians, by activity, 20
Diagnostic radiology
  number of physicians, by activity, 20
  See also Specialties
District of Columbia
  by activity and county, 218
  by activity and county group, 208
  female, by specialty and activity, 157
  by specialty and activity, 103
  See also State data

DOs (Doctors of Osteopathy) *See* Osteopathic physicians
Duke University, physician graduates, by year of graduation, 33
 female, 39
 male, 36
 primary care, 284
East Carolina University, physician graduates, by year of graduation, 33
 female, 39
 male, 36
 primary care, 284
East North Central census division
 by activity and county group, 203
 international medical graduates, by specialty and activity, 72
 by specialty and activity, 87
East South Central census division
 by activity and county group, 203
 international medical graduates, by specialty and activity, 75
 by specialty and activity, 90
East Tennessee State University, physician graduates, by year of graduation, 33
 female, 39
 male, 36
 primary care, 284
Eastern Virginia Medical School, physician graduates, by year of graduation, 33
 female, 39
 male, 36
 primary care, 285
Emergency medicine
 number of physicians, by activity, 20
 See also Specialties
Emory University, physician graduates, by year of graduation, 32
 female, 38
 male, 35
 primary care, 283
Employment status, 394-401
Endocrinology, diabetes and metabolism, number of physicians, by activity, 21
Endovascular surgical neuroradiology, number of physicians, by activity, 21
Epidemiology
 number of physicians, by activity, 21
 See also Specialties
Ethnicity
 race/ethnicity, specialty data, 6-7, 41-43, 320-322

Facial plastic surgery, number of physicians, by activity, 21
Family medicine, number of physicians, by activity, 21
Family practice
 distribution of specialties, subspecialties, 275
 number of physicians, by activity, 21
 specialty, subspecialty data, 279-300
 subspecialties listed, xviii
 See also Specialties

Female physicians
 activity, trends, 398-401
 age, specialty distribution, 11
 by age and state, 49
 age distribution, 2, 45, 49
 board certification, 6, 31
 board certification, primary care, 282
 geographic (state) distribution, 49
 international medical graduates, age, activity distribution, 26
 international medical graduates, age, state of location, 52
 international medical graduates, by state and activity, 58
 international medical graduates, by year of graduation, 40
 international medical graduates, primary care, by age group, 290
 international medical graduates, year of graduation, 7
 major professional activity, age and, 1, 8
 medical school and year of graduation, 38-40
 primary care, by activity, 280
 primary care, by age, 281
 primary care, by state, 289
 primary care, by year of graduation, 286
 primary care specialties, 274, 276
 race/ethnicity and specialties, 43
 specialties, trends, 399-401
 specialty, activity distribution, 28
 specialty, professional activity distribution, 4
 specialty, residency training, 5
 state, specialty and activity, 149-202
 by state and activity, 55
 state and activity data, 46, 55
 total, year of graduation, 6
 trends data, 396-397, 399-401, 407, 412-415
Florida
 by activity and county, 218-219
 by activity and county group, 208
 female, by specialty and activity, 158
 by specialty and activity, 104
 See also State data
Florida, University of, physician graduates, by year of graduation, 32
 female, 38
 male, 35
 primary care, 284
Foot and ankle, orthopedics, number of physicians, by activity, 22
Foreign medical graduates. See International medical graduates
Forensic pathology
 number of physicians, by activity, 21
 See also Specialties
Forensic psychiatry, number of physicians, by activity, 23

Gastroenterology
 number of physicians, by activity, 21
 See also Specialties

Gender. *See* Female physicians; Male physicians

General practice

distribution of specialties, subspecialties, 275

number of physicians, by activity, 21

specialty, subspecialty data, 279-300

See also Specialties

General preventive medicine

number of physicians, by activity, 21

See also Specialties

General surgery

number of physicians, by activity, 21

See also Specialties

Geographic distribution. *See* Census divisions; Census regions; County data; County groups; Metropolitan statistical areas; State data

George Washington University, physician graduates, by year of graduation, 32

female, 38

male, 35

primary care, 283

Georgetown University, physician graduates, by year of graduation, 32

female, 38

male, 35

primary care, 283

Georgia

by activity and county, 219-222

by activity and county group, 208

female, by specialty and activity, 159

by specialty and activity, 105

See also State data

Georgia, Medical College of, physician graduates, by year of graduation, 32

female, 38

male, 35

primary care, 283

Geriatric medicine, number of physicians, by activity, 21

Geriatric psychiatry, number of physicians, by activity, 24

Graduation year. *See* Medical schools

Gynecological oncology, number of physicians, by activity, 21

Gynecology

number of physicians, by activity, 21

See also Obstetrics/gynecology

Hand surgery, number of physicians, by activity, 21

Harvard University, physician graduates, by year of graduation, 32

female, 38

male, 35

primary care, 283

Hawaii

by activity and county, 222

by activity and county group, 212

female, by specialty and activity, 160

by specialty and activity, 106

See also State data

Hawaii, University of, physician graduates, by year of graduation, 32

female, 38

male, 35

primary care, 283

Head and neck surgery, number of physicians, by activity, 21

Hematology, number of physicians, by activity, 21

Hematology/oncology, number of physicians, by activity, 21

Hepatology, number of physicians, by activity, 21

Hispanic-American physicians. *See* Ethnicity

Hospital-based practice

definition, explanation, xvii

trends data, 396, 398

See also Major professional activity

Hospitalist, number of physicians, by activity, 21

Howard University, physician graduates, by year of graduation, 32

female, 38

male, 35

primary care, 283

Idaho

by activity and county, 222

by activity and county group, 211

female, by specialty and activity, 161

by specialty and activity, 107

See also State data

Illinois

by activity and county, 222-224

by activity and county group, 206

female, by specialty and activity, 162

by specialty and activity, 108

See also State data

Illinois, University of, physician graduates, by year of graduation, 32

female, 38

male, 35

primary care, 283

IMGs. *See* International medical graduates

Immunology, number of physicians, by activity, 21

Inactives

definition, explanation of term, xviii

trends data, 398-400

See also Major professional activity

Indiana

by activity and county, 224-226

by activity and county group, 206

female, by specialty and activity, 163

by specialty and activity, 109

See also State data

Indiana University, physician graduates, by year of graduation, 32

female, 38

male, 35

primary care, 283

Infectious disease, number of physicians, by activity, 21

Internal medicine
    distribution of specialties, subspecialties, 275
    number of physicians, by activity, 21, 22
    specialty, subspecialty data, 279-300
    subspecialties listed, xviii
    See also Specialties
International medical graduates
    activity, by specialty, 4, 25
    activity, by state, 56-58
    activity, trends, 397-398
    age, sex distribution, 4-5, 26
    female, year of graduation, 40
    geographic distribution, 46, 50
    male, year of graduation, 37
    primary care, 285, 290-291
    sex distribution, year of graduation, 7
    specialties, trends, 398
    state data, 50
    trends data, 398-400, 408-411
    year of graduation, 34
Interventional cardiology, number of physicians, by activity, 21
Iowa
    by activity and county, 226-227
    by activity and county group, 207
    female, by specialty and activity, 164
    by specialty and activity, 110
    See also State data
Iowa, University of, physician graduates, by year of graduation, 32
    female, 38
    male, 35
    primary care, 283

Jefferson Medical College, physician graduates, by year of graduation, 33
    female, 39
    male, 36
    primary care, 283
Johns Hopkins University, physician graduates, by year of graduation, 32
    female, 38
    male, 35
    primary care, 283

Kansas
    by activity and county, 227-229
    by activity and county group, 207
    female, by specialty and activity, 165
    by specialty and activity, 111
    See also State data
Kansas, University of, physician graduates, by year of graduation, 32
    female, 38
    male, 35
    primary care, 283

Kentucky
    by activity and county, 229-231
    by activity and county group, 209
    female, by specialty and activity, 166
    by specialty and activity, 112
    See also State data
Kentucky, University of, physician graduates, by year of graduation, 32
    female, 38
    male, 35
    primary care, 283

Legal medicine, number of physicians, by activity, 21
Loma Linda University, physician graduates, by year of graduation, 32
    female, 38
    male, 35
    primary care, 283
Louisiana
    by activity and county, 231-232
    by activity and county group, 210
    female, by specialty and activity, 167
    by specialty and activity, 113
    See also State data
Louisiana State University (New Orleans), physician graduates, by year of graduation, 32
    female, 38
    male, 35
    primary care, 283
Louisiana State University (Shreveport), physician graduates, by year of graduation, 32
    female, 38
    male, 35
    primary care, 283
Louisville, University of, physician graduates, by year of graduation, 32
    female, 38
    male, 35
    primary care, 283
Loyola University/Stritch, physician graduates, by year of graduation, 32
    female, 38
    male, 35
    primary care, 283

Maine
    by activity and county, 232
    by activity and county group, 205
    female, by specialty and activity, 168
    by specialty and activity, 114
    See also State data
Major professional activity
    age, sex distribution and, 1, 8
    definition, explanation, categories of, xvii-xviii
    detailed specialty data, 2-4, 15-19
    female physicians, by state and specialty, 149-202
    female physicians, specialty distribution, 28

female physicians, trends, 400, 401, 415
international medical graduates, 397-398, 411
international medical graduates, age, sex distribution, 26
international medical graduates, by specialty, 4, 25
physicians, by county, 213-266
physicians, by state and specialty, 95-148
physicians, metropolitan areas, by specialty, 269-273
physicians, rural areas, by specialty, 268
physicians, specialty data, 63-64
primary care, sex distribution, 280
primary care specialty and metropolitan area, 295-300
specialty, geographic region data, 59-273
trends data, 394-401, 403, 411, 415
Male physicians
    age, specialty distribution, 10
    age distribution, 2, 45, 46, 48
    board certification, 5-6, 30
    board certification, primary care, 276, 282
    geographic (state) distribution, 48
    international medical graduates, age, activity distribution, 26
    international medical graduates, primary care, by age group, 290
    international medical graduates, by year of graduation, 7, 34
    major professional activity, age and, 8
    medical school and year of graduation, 35-37
    primary care, by activity, 280
    primary care, by age, 281
    primary care, by state, 288
    primary care specialties, 274-276
    race/ethnicity and specialties, 42
    state distribution and activity, 54
    total, year of graduation, 7
    trends data, 396-397, 407
Marshall University, physician graduates, by year of graduation, 33
    female, 40
    male, 37
    primary care, 285
Maryland
    by activity and county, 233
    by activity and county group, 208
    county data, xxi
    female, by specialty and activity, 169
    by specialty and activity, 115
    See also State data
Maryland, University of, physician graduates, by year of graduation, 32
    female, 38
    male, 35
    primary care, 283
Massachusetts
    by activity and county, 233
    by activity and county group, 205
    female, by specialty and activity, 170
    by specialty and activity, 116
    See also State data

Massachusetts, University of, physician graduates, by year of graduation, 32
    female, 38
    male, 35
    primary care, 283
Masterfile, AMA Physician, xv
Maternal and fetal medicine, number of physicians, by activity, 22
Mayo Medical School, physician graduates, by year of graduation, 32
    female, 38
    male, 35
    primary care, 283
Medical education, xix-xx
Medical genetics
    number of physicians, by activity, 22, 23
    See also Specialties
Medical management, number of physicians, by activity, 21
Medical microbiology, number of physicians, by activity, 22
Medical oncology, number of physicians, by activity, 22
Medical research
    definition, explanation, xvii
    trends data, 395, 398, 400, 403, 411, 415
    See also Major professional activity
Medical schools
    Canadian school graduates, 34, 37, 40
    female graduates, by year of graduation, 38-40
    graduates, by year of graduation, 32-34
    largest numbers of graduates, 6
    male graduates, by year of graduation, 35-37
    primary care specialties, year of graduation, 286
    year of graduation, 6, 32-34
Medical teaching
    definition, explanation, xvii
    trends data, 393-394, 398, 400, 403, 411, 415
    See also Major professional activity
Medical toxicology
    number of physicians, by activity, 21, 23, 24
Meharry Medical College, physician graduates, by year of graduation, 33
    female, 39
    male, 36
    primary care, 285
Mercer University, physician graduates, by year of graduation, 32
    female, 38
    male, 35
    primary care, 283
Metropolitan statistical areas, 62, 267, 269-273
    definition, explanation, xx
    primary care and, 278
    primary care specialty and activity, 294
    by specialty and activity, 267
    trends data, 416-417

Miami, University of, physician graduates, by year of
  graduation, 32
  female, 38
  male, 35
  primary care, 283
Michigan
  by activity and county, 233-235
  by activity and county group, 206
  female, by specialty and activity, 171
  by specialty and activity, 117
  See also State data
Michigan State University, physician graduates, by year of
  graduation, 32
  female, 38
  male, 35
  primary care, 283
Michigan, University of, physician graduates, by year of
  graduation, 32
  female, 38
  male, 35
  primary care, 283
Middle Atlantic census division
  by activity and county group, 203
  international medical graduates, by specialty and activity,
    71
  by specialty and activity, 86
Minnesota
  by activity and county, 235-236
  by activity and county group, 207
  female, by specialty and activity, 172
  by specialty and activity, 118
  See also State data
Minnesota, University of, physician graduates, by year of
  graduation, 32
  female, 38
  male, 35
  primary care, 283
Minnesota, University of (Duluth), physician graduates, by
  year of graduation, 32
  female, 38
  male, 35
  primary care, 283
Mississippi
  by activity and county, 236-237
  by activity and county group, 209
  female, by specialty and activity, 173
  by specialty and activity, 119
  See also State data
Mississippi, University of, physician graduates, by year of
  graduation, 32
  female, 38
  male, 35
  primary care, 284
Missouri
  by activity and county, 237-239
  by activity and county group, 207
  county data, xxi

female, by specialty and activity, 174
  by specialty and activity, 120
  See also State data
Missouri, University of (Columbia), physician graduates, by
  year of graduation, 32
  female, 38
  male, 35
  primary care, 284
Missouri, University of (Kansas City), physician graduates,
  by year of graduation, 32
  female, 38
  male, 35
  primary care, 284
Molecular genetic pathology, number of physicians, by
  activity, 22
Montana
  by activity and county, 239-240
  by activity and county group, 211
  female, by specialty and activity, 175
  by specialty and activity, 121
  See also State data
Morehouse University, physician graduates, by year of
  graduation, 32
  female, 38
  male, 35
  primary care, 283
Mountain census division
  by activity and county group, 204
  international medical graduates, by specialty and activity,
    77
  by specialty and activity, 92
MSA. See Metropolitan statistical areas
Mt Sinai School of Medicine, physician graduates, by year
  of graduation, 33
  female, 39
  male, 36
  primary care, 284
Musculoskeletal oncology, number of physicians, by activity,
  22
Musculoskeletal radiology, number of physicians, by activity,
  22

Native American physicians. *See* Ethnicity
Nebraska
  by activity and county, 240-241
  by activity and county group, 207
  female physicians, by specialty and activity, 176
  by specialty and activity, 122
  See also State data
Nebraska, University of, physician graduates, by year of
  graduation, 33
  female, 39
  male, 36
  primary care, 284
Neonatal perinatal medicine, number of physicians, by
  activity, 22
Nephrology, number of physicians, by activity, 22

Neurodevelopmental disabilities, number of physicians, by activity, 22

Neurological surgery
  number of physicians, by activity, 22
  See also Specialties

Neurology
  number of physicians, by activity, 22
  See also Specialties

Neuromuscular medicine, number of physicians, by activity, 22

Neuropathology, number of physicians, by activity, 22

Neuropsychiatry, number of physicians, by activity, 22

Neuroradiology, number of physicians, by activity, 24

Nevada
  by activity and county, 242
  by activity and county group, 211
  female, by specialty and activity, 177
  by specialty and activity, 123
  See also State data

Nevada, University of, physician graduates, by year of graduation, 33
  female, 39
  male, 36
  primary care, 284

New England census division
  by activity and county group, 203
  international medical graduates, by specialty and activity, 70
  by specialty and activity, 85

New Hampshire
  by activity and county, 242
  by activity and county group, 205
  female, by specialty and activity, 178
  by specialty and activity, 124
  See also State data

New Jersey
  by activity and county, 242
  by activity and county group, 205
  female, by specialty and activity, 179
  by specialty and activity, 125
  See also State data

New Jersey Medical School (Newark), physician graduates, by year of graduation, 33
  female, 39
  male, 36
  primary care, 284

New Jersey Medical School (Rutgers), physician graduates, by year of graduation, 33
  female, 39
  male, 36
  primary care, 284

New Mexico
  by activity and county, 242-243
  by activity and county group, 211
  female, by specialty and activity, 180
  by specialty and activity, 126
  See also State data

New Mexico, University of, physician graduates, by year of graduation, 33
  female, 39
  male, 36
  primary care, 284

New York
  by activity and county, 243-244
  by activity and county group, 206
  female, by specialty and activity, 181
  by specialty and activity, 127
  See also State data

New York Medical College, physician graduates, by year of graduation, 33
  female, 39
  male, 36
  primary care, 284

New York, State University of (Brooklyn), physician graduates, by year of graduation, 33
  female, 39
  male, 36
  primary care, 284

New York, State University of (Buffalo), physician graduates, by year of graduation, 33
  female, 39
  male, 36
  primary care, 284

New York, State University of (Stony Brook), physician graduates, by year of graduation, 33
  female, 39
  male, 36
  primary care, 284

New York, State University of (Syracuse), physician graduates, by year of graduation, 33
  female, 39
  male, 36
  primary care, 284

New York University, physician graduates, by year of graduation, 33
  female, 39
  male, 36
  primary care, 284

North Carolina
  by activity and county, 244-246
  by activity and county group, 208
  female, by specialty and activity, 182
  by specialty and activity, 128
  See also State data

North Carolina, University of, physician graduates, by year of graduation, 33
  female, 39
  male, 36
  primary care, 284

North Central census region
  international medical graduates, by specialty and activity, 66
  by specialty and activity, 81

North Dakota
  by activity and county, 246
  by activity and county group, 207
  female, by specialty and activity, 183
  by specialty and activity, 129
  See also State data
North Dakota, University of, physician graduates, by year of graduation, 33
  female, 39
  male, 36
  primary care, 284
Northeast census region
  international medical graduates, by specialty and activity, 65
  by specialty and activity, 80
Northeast Ohio University, physician graduates, by year of graduation, 33
  female, 39
  male, 36
  primary care, 284
Northwestern University, physician graduates, by year of graduation, 32
  female, 38
  male, 35
  primary care, 283
Not classified
  definition, explanation of term, xviii
  trends data, 398, 400
  See also Major professional activity
Nuclear cardiology
  number of physicians, by activity, 22
Nuclear medicine
  number of physicians, by activity, 22
  See also Specialties
Nuclear radiology, number of physicians, by activity, 22
Nutrition, number of physicians, by activity, 22

Obstetrics, number of physicians, by activity, 22
Obstetrics/gynecology
  distribution of specialties, subspecialties, 275
  number of physicians, by activity, 22
  specialty, subspecialty data, 279-300
  subspecialties listed, xviii
  See also Specialties
Occupational medicine
  number of physicians, by activity, 22
  See also Specialties
Office-based practice
  definition, explanation, xvii
  trends data, 394-396, 398, 400, 401, 411, 415-417, 424-425
  See also Major professional activity
Ohio, Medical College of, physician graduates, by year of graduation, 33
  female, 39
  male, 36
  primary care, 284

Ohio
  by activity and county, 246-248
  by activity and county group, 206
  female, by specialty and activity, 184
  by specialty and activity, 130
  See also State data
Ohio State University, physician graduates, by year of graduation, 33
  female, 39
  male, 36
  primary care, 284
Oklahoma
  by activity and county, 248-249
  by activity and county group, 210
  female, by specialty and activity, 185
  by specialty and activity, 131
  See also State data
Oklahoma, University of, physician graduates, by year of graduation, 33
  female, 39
  male, 36
  primary care, 284
Oncology, number of physicians, by activity, 22, 23, 24
Ophthalmology
  number of physicians, by activity, 22
  See also Specialties
Oral and maxillofacial surgery, number of physicians, by activity, 22
Oregon
  by activity and county, 249-250
  by activity and county group, 212
  female, by specialty and activity, 186
  by specialty and activity, 132
  See also State data
Oregon, University of, physician graduates, by year of graduation, 33
  female, 39
  male, 36
  primary care, 284
Orthopedic surgery
  number of physicians, by activity, 22
  See also Specialties
Orthopedic surgery of the spine, number of physicians, by activity, 22
Orthopedic trauma, number of physicians, by activity, 23
Orthopedics, number of physicians, by activity, 22
Osteopathic manipulative medicine, number of physicians, by activity, 22
Osteopathic physicians, xiii, 301-392
  activity, by specialty, 301-303, 313-319
  activity, by state, 303, 326-328
  activity, trends, 301-304
  age, sex distribution, 301, 305
  age, by specialty, 301, 306-308
  age, by state of location, 323-325
  female, by age and specialty, 308
  female, by age and state of location, 325

female, by race/ethnicity, 322
female, by specialty and activity, 304, 319
female, by state and activity, 328
geographic distribution, 303-304, 383-389
male, by age and specialty, 307
male, by age and state of location, 324
male, by race/ethnicity, 321
male, by specialty and activity, 304, 318
male, by state and activity, 327
mean age, by specialty and activity, 302, 309-312
metropolitan areas, by specialty and activity, 304, 383, 385-389
primary care DOs, by activity and sex distribution, 304, 390
primary care DOs, by age and sex distribution, 304, 391
primary care DOs, by specialty and state, 304, 392
by race/ethnicity, 320-322
rural areas, by specialty and activity, 384
sex distribution, 301, 305, 318-319, 321-322, 324-325, 327-328, 390-391
state of location and professional activity, 303, 326-382
Other activity
    definition, explanation of term, xviii
    trends data, 394, 398, 400, 403, 411, 415
    See also Major professional activity
Other specialties, 22. See also Specialties
Otolaryngology
    number of physicians, by activity, 23
    See also Specialties
Otology/Neurotology, number of physicians, by activity, 22

Pacific census division
    by activity and county group, 204
    international medical graduates, by specialty and activity, 78
    by specialty and activity, 93
Pacific Islands
    by activity and county, 266
    by activity and county group, 212
    female, by specialty and activity, 202
    by specialty and activity, 148
    See also State data
Pain management
    number of physicians, by activity, 20, 23
    See also Specialties
Pain medicine, number of physicians, by activity, 23
Palliative medicine, number of physicians, by activity, 23
Pathology/anatomy, clinical. *See* Specialties
Patient care activity. *See* Hospital-based practice; Major professional activity; Office-based practice
Pediatric allergy, number of physicians, by activity, 23
Pediatric anesthesiology, number of physicians, by activity, 23
Pediatric cardiology
    number of physicians, by activity, 23
    See also Specialties
Pediatric cardiothoracic surgery, number of physicians, by activity, 23

Pediatric clinical and laboratory immunology, number of physicians, by activity, 23
Pediatric critical care medicine, number of physicians, by activity, 20
Pediatric emergency medicine, number of physicians, by activity, 20, 21, 23
Pediatric endocrinology, number of physicians, by activity, 23
Pediatric gastroenterology, number of physicians, by activity, 23
Pediatric hematology/oncology, number of physicians, by activity, 23
Pediatric infectious disease, number of physicians, by activity, 23
Pediatric medical toxicology, number of physicians, by activity, 23
Pediatric nephrology, number of physicians, by activity, 23
Pediatric ophthalmology, number of physicians, by activity, 23
Pediatric orthopedics, number of physicians, by activity, 22
Pediatric otolaryngology, number of physicians, by activity, 23
Pediatric pathology, number of physicians, by activity, 23
Pediatric psychiatry, number of physicians, by activity, 20
Pediatric pulmonology, number of physicians, by activity, 23
Pediatric radiology, number of physicians, by activity, 23
Pediatric rehabilitation medicine
    number of physicians, by activity, 23, 24
    See also Specialties
Pediatric rheumatology, number of physicians, by activity, 24
Pediatric sports medicine, number of physicians, by activity, 24
Pediatric surgery, number of physicians, by activity, 22, 23
Pediatric urology, number of physicians, by activity, 24
Pediatrics
    distribution of specialties, subspecialties, 275
    number of physicians, by activity, 23-24
    specialty, subspecialty data, 279-300
    subspecialties listed, xviii
    See also Specialties
Pennsylvania
    by activity and county group, 206
    by activity and county, 250-251
    female, by specialty and activity, 187
    by specialty and activity, 133
    See also State data
Pennsylvania, Medical College of, physician graduates, by year of graduation, 33
    female, 39
    male, 36
    primary care, 284
Pennsylvania State University, physician graduates, by year of graduation, 33
    female, 39
    male, 36
    primary care, 284

Pennsylvania, University of, physician graduates, by year of graduation, 33
 female, 39
 male, 36
 primary care, 284
Pharmaceutical medicine, number of physicians, by activity, 23
Phlebology, number of physicians, by activity, 23
Physical medicine and rehabilitation
 number of physicians, by activity, 23
 See also Specialties
Physician characteristics. *See* Age; Ethnicity; Female physicians; International medical graduates; Major professional activity; Male physicians; Medical schools; Specialties
Physician geographic characteristics. *See* Census divisions; Census regions; County data; County groups; Metropolitan statistical areas; State data
Physician Masterfile, AMA, xv
Physician/population ratios, 61
 trends, 401, 403, 418-421, 425
Physicians
 age, sex distribution and specialties, 1-5, 8-9
 geographic distribution, data and tables, 47-58
 geographic distribution, definitions and explanations, 45-46
 race/ethnicity, 41-43
 sex distribution, year of graduation, 7
 specialty and activity, 59, 63
 state distribution and activity, 53
 trends data, 393-425
 See also Female physicians; International medical graduates; Major professional activity; Male Physicians; Specialties
Pittsburgh, University of, physician graduates, by year of graduation, 33
 female, 39
 male, 36
 primary care, 284
Plastic surgery
 number of physicians, by activity, 23, 24
 See also Specialties
Ponce Medical School, physician graduates, by year of graduation, 33
 female, 39
 male, 36
 primary care, 284
Possessions, US. *See* United States Possessions
Primary care specialties, 274-300
 activity and gender, 274-276
 activity and sex distribution, 280
 age and gender, 275-276, 281
 board certification and gender, 276, 282
 Canadian graduates, by state, 293
 country of graduation, 277
 international medical graduates, 277, 290-291
 metropolitan areas, 277-278
 metropolitan areas, by activity, 294-300

school and year of graduation, 276, 283-286
 selected years, 279
 sex distribution, by state, 276-277
 state data, 287-289
 states with largest percentage, 277
 specialties, subspecialties (definition, explanation), xviii-xix
 trends, 274, 279
 US medical school graduates, 292
Procedural dermatology, number of physicians, by activity, 24
Proctology
 number of physicians, by activity, 24
Professional activity. *See* Major professional activity
Psychiatry
 number of physicians, by activity, 22, 23, 24
 See also Specialties
Psychoanalysis, number of physicians, by activity, 24
Psychosomatic medicine, number of physicians, by activity, 24
Public health and general preventive medicine
 number of physicians, by activity, 23
 See also Specialties
Puerto Rico
 by activity and county, 251-252
 by activity and county group, 212
 female, by specialty and activity, 188
 by specialty and activity, 134
 See also State data
Puerto Rico, University of, physician graduates, by year of graduation, 33
 female, 39
 male, 36
 primary care, 284
Pulmonary critical care medicine, number of physicians, by activity, 23
Pulmonary diseases
 number of physicians, by activity, 24
 See also Specialties

Race. *See* Ethnicity
Radiation oncology
 number of physicians, by activity, 24
 See also Specialties
Radiological physics, number of physicians, by activity, 24
Radiology
 number of physicians, by activity, 24
 See also Specialties
Reproductive endocrinology, number of physicians, by activity, 24
Research. *See* Medical research
Residents
 definition, explanation, xvii
 female physicians, 4
 training data definition, explanation, xix
 trends data, 398
 See also Major professional activity

Rheumatology, number of physicians, by activity, 24
Rhode Island
    by activity and county, 252
    by activity and county group, 205
    female, by specialty and activity, 189
    by specialty and activity, 135
    See also State data
Rochester, University of, physician graduates, by year of
    graduation, 33
    female, 39
    male, 36
    primary care, 284
Rural areas
    physicians, by specialty and activity, 268
Rush Medical College, physician graduates, by year of
    graduation, 32
    female, 38
    male, 35
    primary care, 283

St Louis University, physician graduates, by year of
    graduation, 32
    female, 38
    male, 35
    primary care, 284
School of graduation. *See* Medical schools; names of schools
Selective pathology, number of physicians, by activity, 24
Sex data. *See* Female physicians; Male physicians
Sleep medicine, number of physicians, by activity, 24
South Alabama, University of, physician graduates, by year
    of graduation, 32
    female, 38
    male, 35
    primary care, 283
South Atlantic census division
    by activity and county group, 203
    international medical graduates, by specialty and activity,
    74
    by specialty and activity, 89
South Carolina
    by activity and county, 252-253
    by activity and county group, 208
    female, by specialty and activity, 190
    by specialty and activity, 136
    See also State data
South Carolina, Medical College of, physician graduates, by
    year of graduation, 33
    female, 39
    male, 36
    primary care, 284
South Carolina, University of, physician graduates, by year
    of graduation, 33
    female, 39
    male, 36
    primary care, 284

South census region
    international medical graduates, by specialty and activity,
    67
    by specialty and activity, 82
South Dakota
    by activity and county, 253-254
    by activity and county group, 208
    female, by specialty and activity, 191
    by specialty and activity, 137
    See also State data
South Dakota, University of, physician graduates, by year of
    graduation, 33
    female, 39
    male, 36
    primary care, 284
South Florida, University of, physician graduates, by year of
    graduation, 32
    female, 38
    male, 35
    primary care, 283
Southern California, University of, physician graduates, by
    year of graduation, 32
    female, 38
    male, 35
    primary care, 283
Southern Illinois University, physician graduates, by year of
    graduation, 32
    female, 38
    male, 35
    primary care, 283
Specialties
    activity and, 63
    age, sex distribution and, 1-2, 8-14
    board certification (total, male, female physicians), 29-31
    detailed, data, 2-4, 20-24
    detailed, female physicians, by activity, 28
    female physicians, by state and activity, 149-202
    female physicians, trends, 398-399
    geographic data, 59-273
    highest-ranking, by activity, 60
    international medical graduates, by activity, 4, 25
    international medical graduates, trends, 397-399,
        408-411
    largest, 3
    metropolitan areas, by activity, 267, 269-273
    physician/population ratios, 401, 425
    primary care, 274-300
    primary care, definition, explanation, xviii-xix
    race, ethnicity data, 6, 41-43
    rural areas, by activity, 268
    self-designated, definition, explanation, xviii
    state and activity, 95-148
    trends data, 395-396, 398, 399-401, 404-406, 412-414,
        424-425
    See also Primary care specialties
Spinal cord injury, number of physicians, by activity, 24

Sports medicine. *See also* Specialties
number of physicians, by activity, 21, 22, 23, 24
Stanford University, physician graduates, by year of
graduation, 32
female, 38
male, 35
primary care, 283
State data
age, activity, by sex, 46
age distribution, 47
female physicians, 49
female physicians, by activity, 55
female physicians, by specialty and activity, 149-202
international medical graduates, by activity, 56
international medical graduates, primary care, 291
major professional activity, 53-55
male physicians, 48
physician/population ratios, 401, 419-423
primary care, 287-289
primary care, largest percentages, 277
specialty and activity, 95-148
US medical school graduates, primary care, 292
See also Census divisions; Census regions; County data;
County groups; Metropolitan statistical areas; names
of states
State University of New York branches. *See* New York, State
University of
Subspecialties. *See* Primary care specialties
Surgery of the hand, number of physicians, by activity, 21
Surgical critical care, number of physicians, by activity, 20
Surgical oncology, number of physicians, by activity, 24

Teaching. *See* Medical teaching
Temple University, physician graduates, by year of
graduation, 33
female, 39
male, 36
primary care, 284
Tennessee
by activity and county, 254-256
by activity and county group, 209
female, by specialty and activity, 192
by specialty and activity, 138
See also State data
Tennessee, University of, physician graduates, by year of
graduation, 33
female, 39
male, 36
primary care, 285
Terminology. *See* Definitions
Texas
by activity and county, 256-259
by activity and county group, 210
female, by specialty and activity, 193
by specialty and activity, 139
See also State data

Texas A&M University, physician graduates, by year of
graduation, 33
female, 39
male, 36
primary care, 285
Texas Tech University, physician graduates, by year of
graduation, 33
female, 39
male, 36
primary care, 285
Texas, University of (Dallas), physician graduates, by year of
graduation, 33
female, 39
male, 36
primary care, 285
Texas, University of (Galveston), physician graduates, by
year of graduation, 33
female, 39
male, 36
primary care, 285
Texas, University of (Houston), physician graduates, by year
of graduation, 33
female, 39
male, 36
primary care, 285
Texas, University of (San Antonio), physician graduates, by
year of graduation, 33
female, 39
male, 36
primary care, 285
Thoracic surgery
number of physicians, by activity, 24
See also Specialties
Transplant surgery
number of physicians, by activity, 24
See also Specialties
Transplantation medicine, number of physicians, by activity,
24
Trauma surgery, number of physicians, by activity, 24
Trends, 274, 393-425. *See also* Physicians
Tufts University, physician graduates, by year of graduation,
32
female, 38
male, 35
primary care, 283
Tulane University, physician graduates, by year of
graduation, 32
female, 38
male, 35
primary care, 283

Undersea & Hyperbaric medicine, number of physicians, by
activity, 24
Uniformed Services, University of the, physician graduates,
by year of graduation, 32
female, 38
male, 35
primary care, 283

United States Possessions
    by county and activity, 266
    by county group and activity, 204
    international medical graduates, by specialty and activity, 69, 79
    by specialty and activity, 84, 94
Universities. *See* Medical schools; names of universities
Unspecified speciality, number of physicians, by activity, 24
Urgent care medicine, number of physicians, by activity, 24
Urological surgery. *See* Specialties
Urology, number of physicians, by activity, 24
Utah
    by activity and county, 259-260
    by activity and county group, 211
    female, by specialty and activity, 194
    by specialty and activity, 140
    See also State data
Utah, University of, physician graduates, by year of graduation, 33
    female, 39
    male, 36
    primary care, 285

Vanderbilt University, physician graduates, by year of graduation, 33
    female, 39
    male, 36
    primary care, 285
Vascular and interventional radiology, number of physicians, by activity, 24
Vascular medicine
    number of physicians, by activity, 24
    See also Specialties
Vascular neurology
    number of physicians, by activity, 24
Vascular surgery, number of physicians, by activity, 24
Vermont
    by activity and county, 260
    by activity and county group, 205
    female, by specialty and activity, 195
    by specialty and activity, 141
    See also State data
Vermont, University of, physician graduates, by year of graduation, 33
    female, 39
    male, 36
    primary care, 285
Virginia
    by activity and county, 260-262
    by activity and county group, 209
    county data, xx-xxi
    female, by specialty and activity, 196
    by specialty and activity, 142
    See also State data

Virginia, Medical College of, physician graduates, by year of graduation, 33
    female, 39
    male, 36
    primary care, 285
Virginia, University of, physician graduates, by year of graduation, 33
    female, 39
    male, 36
    primary care, 285
Virgin Islands
    by activity and county, 263
    by activity and county group, 212
    female, by specialty and activity, 197
    by specialty and activity, 143
    See also State data

Washington
    by activity and county, 263
    by activity and county group, 212
    female, by specialty and activity, 198
    by specialty and activity, 144
    See also State data
Washington, University of, physician graduates, by year of graduation, 33
    female, 40
    male, 37
    primary care, 285
Washington University, physician graduates, by year of graduation, 32
    female, 38
    male, 35
    primary care, 284
Wayne State University, physician graduates, by year of graduation, 32
    female, 38
    male, 35
    primary care, 284
West census region
    international medical graduates, by specialty and activity, 68
    by specialty and activity, 83
West North Central census division
    by activity and county group, 203
    international medical graduates, by specialty and activity, 73
    by specialty and activity, 88
West South Central census division
    by activity and county group, 204
    international medical graduates, by specialty and activity, 76
    by specialty and activity, 91
West Virginia
    by activity and county, 263-264
    by activity and county group, 209
    female, by specialty and activity, 199
    by specialty and activity, 145
    See also State data

West Virginia University, physician graduates, by year of
    graduation, 34
    female, 40
    male, 37
    primary care, 285
White physicians. *See* Ethnicity
Wisconsin
    by activity and county, 264-265
    by activity and county group, 207
    female, by specialty and activity, 200
    by specialty and activity, 146
    See also State data
Wisconsin, Medical College of, physician graduates, by year
    of graduation, 34
    female, 40
    male, 37
    primary care, 285
Wisconsin, University of, physician graduates, by year of
    graduation, 34
    female, 40
    male, 37
    primary care, 285

Women physicians. *See* Female physicians
Wright State University, physician graduates, by year of
    graduation, 33
    female, 39
    male, 36
    primary care, 284
Wyoming
    by activity and county, 265-266
    by activity and county group, 211
    female, by specialty and activity, 201
    by specialty and activity, 147
    See also State data

Yale University, physician graduates, by year of graduation,
    32
    female, 38
    male, 35
    primary care, 283
Year of graduation. *See* Medical schools